Anatomic Basis
of Neurologic Diagnosis

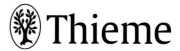

Anatomic Basis
of Neurologic Diagnosis

Cary D. Alberstone, MD
Ventura County Neurosurgical Associates
Oxnard, California

Edward C. Benzel, MD
Chairman
Department of Neurosurgery
Director
Center for Spine Health
Cleveland Clinic
Cleveland, Ohio

Imad M. Najm, MD
Director
Epilepsy Center
Neurological Institute
Cleveland Clinic
Cleveland, Ohio

Michael P. Steinmetz, MD
Assistant Professor
Department of Neurosurgery
Center for Spine Health
Director
Spinal Cord Injury Laboratory
Cleveland Clinic
Cleveland, Ohio

Illustrators
Joseph Kanasz
Michael Norviel

Thieme
New York • Stuttgart

Thieme Medical Publishers, Inc.
333 Seventh Ave.
New York, NY 10001

The artwork for this book was partially underwritten by unrestricted educational grants from the following companies:
Abbott Spine
DePuy AcroMed
Medtronic Sofamor Danek
NuVasive
Zimmer Spine
We thank them for their support of this project.

Executive Editor: Kay D. Conerly
Associate Editor: Ivy Ip
Vice President, Production and Electronic Publishing: Anne T. Vinnicombe
Production Editor: Anne T. Vinnicombe
Vice President, International Marketing and Sales: Cornelia Sculze
Chief Financial Officer: Peter van Woerden
President: Brian D. Scanlan
Compositor: Macmillan Publishing Solutions
Printer: Everbest Printing Co.
Artists: Joseph Kanasz and Michael Norviel

Library of Congress Cataloging-in-Publication Data
Anatomic basis of neurologic diagnosis / Cary D. Alberstone . . . [et al.].
        p. ; cm.
    Includes bibliographical references and index.
    ISBN 978-0-86577-976-1 (alk. paper)
    1. Neurologic examination. 2. Neuroanatomy. I. Alberstone, Cary D.
    [DNLM: 1. Diagnostic Techniques, Neurological. 2. Central Nervous System—anatomy & histology.   WL 141 A535 2009]
    RC348.A53 2009
    616.8'0475—dc22
                                                                2008035366

Important note: Medical knowledge is ever-changing. As new research and clinical experience broaden our knowledge, changes in treatment and drug therapy may be required. The authors and editors of the material herein have consulted sources believed to be reliable in their efforts to provide information that is complete and in accord with the standards accepted at the time of publication. However, in view of the possibility of human error by the authors, editors, or publisher of the work herein or changes in medical knowledge, neither the authors, editors, nor publisher, nor any other party who has been involved in the preparation of this work, warrants that the information contained herein is in every respect accurate or complete, and they are not responsible for any errors or omissions or for the results obtained from use of such information. Readers are encouraged to confirm the information contained herein with other sources. For example, readers are advised to check the product information sheet included in the package of each drug they plan to administer to be certain that the information contained in this publication is accurate and that changes have not been made in the recommended dose or in the contraindications for administration. This recommendation is of particular importance in connection with new or infrequently used drugs.

Some of the product names, patents, and registered designs referred to in this book are in fact registered trademarks or proprietary names even though specific reference to this fact is not always made in the text. Therefore, the appearance of a name without designation as proprietary is not to be construed as a representation by the publisher that it is in the public domain.

Printed in India

5 4 3 2 1

ISBN 978-0-86577-976-1

To my wife, Lisa: Thank you for your patience and your friendship.
And to my children, Lauren and Adam: The nervous system is an extraordinary asset;
use yours to the utmost.
— *Cary Alberstone*

I dedicate this book to Mrs. Benzel (Mary, my wife) for her unending love and
support of my craziness and to our children (Morgan, Jason, Brian, and Matthew)
for their tolerance and their commitment to the team we call family.
— *Ed Benzel*

To my wife, Tania, whose continuous support allowed me to work on this book,
and to my children, Elias, Joseph and Maya, who make our efforts all worthwhile.
— *Imad Najm*

I dedicate this book to my wife, Bettina, and my children, Cameron and Marcus,
for their unending love and support. My family continuously reminds me
why we undertake such endeavors.
— *Michael Steinmetz*

Contents

Foreword

The authors of this volume are a world-class group of clinical neuroscientists from one of the world's greatest medical centers. They have done a masterful job of integrating basic anatomy and neurologic diagnosis based on the patient's signs and symptoms. This is the best book I have seen on the correlation between neuroanatomy and clinical findings during my more than 40 years of clinical practice. In 23 chapters, beginning with neuro-embryology and ending with cerebrospinal fluid, they have covered the full spectrum of regional and system-based neuroanatomy, related syndromes, and differential diagnosis. The presentation of each topic is concise, but it is comprehensive in its overall coverage of neurologic diagnosis. The text in each chapter is supplemented with color illustrations showing the anatomic basis of the patient's signs and symptoms. Students and trainees will benefit from studying this book from cover to cover, and clinicians with advanced knowledge and experience will use it frequently for quick reference.

Albert L. Rhoton Jr., MD
R.D. Keene Family Professor
Professor and Chairman Emeritus
Department of Neurosurgery
University of Florida

Preface

This book is intended for medical students, residents, and practicing clinicians who wish to understand or review the basic anatomic concepts that underlie neurologic diagnosis. The book explains the fundamentals of neuroanatomy and illustrates their clinical application. In keeping with this philosophy, this book emphasizes principles and clinically relevant facts: anatomic details with little or no clinical import are discussed briefly or omitted so as to concentrate on the essentials of neurologic diagnosis.

This fund of knowledge is organized as the clinical neurologist would organize it: by regions and functional systems. Thus, after an introductory chapter on neuroembryology (Part I), Part II of the book comprises a series of chapters on the anatomy of regional parts of the nervous system, including peripheral nerves, plexuses, nerve roots and spinal nerves, spinal cord, brainstem, cranial nerves, cerebellum, thalamus, hypothalamus, basal ganglia, limbic system, and cerebral cortex. These chapters are divided into two sections: the first section describes the basic anatomy of the region, the second section discusses the region's cardinal manifestations in disease.

Part III comprises a series of chapters on functional systems. These include the somatosensory system, visual system, auditory system, vestibular system, ocular motor system, motor system, autonomic system, and consciousness. These chapters are divided into two sections: the first section describes the basic anatomy of the system, the second section describes a practical approach to the patient with a system disorder. Part IV comprises a chapter on the vascular system and a chapter on the cerebrospinal fluid.

To complement and amplify the text we have illustrated the book lavishly with original drawings that convey anatomic and clinical concepts. These unique drawings are rendered so as to illustrate structure, function, and dysfunction in a single view. Thus each drawing illustrates the clinical deficit associated with a described structure, or, conversely, a structure that produces a described clinical deficit.

In introducing clinical material we have eschewed the fashionable "clinical notes" and "clinical correlates" frequently found in neuroanatomy textbooks. The inclusion of such corollaries, which primarily comprise descriptions of randomly selected syndromes, diseases, and diagnostic tests, in our view fails to meet the needs of those who actually require a logical, patient-oriented approach. Discussions of the pathology and clinical presentation of specific disease states are also assiduously avoided so as to put the proper emphasis where it belongs: on patients and their neurologic symptoms.

To that end, this book offers the following features:

- The cardinal manifestations of regional nervous system disturbances facilitate rapid anatomic localization.
- Approaches to common neurologic complaints demonstrate the systematic method of neurologic diagnosis.
- Abundant original drawings summarize key anatomic and clinical concepts.
- Ample tables summarize key points.

In this era of advanced diagnostic technology, the relevance of clinical diagnosis in neurology has not diminished. Indeed, despite recent technological advances made in our approach to the nervous system, particularly in neuroimaging, the signs and symptoms elicited by the clinician at bedside remain paramount in the process of neurologic diagnosis. With no working hypothesis—formulated by history taking and tested by physical examination—to guide ancillary studies, no rational decision can be made regarding which studies to undertake.

In whatever field of medicine or surgery one eventually practices, patients will present with nervous disorders. These patients deserve caring and knowledgeable physicians to accurately diagnose their complaints. The present book provides a rational and practical approach to this humbling task.

Acknowledgments

We wish to thank Christine Moore for her outstanding organizational contributions and Joseph Kanasz and Michael Norviel for their creativity and artistic skills.

Cary D. Alberstone
Edward C. Benzel
Imad M. Najm
Michael P. Steinmetz

I

Development and Developmental Disorders

1 Neuroembryology

Knowledge of nervous system development can provide the foundation for understanding nervous system structure and function. This chapter describes early development of the nervous system and then discusses development of the spinal cord and brain. The main malformations due to abnormal nervous system development are also discussed. **Table 1.1** summarizes the embryonic elements of the nervous system and their derivatives in the adult.

Early Neural Development

See **Fig. 1.1**.

Formation of the nervous system begins during the third week of gestation, when the neural plate develops from a thickening of the embryonic ectoderm. A longitudinal neural groove, bounded by two neural folds, forms along the midline of the plate. Fusion of the neural folds, which meet along the midline, proceeds in both cranial and caudal directions, gradually converting the grooved plate into the *neural tube*, which comes to lie below the surface ectoderm.

The process of neural tube formation (neurulation) occurs simultaneously with the separation of the neuroectoderm from the surface ectoderm, a process termed disjunction. Disjunction results in a separation of the future nervous system from the future skin. Failure to complete the process of disjunction (nondisjunction) and completion of disjunction prior to neural tube closure (premature disjunction) are two sources of spinal dysraphism.

Before the neural tube closes completely during the fourth week of embryonic development, it remains in communication with the amniotic cavity through the anterior and posterior neuropores. The anterior neuropore closes between gestational days 23 and 25; the posterior neuropore closes between gestational days 25 and 27.

Along the lateral margins on either side of the neuroepithelial cells of the neural plate are two strips of cells that pinch off from the neural groove as it forms the neural tube. These *neural crest* cells eventually occupy a dorsolateral position between the surface ectoderm and the neural tube. Most of the peripheral nervous system is derived from the neural crest, including sensory ganglion cells of the cranial and spinal nerves, autonomic ganglia, and Schwann cells. Neural crest cells give origin to the adrenal medulla and melanocytes as well (**Table 1.2**).

Thickening of the neural tube walls gives form to the brain and the spinal cord, whereas the lumen of the tube becomes the ventricular system and the central canal. The neuroepithelial cells that form the walls of the neural tube give origin to neurons and macroglia (i.e., astrocytes, oligodendrocytes, and ependymal cells). The microglia are derived from cells of mesodermal origin that enter the central nervous system (CNS) from the vasculature during development (**Table 1.2**).

Table 1.1 Adult Derivatives of Embryonic Brain Vesicles

Primary Vesicles	Secondary Vesicles	Adult Derivatives	
		Walls	**Cavities**
Forebrain (prosencephalon)	Telencephalon	Cerebral hemispheres	Lateral
	Diencephalon	Thalamus Epithalamus Hypothalamus	Third
Midbrain (mesencephalon)	Mesencephalon	Midbrain	Cerebral aqueduct
Hindbrain (rhombencephalon)	Metencephalon	Pons Cerebellum	Fourth
	Myelencephalon	Medulla	Fourth

Fig. 1.1 Early neural development.

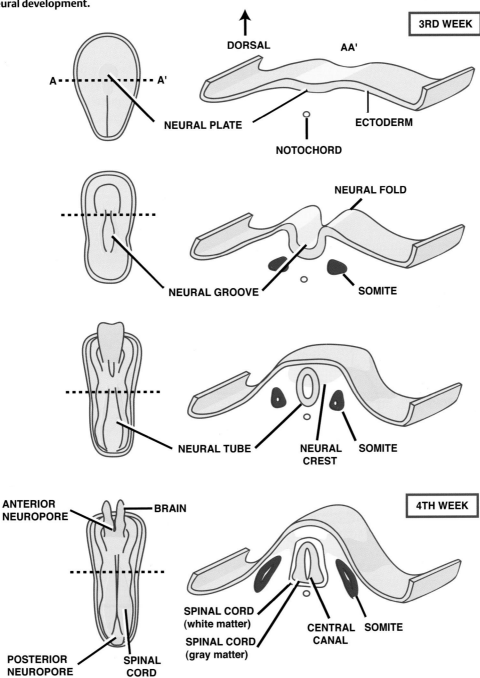

Table 1.2 Comparison of Neural Tube and Neural Crest Derivatives

Neural Tube Derivatives	Neural Crest Derivatives
Ventral horn cells	Cranial ganglia
Preganglionic autonomic neurons	Dorsal root ganglia
Astrocytes, oligodendrocytes, and ependymal cells	Autonomic ganglia
Retina	Schwann cells
Posterior pituitary	Adrenal medulla
Cortical neurons	Melanocytes
Gray nuclei of the brain and spinal cord	

Early Development of the Spinal Cord

See **Fig. 1.2**.

Three layers of cells are formed from the proliferation and differentiation of the thick, pseudostratified neuroepithelium that makes up the wall of the neural tube. Beginning from inner- to outermost, these are the *neuroepithelial layer*, the *mantle layer*, and the *marginal layer*.

On the innermost aspect of the neural tube, the neuroepithelium forms a layer of ciliated columnar cells, the neuroepithelial (or ependymal) layer, that lines the future ventricles and central canal.

The neuroepithelium also gives rise to primitive neurons, called *neuroblasts*, that migrate peripherally to surround the neuroepithelial layer. This so-called mantle layer will later form the gray matter of the spinal cord.

As the neuroblasts in the mantle layer develop into mature neurons with cytoplasmic processes, these processes extend peripherally to form the outermost marginal layer that later becomes the white matter of the spinal cord.

Astrocytes and oligodendrocytes are also derived from precursor blast cells that originate in the neuroepithelial layer and migrate peripherally into the mantle and marginal layers.

Fig. 1.2 **Early development of the spinal cord.**

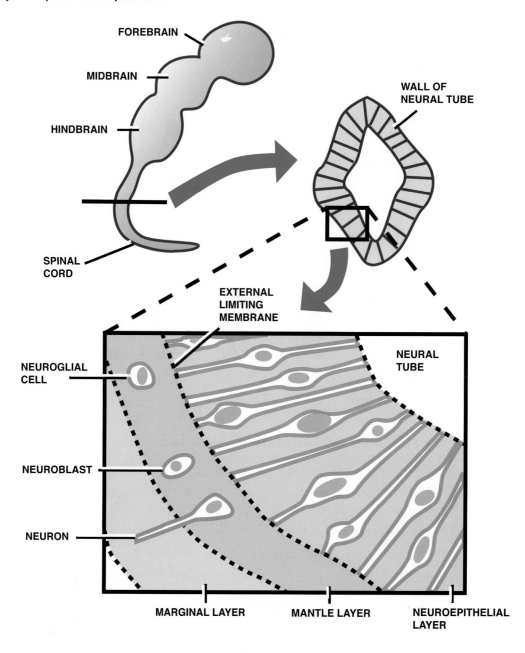

Spinal Gray Matter

See **Fig. 1.3**.

Thickening of the dorsal and ventral aspects of the neural tube produces the *alar* and *basal plates*, respectively. Together, these plates represent the future gray matter of the spinal cord. These dorsal and ventral bulges are separated by a longitudinal groove, the *sulcus limitans*, that develops along the sides of the central cavity.

The alar plate forms the dorsal gray columns, which contain sensory afferent neurons. In cross section, these columns are referred to as the dorsal horns. The basal plate contains somatic and autonomic motor neurons that constitute the *ventral* and *lateral gray columns*, respectively. In cross section, these columns are known as the ventral and lateral horns.

Fig. 1.3 **Spinal gray matter.**

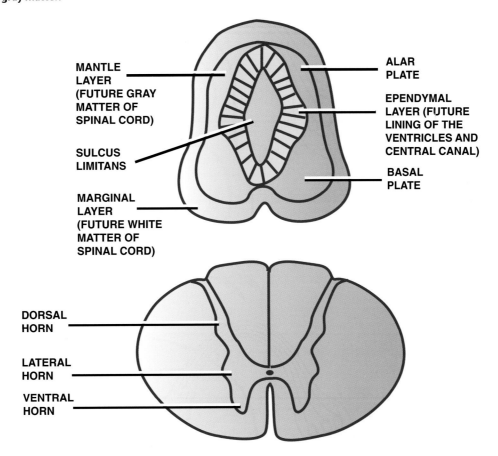

Ventral and Dorsal Roots

See **Fig. 1.4**.

Sensory neurons in the *dorsal root ganglia* are derived from the neural crest. These pseudounipolar neurons project both central and peripheral branches (axons).

The central branches of the dorsal root ganglia enter the spinal cord through the *dorsal sensory roots*. They either synapse in the dorsal gray column (spinothalamic tract) or ascend in the dorsal white column to terminate in the dorsal column nuclei (dorsal column–medial lemniscus tract). Neurons in the dorsal gray column and the dorsal column nuclei are derived from the alar plate.

The peripheral branches of the dorsal root ganglia enter the *spinal nerves*, course peripherally, and terminate as sensory endings in somatic or visceral structures.

Motor neurons in the ventral gray columns are derived from the basal plate. They project axons peripherally into the *ventral motor roots*.

Somatic motor neurons in the ventral motor roots join peripheral branches of the dorsal root ganglia in the region of the intervertebral foramina to form the spinal nerves. Sympathetic motor neurons in the ventral motor roots also join the spinal nerves but exit soon after in the *white communicating ramus* to reach the *paravertebral* and *prevertebral ganglia*.

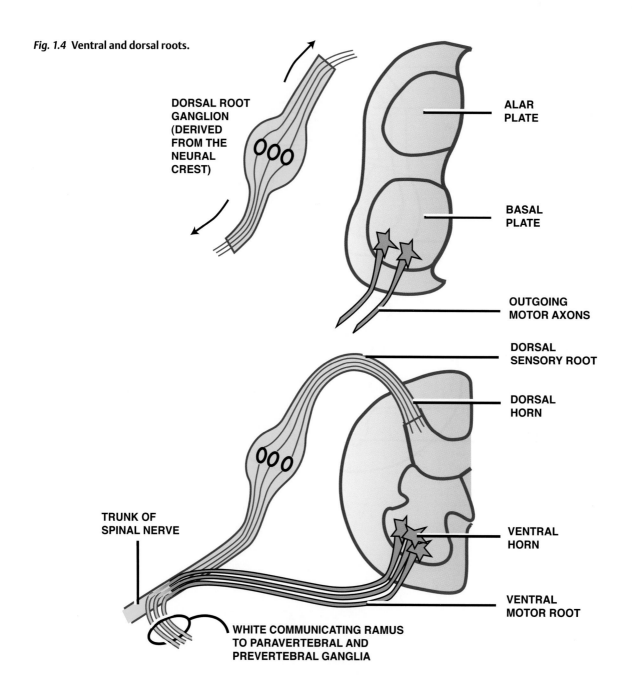

Fig. 1.4 **Ventral and dorsal roots.**

DORSAL ROOT GANGLION (DERIVED FROM THE NEURAL CREST)

ALAR PLATE

BASAL PLATE

OUTGOING MOTOR AXONS

DORSAL SENSORY ROOT

DORSAL HORN

TRUNK OF SPINAL NERVE

VENTRAL HORN

VENTRAL MOTOR ROOT

WHITE COMMUNICATING RAMUS TO PARAVERTEBRAL AND PREVERTEBRAL GANGLIA

Ascent of the Conus Medullaris

See **Fig. 1.5**.

During the early stages of development, the rate of growth of the spinal cord keeps pace with that of the vertebral column; thus, the spinal nerves pass through the intervertebral foramina at their respective level of origin in the spinal cord.

After the third month of embryonic development, however, the rate of growth of the vertebral column exceeds that of the spinal cord so that the end of the spinal cord assumes an increasingly higher position in relation to the vertebral column. In the adult, the caudal end of the spinal cord, called the *conus medullaris*, is positioned at the level of the first lumbar vertebra. The conus med-

ullaris is attached to the periosteum of the coccygeal vertebrae by a long thread of pia mater known as the *filum terminale*. Because of the differential rate of growth of the spinal column and spinal cord, the spinal cord segment does not correlate with the respective vertebral column levels. In the cervical spine, each vertebral level corresponds to the level of the succeeding cord segment (i.e., the sixth cervical spine corresponds to the level of the seventh spinal cord segment). In the upper thoracic spine, the difference is two segments, and in the lower thoracic and upper lumber spine, the difference is three segments.

Because all spinal nerves pass through their corresponding intervertebral foramina, the lumbar and sacral roots are considerably stretched. These lengthy fibers constitute the cauda equina (L. horse's tail).

Fig. 1.5 **Ascent of the conus medullaris.**

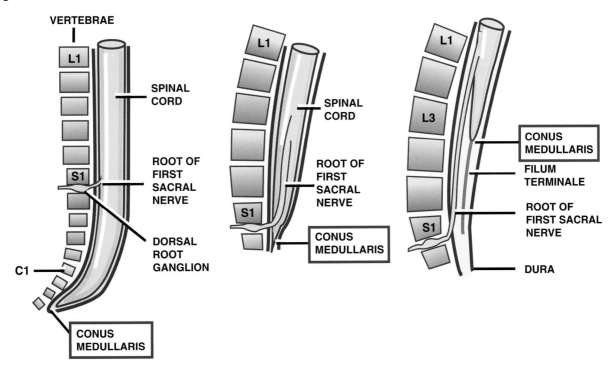

The Brain Vesicles

See **Fig. 1.6**.

During the fourth week of gestation, the rostral neural tube takes the form of three *primary brain vesicles*: the *forebrain* or prosencephalon, the *midbrain* or mesencephalon, and the *hindbrain* or rhombencephalon. During the fifth week, the forebrain divides into the *telencephalon* and *diencephalon*, the midbrain becomes the *mesencephalon*, and the hindbrain divides into the *metencephalon* and the *myelencephalon*, resulting in the formation of five *secondary brain vesicles*.

Fig. 1.6 **Brain vesicles.**

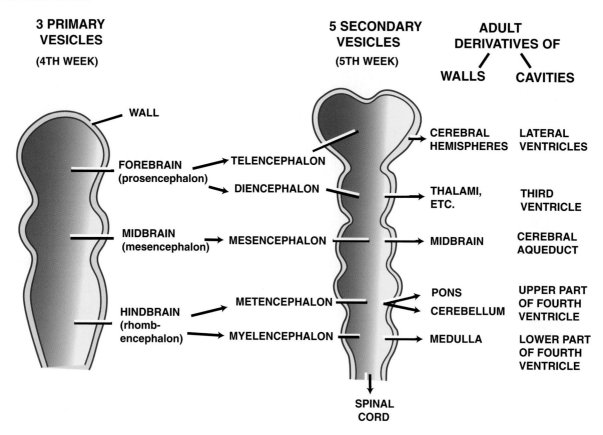

The Brain Flexures

See **Fig. 1.7**.

As the primary brain vesicles develop, the brain flexes, or bends, to form the *cephalic flexure* in the midbrain region, and the *cervical flexure* at the junction of the hindbrain and the spinal cord. A compensatory *pontine flexure* later forms between the cephalic and cervical flexures.

Fig. 1.7 **Brain flexures.**

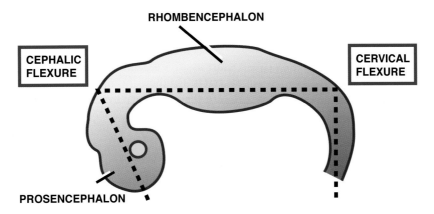

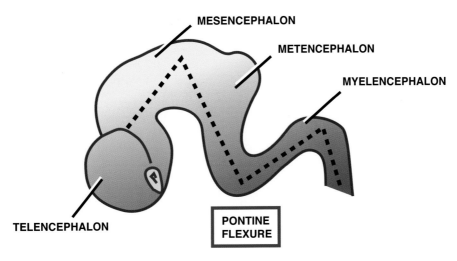

The Rhombencephalon (Hindbrain)

The cervical flexure marks the junction between the spinal cord and the hindbrain. The hindbrain is divided by the pontine flexure into the myelencephalon (the future medulla) and the metencephalon (the future pons and cerebellum).

The central cavity of the hindbrain becomes the fourth ventricle, the dorsal surface of which is bounded by an ependymal roof plate. The roof plate is formed as the fourth ventricle expands, spreading its lateral walls open like the pages of a book.

As a result of this change, the roof plate of the fourth ventricle, which is covered by vascular pia mater, is stretched and greatly thinned. Together, the roof plate and the vascular pia mater constitute the tela choroidea. Invagination of the tela choroidea into the cavity of the fourth ventricle forms the choroid plexus, which is responsible for the secretion of cerebrospinal fluid (CSF). Similar plexuses develop in the third and lateral ventricles.

CSF flows out of the fourth ventricle through two lateral apertures (the foramina of Luschka) and one median aperture (the foramen of Magendie) that are formed as local resorptions of the roof of the fourth ventricle.

Another change produced by the spread of the lateral walls of the fourth ventricle is that the alar plates assume a lateral position in relation to the basal plates. This explains why sensory neurons (derivatives of the alar plates) lie lateral to motor neurons (derivatives of the basal plates) in the pons and medulla, in contrast to their dorsal-ventral relation in the spinal cord.

The Myelencephalon

See **Fig. 1.8**.

The myelencephalon develops into the medulla oblongata. Many of the structural similarities between the medulla and the spinal cord, with which it is continuous, disappear during development as the fourth ventricle expands (see earlier discussion).

Neuroblasts of the alar plate develop into sensory nuclei; neuroblasts of the basal plate develop into motor nuclei. Some neuroblasts of the alar plate migrate ventrally to form isolated areas of gray matter, including the *inferior olivary nuclei*, which are associated with the cerebellum, and the *gracile* and *cuneate nuclei*, which are associated with the dorsal column–medial lemniscus tracts. On the ventralmost aspect of the caudal medulla are the medullary *pyramids*, which contain the corticospinal tracts.

Fig. 1.8 **The myelencephalon.**

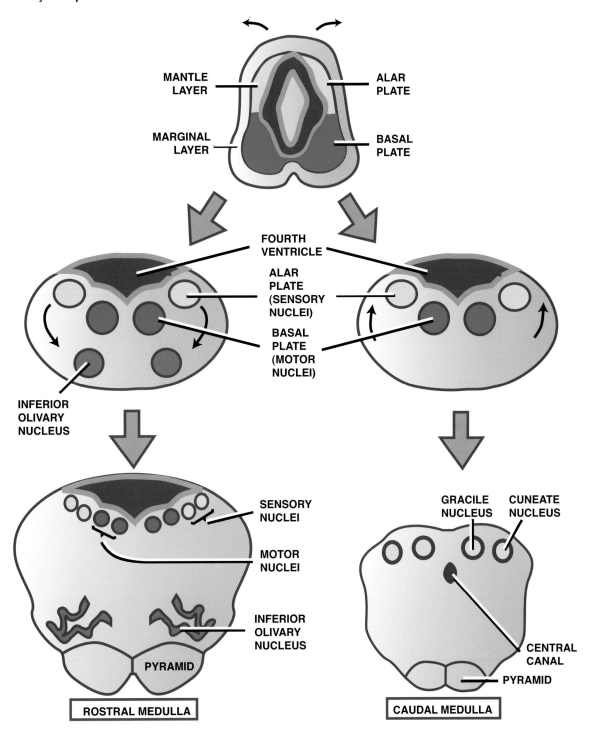

The Metencephalon

See **Fig. 1.9**.

The dorsal part of the metencephalon develops into the cerebellum, and the ventral part develops into the pons.

The *cerebellum* is formed from the fusion of dorsolateral thickenings of the metencephalon that overgrow the roof of the fourth ventricle. These thickenings, or *rhombic lips*, fuse in the midline to form the cerebellar *vermis*, which is flanked on either side by enlarging cerebellar *hemispheres*. Peripherally migrating neuroblasts contribute to the cerebellar *cortex*, whereas those situated centrally differentiate into the deep *intracerebellar nuclei*.

Development of the pons occurs ventral to the cerebellum in the ventral aspect of the metencephalon. The *pontine nuclei*, whose axons project to contralateral cerebellar cortices, come to lie in the ventral pons; the dorsal pons contains the cranial nerve nuclei. As in the myelencephalon, *motor cranial nerve nuclei* are derived from the *basal plate*; *sensory cranial nerve nuclei* are derived from the *alar plate*.

Fig. 1.9 **The metencephalon.**

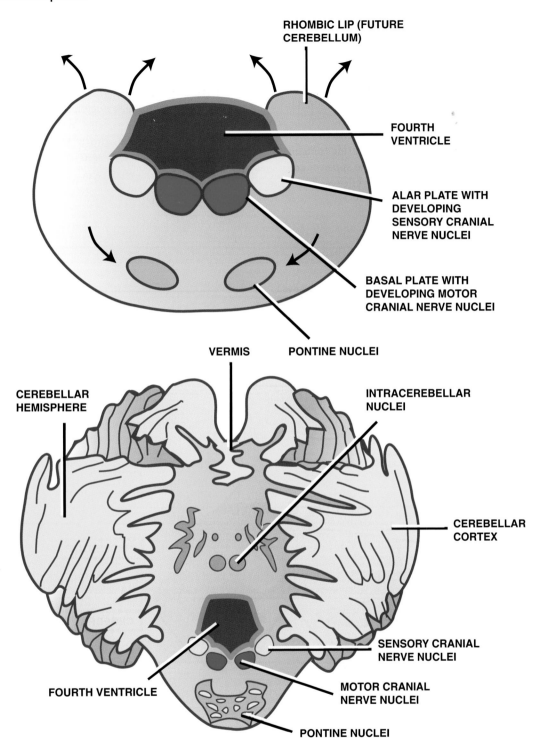

RHOMBIC LIP (FUTURE CEREBELLUM)

FOURTH VENTRICLE

ALAR PLATE WITH DEVELOPING SENSORY CRANIAL NERVE NUCLEI

BASAL PLATE WITH DEVELOPING MOTOR CRANIAL NERVE NUCLEI

VERMIS

PONTINE NUCLEI

CEREBELLAR HEMISPHERE

INTRACEREBELLAR NUCLEI

CEREBELLAR CORTEX

FOURTH VENTRICLE

SENSORY CRANIAL NERVE NUCLEI

MOTOR CRANIAL NERVE NUCLEI

PONTINE NUCLEI

The Mesencephalon

See **Fig. 1.10**.

Of all the parts of the brain, except the caudal hindbrain, the midbrain undergoes the least dramatic change during development. The central cavity of the midbrain forms the *cerebral aqueduct of Sylvius*, which connects the more expansive third and fourth ventricles.

Neuroblasts from the alar plates migrate into the roof, or *tectum*, of the midbrain to form the *inferior colliculi*, which are concerned with audition, and the *superior colliculi*, which are concerned with visual reflexes. These collections of cells produce four bulges on the dorsal surface of the midbrain, known as the quadrigeminal plate. The *central gray* surrounding the aqueduct is also derived from neuroblasts of the alar plates.

Neuroblasts from the basal plates give rise to several groups of neurons in the *tegmentum* of the midbrain, comprising the *oculomotor* (III) and *trochlear* (IV) cranial nerve nuclei, the reticular nuclei, the *red nuclei*, and the *substantia nigra*.

Two *cerebral peduncles* in the ventral midbrain contain cortical fibers descending to the brainstem and spinal cord.

Fig. 1.10 **The mesencephalon.**

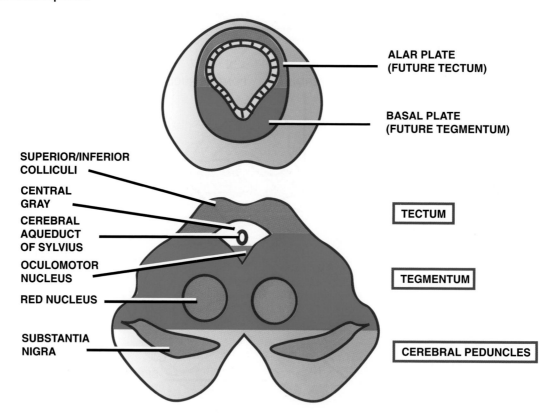

The Prosencephalon (Forebrain)

Early in development, a lateral outgrowth called the optic vesicle appears on each side of the forebrain. These vesicles, which give origin to the retinas and optic nerves, divide the forebrain into rostral and caudal parts, referred to as the telencephalon and diencephalon, respectively. (The optic vesicles themselves are of diencephalic origin.)

The Diencephalon

See **Fig. 1.11**.

The central cavity of the diencephalon becomes the *third ventricle*. As the third ventricle extends into the medial portion of the telencephalon, it is flanked by two larger lateral ventricles.

Three swellings develop in the lateral walls of the third ventricle that give rise to the *epithalamus*, the paired thalami, and the *hypothalamus*. The thalami are situated between the dorsally located epithalamus and the ventrally located hypothalamus. They are separated from the epithalamus by the epithalamic sulcus, and from the hypothalamus by the hypothalamic sulcus.

The epithalamus gives origin to the habenular nuclei and the pineal gland.

The thalami, which expand greatly in the lateral walls of the third ventricle, reduce the ventricle to a thin slit. In many brains, the thalami meet and fuse in the midline to form a gray matter structure called the massa intermedia.

The hypothalamus contains several cell groups related to autonomic and endocrine functions, and a paired group of neurons called the *mammillary bodies* that are visible as rounded swellings on the diencephalon's ventral surface.

More rostrally, two other swellings appear on the ventral surface of the diencephalon. These are the *optic chiasm*, in which the fibers from the medial halves of the retinas cross the midline, and the *infundibulum*, which is the stem of the pituitary gland. The retinas and the pituitary gland are both derived from a combination of surface and neural ectoderm, the latter of which is derived from a downward evagination of the diencephalon.

The Telencephalon

The telencephalon is subject to the most extensive developmental changes in the nervous system. It gives rise to the cerebral hemispheres, the cerebral commissures, the corpus striatum, and the internal capsule.

Early in development, the telencephalon consists of a median portion and two lateral diverticula, the telencephalic vesicles that will develop into the cerebral hemispheres. As mentioned earlier, the median portion of the telencephalon is filled by the rostral extension of the third ventricle. Filling the telencephalic vesicles are the lateral ventricles, which communicate with the third ventricle through the interventricular foramina (Monro).

Fig. 1.11 **The diencephalon.**

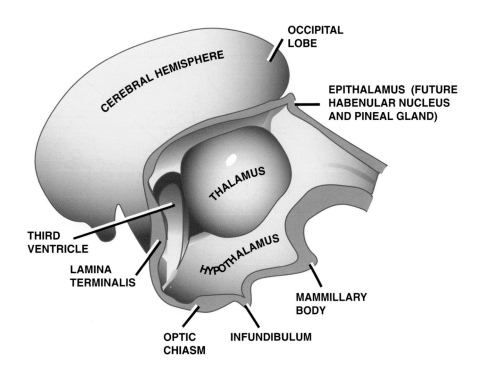

Cerebral Hemispheres

See **Fig. 1.12**.

During the fifth gestational week, the developing cerebral hemispheres expand in several directions, overgrowing the diencephalon, the midbrain, and the hindbrain. Embryonic mesenchyme that is trapped in the longitudinal fissure between the two hemispheres gives rise to the falx cerebri.

The multiple directions through which the cerebral hemispheres expand account for its mature, **C**-shaped, configuration. Thus the *frontal lobe* is formed from anterior growth of the hemispheres; the *parietal lobe* from lateral-superior growth; and the *occipital* and *temporal*

lobes from posterior-inferior growth. The slowly growing *insula* or *insular cortex* overlying the outer surface of the corpus striatum is overgrown by the frontal, parietal, and temporal lobes and thus comes to lie deep in the lateral cerebral sulcus (sylvian fissure).

A complex pattern of sulci and gyri develops in the external surface of the cerebral hemispheres, creating an increase in brain surface without a proportionate increase in the whole brain volume. Internally, the development of the lateral ventricles roughly parallels the development of the hemispheres. The anterior horn thus develops in the frontal lobe, the posterior horn forms into the occipital lobe, and the inferior horn projects to the temporal lobe.

The **C**-shaped pattern of growth assumed by the cerebral hemisphere and the lateral ventricle produces parallel **C**-shaped structures, including the fornix and the caudate nucleus (see later discussion).

Fig. 1.12 **Cerebral hemispheres.**

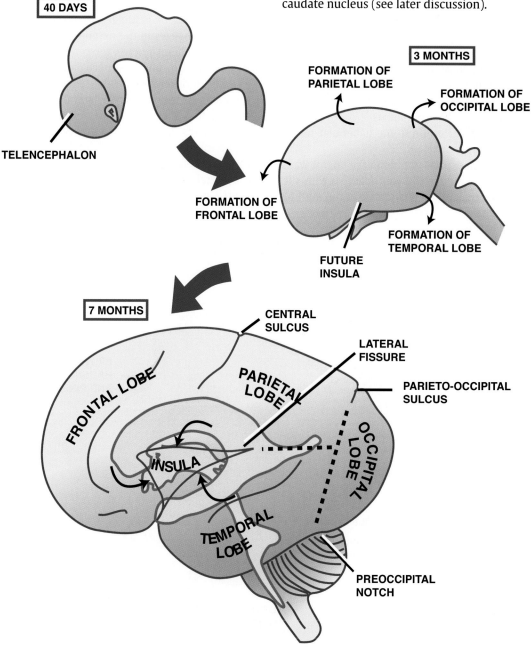

Cerebral Commissures

See **Fig. 1.13**.

These are groups of fibers that interconnect corresponding regions of the two cerebral hemispheres. This function is originally served by the cephalic end of the neural tube, the *lamina terminalis*, which later forms the anterior wall of the third ventricle. Three major commissures develop within (or from) the lamina terminalis.

The *anterior commissure* is the first commissure to form. It connects the olfactory bulbs and temporal lobes of both sides. Forming a **C**-shaped arch that overlies the thalamus, the *fornix*, which develops next, consists of longitudinally oriented fibers that project from the hippo-

campus to the mammillary bodies of the hypothalamus. Commissural fibers of the fornix connect the hippocampal formations of both sides, forming the *hippocampal commissure*. Finally, the *corpus callosum*, the largest of the cerebral commissures, takes the form of an arch over the third ventricle. It connects the neocortices of both sides.

What is left of the lamina terminalis after the development of these commissures is a thin wall called the *septum pellucidum*, which separates the anterior horns of the lateral ventricles. The corpus callosum and the fornix bound the anterior horns of the lateral ventricles from above and below, respectively.

Fig. 1.13 **Cerebral commissures** (Continued on p. 18).

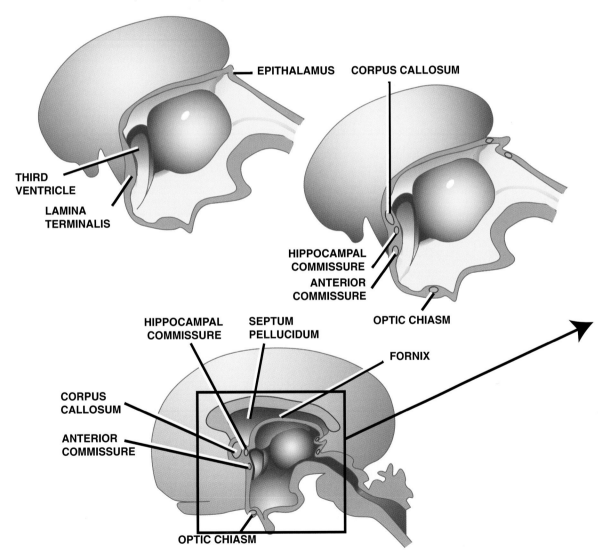

Fig. 1.13 **Cerebral commissures** *(Continued)*

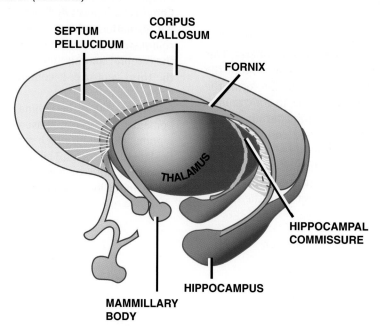

Corpus Callosum

See **Fig. 1.14**.

Because of its clinical importance, the development of the corpus callosum is worthy of a more detailed discussion. Anatomically, the corpus callosum is divided into four sections: the *rostrum*, *genu*, *body*, and *splenium*. Development of the corpus callosum begins at about the seventh week of gestation, when the dorsal aspect of the lamina terminalis thickens into what is known as the commissural plate. Once formed, a groove develops in the commissural plate, which becomes filled with cellular material. This cellular material forms a glial bridge superiorly across the groove, the cellular components of which express surface molecules and secrete chemical messengers that attract and help guide axons across the midline to form the three cerebral commissures.

Development of the entire corpus callosum, however, does not occur simultaneously; rather, it follows a rostral to caudal sequence. This means that arrest of the corpus callosum development prior to its completion results in a normally formed anterior portion but an absent or only partially formed posterior portion. Exceptions to this rostral-caudal sequence of development include the rostralmost portions of the corpus callosum—the rostrum and the anterior part of the genu. Violations of the "front to back" rule may also occur as a result of secondary destructive processes that damage the corpus callosum after it has already fully formed. These processes may lead to an absent or small genu or body and an intact splenium and rostrum.

Fig. 1.14 **Corpus callosum.**

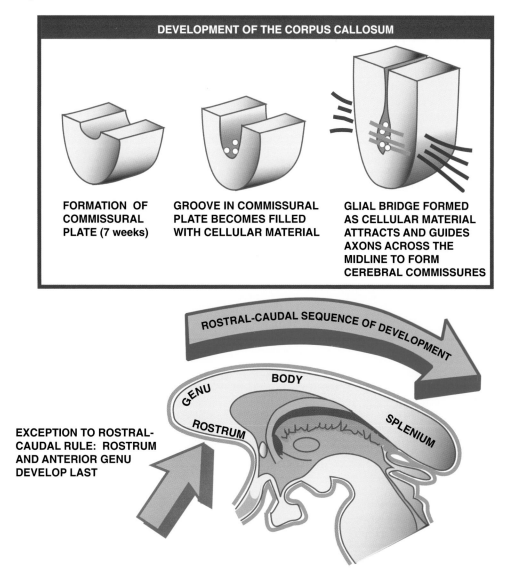

Corpus Striatum and Internal Capsule

See **Figs. 1.15** and **1.16**.

The putamen, the globus pallidus, and the *caudate nucleus* collectively constitute the *corpus striatum*, which represents the main component of the basal ganglia. These structures develop within the thick floor of the cerebral hemispheres, which undergo less lateral growth than the thin cortical walls. As a result, the striatum remains close to the midline of the brain, just lateral to the diencephalon (thalamus) because of posterior expansion.

The topographic anatomy of the corpus striatum is as follows. The *lentiform nucleus* (globus pallidus + puta-men) lies ventrolateral to the caudate, separated by the anterior limb of the *internal capsule*, which contains fibers headed to and from the cortex. The posterior limb of the internal capsule separates the lentiform nucleus from the thalamus.

Functionally and histologically, the putamen is similar to the caudate nucleus, and collectively they are known as the striatum. The striatum receives all of the afferent input to the basal ganglia. The globus pallidus, which is functionally and histologically distinct from the striatum, gives rise to the major efferents from the basal ganglia.

Fig. 1.15 **Corpus striatum and internal capsule.**
The putamen, caudate nucleus, and globus pallidus constitute the corpus striatum. The thalamus is medial. The lentiform nucleus (globus pallidus + putamen) lies ventromedial to the caudate nucleus, separated by the internal capsule.

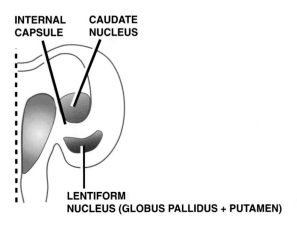

As mentioned, the peculiar **C**-shaped development of the cerebral hemispheres accounts for the configuration of the lateral ventricles. This is also true for the **C**-shaped caudate nucleus, whose head and body form the floor of the anterior horn and body of the lateral ventricle and whose tail forms the roof of the inferior horn.

Two smaller fiber tracts in this area are worthy of mention. The external capsule contains cortical projection fibers that pass lateral in relation to the lentiform nucleus. The extreme capsule separates another nucleus, the calustrum, from the insular cortex.

Fig. 1.16 **C-shaped development of the caudate nucleus**

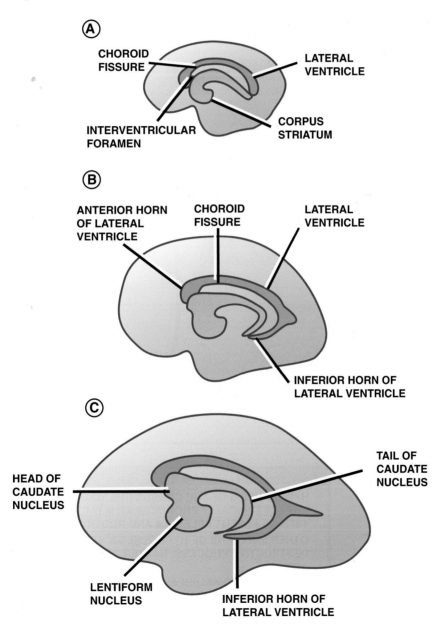

Congenital Malformations

See **Table 1.3**.

Anomalies of the Corpus Callosum

See **Fig. 1.17**.

As mentioned, the corpus callosum develops in a rostral to caudal sequence, with the exception of the rostrum and the anterior portion of the genu, which develop last. Normally, the corpus develops between the eighth and twentieth weeks of gestation, at the same time as the rest of the cerebrum and cerebellum. Developmental arrest of the corpus may result in its partial or complete absence. Because of the normal sequence of its development, partial absence of the corpus almost always presents as an intact genu, a partially or completely formed body, and a small or absent splenium and rostrum. Deviation from this scheme, such as a small or absent genu or body but an intact splenium and rostrum, are evidence of a secondary destructive process, rather than a developmental arrest. An exception is the callosal anomaly associated with holoprosencephaly, in which the corpus demonstrates an intact splenium in the absence of a genu or body.

Because the corpus develops at the same time as the cerebrum and cerebellum, callosal anomalies are often associated with other brain anomalies, such as the Dandy-Walker malformation, disorders of neuronal migration and organization, and encephaloceles. Isolated anomalies of the corpus callosum are usually asymptomatic. Symptoms, when present, are often related to associated brain anomalies. The most common associated symptoms are seizures and mental retardation. Callosal anomalies contribute to several syndrome complexes, such as Aicardi's syndrome, which is an X-linked disorder comprising infantile spasms, callosal agenesis or hypogenesis, chorioretinopathy, and an abnormal electroencephalogram.

Fig. 1.17 **Anomalies of the corpus callosum.**

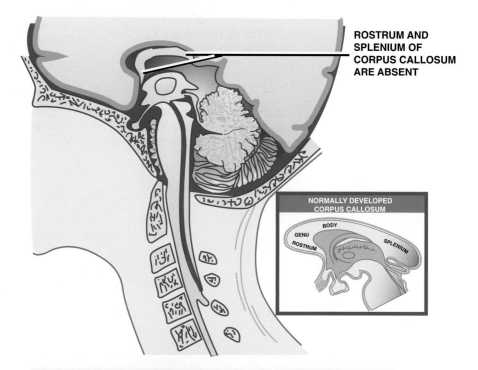

ROSTRUM AND SPLENIUM OF CORPUS CALLOSUM ARE ABSENT

NORMALLY DEVELOPED CORPUS CALLOSUM

BODY
GENU
ROSTRUM
SPLENIUM

CARDINAL FEATURES

- HYPOGENESIS OF THE CORPUS DUE TO DEVELOPMENTAL ARREST TYPICALLY PRODUCES AN INTACT GENU AND BODY WITH AN ABSENT SPLENIUM AND ROSTRUM
- OTHER PATTERNS OF HYPOGENESIS SUGGEST A SECONDARY DESTRUCTIVE PROCESS, RATHER THAN A DEVELOPMENTAL ARREST
- CALLOSAL ANOMALIES ARE FREQUENTLY ASSOCIATED WITH OTHER BRAIN ANOMALIES, SUCH AS DANDY-WALKER MALFORMATION, DISORDERS OF NEURONAL MIGRATION AND ORGANIZATION, AND ENCEPHALOCELES
- SYMPTOMS, WHICH MOST COMMONLY INCLUDE MENTAL RETARDATION, ARE USUALLY THE RESULT OF OTHER BRAIN ANOMALIES

Table 1.3 Congenital Malformations of the Central Nervous System

Anomalous Developmental Process	Congenital Malformation	Structural Defect	Clinical Manifestations
Neural tube closure	Anencephaly	Cranium and cerebral hemispheres absent	Stillborn
	Cranium bifidum	Cranial defect with herniation of meninges (meningocele); meninges and brain (meningoencephalocele); meninges, brain, and ventricles (menin-gohydroen-cephalocele	Varies from no functional impairment to severe motor and mental impairment with seizures
	Spina bifida occulta	Vertebral arch defect	Usually asymptomatic
Spina bifida cystica	Vertebral arch defect with herniation of meninges (meningocele) or meninges and spinal cord (meningomyelocele)	Varies depending on level, from saddle anesthesia to complete motor/sensory loss in the lower extremities and bladder/rectal incontinence	Differentiation and growth of cerebral hemisphere
	Agenesis of corpus callosum	Absence of corpus callosum	May be asymptomatic, mental retardation, seizures, disconnection syndrome
	Microcephaly	Low brain weight and size	Mental retardation
	Lissencephaly	Absence of cortical gyri	Mental retardation and hypotonia or spasticity
Polymicrogyria	Overabundant, undersized cortical gyri	Mental retardation and hypotonia or spasticity	Development of cerebrospinal fluid circulation
	Hydrocephalus	Enlargement of ventricles with increased intracranial pressure	Poor feeding, vomiting, paralysis of upward gaze, spasticity, mental retardation, decreased visual acuity

Intracranial Lipomas

See **Fig. 1.18**.

In normal development, an undifferentiated mesenchyme that surrounds the developing brain gives rise to the leptomeninges and the subarachnoid space. For reasons that are not well understood, abnormal differentiation of this undifferentiated mesenchyme may lead to the formation and deposition of fat in the subarachnoid space. Because of their location in the subarachnoid space, such lipomas typically contain blood vessels and cranial nerves, creating an obstacle to their surgical removal. In decreasing order of frequency, intracranial lipomas are found in the deep interhemispheric fissure, the quadrigeminal plate cistern, the interpeduncular cistern, the cerebellopontine angle cistern, and the sylvian cistern.

Interhemispheric lipomas, also known as lipomas of the corpus callosum, are typically associated with hypogenesis or agenesis of the corpus callosum. There is frequently also evidence of punctate or curvilinear midline calcifications, or the presence of other anomalies, such as encephaloceles and cutaneous lipomas. Rarely do intracranial lipomas exert significant mass effect on surrounding brain structures; thus, the need for surgical intervention is rare as well.

Cephaloceles

A cephalocele is a skull-base or calvarial defect that is associated with herniation of intracranial contents. If the herniated contents contain both meninges and brain tissue, then the malformation is termed a meningoencephalocele; if the herniated contents contain meninges only, then the malformation is termed a meningocele. The pathogenesis of cephaloceles varies depending on their location. Skull-base cephaloceles, which represent defects of endochondral bone, are caused either by failure of induction of bone due to faulty neural tube closure or disunion of basilar ossification centers. Calvarial cephaloceles, which represent defects of membranous bone, are caused either by a defect of bone induction, mass effect and pressure erosion of bone by an expanding intracranial lesion, or failure of neural tube closure. Cephaloceles are also classified according to their location, the most common of which include (1) occipital, (2) frontoethmoidal, (3) parietal, and (4) nasopharyngeal.

Fig. 1.18 **Intracranial lipomas.**

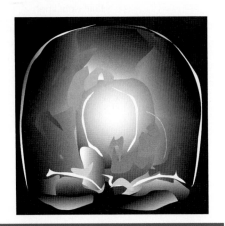

CLASSIC RADIOGRAPHIC APPEARANCE OF CURVILINEAR CALCIFICATION AT MARGINS OF INTERHEMISPHERIC LIPOMA

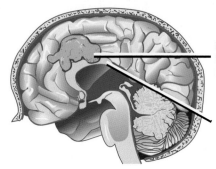

INTER-HEMISPHERIC LIPOMA

HYPOGENESIS OF CORPUS CALLOSUM

CARDINAL FEATURES

- REPRESENT AN ABNORMAL DIFFERENTIATION OF THE UNDIFFERENTIATED MESENCHYME THAT SURROUNDS THE DEVELOPING BRAIN
- THIS ANOMALOUS DEVELOPMENT RESULTS IN THE FORMATION AND DEPOSITION OF FAT IN A SUBARACHNOID SPACE
- THE MOST COMMON LOCATIONS: INTERHEMISPHERIC TISSUE, QUADRIGEMINAL PLATE CISTERN, INTER-PEDUNCULAR CISTERN, CEREBELLOPONTINE ANGLE CISTERN, AND SYLVIAN CISTERN

Occipital Cephaloceles

See **Fig. 1.19**.

The occipital region is the most common location for the development of a cephalocele and is generally associated with a less favorable prognosis, as compared with other locations. Herniated intracranial contents, when present, include supratentorial and infratentorial structures with equal frequency. Evaluation of these lesions should determine whether a dural venous sinus is included in the herniated sac, and which, if any, associated brain anomalies are present. Commonly associated brain anomalies include callosal anomalies, anomalies of neuronal migration, Chiari malformations, and Dandy-Walker malformations. Poor prognostic indicators include hydrocephalus, microcephaly, and the presence of brain tissue in the herniated sac.

Fig. 1.19 Occipital cephalocele.

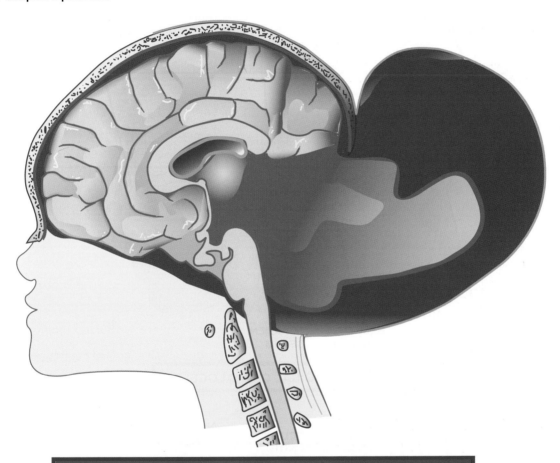

CARDINAL FEATURES

- REPRESENTS THE MOST COMMON LOCATION FOR A CEPHALOCELE
- PROGNOSIS LESS FAVORABLE AS COMPARED WITH OTHER LOCATIONS
- SUPRATENTORIAL AND INFRATENTORIAL STRUCTURES ARE INCLUDED IN THE HERNIA SAC WITH EQUAL FREQUENCY
- ASSOCIATED BRAIN ANOMALIES ARE COMMON
- POOR PROGNOSTIC INDICATORS INCLUDE HYDROCEPHALUS, MICROCEPHALY, AND THE PRESENCE OF BRAIN TISSUE IN THE HERNIA SAC

Frontoethmoidal Cephaloceles

See **Fig. 1.20**.

The underlying developmental anomaly responsible for the development of the frontoethmoidal cephalocele appears to be a failure in the normal regression of a projection of dura that extends from the cranial cavity to the skin through a persistent foramen cecum or fonticulus frontalis. Persistence of this projection of dura may give rise to a dermal sinus tract, which in turn may give origin to a dermoid or epidermoid tumor (see later discussion).

Examination reveals a superficial skin-covered mass or nasal dimple and frequently hypertelorism. Subtypes of frontoethmoidal cephaloceles are identified by the location of the bony defect, which may be between the frontal and nasal bones (*frontonasal cephalocele*); the frontal, nasal, and ethmoidal bones (*frontoethmoidal cephalocele*); or the frontal, lacrimal, and ethmoidal bones extending into the anteromedial portion of the orbit (naso-orbital cephalocele, not shown in figure).

Fig. 1.20 Frontoethmoidal cephaloceles.

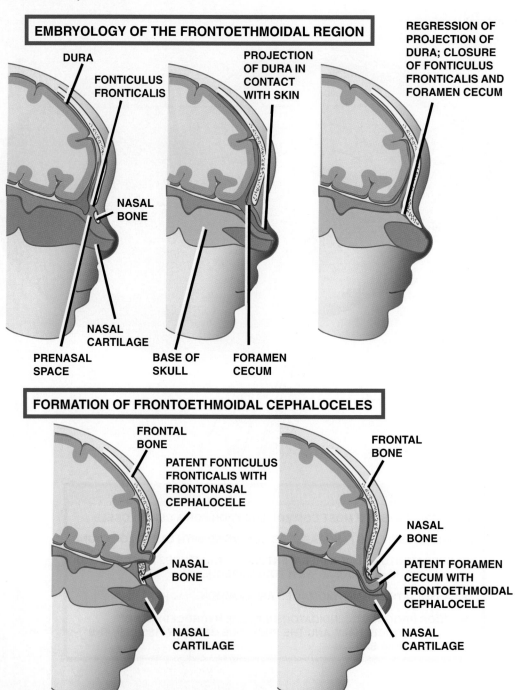

EMBRYOLOGY OF THE FRONTOETHMOIDAL REGION

REGRESSION OF PROJECTION OF DURA; CLOSURE OF FONTICULUS FRONTICALIS AND FORAMEN CECUM

DURA
FONTICULUS FRONTICALIS
PROJECTION OF DURA IN CONTACT WITH SKIN
NASAL BONE
NASAL CARTILAGE
PRENASAL SPACE
BASE OF SKULL
FORAMEN CECUM

FORMATION OF FRONTOETHMOIDAL CEPHALOCELES

FRONTAL BONE
PATENT FONTICULUS FRONTICALIS WITH FRONTONASAL CEPHALOCELE
NASAL BONE
NASAL CARTILAGE

FRONTAL BONE
NASAL BONE
PATENT FORAMEN CECUM WITH FRONTOETHMOIDAL CEPHALOCELE
NASAL CARTILAGE

Parietal Cephaloceles

See **Fig. 1.21**.

Parietal cephaloceles are uncommon. Prognosis is generally poor as a result of their common association with major brain anomalies, including Dandy-Walker malformation, callosal agenesis, Chiari II malformation, and holoprosencephaly. Because of their location, there is an increased incidence of sagittal sinus involvement, which must be specifically investigated. The parietal region is also a common location for atretic cephaloceles, which are small, hairless, midline masses associated with a sharply marginated calvarial defect and a high incidence of midline anomalies, such as porencephalies, interhemispheric cysts, and callosal agenesis.

Fig. 1.21 **Parietal cephalocele.**

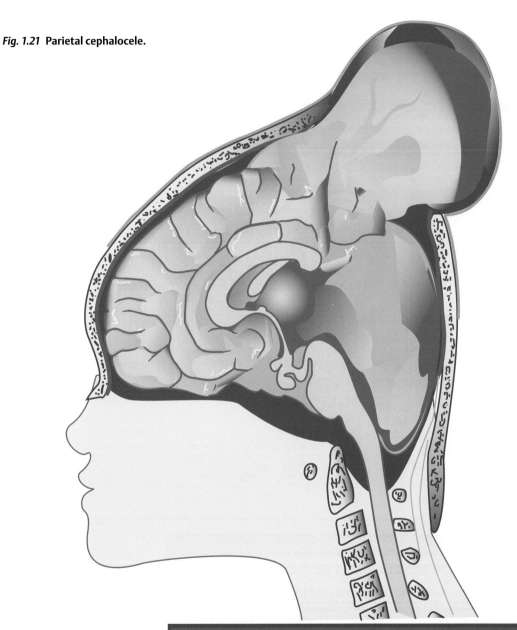

CARDINAL FEATURES
● **UNCOMMON**
● **PROGNOSIS POOR DUE TO ASSOCIATED MAJOR BRAIN ANOMALIES**
● **COMMON LOCATION FOR ATRETIC CEPHALOCELES, WHICH ARE MIDLINE MASSES FREQUENTLY ASSOCIATED WITH MIDLINE ANOMALIES SUCH AS PORENCEPHALIES, INTERHEMISPHERIC CYSTS, AND CALLOSAL AGENESIS**

Nasopharyngeal Cephaloceles

See **Fig. 1.22**.

These lesions are very uncommon. Their clinical significance lies in the fact that they are occult. Whereas the other cephaloceles are evident at birth, these lesions usually do not present until the end of the first decade of life, when they are diagnosed during an evaluation for persistent nasal stuffiness or excessive "mouth breathing." On examination they appear as nasopharyngeal masses that increase in size with a Valsalva maneuver. Associated intracranial anomalies, such as callosal agenesis, are common. In addition, tethering of the hypothalamus and optic chiasm as they extend into the sac may result in both endocrine and visual dysfunction.

Fig. 1.22 **Nasopharyngeal cephalocele.**

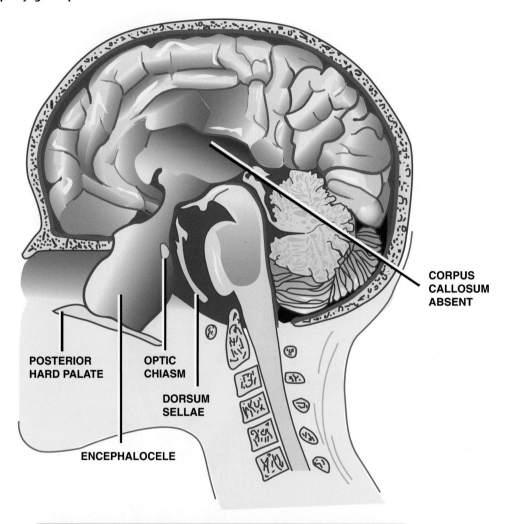

CORPUS
CALLOSUM
ABSENT

POSTERIOR
HARD PALATE

OPTIC
CHIASM

DORSUM
SELLAE

ENCEPHALOCELE

CARDINAL FEATURES
● UNCOMMON AND CLINICALLY OCCULT
● TYPICALLY PRESENT AT END OF FIRST DECADE OF LIFE AS NASAL STUFFINESS OR "MOUTH BREATHING"
● ASSOCIATED BRAIN ANOMALIES SUCH AS CALLOSAL AGENESIS ARE COMMON
● MAY PRODUCE ENDOCRINE OR VISUAL DYSFUNCTION DUE TO TETHERING OF HYPOTHALAMUS OR OPTIC APPARATUS

Dermal Sinuses

See **Fig. 1.23**.

Dermal sinuses are formed during the third to fifth weeks of intrauterine life when a defect occurs in the separation of neuroectoderm (the embryological precursor of nervous tissue) from surface ectoderm (the embryological precursor of skin). The dermal sinus tract thus formed may represent an abnormal communication between the dermis and the intracranial cavity, although the tract may end in subcutaneous tissue or in any tissue plane superficial to the intradural space. Because the primitive ectoderm has the capacity to form both dermal and epidermal tissue, the sinus tract frequently contains elements of both. Thus, a dermal sinus is typically composed of stratified squamous epithelium (epidermal component) as well as hair follicles, sebaceous glands, and sweat glands (dermal component).

The dermal sinus is a midline defect that may be found anywhere between the nasion and coccyx, although it is not commonly found between the glabella and the inion. Associated dermoid or epidermoid cysts may form at any point along the sinus tract, but most commonly they occur at the terminus of the tract. Clinical presentation varies from a benign cutaneous cosmetic blemish to a serious intracranial infection or a tumorlike process due to mass effect from a dermoid or epidermoid cyst. Commonly associated cutaneous stigmata include angiomata, abnormalities of pigmentation, hypertrichosis, abnormal hair pattern, subcutaneous lipomata, and skin tags.

Fig. 1.23 **Dermal sinuses.**

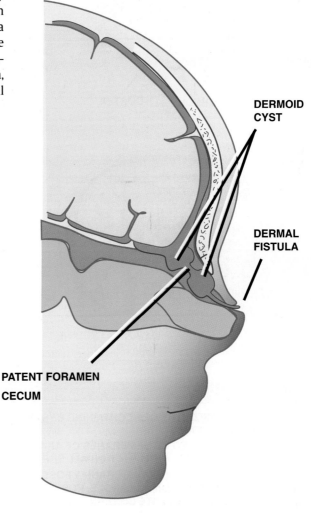

DERMOID CYST

DERMAL FISTULA

PATENT FORAMEN CECUM

Arachnoid Cysts

See **Fig. 1.24**.

Arachnoid cysts are CSF-containing lesions covered by membranes that consist of arachnoid cells and collagen fibers, which are continuous with the normal surrounding arachnoid. The formation of an arachnoid cyst appears to result from an anomalous splitting and duplication of the *endomeninx*, which normally forms a loose extracellular substance in the future CSF-filled subarachnoid space. Approximately two thirds of arachnoid cysts are located in the supratentorial space, most commonly the sylvian cistern, and one third are located in the infratentorial space, the latter fairly evenly divided between the cerebellopontine angle, posterior to the vermis, and superior to the quadrigeminal plate. Other supratentorial locations include suprasellar, interhemispheric, intraventricular, and superficial to the cerebral convexities. The clinical manifestations of arachnoid cysts may be variably attributed to mass effect, intracranial hypertension, or obstructive hydrocephalus. Patients may present with headache, seizure, or neurologic deficit.

Fig. 1.24 Arachnoid cysts.

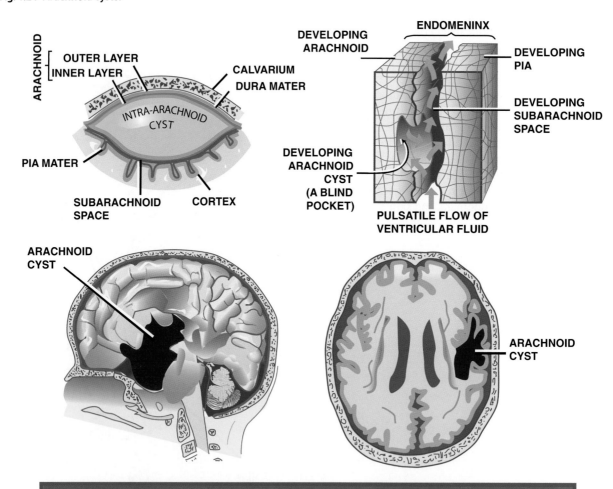

CARDINAL FEATURES

- CHARACTERIZED BY CSF-CONTAINING CYSTS FORMED BY AN ANOMALOUS SPLITTING OF THE ARACHNOID
- CYSTS ARE LINED BY MEMBRANES OF ARACHNOID CELLS AND COLLAGEN FIBERS, WHICH ARE CONTINUOUS WITH THE NORMAL SURROUNDING ARACHNOID
- SYLVIAN CISTERN (MIDDLE CRANIAL FOSSA) IS MOST COMMON LOCATION; OTHERS INCLUDE THE CEREBELLOPONTINE ANGLE, POSTERIOR TO THE VERMIS, AND SUPERIOR TO THE QUADRIGEMINAL PLATE CISTERN
- SYMPTOMS, WHEN PRESENT, ARE DUE TO MASS EFFECT, INTRACRANIAL HYPERTENSION, OR OBSTRUCTIVE HYDROCEPHALUS

Anomalies of Neuronal Migration and Organization

See **Fig. 1.25**.

During the seventh week of intrauterine life, a proliferation of neurons occurs in the subependymal walls of the lateral ventricles, in an area termed the *germinal matrix*. The proliferation of these neurons, which will eventually give rise to the cerebral cortex, is followed by a period of radial migration, which begins at about the eighth week of gestation. This migration of neurons is facilitated by radial glial fibers that extend from the ventricular surface to the pia. These glia provide an avenue for neuronal migration, which follows an orderly, predictable sequence; namely, those neurons destined for the deepest cortical layer (layer 6) migrate early, followed by neurons that will form successively superficial cortical layers. An exception are the neurons that are destined to form the most superficial layer, the molecular layer (layer 1), which apparently migrate first.

Once the neurons arrive in the cerebral cortex, a period of neuronal organization ensues in which the neurons are arranged into a discrete laminar pattern, after which they establish synaptic contacts with other local and remotely located neurons. Defects in the processes of neuronal migration or neuronal organization result in a variety of cerebral anomalies, which share in common that normally formed cortical neurons are residing in abnormal locations or patterns. Specific malformations that fall into this category include lissencephaly, heterotopia, polymicrogyria, and schizencephaly.

Fig. 1.25 **Anomalies of neuronal migration and organization.**

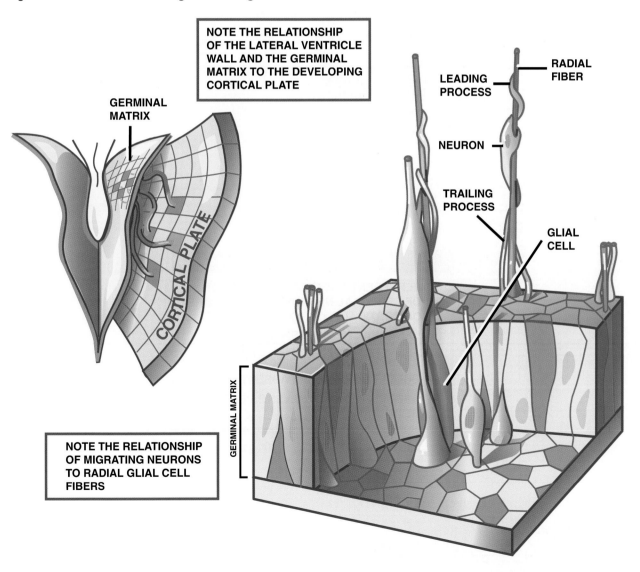

Lissencephaly

See **Fig. 1.26**.

In this condition, defective migration of cerebral neurons results in failure of cortical gyri to develop. Grossly, the cerebral hemispheres are smooth, cortical sulci are absent, and cerebral fissures are shallow. Microscopically, the cortical cell layers are aberrant. Affected children are severely mentally retarded.

Fig. 1.26 **Lissenencephaly.**

SHALLOW
SYLVIAN
FISSURES

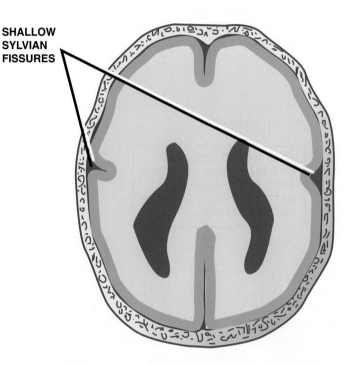

CARDINAL FEATURES
● REPRESENTS DEFECTIVE MIGRATION OF CEREBRAL NEURONS WITH FAILURE OF CORTICAL GYRI TO FORM
● CEREBRAL HEMISPHERES SMOOTH
● CORTICAL CELL LAYERS ABERRANT
● SULCATION OF BRAIN ABSENT
● ASSOCIATED WITH SEVERE MENTAL RETARDATION

Heterotopia

See **Fig. 1.27**.

Heterotopias comprise collections of normal "cortical" neurons that fail to reach the cortex as a result of a defect in radial neuronal migration. These ectopic islands of gray matter may occur in isolation or in association with other brain anomalies. Three subtypes of heterotopia are identified by location and pattern of organization, each of which is associated with a distinctive clinical picture and all of which share in common the presence of a seizure disorder. *Subependymal heterotopia* typically presents with normal motor function, normal development, and the onset of seizures in the second decade of life. *Focal subcortical heterotopia,* depending on its size, presents with normal to severely abnormal developmental delay and motor disturbances in association with a seizure disorder. *Band heterotopia* (also known as diffuse gray matter heterotopia) is typically manifest by moderate to severe developmental delay and medically intractable seizures.

Fig. 1.27 **Heterotopia.**

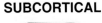

SUBEPENDYMAL   SUBCORTICAL   BAND

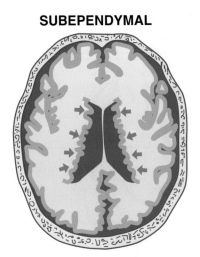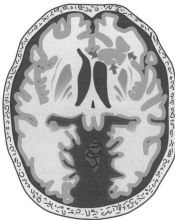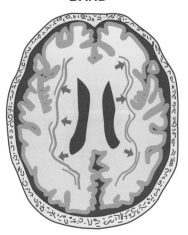

CARDINAL FEATURES

- **DEFINED AS ECTOPIC ISLANDS OF GRAY MATTER ("CORTICAL" NEURONS THAT FAIL TO REACH THE CORTEX)**
- **REPRESENTS A DEFECT IN RADIAL NEURONAL MIGRATION**
- **THREE SUBTYPES: SUBEPENDYMAL, SUBCORTICAL, AND BAND**
- **SEIZURE DISORDER IS THE CLINICAL FEATURE COMMON TO ALL THREE SUBTYPES**

Polymicrogyria

See **Fig. 1.28**.

Polymicrogyria, or cortical dysplasia, as the disorder is also known, represents an anomaly in neuronal organization. It is defined by a defect in the normal six-layered lamination of the cortex and an abnormal distribution of neurons into multiple small gyri. This abnormal cortical cellular organization may affect a variable portion of the cortex in one or both hemispheres. The most common area of involvement is the posterior end of the *sylvian fissure*. Grossly, polymicrogyria may demonstrate an irregular and bumpy surface or may be paradoxically smooth as a result of coalescence of microgyri in the molecular (surface) layer. Clinically, the malformation is associated with variably severe motor and intellectual dysfunction, depending on the extent of cortical involvement. There is a close association between cortical dysplasia and congenital cytomegalovirus infection.

Fig. 1.28 Polymicrogyria.

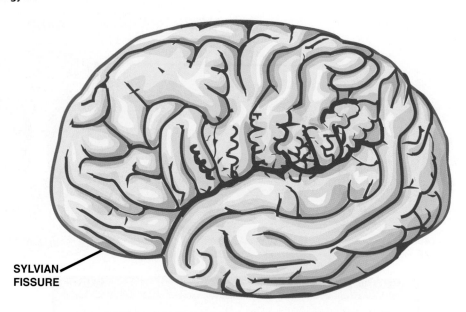

SYLVIAN FISSURE

CARDINAL FEATURES

- AN ANOMALY OF NEURONAL ORGANIZATION
- REPRESENTS ABNORMAL DISTRIBUTION OF NEURONS INTO MULTIPLE SMALL GYRI
- POSTERIOR END OF SYLVIAN FISSURE IS MOST COMMON AREA OF INVOLVEMENT
- CLINICALLY MANIFESTED BY MOTOR AND INTELLECTUAL DYSFUNCTION
- ASSOCIATED WITH CONGENITAL CYTOMEGALOVIRUS

Schizencephaly

See **Fig. 1.29**.

Schizencephaly is characterized by the abnormal development of a gray matter–lined cleft within the cerebral hemisphere that may extend for part of or the entire distance from the pial lining of the cortical surface to the ependymal lining of the lateral ventricle. These clefts are further classified as open or closed lip, depending on whether they extend the entire distance to the ventri-

cle (open) or stop short of the ventricle within the substance of the cerebrum (closed). Histologically, the clefts comprise cortical neurons that do not exhibit the normal six-layered lamination. They most frequently occur in the region of the pre- or postcentral gyri and may be unilateral or bilateral. Bilateral clefts are associated with a significantly worse prognosis. Clinically, the malformation is marked by seizures, hemiparesis, and variable developmental delay, the severity of which is determined by the location, extent, and number of clefts.

Fig. 1.29 Schizencephaly.

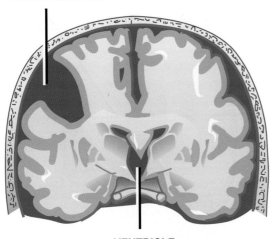 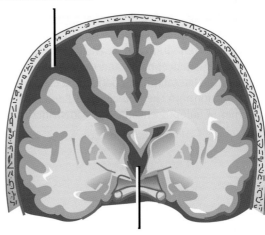

CLOSED LIP SCHIZENCEPHALY

OPEN LIP SCHIZENCEPHALY

VENTRICLE

VENTRICLE

CARDINAL FEATURES

- DEFINED AS AN ABNORMAL DEVELOPMENT OF A GRAY MATTER–LINED CLEFT THAT EXTENDS A VARIABLE DISTANCE FROM THE CORTICAL SURFACE TO THE LATERAL VENTRICLE
- THE CLEFT MAY EXTEND THE ENTIRE DISTANCE FROM THE CORTICAL SURFACE TO THE VENTRICLE (OPEN LIP SCHIZENCEPHALY), OR IT MAY STOP SHORT OF THE VENTRICLE (CLOSED LIP SCHIZENCEPHALY)
- THE PRE- AND POSTCENTRAL GYRI ARE THE MOST COMMON LOCATION OF THE CLEFT, WHICH MAY BE UNILATERAL OR BILATERAL

Holoprosencephaly

Holoprosencephaly refers to a group of related disorders that share in common a failure of differentiation and cleavage of the prosencephalon. By day 32 of normal development, the germinal matrix begins to cleave into superior and inferior portions. The germinal matrix gives rise to all of the neurons of the cerebral hemispheres and the deep cerebral nuclei. In time, the superior portion of the germinal matrix will give rise to neurons that form the telencephalon (the caudate, putamen, and cerebral hemispheres), whereas the inferior portion will give rise to neurons that form the diencephalon (the thalamus, hypothalamus, and globus pallidus).

Almost simultaneously, between days 32 and 34, the lamina terminalis begins to differentiate into the interhemispheric cerebral commissures, the formation of which is associated with the evagination and separation of the cerebral hemispheres, which begin on day 35. A defect in the cleavage processes involving the germinal matrix and the lamina terminalis results in a failure of the transverse differentiation and cleavage of the prosencephalon into the telencephalon and the diencephalon, and a failure of the lateral differentiation and cleavage of the prosencephalon into the two cerebral hemispheres. Three subtypes of holoprosencephaly are identified.

Alobar holoprosencephaly (**Fig. 1.30**) is the most severe form. It is characterized by *fused thalami* and an *absent third ventricle*. There is no interhemispheric fissure, falx cerebri, or corpus callosum. A *holoventricle* is contiguous with a large dorsal cyst, leaving only a small rim of brain anteriorly. Associated anomalies include severe midline facial deformities and hypotelorism, which in its most severe form is manifest by cyclopia.

Fig. 1.30 **Alobar holoprosencephaly.**

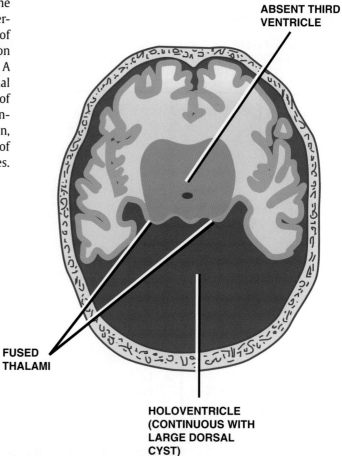

ABSENT THIRD VENTRICLE

FUSED THALAMI

HOLOVENTRICLE (CONTINUOUS WITH LARGE DORSAL CYST)

CARDINAL FEATURES
● MOST SEVERE FORM OF HOLOPROSENCEPHALY, (A FAILURE OF DIFFERENTIATION AND CLEAVAGE OF PROSENCEPHALON)
● FUSED THALAMI WITH ABSENT THIRD VENTRICLE
● ABSENT INTERHEMISPHERIC FISSURE, FALX CEREBRI, AND CORPUS CALLOSUM
● HOLOVENTRICLE IS CONTINUOUS WITH LARGE DORSAL CYST
● ASSOCIATED WITH SEVERE MIDLINE FACIAL DEFORMITIES AND HYPOTELORISM

Semilobar holoprosencephaly (**Fig. 1.31**) represents a less severe malformation than alobar holoprosencephaly. There is present at least a partial separation of the thalami, and thus a *small third ventricle* and a partially formed or absent interhemispheric fissure and falx cerebri. In contrast to the usual hypogenetic corpus callosum, in which genu and body are normally developed but the splenium is absent or small, holoprosencephaly is the one exception that demonstrates an intact splenium but a small or absent genu and body.

Fig. 1.31 **Semilobar holoprosencephaly.**

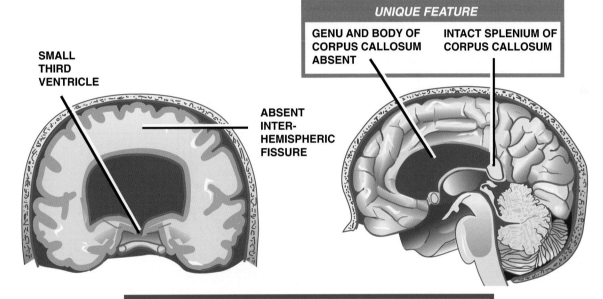

SMALL
THIRD
VENTRICLE

ABSENT
INTER-
HEMISPHERIC
FISSURE

UNIQUE FEATURE

GENU AND BODY OF
CORPUS CALLOSUM
ABSENT

INTACT SPLENIUM OF
CORPUS CALLOSUM

CARDINAL FEATURES

● MODERATELY SEVERE FORM OF HOLOPROSENCEPHALY, (A FAILURE OF DIFFERENTIATION AND CLEAVAGE OF PROSENCEPHALON)

● PARTIAL SEPARATION OF THALAMI WITH SMALL THIRD VENTRICLE

● PARTIALLY FORMED OR ABSENT INTERHEMISPHERIC TISSUE AND FALX CEREBRI

● INTACT SPLENIUM OF CORPUS CALLOSUM (SMALL OR ABSENT GENU AND BODY)

Finally, lobar holoprosencephaly (**Fig. 1.32**) represents a still less severe form of holoprosencephaly. It is characterized by a fully formed third ventricle and an intact corpus callosum. As in all forms of holoprosencephaly, the septum pellucidum is absent, and the frontal lobes are typically hypoplastic.

Fig. 1.32 **Lobar holoprosencephaly.**

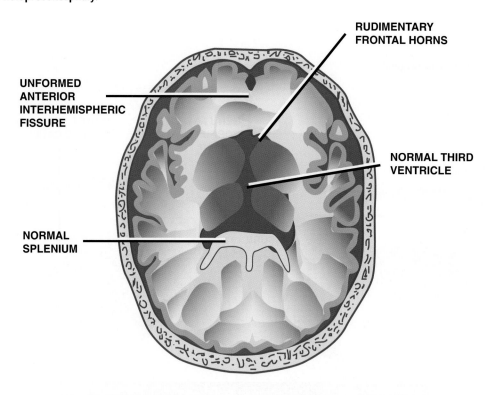

RUDIMENTARY FRONTAL HORNS

UNFORMED ANTERIOR INTERHEMISPHERIC FISSURE

NORMAL THIRD VENTRICLE

NORMAL SPLENIUM

CARDINAL FEATURES
● MILDEST FORM OF HOLOPROSENCEPHALY
● SEPTUM PELLUCIDUM IS ABSENT AND FRONTAL LOBES ARE HYPOPLASTIC, BUT THIRD VENTRICLE AND CORPUS CALLOSUM ARE INTACT

Septo-optic Dysplasia

See **Fig. 1.33**.

Septo-optic dysplasia is characterized by two primary features: (1) hypoplasia of the optic nerves and (2) hypoplasia or absence of the septum pellucidum. Clinically, the malformation exhibits visual disturbances, which may include nystagmus or loss of visual acuity, and an endocrine deficiency that usually involves growth hormone and thyroid-stimulating hormone.

Fig. 1.33 **Septo-optic dysplasia.**

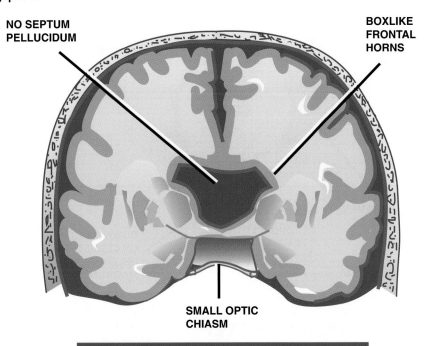

NO SEPTUM PELLUCIDUM

BOXLIKE FRONTAL HORNS

SMALL OPTIC CHIASM

CARDINAL FEATURES
● CHARACTERIZED BY HYPOPLASIA OF OPTIC NERVE AND HYPOPLASIA OR ABSENCE OF SEPTUM PELLUCIDUM
● ASSOCIATED WITH VISUAL DISTURBANCES AND ENDOCRINE DEFICIENCIES

Chiari Malformations

Chiari described three malformations of the hindbrain, which share in common the presence of hydrocephalus. The Chiari I malformation (**Fig. 1.34**) consists of a caudal extension of the cerebellar tonsils below the level of the foramen magnum. These malformations may be asymptomatic or may be associated with symptoms related to syringomyelia, such as cranial nerve palsies and dissociated sensory loss. Headache, neck, and arm pain may develop in the adult.

Fig. 1.34 **Chiari I malformation.**

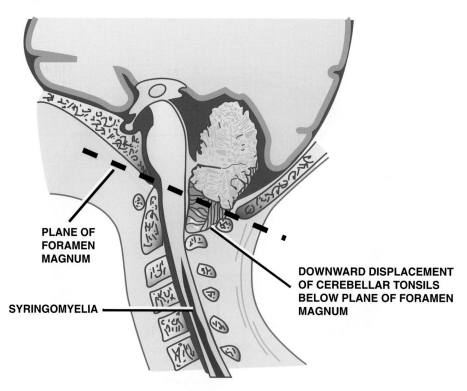

PLANE OF
FORAMEN
MAGNUM

DOWNWARD DISPLACEMENT
OF CEREBELLAR TONSILS
BELOW PLANE OF FORAMEN
MAGNUM

SYRINGOMYELIA

CARDINAL FEATURES
● DEFINED BY A CAUDAL EXTENSION OF CEREBELLAR TONSILS BELOW LEVEL OF FORAMEN MAGNUM
● APPROXIMATELY 50% OF CASES ASSOCIATED WITH SYRINGOMYELIA
● MAY BE ASYMPTOMATIC OR ASSOCIATED WITH HEADACHE, NECK, OR ARM PAIN
● SYMPTOMS OF SYRINGOMYELIA (CRANIAL NERVE PALSIES, DISSOCIATED SENSORY LOSS, OR MYELOPATHY) MAY ALSO OCCUR

The Chiari II malformation (**Fig. 1.35**) is a complex malformation that is invariably associated with myelomeningocele and with multiple other brain anomalies. It has been postulated that the hindbrain findings of the Chiari II malformation may be explained by the development of a normal-sized cerebellum but an abnormally small posterior fossa and a low tentorial attachment. The clinical manifestations of Chiari II malformation are complex and varied. Infants require repair of the myelo-meningocele and shunting of the hydrocephalus. They may exhibit life-threatening bulbar symptoms, such as apnea and bradycardia, and nystagmus is a common clinical finding. In childhood, progressive spastic weakness and appendicular ataxia may develop gradually, adding incrementally to the child's disability. Teenagers may present with insidious onset gait difficulty and truncal ataxia, although by adulthood the symptoms tend to stabilize.

Fig. 1.35 **Chiari II malformation.**

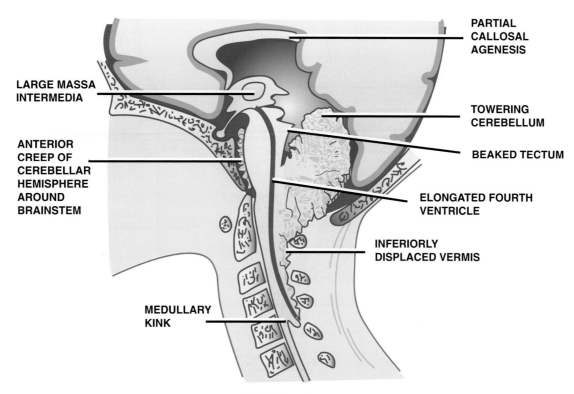

LARGE MASSA INTERMEDIA

ANTERIOR CREEP OF CEREBELLAR HEMISPHERE AROUND BRAINSTEM

MEDULLARY KINK

PARTIAL CALLOSAL AGENESIS

TOWERING CEREBELLUM

BEAKED TECTUM

ELONGATED FOURTH VENTRICLE

INFERIORLY DISPLACED VERMIS

CARDINAL FEATURES
● DEFINED BY INFERIORLY DISPLACED VERMIS AND MULTIPLE ASSOCIATED ANOMALIES
● ASSOCIATED WITH LACUNAR SKULL ("LÜCKENSCHÄDEL"), MYELOMENINGOCELE (100%), SYRINGOMYELIA (50–90%), FENESTRATED FALX, SMALL POSTERIOR FOSSA, HYDROCEPHALUS (90%), AND MULTIPLE BRAIN ANOMALIES (SEE LIST BELOW)
● CLINICAL MANIFESTATIONS ARE COMPLEX AND VARIED (SEE TEXT)

ASSOCIATED BRAIN ANOMALIES	
● INFERIORLY DISPLACED VERMIS	● HETEROTOPIAS
● MEDULLARY KINKING	● POLYMICROGYRIA
● INTERDIGITATED GYRI	● BEAKED TECTUM
● LARGE MASSA INTERMEDIA	● TOWERING CEREBELLUM WITH ANTERIOR CREEP AROUND BRAINSTEM
● PARTIAL CALLOSAL AGENESIS	

Finally, the Chiari III malformation (**Fig. 1.36**), an extremely rare condition, is characterized by herniation of posterior fossa contents through a spina bifida defect at the C1–C2 level. This malformation is rarely compatible with life.

Fig. 1.36 **Chiari III malformation.**

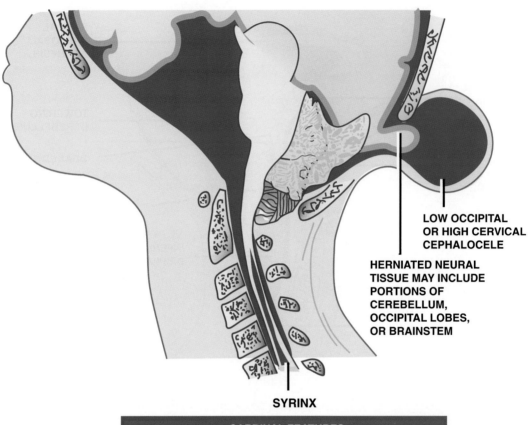

LOW OCCIPITAL
OR HIGH CERVICAL
CEPHALOCELE

HERNIATED NEURAL
TISSUE MAY INCLUDE
PORTIONS OF
CEREBELLUM,
OCCIPITAL LOBES,
OR BRAINSTEM

SYRINX

CARDINAL FEATURES
● RARE CONDITION
● DEFINED BY LOW OCCIPITAL OR HIGH CERVICAL CEPHALOCELE

Dandy-Walker Malformation

See **Fig. 1.37**.

The Dandy-Walker malformation is characterized by an enlarged posterior fossa with an elevated tentorial attachment, hypogenesis or agenesis of the cerebellar vermis, and a cystic dilatation of the fourth ventricle. The presence of a communication between the fourth ventricle and the *cisterna magna* differentiates this malformation from a mega cisterna magna, which exhibits an enlarged posterior fossa but an intact cerebellar vermis and an intact fourth ventricle without communication between the latter and the cisterna magna. The Dandy-Walker variant, which also must be considered in the differential diagnosis of the Dandy-Walker malformation, is defined by hypogenesis of the cerebellar vermis and cystic dilatation of the fourth ventricle but a normal-sized posterior fossa.

Hydrocephalus frequently accompanies the Dandy-Walker malformation, affecting ~90% of patients at the time of diagnosis. The most commonly associated brain anomaly is callosal agenesis, which affects about one third of patients with the malformation. Clinically, the malformation may present with developmental delay, enlarged head circumference, or signs and symptoms of hydrocephalus.

Fig. 1.37 **Dandy-Walker malformation.**

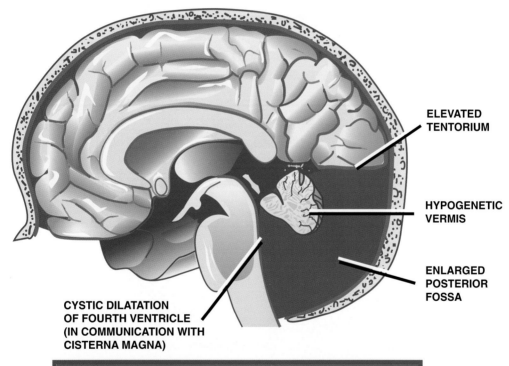

ELEVATED
TENTORIUM

HYPOGENETIC
VERMIS

ENLARGED
POSTERIOR
FOSSA

CYSTIC DILATATION
OF FOURTH VENTRICLE
(IN COMMUNICATION WITH
CISTERNA MAGNA)

CARDINAL FEATURES

- CHARACTERIZED BY (1) AN ENLARGED POSTERIOR FOSSA, (2) AN ELEVATED TENTORIAL ATTACHMENT, (3) HYPOGENESIS OR AGENESIS OF THE CEREBELLAR VERMIS, AND (4) A CYSTIC DILATATION OF THE FOURTH VENTRICLE
- ASSOCIATED WITH HYDROCEPHALUS IN 90% OF CASES
- ASSOCIATED WITH CALLOSAL AGENESIS IN ONE THIRD OF CASES
- MAY BE ASSOCIATED WITH DEVELOPMENTAL DELAY, ENLARGED HEAD CIRCUMFERENCE, OR SIGNS AND SYMPTOMS OF HYDROCEPHALUS

Lhermitte-Duclos Syndrome

See **Fig. 1.38**.

Lhermitte-Duclos syndrome, also known as diffuse hypertrophy of the cerebellar cortex or dysplastic cerebellar gangliocytoma, is defined by a focal hypertrophy of the cerebellar cortex. Histologically, the affected cortex demonstrates a thick layer of abnormal ganglion cells that occupy the granular layer, a thick hypermyelinated marginal layer, and a thin Purkinje layer. Grossly, the disorder may extend into the vermis or, rarely, into the contralateral hemisphere. Mass effect, if present, may produce cerebellar symptoms, although many affected individuals are asymptomatic.

Fig. 1.38 **Lhermitte-Duclos syndrome.**

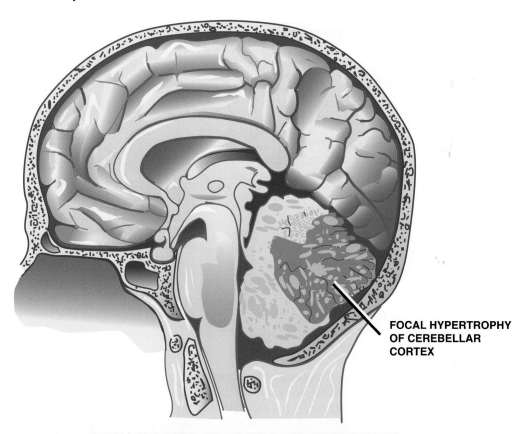

FOCAL HYPERTROPHY
OF CEREBELLAR
CORTEX

CARDINAL FEATURES

- **CHARACTERIZED BY A FOCAL HYPERTROPHY OF THE CEREBELLAR CORTEX**
- **HISTOLOGICALLY MARKED BY A THICK LAYER OF GANGLION CELLS THAT OCCUPY THE GRANULAR LAYER, A THICK HYPERMYELINATED MARGINAL LAYER, AND A THIN PURKINJE LAYER**
- **MAY BE ASYMPTOMATIC OR PRODUCE BRAINSTEM OR CEREBELLAR SYMPTOMS DUE TO MASS EFFECT**

The Phakomatoses

The phakomatoses represent a group of congenital disorders that share in common a defect in the development of ectodermal structures, including the nervous structures, the skin, the retina, and the globe. Four major malformations are identified: neurofibromatosis, tuberous sclerosis, Sturge-Weber syndrome, and von Hippel-Lindau disease.

Neurofibromatosis

There are two types of neurofibromatosis, type 1 and type 2, that are distinguished on the basis of their pathological and clinical manifestations. Neurofibromatosis type 1 (NF1), known as von Recklinghausen's disease, is an autosomal dominant disorder that affects ~1 in 3000 to 5000 people. Genetic analysis has linked the disease to the long arm of chromosome 17. Diagnostic criteria of NF1 have been established by a National Institutes of Health (NIH) Consensus Development Conference. The major intracranial lesions associated with the disease are optic gliomas, other cerebral astrocytomas, sphenoid wing dysplasia, and plexiform neurofibromas. Spinal manifestations include scoliosis, nerve sheath tumors, and lateral meningoceles.

Neurofibromatosis type 2 (NF2) is an autosomal dominant disorder associated with an abnormality of chromosome 22. Its most distinctive feature is the almost invariable appearance of bilateral acoustic schwannomas. Other intracranial tumors, particularly meningiomas, may occur in multiple numbers. Spinal manifestations include multiple extramedullary schwannomas and meningiomas, as well as intramedullary spinal cord ependymomas. Absent or minimal in size or number are many of the common features of NF1, including café au lait spots, cutaneous neurofibromas, optic gliomas, skeletal dysplasias, and Lisch nodules. Diagnostic criteria for NF2 have been established by the NIH Consensus Development Conference.

Tuberous Sclerosis

Tuberous sclerosis, or Bourneville's disease, as the disorder is also known, is an autosomal dominant disease that affects ~1 in 100,000 people. It is classically characterized by the triad of mental retardation, epilepsy, and adenoma sebaceum, although the triad is present in only about half of patients with tuberous sclerosis. The disorder predominantly consists of hamartomatous lesions involving the brain, the eye, and the visceral organs. Cutaneous manifestations, which are also common, include adenoma sebaceum, which is an angiofibroma involving the face, and ash leaf macules, which are depigmented nevi that tend to involve the trunk and extremities. Associated brain lesions comprise a variety of hamartomatous lesions, including subependymal hamartomas, giant cell tumors, cortical "tubers," and white matter lesions. Hamartoma lesions also involve the kidneys (angiomyolipoma), the heart (rhabdomyoma), the lungs (lymphangiomyoma), and the eye (retinal hamartoma).

Subependymal hamartomas, which tend to reside along the ventricular surface of the caudate nucleus, are the most common associated brain lesions. Subependymal giant cell tumors are distinguished from subependymal hamartomas by their intense contrast enhancement on magnetic resonance imaging (MRI), their larger size, their tendency to enlarge, and their propensity to occur near the foramen of Monro, an obstruction of which may result in hydrocephalus. Cortical tubers are characteristic hamartomas made of bizarre giant cells, fibrillary gliosis, and disordered myelin sheaths that appear as smooth, slightly raised subcortical nodules.

Sturge-Weber Syndrome

Sturge-Weber syndrome is a typically nonfamilial congenital malformation that is characterized by angiomatosis involving the face, the choroid of the eye, and the leptomeninges. The facial angioma, a port wine–colored nevus, typically follows the distribution of the ophthalmic division of the trigeminal nerve. Localized atrophy and calcification of the cerebral cortex ipsilateral to the facial nevus is another common lesion, whose etiology is apparently independent of the angiomatous malformations of the leptomeninges. Clinically, affected patients present with seizures, hemiparesis, and a homonymous hemianopsia, any one or all of which may be progressive. Mental retardation is another common finding.

Von Hippel-Lindau Disease

Von Hippel-Lindau disease is an autosomal dominant disorder that is characterized by retinal angiomas, cerebellar and spinal cord hemangioblastomas, renal cell carcinoma, pheochromocytomas, angiomas of the liver and kidney, and cysts of the pancreas, kidney, liver, and epididymis. The genetic basis of the disease has been localized to chromosome 3. Sufficient criteria to establish the diagnosis require one of several combinations of lesions: either more than one hemangioblastoma of the central nervous system (CNS), or one hemangioblastoma with a visceral manifestation of the disease, or one manifestation of the disease and a known family history. Affected patients most commonly present with decreasing visual acuity or pain in the eye, often followed by cerebellar symptoms or symptoms associated with increasing intracranial pressure.

Spinal Dysraphism

Spinal dysraphism comprises a group of congenital malformations that share in common a developmental defect in neurulation (neural tube closure). It is an umbrella term that encompasses all forms of spina bifida, both open and closed, which demonstrate, at the least, bony spinal defects, including splaying of the pedicles and laminae. These malformations range from closed spinal lesions, with or without cutaneous manifestations, to open spinal lesions in which the neural elements are dorsally exposed to the environment.

Spina Bifida Occulta

Spina bifida occulta is a radiological diagnosis, which is without external signs of a developmental anomaly. It is characterized by the absence of one or more spinous processes associated with hypogenesis of the vertebral arch, most commonly at the L5 and S1 levels. There is no evidence of cutaneous manifestations or of central or peripheral nervous system involvement. The incidence in the general population is ~20 to 30%.

Meningocele

Meningocele is an uncommon lesion that is marked by a cystic, skin- or membrane-covered, midline dorsal mass. The mass consists of a meningeal sac containing only CSF that is in continuity with the CSF of the spinal canal. No neural elements are contained within the lesion, and hydrocephalus is a rare complication.

The etiology of the meningocele is unclear. However, the malformation appears to represent a postneurulation defect that develops after the normal disjunction of the neuroectoderm from the cutaneous ectoderm and after the normal closure of the neural tube. It is thought that the meningocele results instead from a defect in the development of the overlying mesenchymal tissues and the cutaneous ectoderm. This distinguishes the meningocele from the myelomeningocele, which represents a true defect in neurulation.

Myelomeningocele

See **Fig. 1.39**.

Myelomeningocele is a much more common malformation than meningocele. It is apparently caused by a defect in disjunction, which is the process whereby the neuroectoderm and cutaneous ectoderm normally separate during neurulation. It has been postulated that this defect is caused by a lack of expression of complex carbohydrate molecules on the surface of the neuroectoderm cells. As a result, there is a localized failure of fusion of the neural folds, which remain in continuity with the cutaneous ectoderm at the surface of the skin (nondisjunction).

The dorsally exposed neural tissue, which is known as the *neural placode*, is made up of cells that would normally form the ependymal lining of the neural tube. Because the placode remains dorsal and attached to the skin, the mesenchymal elements are unable to migrate medially and fuse. This leads to the development of several vertebral anomalies, including absence of the spinous processes and laminae, reduction in the antero–posterior size of the vertebral bodies, increased interpedicular distance, and large laterally extending transverse processes. These anomalies, in turn, lead to kyphoscoliotic deformities in approximately one third of patients with myelomeningocele.

The neurologic sequelae of myelomeningocele include sensory and motor changes below the level of the lesion with or without fecal and urinary incontinence. Other malformations or sequelae that may produce early or delayed neurologic deterioration are Chiari malformation (which is present in 100% of patients), hydrocephalus, and tethered spinal cord. The diagnosis of myelomeningocele is always evident at birth and is usually repaired within 48 hours (**Table 1.4**).

Fig. 1.39 **Myelomeningocele.**

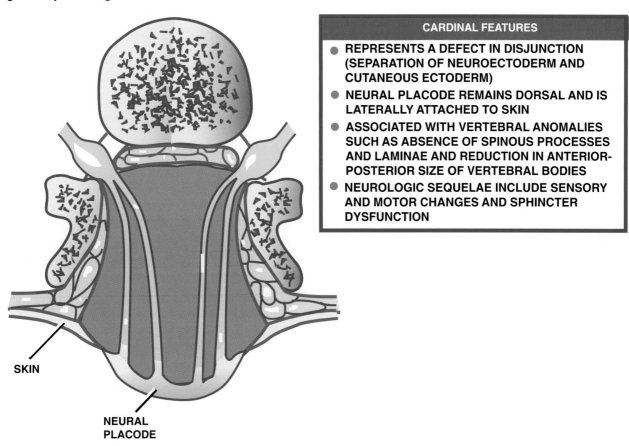

CARDINAL FEATURES

- REPRESENTS A DEFECT IN DISJUNCTION (SEPARATION OF NEUROECTODERM AND CUTANEOUS ECTODERM)
- NEURAL PLACODE REMAINS DORSAL AND IS LATERALLY ATTACHED TO SKIN
- ASSOCIATED WITH VERTEBRAL ANOMALIES SUCH AS ABSENCE OF SPINOUS PROCESSES AND LAMINAE AND REDUCTION IN ANTERIOR-POSTERIOR SIZE OF VERTEBRAL BODIES
- NEUROLOGIC SEQUELAE INCLUDE SENSORY AND MOTOR CHANGES AND SPHINCTER DYSFUNCTION

SKIN

NEURAL PLACODE

Table 1.4 Neurologic Syndromes with Myelomeningoceles

Lesion Level	Spinal-Related Disability
Above L3	Complete paraplegia and dermatomal para-anesthesia
	Bladder/rectal incontinence
	Nonambulatory
L4 and below	Same as for above L3 except preservation of hip flexors, hip abductors, knee extensors
	Ambulatory with aids, bracing, orthopedic surgery
S1 and below	Same as for L4 and below except preservation of feet dorsiflexors and partial preservation of hip extensors and knee flexors
	Ambulatory with minimal aids
S3 and below	Normal lower extremity motor function
	Saddle anesthesia
	Variable bladder/rectal incontinence

Spinal Lipomas

Spinal lipomas are skin-covered dorsal masses of fat and connective tissue that are in continuity with the leptomeninges or spinal cord. These lesions occur as a result of premature disjunction, which refers to the *premature* (not incomplete) separation of neuroectoderm from cutaneous ectoderm during the process of neurulation. As a result of premature disjunction, there is a migration of mesenchymal tissue into the ependymal-lined central canal of the neural tube, which has not yet closed, and to which the mesenchymal tissue does not normally have access. This mesenchymal tissue, which during normal development has contact with the *surface* of the neural tube and differentiates into meningeal tissue, bone, and paraspinal muscles, is apparently induced by its contact with the *central canal* of the neural tube to differentiate into fat (**Fig. 1.40**).

Fig. 1.40 **Intradural lipoma.**

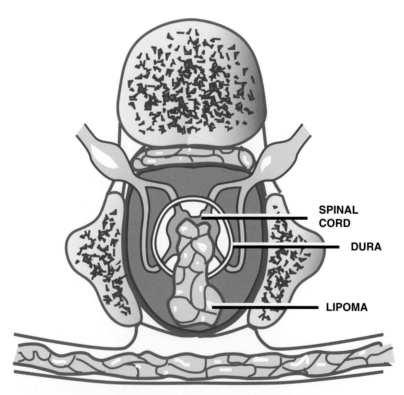

SPINAL CORD

DURA

LIPOMA

CARDINAL FEATURES
● REPRESENTS A PREMATURE SEPARATION OF NEURO-ECTODERM FROM CUTANEOUS ECTODERM (PREMATURE DISJUNCTION)
● MOST COMMONLY OCCURS IN THE THORACIC REGION
● IN THE ADULT, MAY PRESENT WITH SIGNS AND SYMPTOMS OF SPINAL CORD COMPRESSION

Three categories of spinal lipomas are identified: (1) intradural lipomas (4%), (2) lipomyelomeningoceles (84%), and (3) fibrolipomas of the filum terminale (12%). Intradural lipomas, which most commonly occur in the thoracic region, typically present with signs and symptoms of spinal cord compression in the adult. Fibrolipomas of the filum terminale (**Fig. 1.41**) appear to represent an etiologically separate group of disorders that take origin from an abnormality of the caudal cell mass (disorder of secondary neurulation). They are often asymptomatic but may present with symptoms of a tethered spinal cord.

Fig. 1.41 **Fibrolipoma of the filum terminale.**

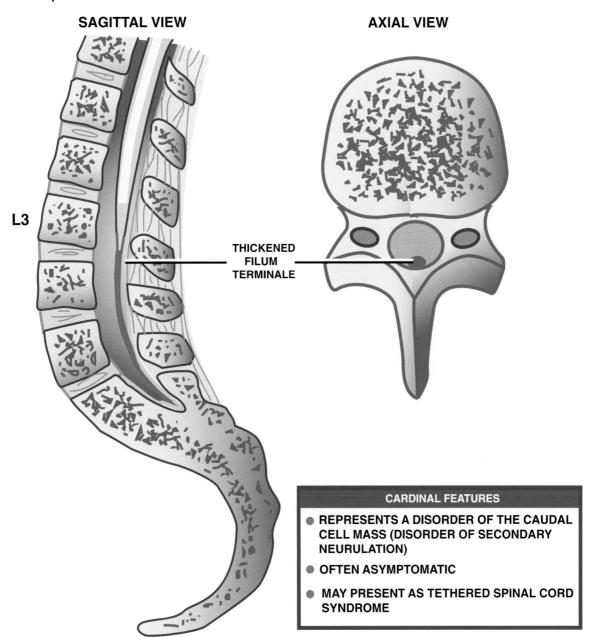

SAGITTAL VIEW

AXIAL VIEW

L3

THICKENED FILUM TERMINALE

CARDINAL FEATURES

- REPRESENTS A DISORDER OF THE CAUDAL CELL MASS (DISORDER OF SECONDARY NEURULATION)
- OFTEN ASYMPTOMATIC
- MAY PRESENT AS TETHERED SPINAL CORD SYNDROME

Finally, lipomyelomeningoceles (**Fig. 1.42**) present as soft, subcutaneous, skin-covered lumbosacral masses. They are the most common form of spinal lipomas. These lesions extend between the dorsal surface of the neural placode and the subcutaneous fat through a bony spina bifida. At the level of the lipoma, the dura is deficient in the dorsal midline, allowing its free medial edges to attach to the neural placode. This places the neural placode in an extradural space, where it attaches to the lipoma, which is continuous with the subcutaneous tissue. The junction between the neural placode and the lipoma may occur within, partly within, or outside (dorsal to) the spinal canal.

As the neural placode herniates dorsally through the bony spina bifida, it typically rotates. This projects the dorsal surface of the neural placode laterally or dorsolaterally, rather than straight dorsally. At the same time, the nerve roots on each side assume asymmetric lengths, such that the nerve roots arising on the superficial side of the rotated spinal cord grow longer than those that arise on the deep side of the rotated spinal cord. The clinical significance of this asymmetry is that the shorter roots may be so short as to tether the spinal cord inferiorly. In summary, the anatomy of the lipomyelomeningocele is similar to that of the myelomeningocele except that the former is skin covered and is marked by a lipoma that is attached to the dorsal surface of the placode. The lesions most commonly occur in the lumbosacral region, where they typically act to tether the spinal cord.

Clinically, those lesions that exhibit a soft lumbosacral mass are usually brought to medical attention early, often before the age of 6 months. The majority of children who do not undergo early repair develop progressive neurologic symptoms, such as sensory loss, weakness, bladder dysfunction, and leg pain. Orthopedic foot deformities are also common. Sacral anomalies and segmentation anomalies are present in nearly 50% of patients.

Fig. 1.42 **Lipomyelomeningocele.**

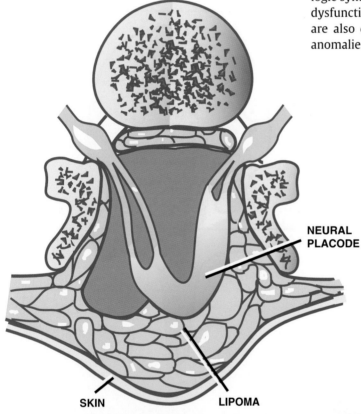

NEURAL
PLACODE

SKIN

LIPOMA

CARDINAL FEATURES
● **SIMILAR TO A MYELOMENINGOCELE, EXCEPT THAT (1) IT IS SKIN COVERED, AND (2) IT CONTAINS A LIPOMA THAT IS ATTACHED TO THE DORSAL SURFACE OF THE PLACODE**
● **MOST COMMON LOCATION IS LUMBOSACRAL REGION**
● **FREQUENTLY ASSOCIATED WITH A TETHERED SPINAL CORD, WHICH MAY RESULT IN PROGRESSIVE SENSORY LOSS, LOWER EXTREMITY WEAKNESS, BLADDER DYSFUNCTION, AND LEG PAIN**
● **OFTEN ASSOCIATED WITH ORTHOPEDIC FOOT DEFORMITIES, SACRAL ANOMALIES, AND SEGMENTATION ANOMALIES**

Split Cord Malformations

See **Fig. 1.43**.

Split cord malformation comprises several anomalies of the spinal cord that share in common an abnormal division of the cord and, at least according to one theory, an embryopathy that originates in a disorder of notochord formation.

In normal development, the formation of the notochord proceeds as follows. During the second week of gestation, the embryo consists of a two-layered disk containing primitive ectoderm dorsally and primitive endoderm ventrally. During the third week of gestation, a local proliferation of cells occurs in the dorsal midline, forming a thickening that is known as Hensen's node. Subsequent migration of these proliferating cells results in separation of the ectoderm from the endoderm and eventual formation of the notochord. According to this theory, failure of the ectoderm to completely separate from the endoderm forces the notochord to split or to deviate around the adhesion between the two layers. This theory attempts to account for both the various spinal anomalies associated with split cord malformation and the commonly associated intestinal duplications and diverticula.

Anatomically, a split cord is defined by a fissure that separates the two halves of the spinal cord for one or more segments. It is typically accompanied by a bony spicule or fibrocartilaginous septum that arises from the dorsal surface of the vertebral body. The *hemicords* reunite distally to reconstitute a single cord structure. Each hemicord contains its own set of ventral and dorsal roots, which may not be equal in number. An arachnoid-dural sleeve may envelop the two hemicords individually or as a whole, which in the latter case predicts the absence of a bony septum.

Clinically, a split cord may present at any age. It is associated with cutaneous manifestations, such as nevi, hypertrichosis, lipomas, dimples, and hemangiomas, in more than 50% of affected patients. Orthopedic foot problems, predominantly club foot, occur at about the same rate. Neurologic symptoms, when present, are usually the result of a tethered cord.

Fig. 1.43 **Diastematomyelia.**

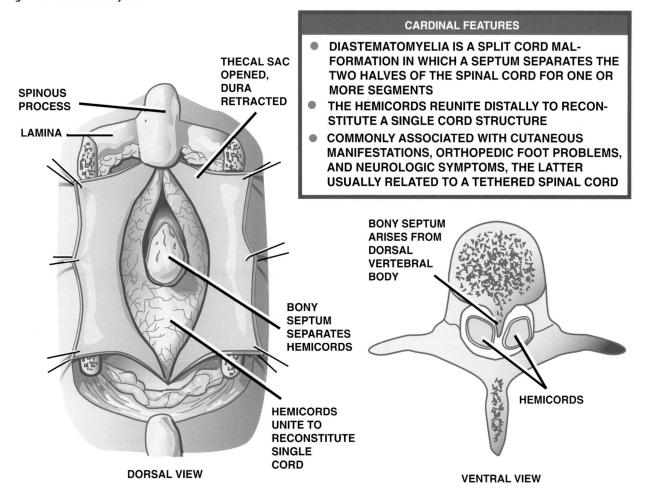

CARDINAL FEATURES

● DIASTEMATOMYELIA IS A SPLIT CORD MALFORMATION IN WHICH A SEPTUM SEPARATES THE TWO HALVES OF THE SPINAL CORD FOR ONE OR MORE SEGMENTS

● THE HEMICORDS REUNITE DISTALLY TO RECONSTITUTE A SINGLE CORD STRUCTURE

● COMMONLY ASSOCIATED WITH CUTANEOUS MANIFESTATIONS, ORTHOPEDIC FOOT PROBLEMS, AND NEUROLOGIC SYMPTOMS, THE LATTER USUALLY RELATED TO A TETHERED SPINAL CORD

SPINOUS PROCESS

LAMINA

THECAL SAC OPENED, DURA RETRACTED

BONY SEPTUM SEPARATES HEMICORDS

HEMICORDS UNITE TO RECONSTITUTE SINGLE CORD

DORSAL VIEW

BONY SEPTUM ARISES FROM DORSAL VERTEBRAL BODY

HEMICORDS

VENTRAL VIEW

Caudal Agenesis

See **Fig. 1.44**.

Caudal agenesis includes a group of caudal malformations that demonstrate partial or complete absence of either or both lumbar and sacral vertebrae, combined with the absence of corresponding segments of the caudal neural tube. Commonly associated vertebral anomalies include hemivertebrae, wedge-shaped vertebrae, fused vertebrae, sacralization of lumbar vertebrae, spina bifida, midline bony septa, and abnormal rib articulations.

The distal spinal cord is absent, and the terminus of the remaining cord ends in a dysplastic glial nodule. Although motor deficits correspond to the level of the lesion, sensory deficits may be conspicuously absent, perhaps because the neural crest cells are relatively spared. (The neural crest cells are the precursors of the dorsal root ganglia.) Affected patients have myelomeningoceles in ~50% of cases.

Fig. 1.44 **Caudal agenesis.**

Associated nonneurologic anomalies are common in caudal agenesis. They include limb malformations, such as flattened buttocks, gluteal atrophy, and equinovarus deformities, and visceral malformations, such as tracheoesophageal fistulas, Meckel's diverticulum, cloacal exstrophy, omphalocele, intestinal malrotations, renal agenesis, horseshoe kidney, ureteral and bladder duplications, and anomalies of the external genitalia.

Several theories have been proposed to explain the cause of caudal agenesis and its associated malformations, but no consensus about its embryogenesis has been reached.

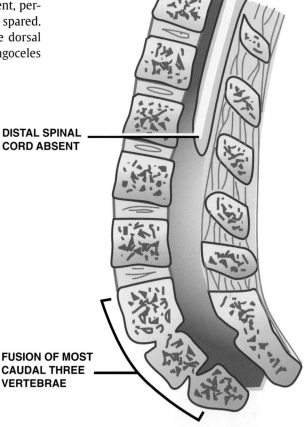

DISTAL SPINAL
CORD ABSENT

FUSION OF MOST
CAUDAL THREE
VERTEBRAE

CARDINAL FEATURES

- REFERS TO A GROUP OF MALFORMATIONS THAT ARE MARKED BY PARTIAL OR COMPLETE ABSENCE OF LUMBAR AND/OR SACRAL VERTEBRAE AND ASSOCIATED NEURAL ELEMENTS
- MOTOR DEFICITS CORRESPOND TO LEVEL OF LESION; SENSATION MAY BE SPARED DUE TO PRESERVATION OF NEURAL CREST CELLS (PRECURSORS OF DORSAL ROOT GANGLION)
- ASSOCIATED VERTEBRAL ANOMALIES INCLUDE HEMI-VERTEBRAE, WEDGE-SHAPED VERTEBRAE, FUSED VERTEBRAE, SACRALIZATION OF LUMBAR VERTEBRAE, AND SPINA BIFIDA
- INCIDENCE OF ASSOCIATED MYELOMENINGOCELE IS 50%

II
Regional Anatomy and Related Syndromes

2 Peripheral Nerves

This chapter discusses the functional anatomy and clinical correlation of the peripheral nerves of the upper and lower extremities. The discussion is limited to those nerves that are susceptible to "entrapment" neuropathies in which the involved nerve is lesioned by extrinsic compression. For each nerve described, there is a discussion of its origin, course, and motor and sensory innervation, as well as the clinical syndrome or syndromes with which the nerve is most closely associated.

A significant number of these syndromes may be amenable to surgical treatment. Therefore, accurate and timely clinical diagnosis is imperative. Important nerves not covered in this chapter, because they are not associated with common entrapment syndromes, are noted at the beginning of the two major sections.

Upper Extremity

The nerves of the upper extremity discussed in the following sections include the radial, the median, and the ulnar nerves. Omitted from the discussion are (1) the axillary nerve, which supplies the deltoid muscle and the skin overlying the muscle, and (2) the musculocutaneous nerve, which supplies the biceps and the brachialis muscles and the skin overlying the radial aspect of the forearm.

Radial Nerve

Anatomy

See **Fig. 2.1**.

The radial nerve receives contributions from the C5–C8 spinal nerves. These contributions pass through the upper, middle, and lower trunks and posterior cord of the brachial plexus. The radial nerve supplies the extensor muscles of the arm and forearm as well as the skin covering them.

Radial Nerve in the Upper Arm

As it winds around the humerus, or just proximal to this section, the radial nerve supplies the *triceps muscle*. After its course in the spiral groove, it then supplies the *brachioradialis* and the *extensor carpi radialis longus* and *brevis* muscles. The nerve then bifurcates into a superficial (sensory) branch and a deep (motor) branch.

Radial Nerve in the Forearm

The *superficial branch* passes distally into the hand, where it supplies the skin of the radial aspect of the dorsum of the hand and the dorsum of the first four fingers. The sensory autonomous zone of the radial nerve is the skin over the first interosseous space.

The *deep branch* of the radial nerve passes deep through the fibrous arch of the supinator muscle (the *arcade of Frohse*) to enter the posterior compartment of the forearm. The nerve continues in this compartment as the purely motor *posterior interosseous nerve*, which innervates the remaining wrist and finger extensors. These include the following: (1) *supinator*, a forearm supinator; (2) *extensor digitorum*, an extensor of the second through the fifth metacarpophalangeal joints; (3) *extensor digiti minimi*, an extensor of the fifth metacarpophalangeal joint; (4) *extensor carpi ulnaris*, an ulnar extensor of the wrist; (5) *abductor pollicis longus*, an abductor of the carpometacarpal joint of the thumb; (6) *extensor pollicis longus*, an extensor of the interphalangeal joint of the thumb; (7) *extensor pollicis brevis*, an extensor of the metacarpophalangeal joint of the thumb; and (10) *extensor indicis*, an extensor of the second finger.

Fig. 2.1 **Radial nerve anatomy.**

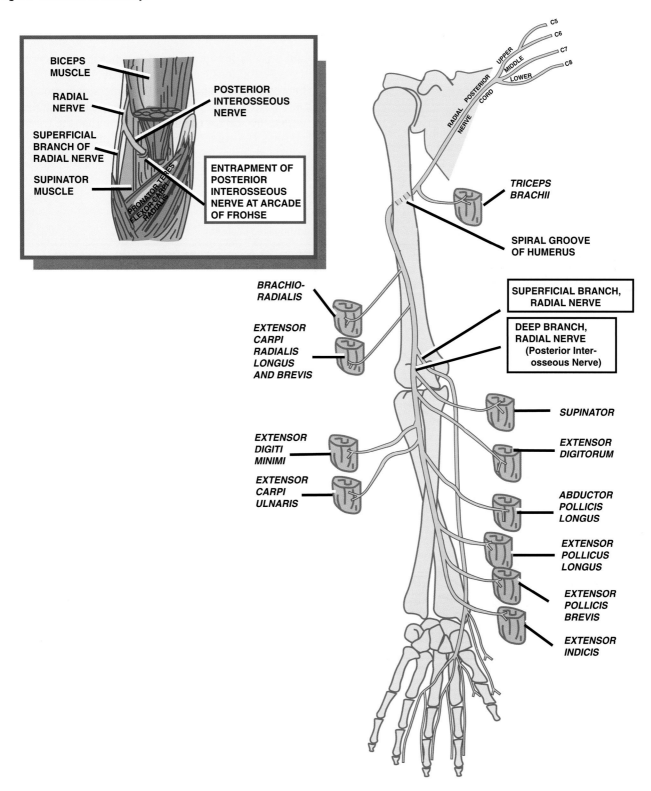

Clinical Syndromes

Two of the most common clinical syndromes of the radial nerve are radial nerve palsy and the posterior interosseous nerve syndrome.

Radial Nerve Palsy

See **Fig. 2.2**.

This syndrome may be caused by a humeral fracture or a lesion due to prolonged pressure on the nerve. The term *radial nerve palsy* refers to the latter mechanism of injury, also known as Saturday night palsy because it is classically associated with a drunkard who falls asleep with his arm hyperabducted across a park bench. The site of compression in either case is in the region of the spiral groove. The syndrome consists of a wrist drop, inability to extend the fingers, weakness of the supinator muscle, and sensory loss involving the radial nerve–innervated areas of the forearm and hand. Wrist drop is the most impressive and typical sign. Weakness of supination is only partial because supination may be accomplished with either biceps or supinator. Note that the triceps is preserved in these lesions because the branches of the radial nerve that innervate the triceps originate proximal to the spiral groove.

Fig. 2.2 **Radial nerve palsy.** Functions or responses marked with an "X" are impaired or absent.

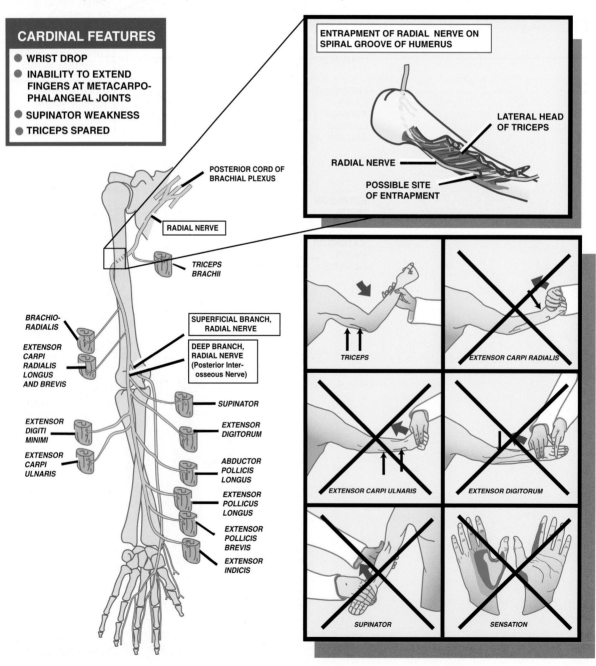

Posterior Interosseous Nerve Syndrome

See **Fig. 2.3**.

The posterior interosseous nerve (PIN) syndrome is the most common syndrome caused by compression at the arcade of Frohse. As the PIN passes under the *arcade of Frohse*, a fibrous arch at the origin of the supinator muscle, the nerve may be pathologically constricted. The cardinal features of this syndrome are an inability to extend the fingers at the metacarpophalangeal joint, the absence

of wrist drop, and normal sensation. Because the finger extensors at the interphalangeal joint are median and ulnar innervated, the patient is able to extend the fingers at this joint. Branches to the supinator muscle are given off proximal to the nerve entering the arcade of Frohse, causing the supinator muscle to be spared. Although no wrist drop is present because the extensor carpi radialis is preserved, the extensor carpi ulnaris is a PIN-innervated muscle, and thus any attempt to extend the wrist results in a radial deviation of the hand. Because the PIN is a pure motor nerve, sensation in this syndrome is entirely normal.

Fig. 2.3 **Posterior interosseous nerve syndrome.** Functions or responses marked with an "X" are impaired or absent.

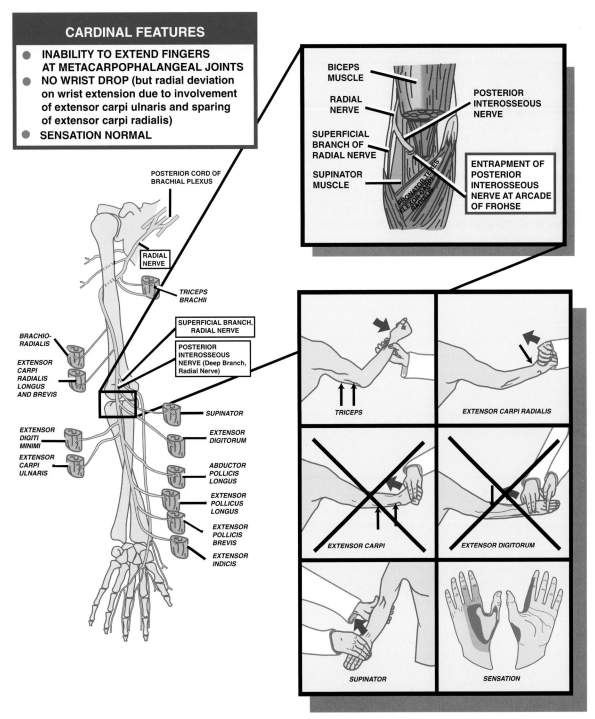

Median Nerve

Anatomy

See **Fig. 2.4**.

The median nerve receives contributions from the C6 to T1 spinal nerves. These pass through the upper, middle, and lower trunks and the lateral and medial cords of the brachial plexus. There are no median nerve branches that originate proximal to the elbow.

Median Nerve at the Elbow

At the elbow, the median nerve lies behind the bicipital aponeurosis (lacertus fibrosus), providing supply to the following muscles: (1) *pronator teres*, a forearm pronator; (2) *flexor carpi radialis*, a radial wrist flexor; (3) *palmaris longus*, a wrist flexor; and (4) *flexor digitorum superficialis*, a flexor at the interphalangeal joint for the second, third, fourth, and fifth fingers.

Median Nerve in the Forearm

From beneath the lacertus fibrosus, the nerve then passes into the forearm between the two heads of the median-innervated pronator teres muscle. As it passes deep to the pronator teres muscle, the median nerve gives off the *anterior interosseous nerve*. The anterior interosseous nerve is a purely motor branch, which supplies the (1) *flexor pollicis longus*, (2) *pronator quadratus*, and (3) *flexor digitorum profundus I* and *II*.

Median Nerve in the Hand

The median nerve then continues deep to the flexor retinaculum through the so-called carpal tunnel to innervate the LOAF muscles of the hand. These include the (1) *lumbricals I* and *II*, (2) *opponens pollicis*, (3) *abductor pollicis brevis*, and (4) *flexor pollicis brevis*.

Sensory branches also originate from the median nerve as it emerges from the carpal tunnel. These palmar digital nerves supply the skin of the palmar aspect of the thumb, second, third, and half of the fourth fingers; the radial aspect of the palm; and the dorsal aspect of the distal and middle phalanges of the second, third, and half of the fourth fingers.

A palmar cutaneous branch originates from the median nerve just proximal to the carpal tunnel, where it crosses the wrist to enter the hand superficial to the flexor retinaculum. It supplies the skin over the median eminence and the proximal palm on the radial aspect of the hand.

Fig. 2.4 **Median nerve anatomy.**

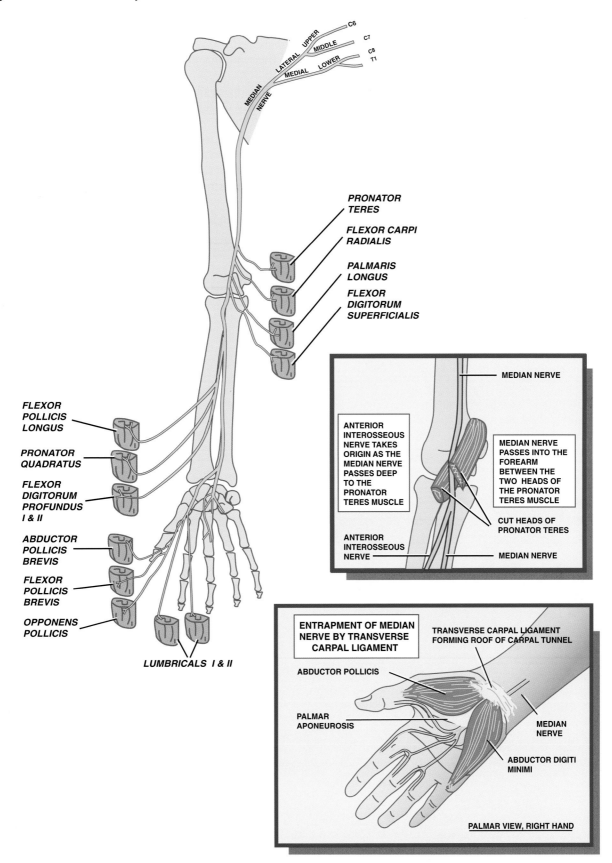

Clinical Syndromes

Three major entrapment syndromes involving the median nerve and its branches are described: (1) the pronator teres syndrome, (2) the anterior interosseous nerve syndrome, and (3) the carpal tunnel syndrome.

Pronator Teres Syndrome

See **Fig. 2.5**.

The pronator teres syndrome results from entrapment of the median nerve as it passes between the two heads of the pronator teres muscle and under the fibrous arch of the flexor digitorum superficialis. Compression may be caused by (1) a thickened lacertus fibrosus (an aponeurosis that overlies the median nerve just proximal to the passage of the nerve between the two heads of the pronator teres), (2) a hypertrophied pronator teres muscle, or (3) a tight fibrous band of the flexor digitorum superficialis.

The syndrome is characterized by pain in the forearm. In addition, weakness in the hand grip and numbness and tingling in the index finger and thumb are characteristically present. The symptoms are similar to those of carpal tunnel syndrome (see p. 64), but nocturnal exacerbation of pain is conspicuously absent. In advanced cases, the hand assumes a "benediction attitude" due to impairment of flexion in the radial three digits. Findings on muscle testing will vary depending on the degree of compression, but often there is no measurable weakness in the median nerve–innervated muscles.

Fig. 2.5 **Pronator teres syndrome.** Functions or responses marked with an "X" are impaired or absent.

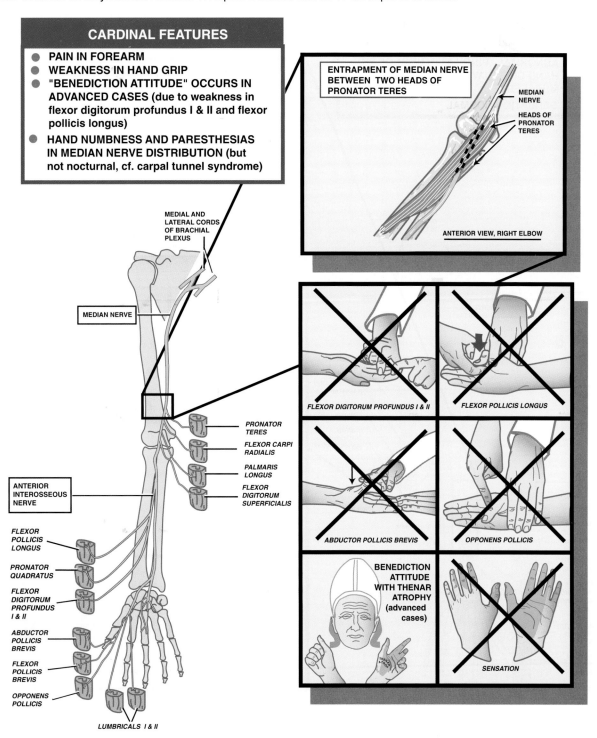

CARDINAL FEATURES

- PAIN IN FOREARM
- WEAKNESS IN HAND GRIP
- "BENEDICTION ATTITUDE" OCCURS IN ADVANCED CASES (due to weakness in flexor digitorum profundus I & II and flexor pollicis longus)
- HAND NUMBNESS AND PARESTHESIAS IN MEDIAN NERVE DISTRIBUTION (but not nocturnal, cf. carpal tunnel syndrome)

MEDIAL AND LATERAL CORDS OF BRACHIAL PLEXUS

MEDIAN NERVE

ANTERIOR INTEROSSEOUS NERVE

FLEXOR POLLICIS LONGUS

PRONATOR QUADRATUS

FLEXOR DIGITORUM PROFUNDUS I & II

ABDUCTOR POLLICIS BREVIS

FLEXOR POLLICIS BREVIS

OPPONENS POLLICIS

LUMBRICALS I & II

PRONATOR TERES

FLEXOR CARPI RADIALIS

PALMARIS LONGUS

FLEXOR DIGITORUM SUPERFICIALIS

ENTRAPMENT OF MEDIAN NERVE BETWEEN TWO HEADS OF PRONATOR TERES

MEDIAN NERVE

HEADS OF PRONATOR TERES

ANTERIOR VIEW, RIGHT ELBOW

FLEXOR DIGITORUM PROFUNDUS I & II

FLEXOR POLLICIS LONGUS

ABDUCTOR POLLICIS BREVIS

OPPONENS POLLICIS

BENEDICTION ATTITUDE WITH THENAR ATROPHY (advanced cases)

SENSATION

Fig. 2.6 **Anterior interosseous nerve syndrome.** Functions or responses marked with an "X" are impaired or absent.

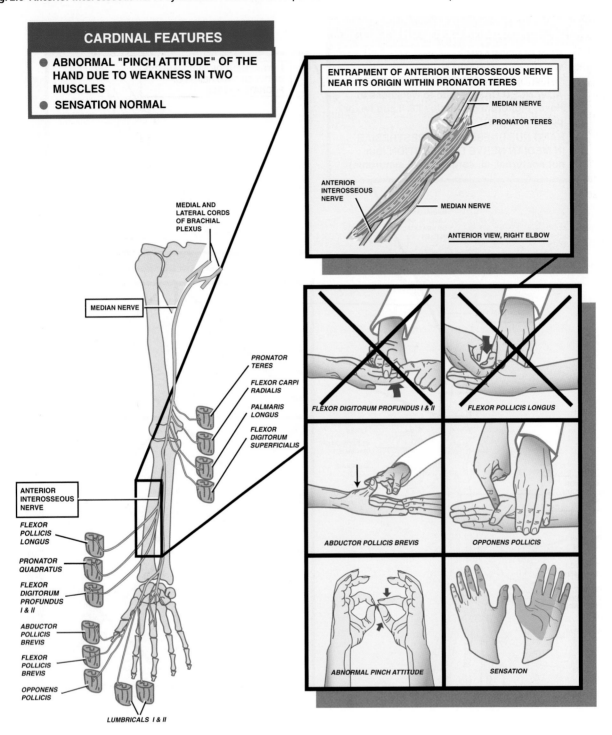

Anterior Interosseous Nerve Syndrome

See **Figs. 2.6** and **2.7**.

The anterior interosseous nerve syndrome is most commonly due to a constricting band causing an entrapment neuropathy near the origin of the nerve. Clinically, it is characterized by weakness in two muscles: (1) the flexor digitorum profundus I and II and (2) the flexor pollicis longus. Its most singular feature, due to weakness in these muscles, is an abnormal "pinch attitude" of the hand. This attitude is characterized by an extension or hyperextension of the terminal phalanges of the thumb and index finger when the thumb and index finger are opposed. Weakness in the pronator quadratus muscle is usually clinically insignificant because of simultaneous contraction of the more powerful pronator teres muscle during pronation motion of the forearm. Sensation in the anterior interosseous nerve syndrome is entirely normal.

Fig. 2.7 **Abnormal pinch attitude.**

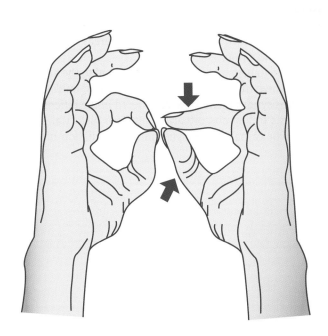

ABNORMAL PINCH ATTITUDE

Carpal Tunnel Syndrome

See **Fig. 2.8**.

Carpal tunnel syndrome is caused by compression of the median nerve as it passes through the carpal tunnel. The carpal tunnel is formed by the transverse carpal ligament, or flexor retinaculum, which stretches transversely across the concavity of the carpal bones.

Clinically, the syndrome is characterized by both sensory and motor symptoms of the hand.

The most common presenting symptom of the syndrome is pain and paresthesias in the wrist and hand, which classically worsen at night, awakening the patient from sleep. These "positive" sensory symptoms are typically associated with "negative" symptoms, involving sensory loss in the distribution of the palmar digital branches of the median nerve (i.e., the radial palm, the palmar aspect of the first three and a half fingers, and the dorsal aspect of the terminal phalanges of the second, third, and half of the fourth fingers). Sensory loss is easiest to discern along the volar tips of the index and middle fingers, which are the autonomous areas for median nerve distribution.

Although pain is most frequently limited to the hand, it may involve the forearm, the elbow, or the shoulder, and thus this syndrome must be considered in the differential diagnosis of any obscure arm pain. Two historical clues that favor carpal tunnel syndrome are radiation of arm pain from distal to proximal and a tendency for the patient to rub or shake the hand to alleviate the pain because pain of more proximal origin such as the cervical spine or the thoracic outlet is usually exacerbated by motion.

Motor involvement, which usually occurs late in the course of the disease process, comprises weakness and atrophy in the four LOAF muscles of the hand: (1) the lumbricals, (2) the opponens pollicis, (3) the abductor pollicis brevis, and (4) the flexor pollicis brevis. Examination may thus reveal weakness in the abduction, opposition, and flexion of the thumb. It should be emphasized, however, that patients with carpal tunnel syndrome most commonly present with sensory complaints, and only rarely do they present with the complaint of weakness or muscle atrophy.

Paradoxically, those patients with pain may demonstrate no weakness, whereas a smaller group of patients may demonstrate weakness but do not complain of pain. In testing for weakness, the abductor pollicis brevis is the easiest of the thenar muscles to test in a reliable way.

Finally, *Phalen's test* may be used to corroborate the diagnosis. It is done by asking the patient to forcibly dorsiflex the affected hand for 60 seconds. A positive test will reproduce the patient's symptoms, although a false-positive test will occur in normal individuals if this position is maintained for too long.

Fig. 2.8 **Carpal tunnel syndrome.** Functions or responses marked with an "X" are impaired or absent.

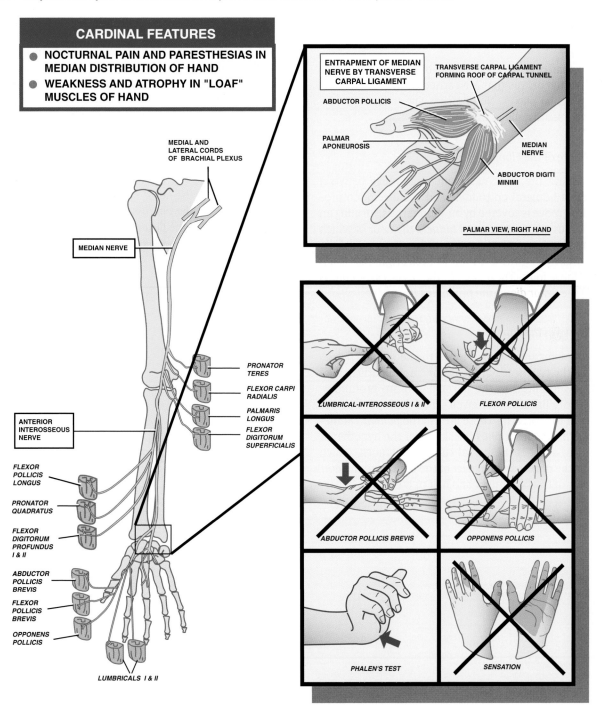

CARDINAL FEATURES
- NOCTURNAL PAIN AND PARESTHESIAS IN MEDIAN DISTRIBUTION OF HAND
- WEAKNESS AND ATROPHY IN "LOAF" MUSCLES OF HAND

MEDIAL AND LATERAL CORDS OF BRACHIAL PLEXUS

MEDIAN NERVE

ANTERIOR INTEROSSEOUS NERVE

FLEXOR POLLICIS LONGUS

PRONATOR QUADRATUS

FLEXOR DIGITORUM PROFUNDUS I & II

ABDUCTOR POLLICIS BREVIS

FLEXOR POLLICIS BREVIS

OPPONENS POLLICIS

LUMBRICALS I & II

PRONATOR TERES

FLEXOR CARPI RADIALIS

PALMARIS LONGUS

FLEXOR DIGITORUM SUPERFICIALIS

ENTRAPMENT OF MEDIAN NERVE BY TRANSVERSE CARPAL LIGAMENT

TRANSVERSE CARPAL LIGAMENT FORMING ROOF OF CARPAL TUNNEL

ABDUCTOR POLLICIS

PALMAR APONEUROSIS

MEDIAN NERVE

ABDUCTOR DIGITI MINIMI

PALMAR VIEW, RIGHT HAND

LUMBRICAL-INTEROSSEOUS I & II

FLEXOR POLLICIS

ABDUCTOR POLLICIS BREVIS

OPPONENS POLLICIS

PHALEN'S TEST

SENSATION

Ulnar Nerve

Anatomy

See **Fig. 2.9**.

The ulnar nerve receives contributions from C7, C8, and T1 spinal nerves that are carried in the medial cord of the brachial plexus. No branches are given off as the nerve courses distally in the arm.

Ulnar Nerve at the Elbow

At the elbow, the ulnar nerve enters a groove between the medial humeral epicondyle and the olecranon process. This groove is covered by an aponeurosis, forming an osseofibrous canal (the *cubital tunnel*), the floor of which is formed by the medial ligament of the elbow joint. Two motor branches of the ulnar nerve take origin just distal to the elbow joint. These are (1) the *flexor carpi ulnaris* and (2) the *flexor digitorum profundus III* and *IV*.

Ulnar Nerve in the Forearm

After supplying these two muscles, the nerve then passes between the two heads of the flexor carpi ulnaris to take its place superficial to the flexor digitorum profundus. Two sensory branches are given off as the nerve courses distally in the forearm. These are (1) the *palmar cutaneous branch*, which supplies the skin over the hypothenar eminence; and (2) the *dorsal cutaneous branch*, which supplies the dorsal ulnar aspect of the hand, and the dorsal aspect of the fifth finger and half of the fourth finger.

Ulnar Nerve in the Hand

The ulnar nerve then passes into the hand through *Guyon's canal*, which is formed by the volar carpal ligament (roof), the transverse carpal ligament (floor), the pisiform bone (medial wall), and the hook of the hamate bone (lateral wall). Proximal in the canal the ulnar nerve gives off the *superficial sensory branch*. This sensory branch supplies the skin of the distal part of the ulnar aspect of the palm and the palmar aspect of the fifth and half of the fourth finger. The ulnar nerve then continues in the canal as the *deep motor branch*, which supplies the following muscles: (1) the *abductor digiti minimi*, (2) the *opponens digiti minimi*, (3) the *flexor digiti minimi*, (4) the *lumbricals III* and *IV*, (5) the *interosseous muscles*, (6) the *adductor pollicis*, and (7) the *flexor pollicis brevis*.

Fig. 2.9 **Ulnar nerve anatomy.**

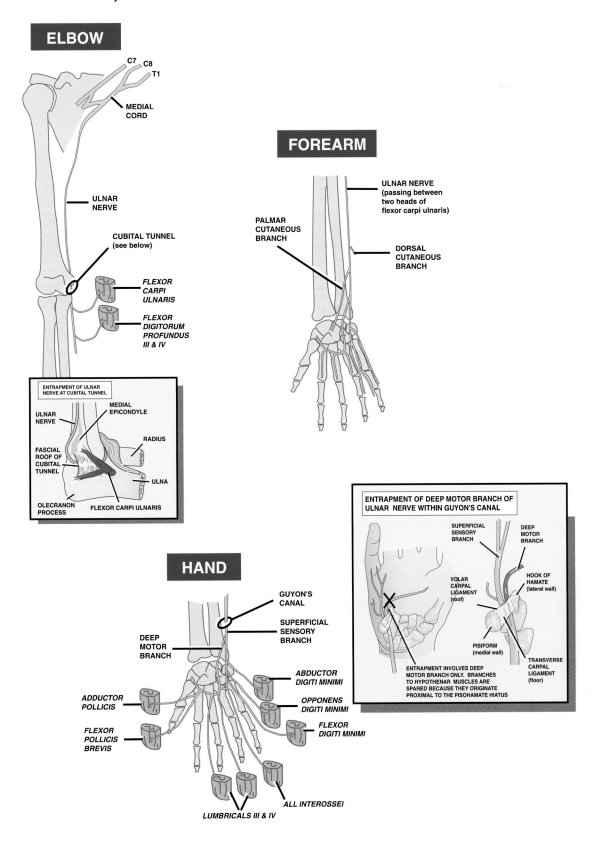

ELBOW

C7 C8 T1

MEDIAL CORD

ULNAR NERVE

CUBITAL TUNNEL (see below)

FLEXOR CARPI ULNARIS

FLEXOR DIGITORUM PROFUNDUS III & IV

ENTRAPMENT OF ULNAR NERVE AT CUBITAL TUNNEL

MEDIAL EPICONDYLE

ULNAR NERVE

RADIUS

FASCIAL ROOF OF CUBITAL TUNNEL

ULNA

OLECRANON PROCESS

FLEXOR CARPI ULNARIS

FOREARM

ULNAR NERVE (passing between two heads of flexor carpi ulnaris)

PALMAR CUTANEOUS BRANCH

DORSAL CUTANEOUS BRANCH

HAND

GUYON'S CANAL

SUPERFICIAL SENSORY BRANCH

DEEP MOTOR BRANCH

ABDUCTOR DIGITI MINIMI

ADDUCTOR POLLICIS

OPPONENS DIGITI MINIMI

FLEXOR POLLICIS BREVIS

FLEXOR DIGITI MINIMI

ALL INTEROSSEI

LUMBRICALS III & IV

ENTRAPMENT OF DEEP MOTOR BRANCH OF ULNAR NERVE WITHIN GUYON'S CANAL

SUPERFICIAL SENSORY BRANCH

DEEP MOTOR BRANCH

VOLAR CARPAL LIGAMENT (roof)

HOOK OF HAMATE (lateral wall)

PISIFORM (medial wall)

TRANSVERSE CARPAL LIGAMENT (floor)

ENTRAPMENT INVOLVES DEEP MOTOR BRANCH ONLY. BRANCHES TO HYPOTHENAR MUSCLES ARE SPARED BECAUSE THEY ORIGINATE PROXIMAL TO THE PISOHAMATE HIATUS

Clinical Syndromes

The two major clinical syndromes involving the ulnar nerve are (1) the cubital tunnel syndrome and (2) Guyon's canal syndrome. Note the diagnostic importance of the dorsal cutaneous nerve, which is included as part of the cubital tunnel syndrome but is spared in Guyon's canal syndrome.

Cubital Tunnel Syndrome

See **Fig. 2.10**.

The cubital tunnel syndrome is frequently caused by compression of the ulnar nerve within the cubital tunnel. Most commonly it is due to constriction of the nerve by the overlying aponeurosis. The cardinal features of cubital tunnel syndrome are (1) numbness and tingling of the ulnar aspect of the hand; (2) weakness variously described as impairment of hand grip, clumsiness, or difficulty buttoning shirts; and (3) atrophy, most marked in the hypothenar eminence and the first interosseous space (most noticeable on the dorsal aspect of the hand). Sensory loss is most easily observed in the distal two phalanges of the little finger, which is the autonomous zone of the ulnar nerve.

Two additional signs of ulnar neuropathy are (1) a claw hand deformity and (2) Froment's sign. A *claw hand* deformity results from the simultaneous hyperexten-sion at the metacarpophalangeal joints and flexion at the interphalangeal joints. Hyperextension at the metacarpophalangeal joints is due to weakness in the interossei muscles, which results in unopposed action of the extensor digitorum muscles. Flexion at the interphalangeal joints is due to the passive tethering pull of the flexor digitorum muscle, which occurs when the metacarpophalangeal joints are in hyperextension.

Froment's sign is due to weakness in the adductor pollicis muscle. It may be detected by asking an affected individual to grasp a piece of paper between the thumb and index finger while the examiner attempts to pull the paper away. The patient may attempt to compensate for the inability to adduct the thumb by extending the proximal and flexing the distal thumb phalanges (Froment's sign).

Although branches to the flexor carpi ulnaris and flexor digitorum profundus muscles originate within the cubital tunnel, these muscles are rarely involved in cubital tunnel syndrome, probably because they are situated deeply within the nerve and are therefore spared the compressive effects of the more superficially located fibers.

In contrast to carpal tunnel syndrome in which pain is a prominent symptom, cubital tunnel syndrome is less frequently associated with pain. Likewise, weakness and atrophy, which tend to occur late in the course of carpal tunnel syndrome, typically occur early in cubital tunnel syndrome.

Fig. 2.10 **Cubital tunnel syndrome.** Functions or responses marked with an "X" are impaired or absent.

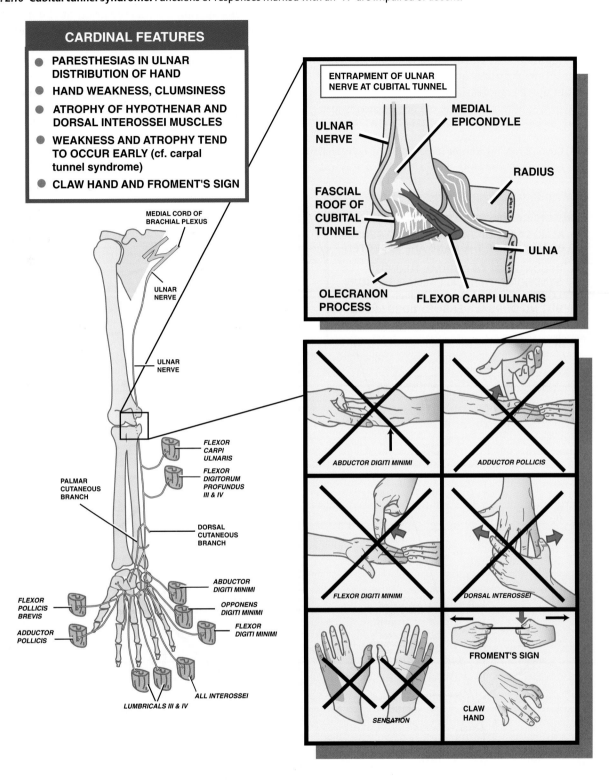

CARDINAL FEATURES

- PARESTHESIAS IN ULNAR DISTRIBUTION OF HAND
- HAND WEAKNESS, CLUMSINESS
- ATROPHY OF HYPOTHENAR AND DORSAL INTEROSSEI MUSCLES
- WEAKNESS AND ATROPHY TEND TO OCCUR EARLY (cf. carpal tunnel syndrome)
- CLAW HAND AND FROMENT'S SIGN

ENTRAPMENT OF ULNAR NERVE AT CUBITAL TUNNEL

ULNAR NERVE

MEDIAL EPICONDYLE

RADIUS

FASCIAL ROOF OF CUBITAL TUNNEL

ULNA

OLECRANON PROCESS

FLEXOR CARPI ULNARIS

MEDIAL CORD OF BRACHIAL PLEXUS

ULNAR NERVE

ULNAR NERVE

PALMAR CUTANEOUS BRANCH

FLEXOR CARPI ULNARIS

FLEXOR DIGITORUM PROFUNDUS III & IV

DORSAL CUTANEOUS BRANCH

ABDUCTOR DIGITI MINIMI

OPPONENS DIGITI MINIMI

FLEXOR DIGITI MINIMI

FLEXOR POLLICIS BREVIS

ADDUCTOR POLLICIS

ALL INTEROSSEI

LUMBRICALS III & IV

ABDUCTOR DIGITI MINIMI

ADDUCTOR POLLICIS

FLEXOR DIGITI MINIMI

DORSAL INTEROSSEI

FROMENT'S SIGN

SENSATION

CLAW HAND

Guyon's Canal Syndrome

See **Fig. 2.11**.

There are multiple causes of Guyon's canal syndrome, including trauma and extrinsic compression. The syndrome has been classified into three different types, based on the site of compression.

In the type 1 syndrome, the site of compression is just proximal to or within Guyon's canal (**Fig. 2.11A**). Almost all of the motor and sensory branches of the hand are affected. Motor sparing includes the flexor carpi ulnaris and the flexor digitorum muscles. However, these muscles are also spared in the cubital tunnel syndrome (see earlier discussion). Therefore, they provide no diagnostic utility. Sensory sparing includes the dorsal aspect of the hand because the dorsal cutaneous branch originates in the distal forearm. The preservation of this branch helps distinguish this syndrome from cubital tunnel syndrome.

Fig. 2.11 (A) Guyon's canal syndrome (type 1). (B) Guyon's canal syndrome (type 2). (C) Guyon's canal syndrome (type 3). Functions or responses marked with an "X" are impaired or absent.

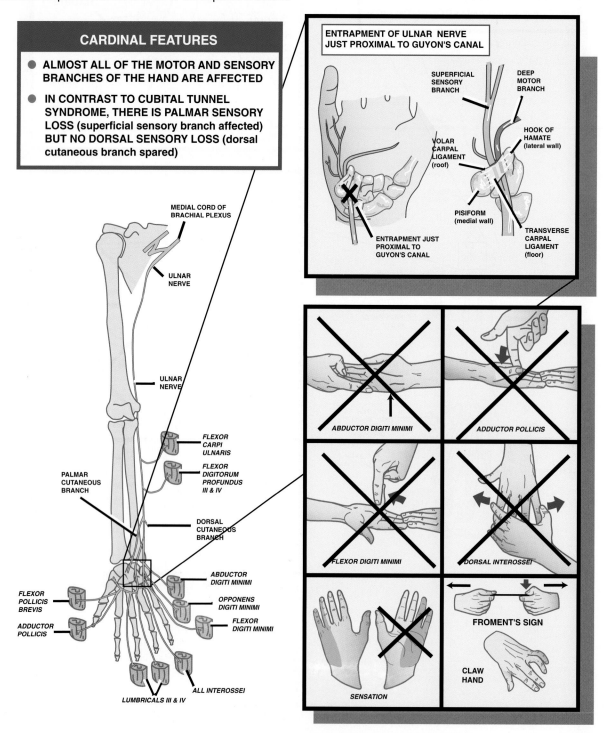

A

In the type 2 syndrome, the site of compression is at the proximal part of the terminal motor branch within Guyon's canal, distal to the takeoff of the superficial terminal cutaneous branch. In this pure motor syndrome, sensation is preserved, as is the innervation of many of the hypothenar muscles because of their more proximal origin. The interossei and adductor pollicis muscles are most frequently affected (**Fig. 2.11B**).

Fig. 2.11 (Continued)

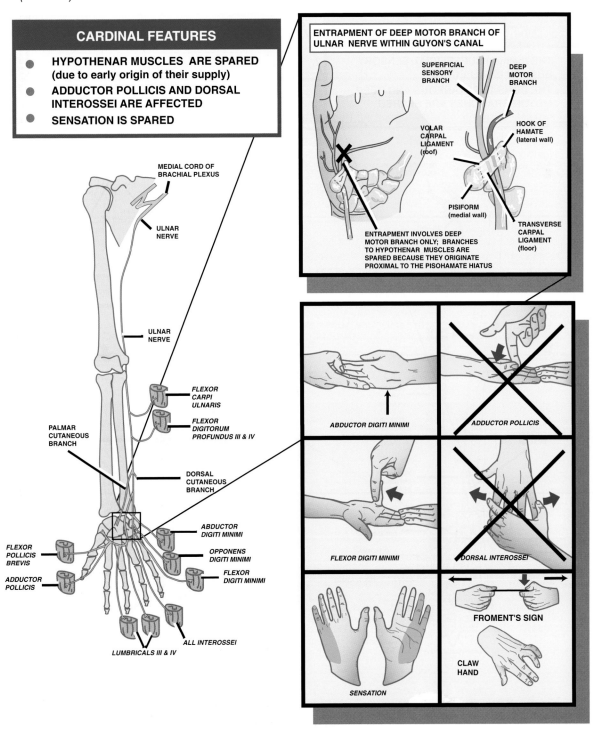

B

In the type 3 syndrome, the rarest of the three, the site of compression is at the distal end of Guyon's canal. The terminal motor branch is preserved in this syndrome, and the syndrome is thus purely sensory (**Fig. 2.11C**).

Fig. 2.11 (Continued)

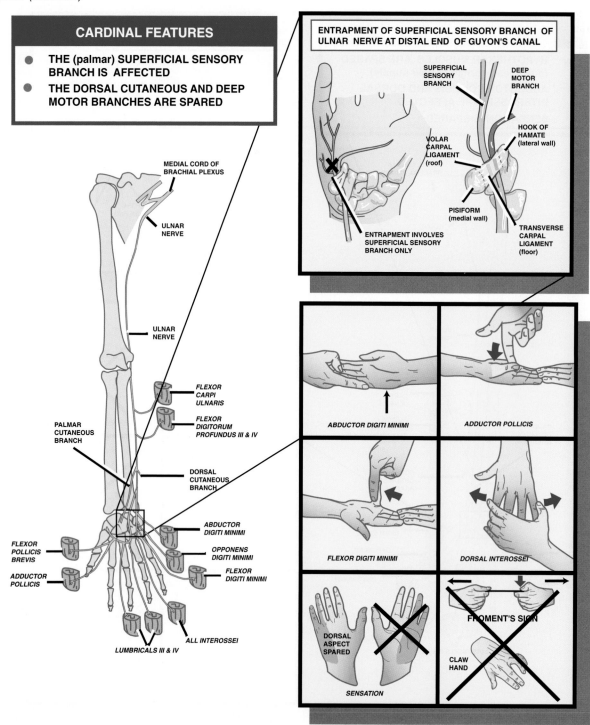

C

Lower Extremity

The major nerves of the thigh are the femoral nerve (ventrally) and the sciatic nerve (dorsally). The leg and foot are mainly supplied by the terminal branches of the sciatic nerve, the peroneal nerve (ventrally), and the tibial nerve (dorsally). Other important nerves of the lower extremity discussed in this chapter include two purely sensory nerves, the lateral femoral cutaneous nerve and the saphenous nerve. Important nerves that are not discussed include the superior and inferior gluteal nerves (which supply the gluteal muscles), the femoral nerve (which supplies the quadriceps femoris muscles), and the obturator nerve (which supplies the adductor muscles).

Lateral Femoral Cutaneous Nerve

The lateral femoral cutaneous nerve, a direct branch of the lumbar plexus, provides sensory innervation to the skin of the ventrolateral aspect of the thigh.

Fig. 2.12 **Lateral femoral cutaneous nerve anatomy.**

Anatomy

See **Fig. 2.12**.

The lateral femoral cutaneous nerve is a purely sensory nerve derived from the second and third lumbar nerves of the lumbar plexus. It emerges from the lateral aspect of the *psoas muscle* to run obliquely forward and inferiorly across the *iliacus muscle*. After passing across the iliac fossa just medial to the anterior superior iliac spine, the nerve enters the thigh beneath the *inguinal ligament*. It then pierces the fascia lata of the lateral thigh, where it terminates.

The distribution of the sensory supply of the lateral femoral cutaneous nerve comprises the skin of the ventrolateral aspect of the thigh.

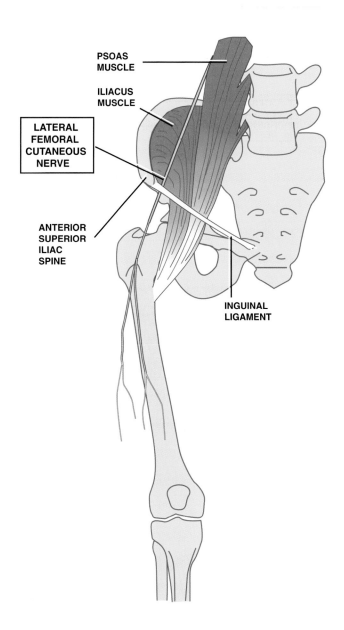

PSOAS MUSCLE

ILIACUS MUSCLE

LATERAL FEMORAL CUTANEOUS NERVE

ANTERIOR SUPERIOR ILIAC SPINE

INGUINAL LIGAMENT

Syndrome of the Lateral Femoral Cutaneous Nerve of the Thigh

See **Fig. 2.13**.

The syndrome of the lateral femoral cutaneous nerve of the thigh, or meralgia paresthetica, as the syndrome is also known, is caused by compression of this nerve in the inguinal region, usually as a result of a fascial band. Clinically, the syndrome is characterized by paresthesias involving the ventrolateral aspect of the thigh. These are variously described as a disagreeable numbness or as a sensation of burning, stinging, tingling, or "pins and needles." The syndrome is most common among obese individuals whose abdominal girth may produce excessive traction or strain on the inguinal ligament. There are no associated motor signs or symptoms.

Fig. 2.13 **Syndrome of the lateral femoral cutaneous nerve (meralgia paresthetica).**

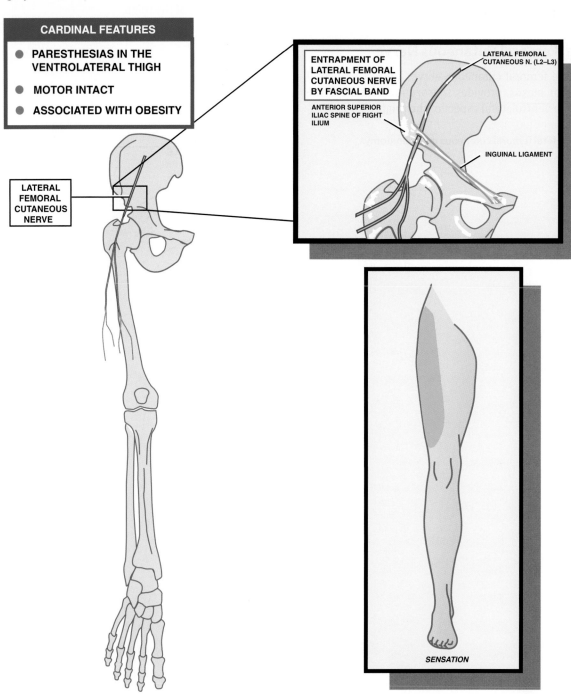

CARDINAL FEATURES

- PARESTHESIAS IN THE VENTROLATERAL THIGH
- MOTOR INTACT
- ASSOCIATED WITH OBESITY

LATERAL FEMORAL CUTANEOUS NERVE

ENTRAPMENT OF LATERAL FEMORAL CUTANEOUS NERVE BY FASCIAL BAND

ANTERIOR SUPERIOR ILIAC SPINE OF RIGHT ILIUM

LATERAL FEMORAL CUTANEOUS N. (L2–L3)

INGUINAL LIGAMENT

SENSATION

Saphenous Nerve

The saphenous nerve, a branch of the femoral nerve, provides sensory innervation to the ventromedial aspect of the knee, leg, and foot.

Anatomy

See **Fig. 2.14**.

   The saphenous nerve is a purely sensory branch of the femoral nerve. It originates just below the *inguinal ligament*, enters the *adductor canal* (Hunter's canal), crosses the femoral artery from lateral to medial, and exits the canal by piercing its roof. The nerve then courses distally, dividing into two terminal branches: (1) an *infrapatellar branch*, which supplies the ventromedial aspect of the knee, and (2) the *descending branch*, which supplies the ventromedial aspect of the leg and ankle.

Fig. 2.14 **Saphenous nerve anatomy.**

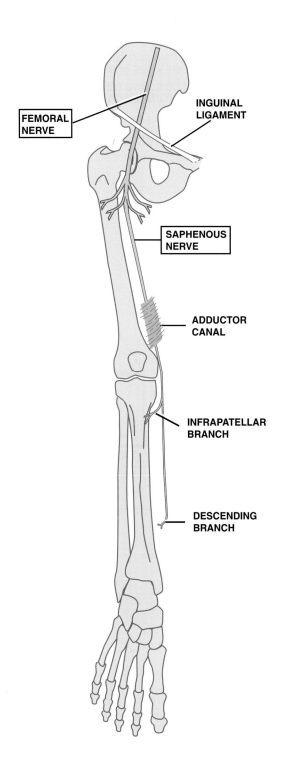

Saphenous Nerve Entrapment Syndrome

See **Fig. 2.15**.

The site of compression of the saphenous nerve occurs at its point of exit from the adductor canal. One of the cardinal features of the syndrome is intense pain along the medial aspect of the knee. Typically, there is also numbness along the medial aspect of the knee or leg or both. No motor signs or symptoms are present.

Fig. 2.15 Saphenous nerve entrapment syndrome.

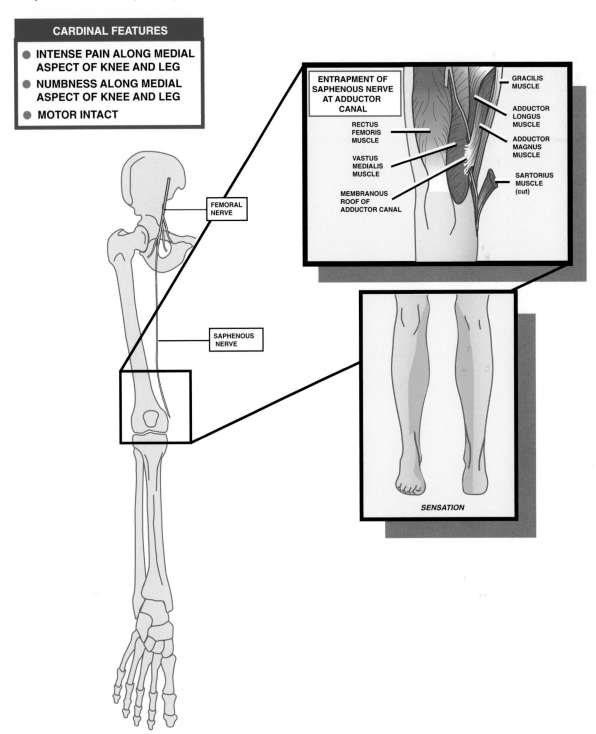

Sciatic Nerve

The sciatic nerve, a direct branch of the lumbosacral plexus, is the largest peripheral nerve in the body. Via its terminal branches, the common peroneal and tibial nerves, the sciatic nerve supplies the hamstring muscles and all of the muscles below the knee. It also provides sensory innervation to the skin of the dorsolateral leg and foot.

Anatomy

See **Fig. 2.16**.

The *sciatic nerve* is a mixed nerve derived from the fourth and fifth lumbar and the first, second, and third sacral spinal segments. The nerve leaves the pelvis through the greater sciatic foramen beneath the tendinous origin of the *piriformis* muscle. It courses laterally and downward, deep to the gluteus maximus muscle, to innervate the *semitendinous, semimembranous, biceps femoris,* and *adductor magnus* muscles. The nerve then proceeds downward in the dorsal thigh to reach the popliteal fossa, where it divides into its two terminal branches, the *tibial nerve* and the *common peroneal nerve*, which supply all the muscles of the leg and foot.

Fig. 2.16 **Sciatic nerve anatomy.**

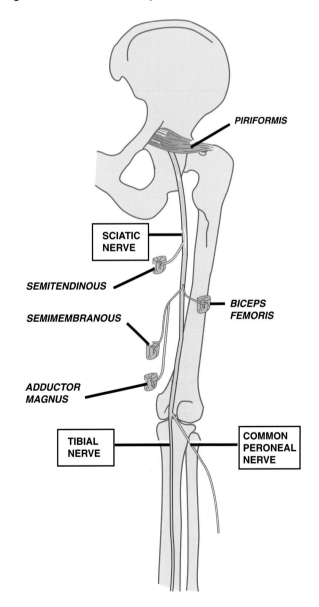

Piriformis Syndrome

See **Fig. 2.17**.

The site of compression in the piriformis syndrome is the proximal segment of the *sciatic nerve* that passes underneath the *piriformis muscle*. The cardinal features of the piriformis syndrome are (1) weakness in any or all of the knee flexors, ankle flexors or extensors, and foot intrinsics; and (2) sensory loss that may involve all of the foot. The clinical picture may be confused by a lumbosacral radiculopathy related to degenerative spine disease.

Fig. 2.17 **Piriformis syndrome.**

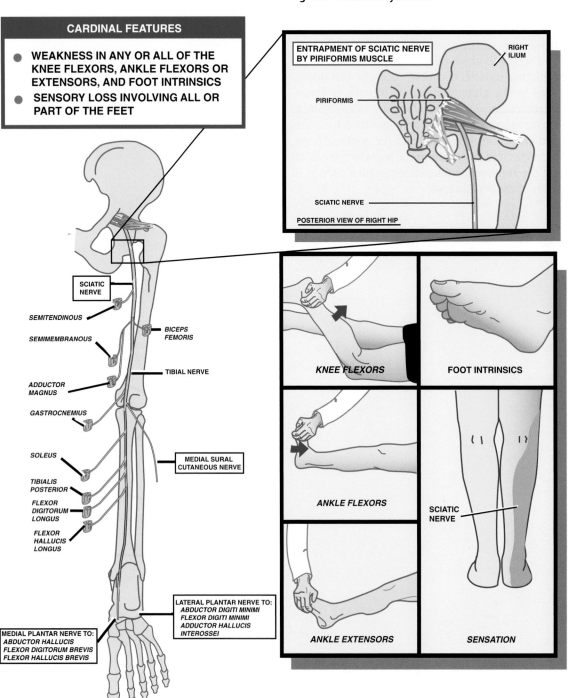

Peroneal Nerve

The peroneal nerve is a terminal branch of the sciatic nerve. It provides motor innervation to the muscles of the anterior compartment of the leg and foot (dorsiflexors and foot evertors) and sensory innervation to the skin of the lower lateral leg and the dorsum of the foot.

Anatomy

See **Fig. 2.18**.

The *common peroneal nerve* (L4, L5, S1, S2) is one of two terminal branches of the sciatic nerve that takes origin in the popliteal fossa. The nerve courses laterally in the popliteal fossa, winding around the neck of the fibula and dividing into the superficial and deep peroneal nerves.

The *superficial peroneal nerve* provides motor innervation to the *peroneus longus* and *brevis* muscles (evertors of the foot) and sensory innervation to the lower lateral leg and the dorsum of the foot (except for the first dorsal web space).

The *deep peroneal nerve* descends deep in the anterior compartment of the leg and provides motor innervation to the following four dorsiflexors of the foot and toes: (1) the *tibialis anterior*, a dorsiflexor and evertor of the foot; (2) the *extensor hallucis longus*, an extensor of the great toe and dorsiflexor of the foot; (3) the *extensor digitorum longus*, an extensor of the four lateral toes and dorsiflexor of the foot; and (4) the *extensor digitorum brevis*, an extensor of the great toe and the three medial toes.

Just proximal to the ankle, the nerve becomes superficial and divides into medial and lateral branches. The lateral (motor) branch innervates the extensor digitorum brevis, and the medial (sensory) branch supplies the skin over the first dorsal web space.

Fig. 2.18 **Peroneal nerve anatomy.**

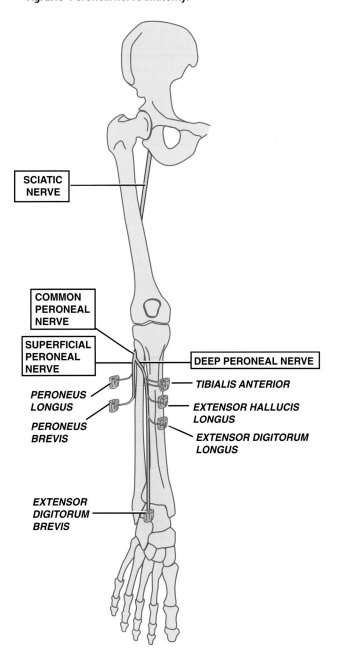

Peroneal Nerve Syndrome

See **Fig. 2.19**.

The most frequent site of compression of the peroneal nerve is at the fibular head. In this location the nerve is superficial and thus susceptible to injury. Most commonly this is due to prolonged extrinsic pressure such as may occur to a patient in the lateral decubitus position who is improperly padded during surgery. The most frequently affected nerve is the deep peroneal nerve, although this same mechanism may involve the common or superficial peroneal nerves.

Fig. 2.19 **Common peroneal nerve syndrome.** Functions or responses marked with an "X" are impaired or absent.

The clinical presentation of the peroneal nerve syndrome is dependent on the particular nerve affected: (1) *Common peroneal nerve* involvement results in weakness of foot aversion and of toe and foot dorsiflexion. In addition, there is sensory loss involving the dorsum of the foot and toes and the lateral aspect of the lower leg. (2) *Deep peroneal nerve* involvement results in weakness of foot and toe dorsiflexion as well as sensory loss involving the first dorsal web space of the foot. (3) *Superficial peroneal nerve* involvement results in weakness of foot aversion as well as sensory loss in the distribution of the lateral aspect of the leg and the dorsum of the foot and toes (except for the first dorsal web space).

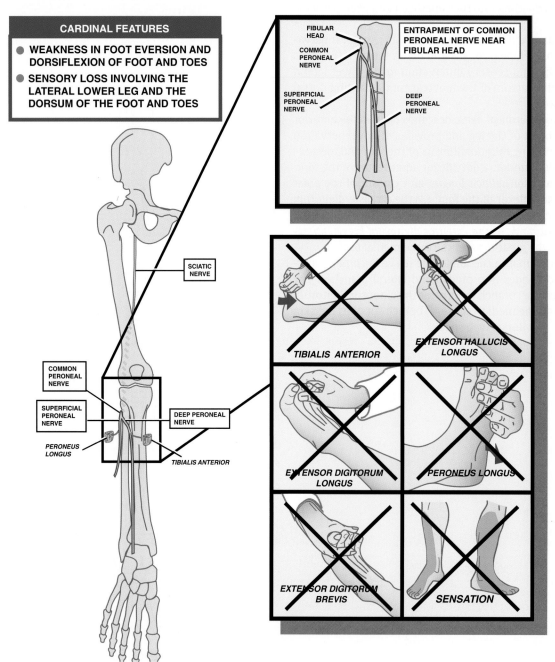

CARDINAL FEATURES
- WEAKNESS IN FOOT EVERSION AND DORSIFLEXION OF FOOT AND TOES
- SENSORY LOSS INVOLVING THE LATERAL LOWER LEG AND THE DORSUM OF THE FOOT AND TOES

ENTRAPMENT OF COMMON PERONEAL NERVE NEAR FIBULAR HEAD

FIBULAR HEAD
COMMON PERONEAL NERVE
SUPERFICIAL PERONEAL NERVE
DEEP PERONEAL NERVE

SCIATIC NERVE
COMMON PERONEAL NERVE
SUPERFICIAL PERONEAL NERVE
PERONEUS LONGUS
DEEP PERONEAL NERVE
TIBIALIS ANTERIOR

TIBIALIS ANTERIOR
EXTENSOR HALLUCIS LONGUS
EXTENSOR DIGITORUM LONGUS
PERONEUS LONGUS
EXTENSOR DIGITORUM BREVIS
SENSATION

Tibial Nerve

The tibial nerve is a terminal branch of the sciatic nerve. It provides motor innervation to the muscles of the posterior compartment of the leg and foot (plantar flexors and foot invertors) and sensory innervation to the skin of the heel and sole.

Anatomy

See **Fig. 2.20**.

The tibial nerve, one of the two terminal branches of the sciatic nerve, carries fibers derived from the fourth and fifth lumbar and the first, second, and third sacral nerve roots. It continues the line of the sciatic nerve through the popliteal fossa, coursing distally in the dorsal aspect of the leg. In the distal popliteal fossa it gives off a branch, the *medial sural cutaneous nerve*, which supplies the skin on the calf. This branch joins the lateral sural cutaneous nerve (a branch of the *common peroneal*) at the level of the Achilles tendon, and together they form the sural nerve. The sural nerve supplies the skin on the lateral heel and the lateral aspect of the foot and small toe.

Also in the popliteal fossa, the tibial nerve gives off branches to the *gastrocnemius* and then the *soleus* muscles—both plantar flexors of the foot. The nerve courses distally in a plane between the gastrocnemius and soleus muscles dorsally and the tibialis posterior ventrally. This segment of the nerve in the upper third of the leg provides motor innervation to three muscles: (1) the *tibialis posterior*, an invertor of the foot; (2) the *flexor digitorum longus*, a plantar flexor of the toes; and (3) the *flexor hallucis longus*, a plantar flexor of the great toe.

At the level of the ankle, the tibial nerve passes caudal and dorsal to the medial malleolus and under the flexor retinaculum (*tarsal tunnel*). A *medial calcaneal branch* variably originates proximal to, distal to, or within the tarsal tunnel. It is a purely sensory branch that supplies the skin of the medial heel.

In the distal portion of the tarsal tunnel, the nerve gives off two terminal branches: (1) the *medial plantar nerve*, which innervates the medial intrinsic muscles of the foot and the skin over the medial three and a half toes; and (2) the *lateral plantar nerve*, which innervates the lateral intrinsic muscles of the foot and the skin over the lateral one and a half toes. Note that the anatomy is analogous to the median and ulnar nerve innervation of the hand.

The tarsal tunnel, like the carpal tunnel, is a fibro-osseous canal. It is formed by the flexor retinaculum (roof) and the calcaneus and medial malleolus (floor).

Fig. 2.20 **Tibial nerve anatomy.**

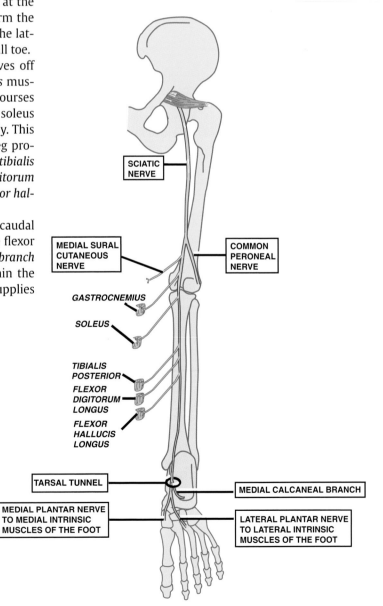

Tarsal Tunnel Syndrome

See **Fig. 2.21**.

Any pathological process, such as trauma or inflammation, that compromises the space available for the neural elements in the tarsal tunnel may result in tarsal tunnel syndrome. The cardinal symptoms of this syndrome are burning pain and paresthesias in the area involved, which varies depending on the nerve or nerves affected. This may include any one or a combination of the heel (calcaneal nerve), the medial sole (medial plantar nerve), or the lateral sole (lateral plantar nerve). In addition, there is weakness in the foot intrinsics.

Fig. 2.21 Tarsal tunnel syndrome.

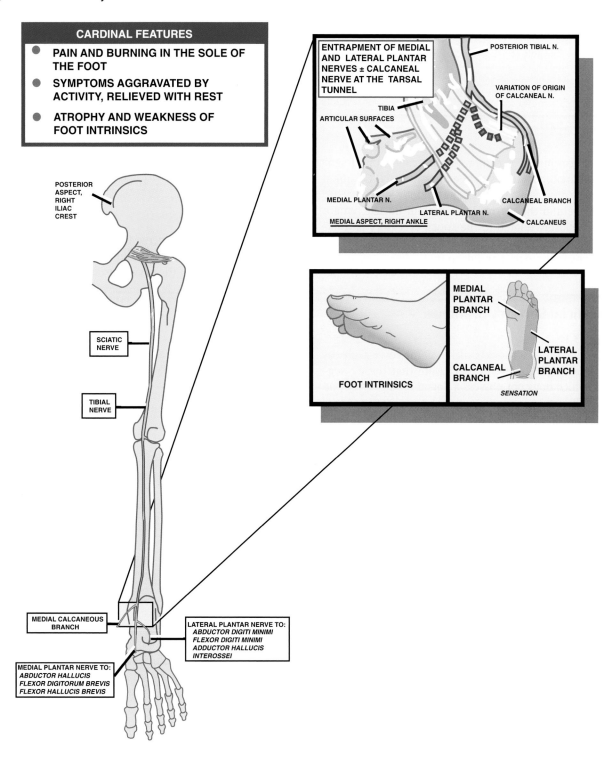

CARDINAL FEATURES

- PAIN AND BURNING IN THE SOLE OF THE FOOT
- SYMPTOMS AGGRAVATED BY ACTIVITY, RELIEVED WITH REST
- ATROPHY AND WEAKNESS OF FOOT INTRINSICS

POSTERIOR ASPECT, RIGHT ILIAC CREST

SCIATIC NERVE

TIBIAL NERVE

MEDIAL CALCANEOUS BRANCH

MEDIAL PLANTAR NERVE TO:
ABDUCTOR HALLUCIS
FLEXOR DIGITORUM BREVIS
FLEXOR HALLUCIS BREVIS

LATERAL PLANTAR NERVE TO:
ABDUCTOR DIGITI MINIMI
FLEXOR DIGITI MINIMI
ADDUCTOR HALLUCIS
INTEROSSEI

ENTRAPMENT OF MEDIAL AND LATERAL PLANTAR NERVES ± CALCANEAL NERVE AT THE TARSAL TUNNEL

POSTERIOR TIBIAL N.

VARIATION OF ORIGIN OF CALCANEAL N.

TIBIA
ARTICULAR SURFACES

MEDIAL PLANTAR N.

LATERAL PLANTAR N.

CALCANEAL BRANCH

CALCANEUS

MEDIAL ASPECT, RIGHT ANKLE

FOOT INTRINSICS

MEDIAL PLANTAR BRANCH

LATERAL PLANTAR BRANCH

CALCANEAL BRANCH

SENSATION

3 Plexuses

Cervical Plexus

The cervical plexus is composed of a collection of sensory and motor branches derived from the C1–C4 spinal nerves. It comprises a series of anastomotic loops that are located behind the sternocleidomastoid muscle, where they are closely related to the spinal accessory and hypoglossal nerves. The plexus may be divided into superficial sensory branches and deep motor branches as follows.

Superficial Sensory Branches

See **Fig. 3.1**.

The superficial sensory branches of the cervical plexus comprise the following nerves. (Note that the C1 segment, which does not possess a dorsal root, provides no sensory branches.)

Greater Occipital Nerve (C2)

The *greater occipital nerve* is derived from the C2 spinal root. It supplies the skin of the posterior scalp.

Lesser Occipital Nerve (C2)

The *lesser occipital nerve* is derived from the C2 spinal root. It supplies the skin overlying the mastoid process, extending just above and below the mastoid process, to include part of the lateral head and part of the lateral neck.

Great Auricular Nerve (C2–C3)

The *great auricular nerve* is derived from the C2–C3 spinal roots. It supplies the skin overlying the external ear, the parotid gland, and the angle of the mandible.

Transverse Cervical Nerve (C2–C3)

The *transverse cervical nerve* is derived from the C2–C3 spinal roots. It supplies the skin overlying the anterior and lateral aspects of the neck from the body of the mandible to the sternum.

Supraclavicular Nerves (C3–C4)

The *supraclavicular nerves* are derived from the C3–C4 spinal roots. They supply the skin just above and below the clavicle.

Fig. 3.1 **Superficial sensory branches of cervical plexus.**

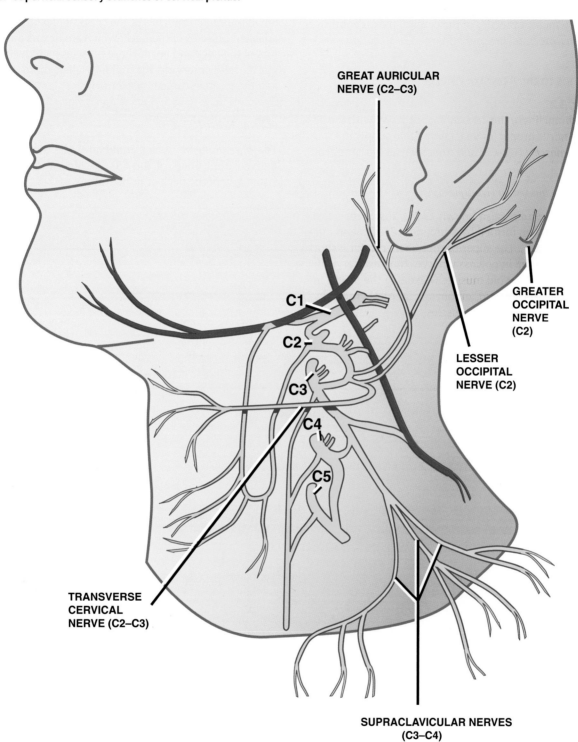

GREAT AURICULAR
NERVE (C2–C3)

GREATER
OCCIPITAL
NERVE
(C2)

LESSER
OCCIPITAL
NERVE (C2)

C1

C2

C3

C4

C5

TRANSVERSE
CERVICAL
NERVE (C2–C3)

SUPRACLAVICULAR NERVES
(C3–C4)

Deep Motor Branches

The deep motor branches of the cervical plexus comprise the following branches and nerves.

Branches to the Accessory Nerve

See **Fig. 3.2**.

The branches to the *accessory nerve* travel with the accessory nerve proper (cranial nerve XI) to supply the *sternocleidomastoid* (C2–C3) and *trapezius* (C3–C4) muscles.

Ansa Cervicalis (Ansa Hypoglossi)

The *ansa cervicalis* (also known as the ansa hypoglossi) comprises a loop formed by a superior (C1–C2) and *inferior root* (C2–C3). The superior root fibers run for a short distance with the hypoglossal nerve. The ansa cervicalis supplies the infrahyoid muscles (flexors of the head), including the sternohyoid, omohyoid, sternothyroid, thyrothyroid, and geniohyoid muscles.

Branches to Adjacent Neck Muscles

Small muscular branches of the cervical plexus innervate adjacent muscles of the neck, which are flexors and rotators of the neck and head. These muscles include the longus muscles anteriorly, the middle scalene more laterally, and the levator scapulae posteriorly.

Phrenic Nerve (C3–C5)

The *phrenic nerve*, which innervates the diaphragm, is derived from fibers of the C3–C5 spinal roots that join either low in the neck or in the thorax.

Fig. 3.2 Deep motor branches of cervical plexus.

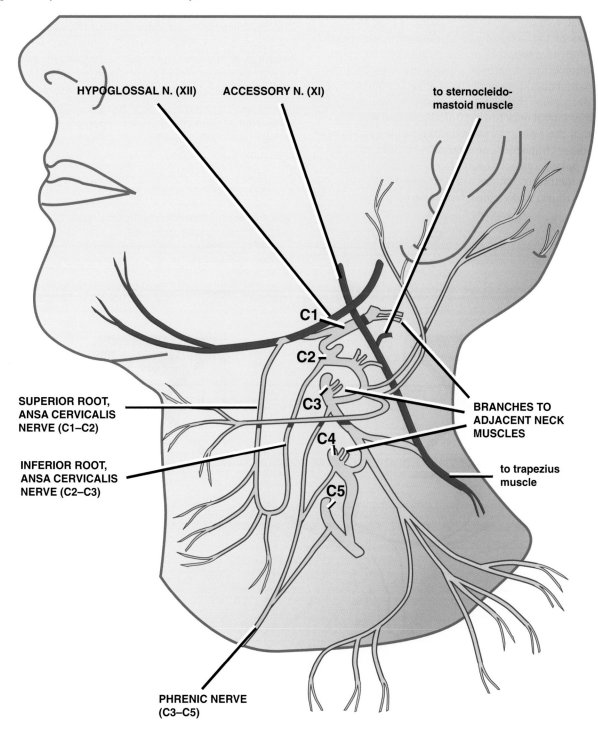

HYPOGLOSSAL N. (XII)

ACCESSORY N. (XI)

to sternocleido-
mastoid muscle

C1

C2

C3

C4

C5

SUPERIOR ROOT,
ANSA CERVICALIS
NERVE (C1–C2)

INFERIOR ROOT,
ANSA CERVICALIS
NERVE (C2–C3)

BRANCHES TO
ADJACENT NECK
MUSCLES

to trapezius
muscle

PHRENIC NERVE
(C3–C5)

Lesions of the Cervical Plexus

See **Fig. 3.3**.

Injuries of the cervical plexus produce a variety of clinical deficits, depending on the location of the lesion. Interruption of the superficial sensory branches may result in partial numbness of the head or neck. Interruption of the deep motor branches may result in weakness of forward or lateral neck flexion (infrahyoid and scalenes), rotation of the head (sternocleidomastoid), elevation of the shoulder (trapezius), or rotation of the scapula (levator scapulae). Typical causes of cervical plexus lesions include penetrating wounds, surgical injury (e.g., carotid endarterectomy), and various mass lesions.

Injuries to the phrenic nerve most commonly occur distal to the cervical plexus in or around the mediastinum. Unilateral lesions result in paralysis of the diaphragm on the affected side. Frequently this is tolerated while the patient is at rest but may result in dyspnea on exertion. On the other hand, bilateral lesions are usually associated with severe ventilatory compromise at rest, unless the phrenic nerve receives an anastomotic branch from the subclavian nerve. Typical causes of phrenic nerve lesions include penetrating injury, surgical injury, and intrathoracic masses.

Fig. 3.3 Lesions of cervical plexus. Functions or responses marked with an "X" are impaired or absent.

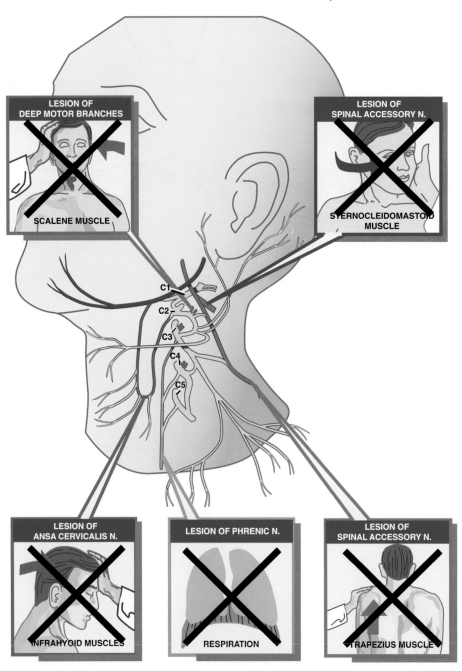

Brachial Plexus

See **Fig. 3.4.**

The brachial plexus comprises an intermingling of fibers derived from the ventral rami of the C5–T1 spinal nerves. In proximal to distal order, the brachial plexus may be divided into five components: (1) roots, (2) trunks, (3) divisions, (4) cords, and (5) branches.

In the posterior triangle of the neck, the C5 and C6 spinal roots join to form the upper trunk, the C7 spinal root continues as the *middle trunk*, and the C8 and T1 spinal roots join to form the *lower trunk*. The posttriangle is defined anteriorly by the sternocleiodomastoid muscle, posteriorly by the trapezius, and inferiorly by the mid-dle third of the clavicle. More distally in the neck, in the supraclavicular fossa, each of the three trunks gives rise to an *anterior* and a *posterior division*. Behind the axillary artery, the three posterior divisions are united to form the *posterior cord*. The anterior divisions of the upper and middle trunk unite to form the *lateral cord*. And the anterior division of the lower trunk continues as the *medial cord*. The cords of the plexus leave the posterior triangle of the neck and enter the axilla through the outlet between the first rib and the clavicle (thoracic outlet). In the axilla, the cords give rise to the terminal branches of the plexus, the peripheral nerves. Along its ~15 cm course, the major components of the plexus give rise to many other important branches (peripheral nerves).

Fig. 3.4 **Brachial plexus.**

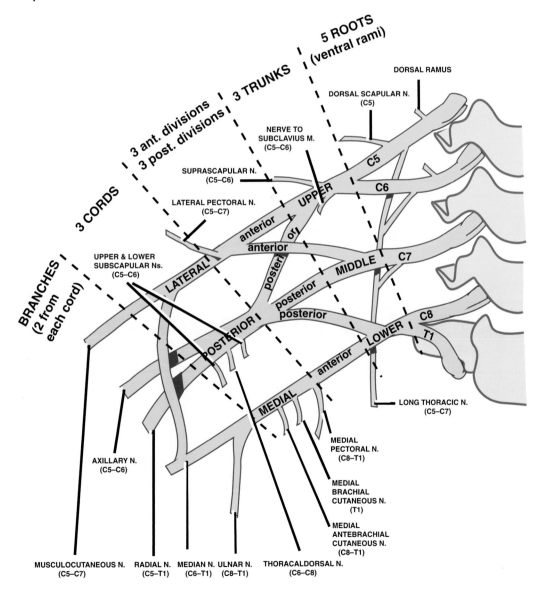

Branches from the Roots

See **Fig. 3.5**.

Dorsal Scapular Nerve

The *dorsal scapular nerve* arises from C5. It supplies the levator scapulae and the rhomboid muscles.

Long Thoracic Nerve

The *long thoracic nerve* arises from C5–C7. It supplies the serratus anterior muscle.

Fig. 3.5 **Branches from the roots of brachial plexus.**

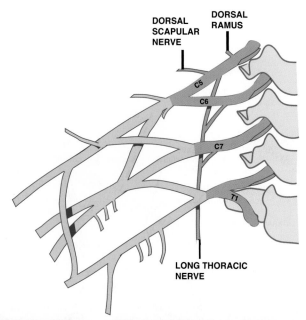

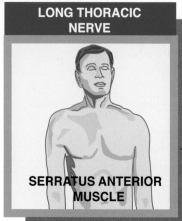

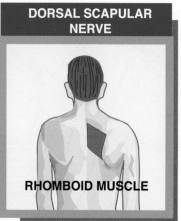

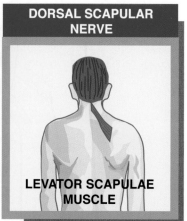

Branches from the Trunks

See **Fig. 3.6**.

Nerve to the Subclavius

The *nerve to the subclavius* arises from the upper trunk of the brachial plexus. It supplies the subclavius muscle. Of clinical importance, this nerve may contain accessory nerve fibers that join the phrenic nerve in the superior mediastinum.

Suprascapular Nerve

The *suprascapular nerve* arises from the upper trunk of the brachial plexus. It supplies the supraspinatus and infraspinatus muscles.

Fig. 3.6 **Branches from the trunks of brachial plexus.**

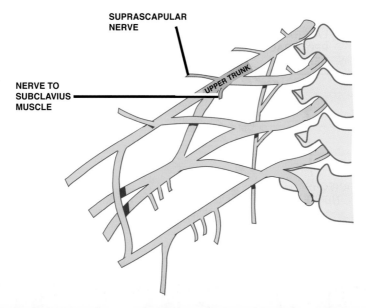

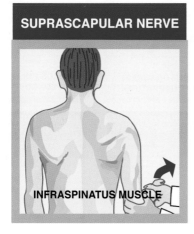
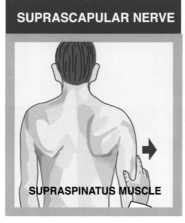
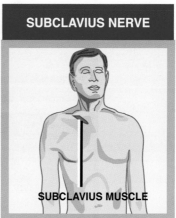

Branches from the Divisions

There are no branches that arise from the divisions of the brachial plexus.

Branches from the Cords

Lateral Cord

See **Fig. 3.7**.

There are three branches that arise from the lateral cord, namely, the *lateral pectoral nerve*, the *musculocutaneous nerve*, and the *lateral root of the median nerve*.

1. The lateral pectoral nerve supplies the pectoralis major muscle.

2. The musculocutaneous nerve supplies the corachobrachialis muscle in the axilla and the biceps and brachialis muscles in the upper arm. In the forearm the musculocutaneous nerve gives rise to a sensory branch, the lateral cutaneous nerve of the forearm.

3. The lateral root of the median nerve is a direct continuation of the lateral cord of the brachial plexus. It is joined by the medial root to form the median nerve trunk. No branches of the median nerve are given off in the axilla.

Fig. 3.7 **Branches from lateral cord of brachial plexus.**

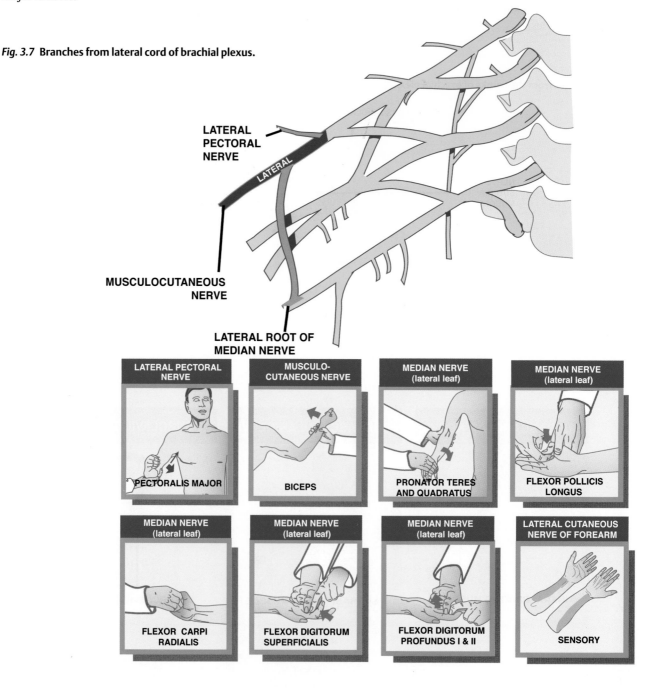

Medial Cord

See **Fig. 3.8**.

There are five branches of the medial cord, namely, the *medial pectoral nerve*, the *medial brachial cutaneous nerve*, the *medial antebrachial cutaneous nerve*, the *ulnar nerve*, and the *medial root of the median nerve*.

1. The medial pectoral nerve supplies the pectoralis major and minor muscles.

2. The medial brachial cutaneous nerve supplies the skin on the medial aspect of the arm.

3. The medial antebrachial cutaneous nerve supplies the skin on the medial aspect of the forearm.

4. The ulnar nerve gives off no major branches in the axilla or the upper arm. In the forearm and hand it gives off both sensory and muscular branches. Both the motor and sensory branches of the ulnar nerve are described in Chapter 2.

5. The medial root of the median nerve is joined by the lateral root to form the median nerve trunk. No branches of the median nerve are given off in the axilla.

Fig. 3.8 **Branches from medial cord of brachial plexus.**

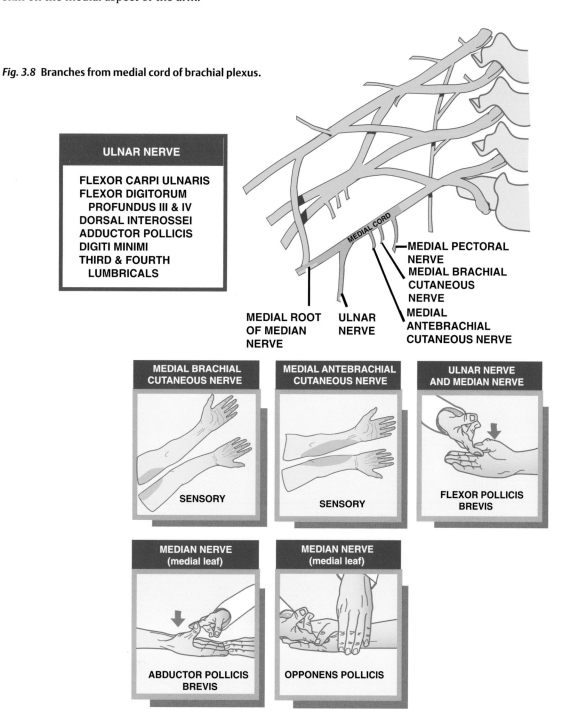

Posterior Cord

See **Fig. 3.9**.

There are three branches of the posterior cord that are given off before its two terminal branches, namely, the *upper subscapular nerve*, the *thoracodorsal nerve*, and the *lower subscapular nerve*. The terminal branches of the posterior cord are the *axillary nerve* and the *radial nerve*.

1. The upper subscapular nerve supplies the upper part of the subscapularis muscle.

2. The thoracodorsal nerve supplies the latissimus dorsi muscle.

3. The lower subscapular nerve supplies the lower part of the subscapularis muscle.

4. The axillary nerve is one of the terminal branches of the posterior cord. It supplies the deltoid muscle and the skin overlying the muscle.

5. The radial nerve is the direct continuation of the posterior cord of the brachial plexus. It is the largest branch of the brachial plexus and lies behind the axillary artery. In the axilla, the radial nerve gives branches to the triceps muscle and supplies the skin on the middle of the back of the arm. Both the motor and sensory branches of the radial nerve are described in Chapter 2.

Fig. 3.9 Branches from posterior cord of brachial plexus.

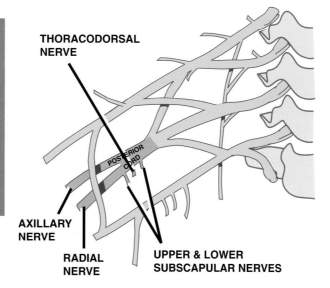

RADIAL NERVE

EXTENSOR MUSCLES OF ARM AND FOREARM, TRICEPS MUSCLE, BRACHIORADIALIS MUSCLE, EXTENSOR CARPI RADIALIS LONGUS MUSCLE, AND BREVIS MUSCLE

DEEP MOTOR BRANCH INNERVATES SUPINATOR, EXTENSOR DIGITORUM, EXTENSOR DIGITI MINIMI, EXTENSOR CARPI ULNARIS, ABDUCTOR POLLICIS LONGUS, EXTENSOR POLLICIS LONGUS AND BREVIS, AND THE EXTENSOR INDICIS MUSCLES

THORACODORSAL NERVE

POSTERIOR CORD

AXILLARY NERVE

RADIAL NERVE

UPPER & LOWER SUBSCAPULAR NERVES

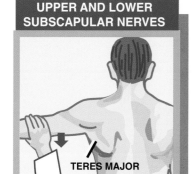

UPPER AND LOWER SUBSCAPULAR NERVES

TERES MAJOR

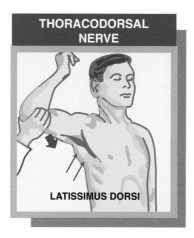

THORACODORSAL NERVE

LATISSIMUS DORSI

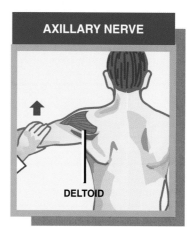

AXILLARY NERVE

DELTOID

Lesions of the Brachial Plexus

Partial lesions of the brachial plexus are far more common than complete lesions. The two most commonly described partial lesions are traumatic lesions involving the upper and lower trunks. These are known as the Erb-Duchenne type and the Dejerine-Klumpke type, respectively. Other traumatic lesions of the brachial plexus may involve the entire plexus or may be isolated to the lateral, medial, or posterior cords. Several nontraumatic lesions have also been described. These include the thoracic outlet syndrome, the apical lung tumor syndrome, radiation brachial plexopathy, and neuralgic amyotrophy.

Lesions of the Upper Brachial Plexus (Erb-Duchenne Type)

See **Fig. 3.10**.

Lesions of the upper brachial plexus typically comprise traction injuries of the C5 and C6 nerve roots. They are frequently associated with excessive lateral displacement of the head to the opposite side or downward displacement of the ipsilateral shoulder, such as may occur during a difficult delivery or a fall or blow on the shoulder. Isolated lesions of the upper plexus primarily affect function of the shoulder and the elbow. The cardinal features of this syndrome are as follows:

1. Impairment of shoulder abduction (due to deltoid and supraspinatus involvement)
2. Impairment of elbow flexion (due to biceps, brachioradialis, and brachialis involvement)
3. Impairment of external rotation of the arm (due to infraspinatus involvement)
4. Impairment of forearm supination (due to biceps involvement)
5. Sensory loss limited to skin over deltoid muscle
6. Depressed or absent biceps and brachioradialis reflexes

The posture of the extremity in upper plexus injuries is characteristic: the upper arm is internally rotated and adducted; the forearm is extended and pronated. The palm in this position faces out and backward, presenting the limb in the so-called policeman's tip or waiter's tip posture.

Fig. 3.10 Upper brachial plexus syndrome.

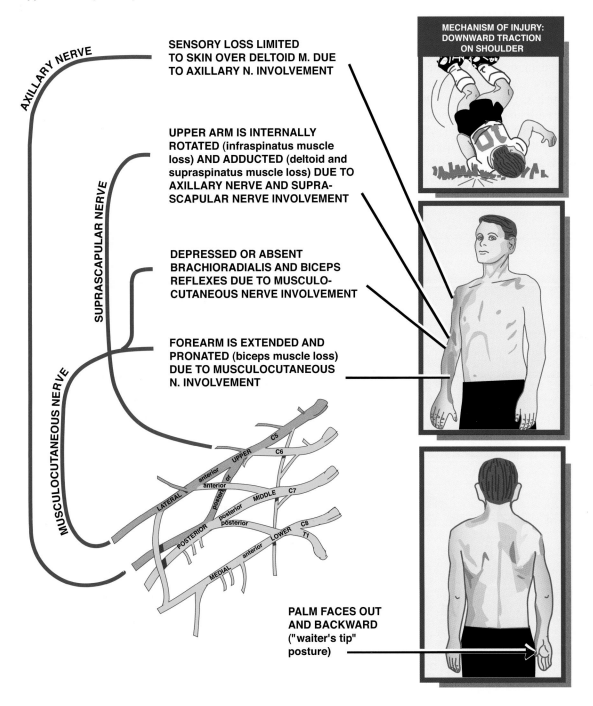

SENSORY LOSS LIMITED
TO SKIN OVER DELTOID M. DUE
TO AXILLARY N. INVOLVEMENT

UPPER ARM IS INTERNALLY
ROTATED (infraspinatus muscle
loss) AND ADDUCTED (deltoid and
supraspinatus muscle loss) DUE TO
AXILLARY NERVE AND SUPRA-
SCAPULAR NERVE INVOLVEMENT

DEPRESSED OR ABSENT
BRACHIORADIALIS AND BICEPS
REFLEXES DUE TO MUSCULO-
CUTANEOUS NERVE INVOLVEMENT

FOREARM IS EXTENDED AND
PRONATED (biceps muscle loss)
DUE TO MUSCULOCUTANEOUS
N. INVOLVEMENT

MECHANISM OF INJURY:
DOWNWARD TRACTION
ON SHOULDER

PALM FACES OUT
AND BACKWARD
("waiter's tip"
posture)

Lesions of the Lower Brachial Plexus (Dejerine-Klumpke Type)

See **Fig. 3.11.**

Lesions of the lower brachial plexus typically comprise traction injuries involving the C8 and T1 roots. They are frequently associated with excessive abduction of the arm, such as may occur to a motorcyclist who falls on his side with his arm outstretched. Isolated lesions of the lower brachial plexus primarily affect the functions subserved by the ulnar nerve. The cardinal feature of the syndrome is a claw hand deformity associated with sensory loss in the ulnar distribution of the hand and forearm. The claw hand deformity results as follows.

The fingers are extended at the metacarpophalangeal joints (due to unopposed action of the radial innervated extensor digitorum muscles) and flexed at the interphalangeal joints (due to unopposed action of the primarily median innervated flexor digitorum superficialis and profundus muscles). The lumbricals and interossei muscles, which are primarily ulnar innervated, normally provide flexion at the metacarpophalangeal joints and extension at the interphalangeal joints.

An ipsilateral Horner syndrome may also be evident due to the presence of sympathetic fibers destined for the superior cervical ganglion in the first thoracic root. The deep tendon reflexes of the triceps, biceps, and brachioradialis muscles are all intact.

Fig. 3.11 **Lower brachial plexus syndrome.**

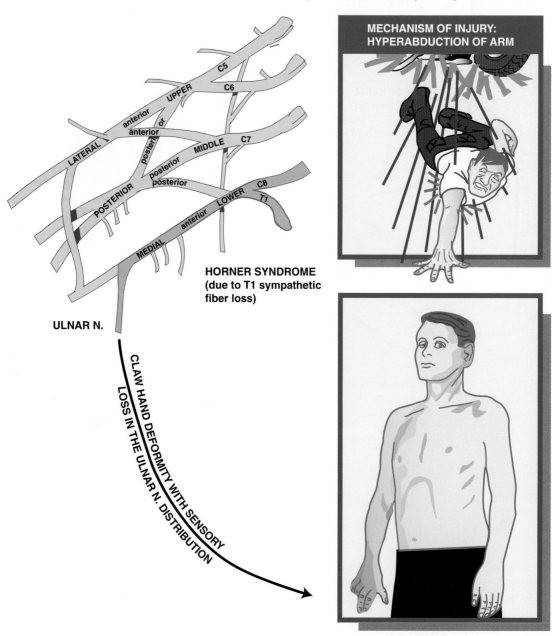

Complete Brachial Plexus Lesions

Complete brachial plexus lesions are unusual. Typically, they are associated with high-speed vehicular accidents. Clinically, they result in a completely paralyzed, asensate, areflexic limb.

Lesions of the Lateral Cord

See **Fig. 3.12**.

Lesions of the lateral cord primarily affect the musculocutaneous nerve and the lateral head of the median nerve. Musculocutaneous nerve palsy results in impairment of elbow flexion and forearm supination due to paresis of the biceps, brachialis, and coracobrachialis muscles.

Median nerve palsy produces:

1. Impairment of forearm pronation (due to involvement of the pronator teres)

2. Impairment of radial wrist flexion (due to involvement of the flexor carpi radialis)

3. Impairment of wrist flexion (due to impairment of the palmaris longus)

4. Impairment of proximal interphalangeal flexion (due to impairment of the flexor digitorum superficialis)

5. Impairment of flexion of the distal phalanx of the thumb (due to impairment of the flexor pollicis longus)

6. Impairment of flexion of the distal phalanges of the second and third digits (due to involvement of the flexor digitorum profundus I and II)

7. Impairment of forearm pronation (due to involvement of the pronator quadratus)

In addition to these motor deficits, sensory loss may occur on the lateral aspect of the forearm (due to involvement of the lateral cutaneous nerve of the forearm, a branch of the musculocutaneous nerve). The biceps reflex is absent or depressed.

Fig. 3.12 **Lateral cord lesion.**

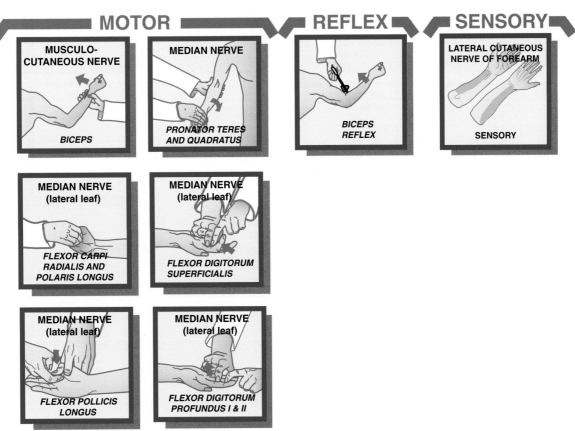

Lesions of the Medial Cord

See **Fig. 3.13**.

Lesions of the medial cord primarily affect the ulnar nerve and the medial head of the median nerve.

Ulnar nerve palsy produces:

1. Impairment of ulnar wrist flexion (due to involvement of the flexor carpi ulnaris)

2. Impairment of flexion of the distal phalanges of the fourth and fifth digits (due to impairment of the flexor digitorum profundus III and IV)

3. Impairment of finger abduction (due to involvement of the interossei)

Median nerve palsy produces:

1. Impairment of abduction of the thumb (due to involvement of the abductor pollicis brevis)

2. Impairment of opposition of the thumb (due to involvement of the opponens pollicis)

3. Impairment of flexion of the proximal phalanx of the thumb (due to involvement of the superficial head of the flexor pollicis brevis)

In addition to these motor deficits, sensory loss may occur on the medial aspect of the arm and forearm (due to involvement of the medial cutaneous nerve, a branch of the medial cord). The deep tendon reflexes of the arm remain intact.

Fig. 3.13 **Medial cord lesion.**

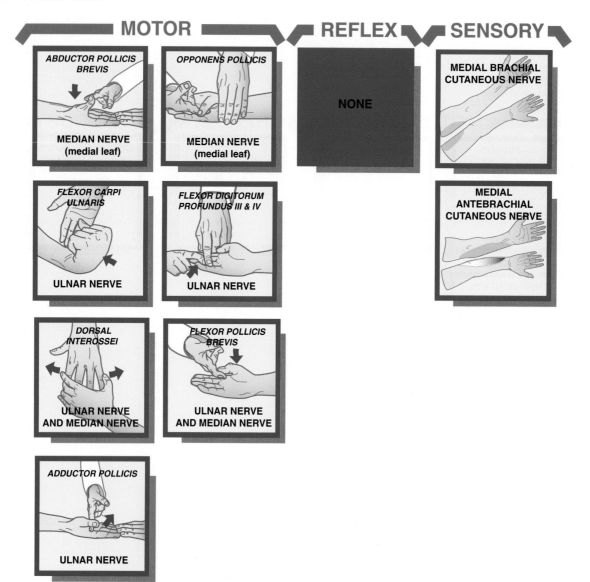

Lesions of the Posterior Cord

See **Fig. 3.14**.

Lesions of the posterior cord primarily affect the subscapular, thoracodorsal, axillary, and radial nerves. Subscapular nerve palsy results in impairment of internal rotation of the humerus (due to involvement of the teres major and subscapularis muscles). Thoracodorsal nerve palsy results in impairment of adduction of the elevated arm (due to involvement of the latissimus dorsi muscle). Axillary nerve palsy results in impairment of arm abduction (due to involvement of the deltoid muscle).

Radial nerve palsy produces:

1. Impairment of elbow extension (due to involvement of the triceps)
2. Impairment of wrist extension (due to involvement of the extensor carpi radialis and ulnaris)
3. Impairment of forearm supination (due to involvement of the supinator)
4. Impairment of finger extension (due to involvement of the extensor digitorum)

The distribution of sensory loss includes the entire extensor surface of the arm and forearm as well as the dorsum of the hand and first four fingers. The triceps reflex is absent or depressed.

Fig. 3.14 **Posterior cord lesion.**

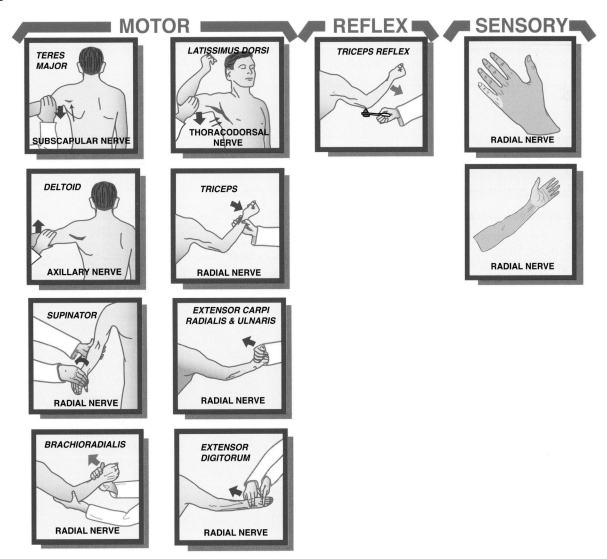

Thoracic Outlet Syndrome

See **Fig. 3.15**.

The thoracic outlet syndrome may involve compression of the *subclavian artery* or vein (vascular thoracic outlet syndrome) or the medial cord or lateral trunk of the *brachial plexus* (neurogenic thoracic outlet syndrome). In all three forms there is prominent shoulder and arm pain. The compression is usually due to several anatomic anomalies in the region. The most common abnormality is an incomplete cervical rib, with a fascial band extending from the tip to the first rib. Other anomalies include an elongated C7 transverse process, a complete cervical rib, and anomalous insertions of the anterior and medial *scalene muscles*.

The clinical syndrome is characterized predominantly by shoulder and arm pain. There may be slight wasting and weakness of the hypothenar, interosseous, adductor pollicis, and deep flexor muscles of the fourth and fifth fingers. Reflexes are usually preserved. In advanced cases, flexor muscles of the forearm may be affected. A majority of patients complain of numbness and tingling along the medial aspect of the forearm and hand.

Fig. 3.15 **Thoracic outlet syndrome.**

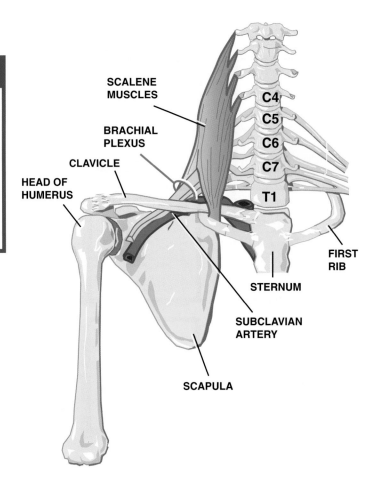

CARDINAL FEATURES

- **SHOULDER AND ARM PAIN**
- **SLIGHT WASTING AND WEAKNESS OF THE HYPOTHENAR, INTEROSSEOUS, ADDUCTOR POLICIS, AND DEEP FLEXOR MUSCLES OF THE FOURTH AND FIFTH FINGERS**
- **NUMBNESS AND TINGLING ALONG THE MEDIAL ASPECT OF THE FOREARM AND HAND**

Apical Lung Tumor Syndrome

See **Fig. 3.16**.

The apical lung tumor syndrome is cause by a Pancoast's tumor. The tumor is usually squamous cell carcinoma in the superior sulcus of the lung. As the tumor enlarges, it may compress or envelope the lower *brachial plexus,* leading to symptoms similar to the thoracic outlet syndrome (see earlier discussion). Because the posterior cord may be involved, there may also be weakness of the triceps along with the characteristic weakness and atrophy of the muscles of the hand. Of note, the neurologic signs and symptoms may occur long before the tumor becomes identified.

Fig. 3.16 **Apical lung tumor syndrome.**

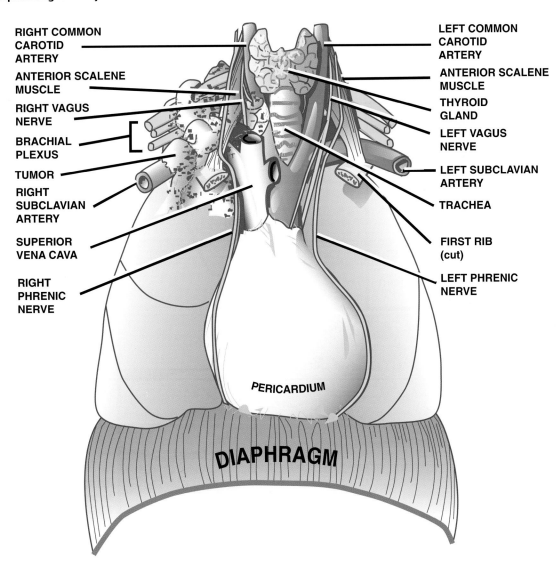

Radiation Plexopathy

See **Fig. 3.17**.

This syndrome is most commonly caused by irradiation of the axilla for carcinoma of the breast, especially when the radiation dose exceeds 6000 rads. Pathologically, there is a delayed but progressive loss of myelin in the brachial plexus, with obliteration of the vasculature and marked fibrosis.

The clinical picture is one of delayed-onset intrinsic hand weakness, associated with distal paresthesias and sensory loss. Atrophy, if present, may be masked by lymphedema. Pain is an inconstant feature. However, severe pain as a presenting symptom may point to malignant infiltration of the plexus, which is an important, and often difficult, differential distinction. The typical latency for the development of symptoms after irradiation is approximately 1 year, although the latent period has reportedly varied between 0 and 34 years.

The natural history of this plexopathy is also variable, with some reports of the process plateauing for varying periods. All too often, however, an inexorable downhill course leads ultimately to a floppy, anesthetic, swollen, and often painful appendage.

Fig. 3.17 **Radiation plexopathy.**

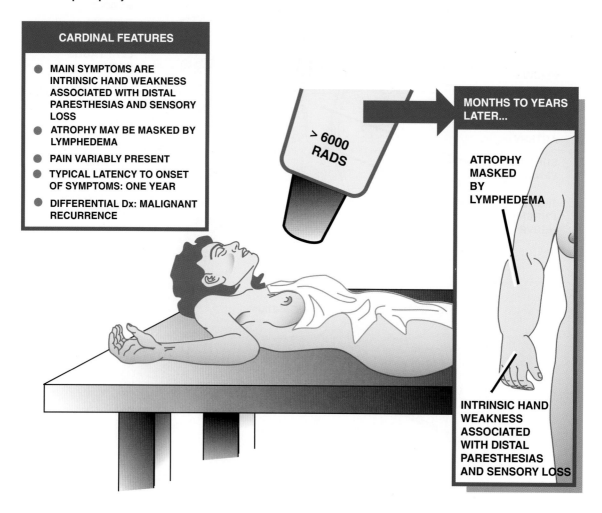

CARDINAL FEATURES

- MAIN SYMPTOMS ARE INTRINSIC HAND WEAKNESS ASSOCIATED WITH DISTAL PARESTHESIAS AND SENSORY LOSS
- ATROPHY MAY BE MASKED BY LYMPHEDEMA
- PAIN VARIABLY PRESENT
- TYPICAL LATENCY TO ONSET OF SYMPTOMS: ONE YEAR
- DIFFERENTIAL Dx: MALIGNANT RECURRENCE

> 6000 RADS

MONTHS TO YEARS LATER...

ATROPHY MASKED BY LYMPHEDEMA

INTRINSIC HAND WEAKNESS ASSOCIATED WITH DISTAL PARESTHESIAS AND SENSORY LOSS

Neuralgic Amyotrophy

See **Fig. 3.18**.

This idiopathic disorder, which is also known as Parsonage-Turner syndrome, is characterized clinically by the abrupt onset of shoulder girdle or scapular pain, followed by prominent weakness and atrophy of the upper arm muscles, especially those about the shoulder girdle. Movement or activity of the shoulder muscles tends to aggravate the pain, which is usually quite severe. The onset of neuralgic amyotrophy is often heralded by some antecedent illness or event, such as an infectious process or the administration of a vaccine.

Pain generally persists for a period of hours to approximately 2 weeks, then abates. Weakness and atrophy usually appear about the time the pain diminishes and may progress over a period of a week or longer. Unlike the pain, the period of weakness and atrophy may be prolonged (even as long as a year or more) and will ultimately determine prognosis. The pattern of weakness and atrophy in individual cases is quite variable and often patchy. In rare cases, the symptoms are bilateral.

Fig. 3.18 **Neuralgic amyotrophy (Parsonage-Turner syndrome).**

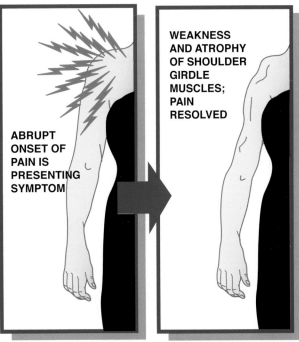

CARDINAL FEATURES

- ABRUPT ONSET OF SHOULDER GIRDLE/SCAPULAR PAIN
- PROMINENT WEAKNESS AND ATROPHY USUALLY APPEARS ABOUT THE TIME PAIN DIMINISHES
- MOVEMENT OF SHOULDER MUSCLES AGGRAVATES PAIN

ABRUPT ONSET OF PAIN IS PRESENTING SYMPTOM

WEAKNESS AND ATROPHY OF SHOULDER GIRDLE MUSCLES; PAIN RESOLVED

Lumbosacral Plexus

The lumbosacral plexus provides innervation to the pelvic girdle and the lower limb. The plexus is composed of an intermingling of the ventral rami between the T12 and the S4 spinal nerves. For the purpose of description, the following discussion divides the plexus into separate lumbar and sacral components.

Anatomy of the Lumbar Plexus

See **Figs. 3.19** to **3.22**.

The lumbar plexus comprises a union of the ventral rami of the L1–L4 spinal nerves, with a small contribution from T12. It is located within the psoas muscle, anterior to the transverse processes of the lumbar vertebrae. The

upper part of the plexus, T12–L2, produces three nerves with sensory branches (the *iliohypogastric, ilioinguinal,* and *genitofemoral nerves*), each of which supplies sensation to the skin around the pelvic girdle. The *lower part* of the plexus, L2–L4, produces two mixed nerves (the *femoral* and *obturator nerves*), which innervate the muscles of the anterior thigh and the skin over the anterior and medial aspects of the thigh and the medial aspect of the lower leg, and one sensory nerve (the *lateral femoral cutaneous nerve*), which supplies sensation to the skin over the lateral thigh.

After leaving the psoas muscle, the upper nerves of the lumbar plexus each run parallel to the lower intercostal nerves, where they help supply the transverse and oblique abdominal muscles. As they continue along their course, the nerves provide the following sensory supply.

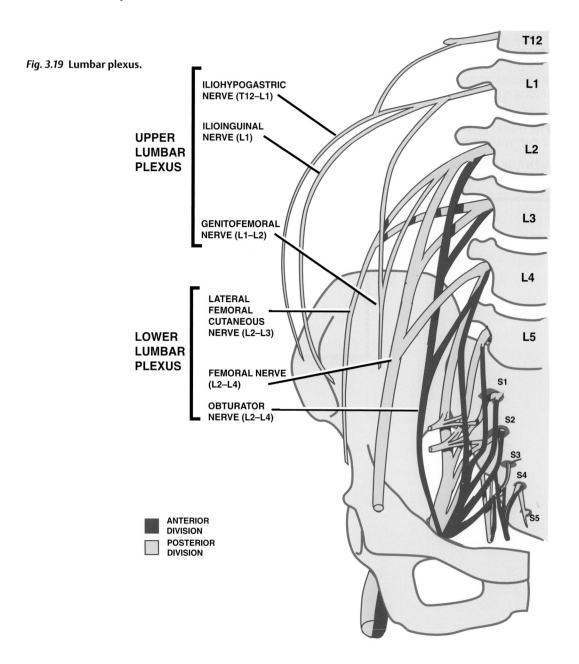

Fig. 3.19 **Lumbar plexus.**

Iliohypogastric Nerve (T12–L2)

See **Fig. 3.20**.

The iliohypogastric nerve divides into two cutaneous branches, an *anterior* and a *lateral*. The anterior branch supplies the skin over the anterior abdominal wall above the pubis, whereas the lateral branch supplies the skin over the outer buttock and hip.

Ilioinguinal Nerve (L1)

See **Fig. 3.20**.

The ilioinguinal nerve supplies the skin of the medial thigh below the inguinal ligament, as well as the skin of the symphysis pubis and the external genitalia.

Genitofemoral Nerve (L1–L2)

See **Fig. 3.20**.

The genitofemoral nerve is divided into two branches, a *genital branch*, which supplies the skin of the scrotum, and a *femoral branch*, which supplies the skin over the femoral triangle. This nerve also supplies motor innervation to the cremaster muscle.

The lower part of the lumbar plexus is derived from L2–L4. It contains the following motor and sensory nerves.

Fig. 3.20 **Upper lumbar plexus.**

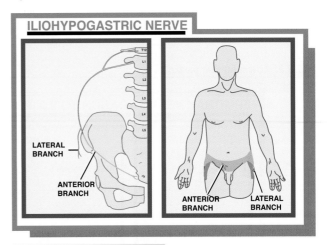

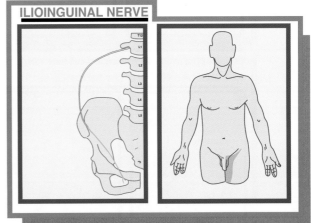

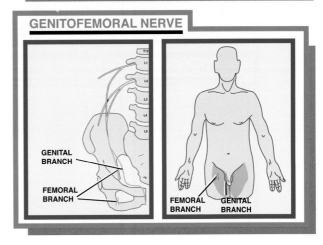

Femoral Nerve (L2–L4)

See **Fig. 3.21**.

The femoral nerve is a mixed motor/sensory nerve that arises within the psoas muscle. The nerve runs in the groove between the psoas and iliacus muscles (extensors of the hip), which it supplies with muscular branches. It then descends behind the inguinal ligament to enter the femoral triangle of the thigh, where it divides into anterior and posterior divisions.

The *anterior division* supplies a muscular branch to the *sartorius muscle* (external rotator of the thigh) and a sensory branch to the skin of the anterior and medial aspects of the thigh (*anterior cutaneous nerve of the thigh*).

The *posterior division* supplies a muscular branch to the *quadriceps femoris muscle* (extensor of the leg) and a sensory branch to the skin over the medial aspect of the leg and foot (*saphenous nerve*).

To summarize its functions, the femoral nerve is responsible for (1) extension at the hip, (2) external rotation of the thigh, (3) extension of the leg, and (4) sensation of the anteromedial thigh and medial leg and foot.

Fig. 3.21 **Lower lumbar plexus.**

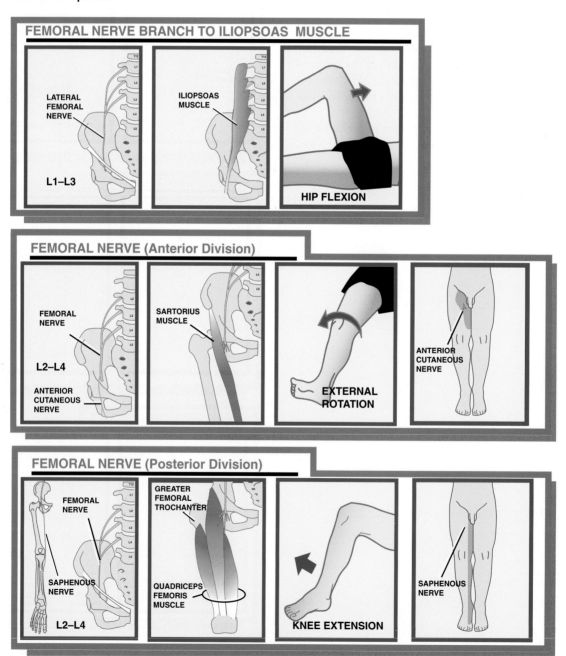

Obturator Nerve (L2–L4)

See **Fig. 3.22**.

The obturator nerve is a mixed motor/sensory nerve that arises within the psoas muscle, passes through the obturator canal, and descends into the medial thigh. Its major contribution is its motor innervation of the adductor muscles of the thigh, although it also supplies the skin over part of the medial aspect of the thigh.

Lateral Femoral Cutaneous Nerve (L2–L3)

See **Fig. 3.22**.

The lateral femoral cutaneous nerve is a purely sensory nerve that arises within the psoas muscle, passes behind the inguinal ligament, and descends into the thigh. It supplies the skin of the anterior thigh and the upper half of the lateral aspect of the thigh.

Fig. 3.22 **Lower lumbar plexus.**

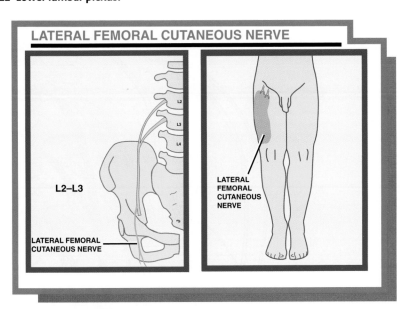

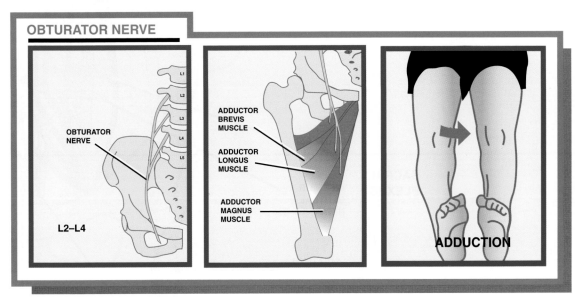

Anatomy of the Sacral Plexus

See **Fig. 3.23**.

The sacral plexus comprises an intermingling of fibers from the L4–S4 spinal nerves. Unlike the lumbar plexus, which is formed in the abdomen, the sacral plexus is formed in the pelvis. Four nerves or groups of nerves are produced by this plexus: (1) the purely motor gluteal nerves, (2) the purely sensory posterior femoral cutaneous nerve, (3) the mixed motor/sensory pudendal nerve, and (4) the mixed motor/sensory sciatic nerve. The functional anatomy of these nerves or groups of nerves is as follows.

Fig. 3.23 **Sacral plexus.**

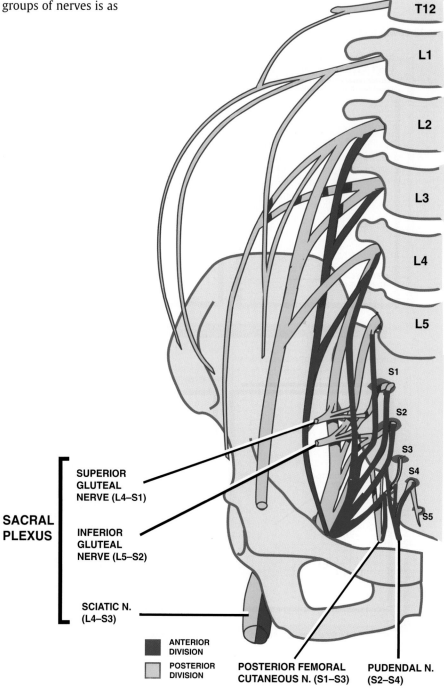

SACRAL PLEXUS

SUPERIOR GLUTEAL NERVE (L4–S1)

INFERIOR GLUTEAL NERVE (L5–S2)

SCIATIC N. (L4–S3)

ANTERIOR DIVISION

POSTERIOR DIVISION

POSTERIOR FEMORAL CUTANEOUS N. (S1–S3)

PUDENDAL N. (S2–S4)

T12

L1

L2

L3

L4

L5

S1

S2

S3

S4

S5

Gluteal Nerves (L4–S2)

See **Fig. 3.24**.

The superior and inferior gluteal nerves are purely motor nerves that leave the pelvis via the greater sciatic notch to supply the muscles of the buttocks. The *superior gluteal nerve* (L4–S1) passes above the piriformis muscle to supply the *gluteus medius, gluteus minimus*, and *tensor fasciae latae muscles*, which are abductors and internal rotators of the thigh. The *inferior gluteal nerve* (L5–S2) passes below the piriformis muscle to supply the *gluteus maximus muscle*, which is the major extensor of the hip.

Fig. 3.24 **Sacral plexus.**

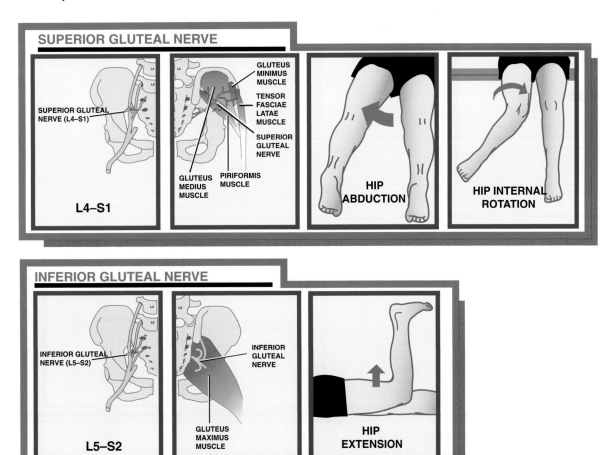

Posterior Femoral Cutaneous Nerve (S1–S3)

See **Fig. 3.25**.

This purely sensory nerve leaves the pelvis to enter the buttock via the greater sciatic notch. It supplies the skin of the posterior thigh and popliteal fossa.

Pudendal Nerve (S2–S4)

See **Fig. 3.25**.

This mixed nerve leaves the pelvis to enter the perineum via the greater sciatic notch. It supplies motor branches to the perineal muscles and external anal sphincter, and sensory branches to the skin of the perineum, penis (or clitoris), scrotum (or labia majus), and anus.

Sciatic Nerve (L4–S3)

See **Fig. 3.25**.

The sciatic nerve and its terminal branches, the common peroneal and tibial nerves, are described in Chapter 2. Together these nerves provide flexion of the leg, all the movements of the foot, and sensation to the skin of the posterior thigh and the skin of the dorsolateral leg and foot.

Fig. 3.25 **Sacral plexus.**

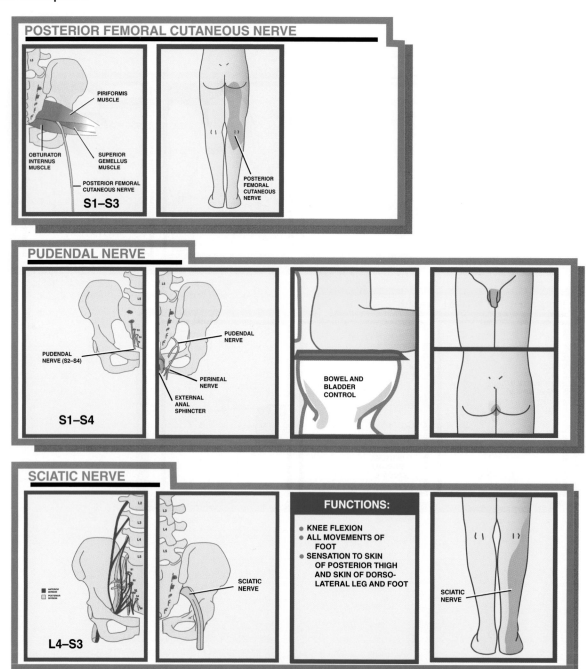

Lesions of the Lumbosacral Plexus

See **Fig. 3.26**.

Lesions of the lumbosacral plexus are unusual, particularly as a consequence of trauma. More commonly the cause is a neoplastic process, postradiation plexopathy, or surgical injury. Because the lumbar plexus is located in the abdomen, and the sacral plexus is located in the pelvis, lesions of the lumbosacral plexus may be isolated to one or the other of these, as follows.

Fig. 3.26 **Lumbosacral plexus.**

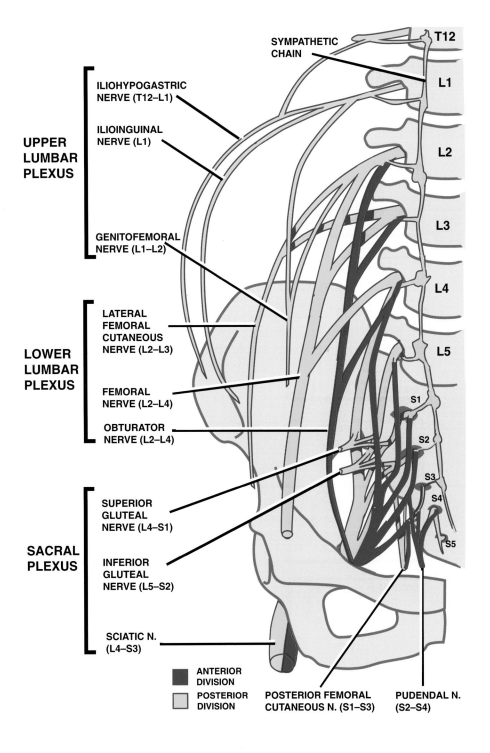

SYMPATHETIC CHAIN

T12

L1

UPPER LUMBAR PLEXUS

ILIOHYPOGASTRIC NERVE (T12–L1)

ILIOINGUINAL NERVE (L1)

L2

GENITOFEMORAL NERVE (L1–L2)

L3

L4

LOWER LUMBAR PLEXUS

LATERAL FEMORAL CUTANEOUS NERVE (L2–L3)

L5

FEMORAL NERVE (L2–L4)

OBTURATOR NERVE (L2–L4)

S1

S2

SACRAL PLEXUS

SUPERIOR GLUTEAL NERVE (L4–S1)

S3

S4

INFERIOR GLUTEAL NERVE (L5–S2)

S5

SCIATIC N. (L4–S3)

ANTERIOR DIVISION

POSTERIOR DIVISION

POSTERIOR FEMORAL CUTANEOUS N. (S1–S3)

PUDENDAL N. (S2–S4)

Lesions of the Lumbar Plexus

See **Fig. 3.27**.

Lesions of the lumbar plexus are also usually incomplete. However, for the purpose of this discussion, a complete lesion is described.

Motor signs are limited to the muscles supplied by the femoral and obturator nerves. As a result of *femoral nerve* (L2–L4) involvement, signs of weakness are present in hip flexion (iliopsoas), leg extension (quadriceps), and thigh rotation (sartorius). As a result of *obturator nerve* (L2–L4) involvement, thigh adduction (adductor muscles) is also impaired.

Sensory loss may include all or part of the following areas:

1. The inguinal region and the genitalia (iliohypogastric, ilioinguinal, and *genitofemoral* nerves)

2. The lateral thigh (*lateral femoral cutaneous nerve*)

3. The anterior and medial thigh (*femoral* and *obturator nerves*)

4. The medial leg and foot (*saphenous nerve*, a branch of the femoral nerve)

Finally, the patellar reflex (femoral nerve) and the cremasteric reflex (genitofemoral nerve) may be absent or depressed.

Fig. 3.27 **Neurologic tests for lumbar plexus lesion.**

MOTOR

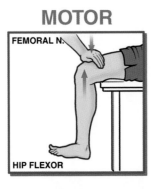

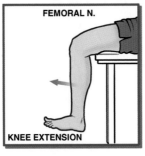

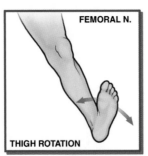

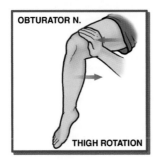

REFLEX

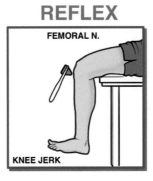

SENSORY

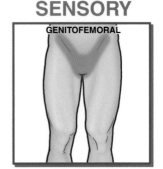

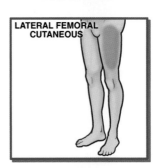

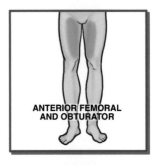

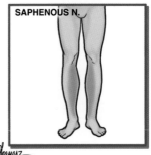

Lesions of the Sacral Plexus

See **Fig. 3.28**.

Lesions of the sacral plexus are usually incomplete. A complete lesion may be characterized as follows.

The motor signs of a sacral plexus lesion reflect the involvement of the muscles supplied by the gluteal nerves and the sciatic nerve and its branches. Thus, the syndrome is characterized by weakness in the following muscles: (1) the abductors and internal rotators of the thigh (*superior gluteal nerve*), (2) the hip extensors (*infe-rior gluteal nerve*), (3) the knee flexors (*sciatic nerve*), and (4) all of the muscles of the leg and foot (*sciatic nerve* and its branches).

The sensory signs of a sacral plexus lesion include sensory loss of the posterior thigh and most of the leg and foot (except for their medial aspects).

The Achilles reflex (S1) may be absent or depressed as a result of sciatic nerve involvement.

Bowel and bladder control is frequently compromised as a result of *pudendal nerve* involvement.

Fig. 3.28 Neurologic tests for sacral plexus lesion.

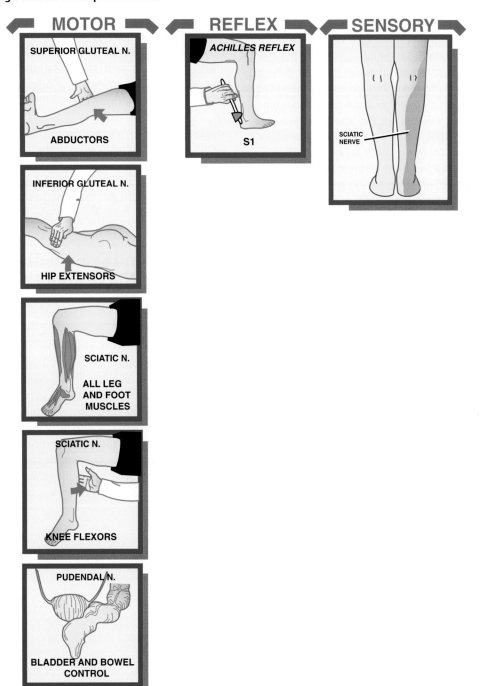

4 Nerve Roots and Spinal Nerves

A ventral and dorsal nerve root exits the spinal cord at each segmental level, carrying motor and sensory fibers, respectively. The nerve roots in each pair unite and combine with autonomic fibers to form a spinal nerve, which exits the vertebral column through the intervertebral foramen to give rise to nerve plexuses and peripheral nerves. There are 8 cervical nerves, 12 thoracic nerves, 5 lumbar nerves, 5 sacral nerves, and 1 coccygeal nerve. The most clinically significant spinal nerves are the C5–T1 segments, which together form the brachial plexus, providing innervation to the upper extremities, and the T12–S4 segments, which together form the lumbosacral plexus, providing innervation to the lower extremities. A group of muscles that is innervated by a single spinal nerve is termed a myotome, and the area of skin that receives sensory innervation from a single spinal nerve is termed a dermatome. This strict organization of clinically relevant motor and sensory innervation patterns provides an excellent opportunity for neurologic diagnosis. After a brief discussion of the anatomy of the nerve root and spinal nerve, this chapter presents the motor, sensory, and reflex examination of lesions affecting the nerve roots and spinal nerves.

Anatomy of the Nerve Roots and Spinal Nerves

At each segmental level, a dorsal nerve root is formed that contains afferent sensory fibers. The cell bodies of these fibers, which enter the spinal cord through the dorsolateral sulcus, are located in an adjacent dorsal root ganglion. Likewise, ventral efferent fibers, which originate in the cell bodies of the ventral gray horn, exit the spinal cord in a ventral nerve root. The dorsal and ventral nerve roots unite to form a spinal nerve, which exits the vertebral column through its corresponding intervertebral foramen.

After emerging from the foramen, the spinal nerve divides into dorsal and ventral rami. The small dorsal ramus turns back to supply the skin of the dorsal aspect of the trunk and the longitudinal muscles of the axial skeleton. The larger ventral ramus supplies sensory and motor innervation to the limbs, the nonaxial skeleton, and the skin of the lateral and ventral aspects of the neck and trunk. The ventral ramus also communicates with the sympathetic chain via the white and gray rami communicantes.

Principles of Nerve Root and Spinal Nerve Localization

The unique character of the nerve roots and spinal nerves lies in their segmental pattern of organization. This distinguishes lesions involving these structures from lesions involving the peripheral nerves and nerve plexuses. The diagnosis of lesions of the nerve roots and spinal nerves thus rests on an orderly evaluation of pertinent myotomes and dermatomes (i.e., a directed motor, sensory, and reflex examination). Every muscle that is innervated by a single spinal nerve or group of spinal nerves need not be examined, or even learned. Rather, it is important to develop a directed examination that identifies a lesion as segmental in character and that correctly localizes the segmental level. The balance of this chapter provides the anatomic basis and the examination methods needed to accomplish this.

Anatomy and Examination of Spinal Nerve and Nerve Root Lesions

C1 to C4 Lesions

See **Fig. 4.1**.

Lesions involving the C1 to C4 nerve roots are especially difficult to evaluate. These nerve roots supply innervation to the muscles and skin of the neck and the head. Significantly, they also contribute to the diaphragm (C3–C5). Because of the difficulty in examining the head and neck muscles, the best method of evaluating this group of nerve roots is to examine their sensory distribution.

Fig. 4.1 **C2–C4 dermatomes.**

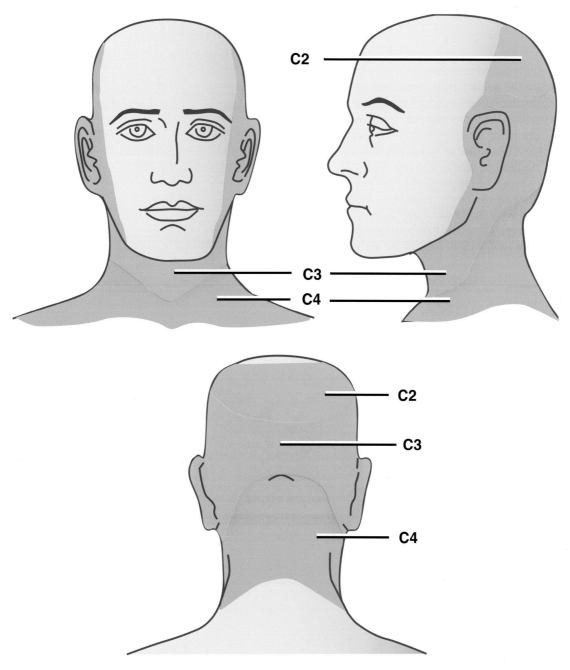

C5 Lesions

See **Fig. 4.2**.

Motor

The most readily tested muscles that derive from the C5 nerve root are the deltoid and biceps muscles. The deltoid muscle receives pure C5 supply and is innervated by the axillary nerve. The biceps muscle is supplied by both C5 and C6 and is innervated by the musculocutaneous nerve. The most important action of the deltoid muscle is shoulder abduction, which it shares with the supraspinatus muscle (C5, C6; suprascapular nerve). The most important action of the biceps muscle is elbow flexion, which it shares with the brachialis muscle (C5; musculocutaneous nerve). Therefore, to test the motor integrity of the C5 nerve root, examine shoulder abduction and elbow flexion.

Sensory

The C5 nerve root supplies the lateral aspect of the arm (axillary nerve). The purest portion of its sensory innervation is a patch of skin on the lateral aspect of the deltoid muscle.

Reflexes

The *biceps reflex* is primarily dependent on the integrity of C5, although it is also partly supplied by C6. Because it receives supply from two segmental levels, compare the biceps reflex on each side; an asymmetry may be indicative of a C5 root lesion.

Fig. 4.2 **Neurologic tests for C5 lesion.**

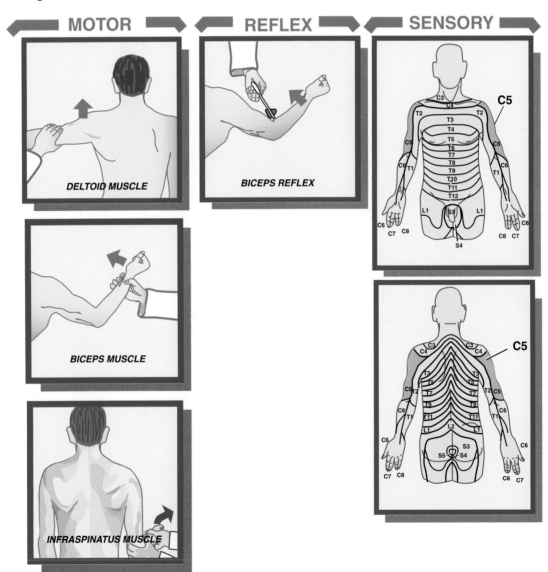

C6 Lesions

See **Fig. 4.3**.

Motor

The wrist extensor group and the biceps muscle both receive their major supply from the C6 nerve root, via the radial nerve and musculocutaneous nerve, respectively. However, the wrist extensor group is also partly innervated by the C7 root (ulnar nerve), and the biceps muscle is also partly innervated by the C5 root (musculocutaneous nerve).

Weakness in wrist extension due to isolated C6 compromise results in ulnar deviation during wrist extension.

As mentioned, the biceps muscle receives motor innervation from both the C5 and C6 nerve roots. The recommended test of biceps muscle function is elbow flexion.

Unilateral weakness of elbow flexion may be indicative of injury to the C6 nerve root.

Sensory

The C6 dermatome comprises the lateral forearm, the thumb, the index finger, and one half of the middle finger.

Reflexes

The deep tendon reflexes of the upper extremity that receive supply from C6 include the biceps reflex (C5–C6) and the brachioradialis reflex (C6). Because the *brachioradialis reflex* receives pure C6 innervation, it is the best reflex to use to test the C6 nerve root.

Fig. 4.3 **Neurologic tests for C6 lesion.**

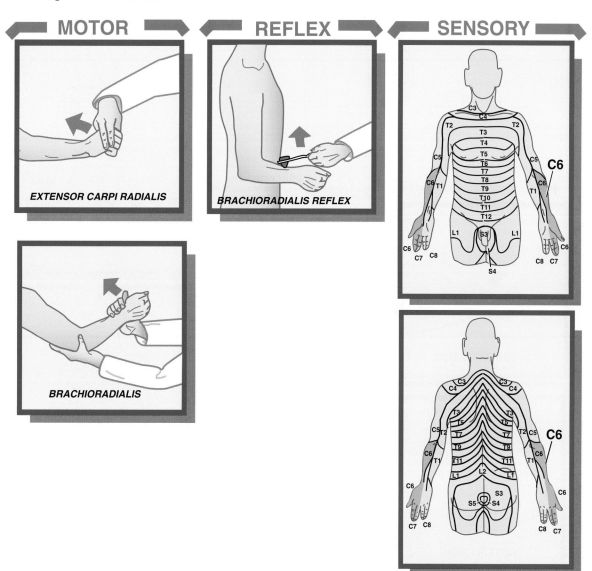

MOTOR — REFLEX — SENSORY

EXTENSOR CARPI RADIALIS

BRACHIORADIALIS REFLEX

BRACHIORADIALIS

C7 Lesions

See **Fig. 4.4**.

Motor

The triceps muscle (radial nerve), wrist flexors (median and ulnar nerves), and finger extensors (radial nerve) are all predominantly innervated by C7. To examine the integrity of the C7 nerve root, test each of these three groups of muscles.

Elbow extension is the best test of the triceps muscle. A C7 lesion results, then, in weakness of elbow extensions. Wrist flexion is primarily due to the flexor carpi radialis (C7; median nerve) and, to a lesser degree, the flexor carpi ulnaris (C8; ulnar nerve). With C7 lesions, wrist flexion results in an ulnarward deviation.

Sensory

C7 supplies sensory innervation to the middle finger. However, because the middle finger may also receive supply from C6 or C8, sensory evaluation of the C7 nerve root is not reliable.

Reflex

The *triceps reflex* receives innervation from the C7 component of the radial nerve and is a reliable test of C7 function.

Fig. 4.4 **Neurologic tests for C7 lesion.**

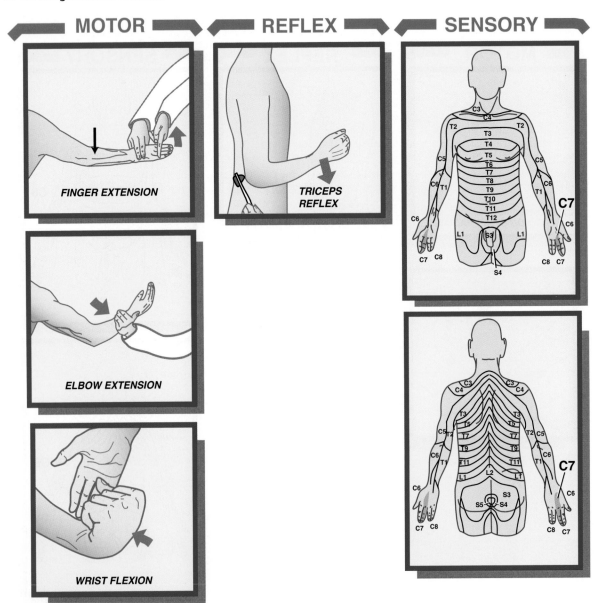

C8 Lesions

See **Fig. 4.5**.

Motor

The muscles of finger flexion (median and ulnar nerves) are supplied by C8. To evaluate the motor innervation of C8, test finger flexion.

Sensory

The sensory innervation supplied by C8 includes the ring and little fingers of the hand and the distal half of the medial aspect of the forearm.

Fig. 4.5 **Neurologic tests for C8 lesion.**

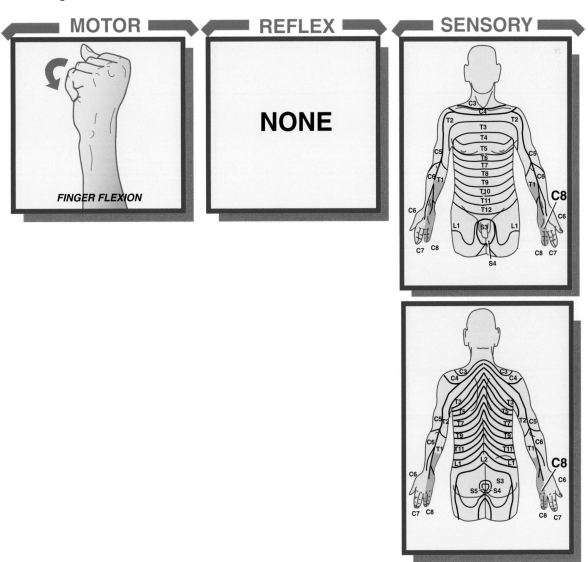

T1 Lesions

See **Fig. 4.6**.

Motor

Finger abduction (T1; ulnar nerve) and *finger adduction* (C8, T1; ulnar nerve) both receive supply from the C8 nerve root. To test finger adduction, place a piece of paper between two of the patient's extended fingers and attempt to pull the paper away. Compare the strength of finger adduction on both sides.

Sensory

The sensory innervation of T1 includes the upper half of the medial forearm and the medial portion of the arm.

Fig. 4.6 **Neurologic tests for T1 lesion.**

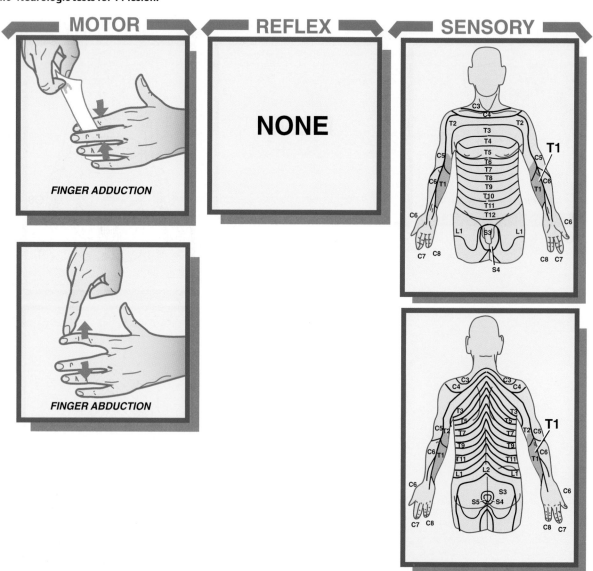

T2–T12 lesions

See **Fig. 4.7**.

Lesions of T2 to T12 are discussed together in this section because they are primarily evaluated by sensory testing (i.e., dermatomal identification).

Motor

Muscles that are innervated by the T2 to T12 nerve roots comprise the intercostals and the rectus abdominal muscles. The intercostal muscles, although they are innervated segmentally, are difficult to examine individually. Asymmetric weakness of the rectus abdominal muscles may be identified by the presence of *Beevor's sign*. Beevor's sign is present when the umbilicus of the patient is drawn up or down, or to one side or the other, when the patient is a quarter way through a sit-up.

Sensory

Sensory examination is performed in the usual manner, with particular attention directed to the identification of dermatomal involvement. Useful reference points include the nipples (T4), the xyphoid process (T6), the umbilicus (T10), and the inguinal ligament (T12). Note the oblique angles assumed by the dermatomes of the trunk.

Fig. 4.7 **Neurologic tests for T2–12 lesion.**

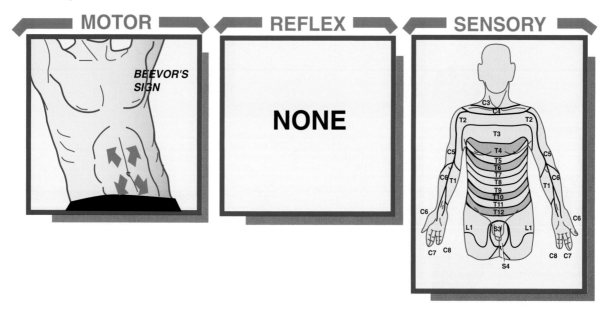

L1–L3 Lesions

See **Fig. 4.8**.

Motor

No specific muscles receive supply from the individual segmental nerve roots between the L1 and L3 levels, but important muscles are innervated by a combination of nerve roots at these levels. These include the *iliopsoas* (L1–L3), the *quadriceps* (L2–L4; femoral nerve), and the *adductor muscles* (L2–L4; obturator nerve).

Sensory

Sensory testing is especially important in this region because of the lack of specificity in muscle testing. The L1 dermatome comprises an oblique band just below the inguinal ligament; the L3 dermatome comprises an oblique band just above the knee; and the L2 dermatome comprises an oblique band located between L1 and L3.

Fig. 4.8 **Neurologic tests for L1–L3 lesion.**

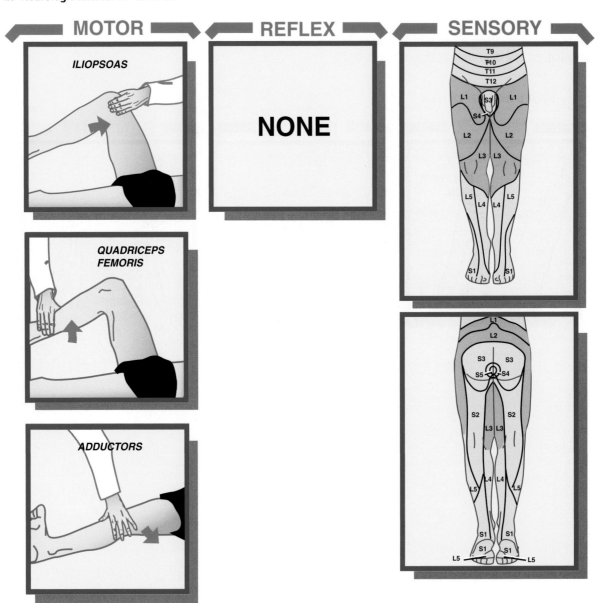

L4 Lesions

See **Fig. 4.9**.

Motor

The *tibialis anterior muscle* receives its predominant supply from the L4 nerve root (deep peroneal nerve). This muscle is responsible for dorsiflexion and inversion of the foot, and may be tested by asking patients to walk on their heels, or by manually resisting dorsiflexion and inversion of the foot. The latter L4 function may be helpful in distinguishing an L4 radiculopathy from a peroneal nerve palsy because the peroneal nerve does not innervate the foot invertor (*tibialis posterior* muscle; tibial nerve).

Sensory

The L4 dermatome covers the medial side of the leg below the knee. Its anterior boundary with the L5 dermatome is marked by the sharp crest of the tibia.

Reflex

The *patellar reflex* receives its predominant supply from the L4 nerve root. An L4 injury, however, may not completely eradicate the reflex because it receives a smaller supply from L2 and L3.

Fig. 4.9 Neurologic tests for L4 lesion.

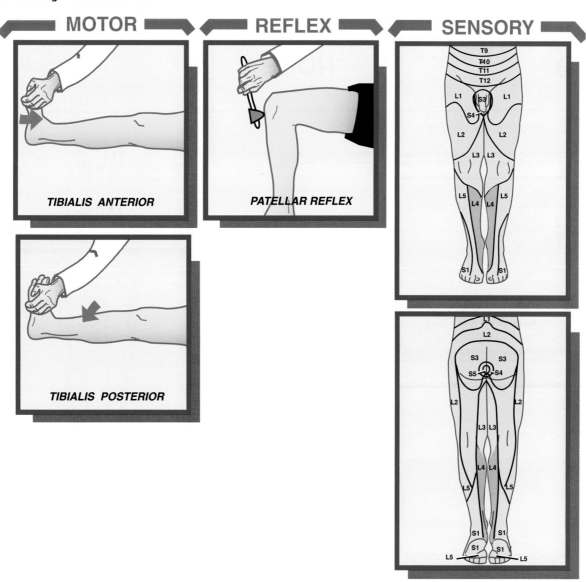

L5 Lesions

See **Fig. 4.10**.

Motor

The L5 nerve root innervates the *extensor hallucis longus* (L5; deep peroneal nerve), the *extensor digitorum* (L5; deep peroneal nerve), and the *gluteus medius* (L5; superior gluteal nerve). The extensor hallucis longus is responsible for dorsiflexion of the big toe, the extensor digitorum is responsible for dorsoflexion of the lateral four toes, and the gluteus medius is responsible for abduction of the hip. Testing of the latter muscle may be especially important in the differentiation of a peroneal nerve palsy from an L5 nerve root injury.

Reflex

There is no deep tendon reflex to test the integrity of the L5 nerve root.

Fig. 4.10 **Neurologic tests for L5 lesion.**

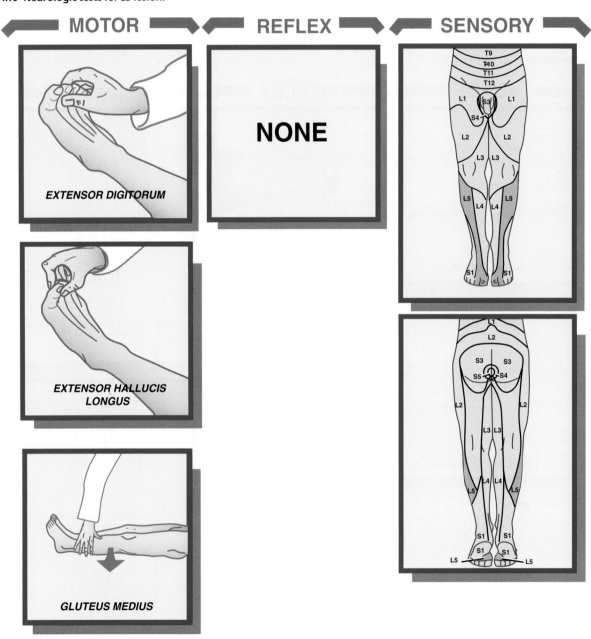

S1 Lesions

See **Fig. 4.11**.

Motor

The S1 nerve root innervates the *peroneus longus* and *brevis* (S1; superficial peroneal nerve), the *gastrocnemius–soleus* muscles (S1, S2; tibial nerve), and the *gluteus maximus* (S1; inferior gluteal nerve). The peronei muscles are evertors of the ankle and foot, the gastrocnemius–soleus group are extensors of the foot, and the gluteus maximus is an extensor of the hip.

Sensory

The S1 dermatome covers the lateral aspect and part of the plantar aspect of the foot.

Reflex

The *Achilles reflex* is innervated by S1.

Fig. 4.11 Neurologic tests for S1 lesion.

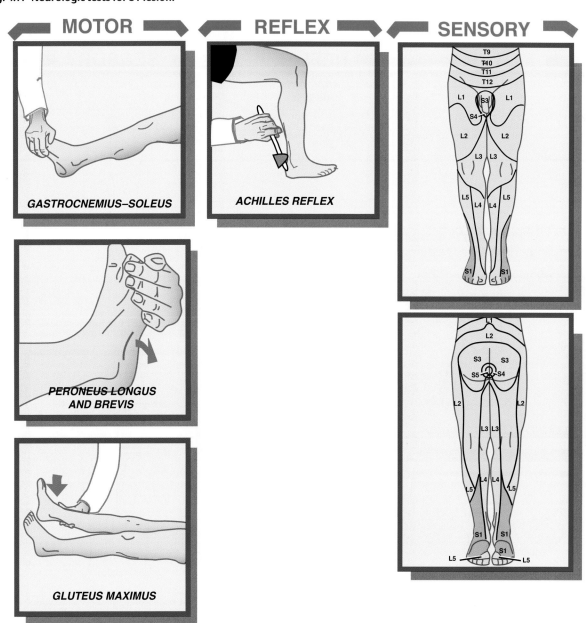

S2–S4 Lesions

See **Fig. 4.12**.

Motor

The muscles that are innervated by the S2–S4 nerve roots comprise the intrinsic muscles of the foot. These muscles are not easily amenable to examination.

Sensory

From outside to in, the dermatomes supplied by the S2–S4 nerve roots comprise progressively smaller concentric rings around the anus.

Reflex

The *anal wink reflex* is supplied by the S2–S4 nerve roots. This reflex consists of contraction of the anal sphincter muscle in response to stimulation of the perianal skin.

Anal Sphincter

The anal sphincter is supplied by the S2-S4 nerve roots. Rectal examination may provide information regarding the integrity of the tone of the anal sphincter.

Fig. 4.12 **Neurologic tests for S2–S4 lesion.**

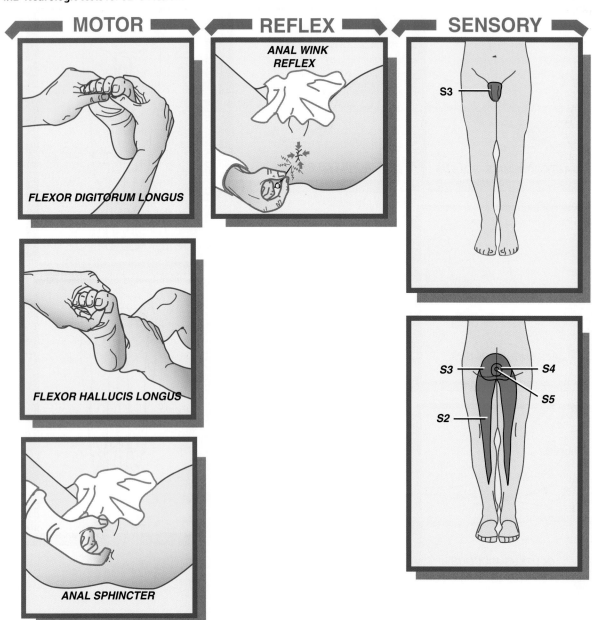

Nerve Root Syndromes

Cervical Disk Disease

See **Fig. 4.13**.

Herniated cervical disks may cause cervical radiculopathy by impinging upon the nerve root that passes across the disk space. Typically, this results in neck and arm pain in a radicular distribution (i.e., pain that is in the distribution of a single nerve root). Paresthesias (i.e., a sense of "tingling" in the distribution of a nerve) may accompany pain but are usually more distal in the extremity. Weakness may also develop and, if chronic, may be associated with atrophy and fasciculations. Examination may reveal loss of the stretch reflex (e.g., biceps reflex) in the corresponding myotome. Almost invariably the symptoms are unilateral.

Typically, impingement of a cervical nerve by a herniated disk occurs laterally in the spinal canal at the level of the disk space, just proximal to where the nerve exits the spinal canal through the neural foramen. The first cervical nerve exits the spinal canal between the occiput and C1, the second nerve exits between C1 and C2, the third nerve exits between C2 and C3, and so on. The eighth cervical nerve exits between C7 and T1.

This anatomy dictates that a herniated C3–C4 disk impinges upon the C4 nerve, a herniated C4–C5 disk impinges upon the C5 nerve, a herniated C5–C6 disk impinges upon the C6 nerve, and so on. The symptoms related to the various cervical radiculopathies are distinctive. The cardinal features of the cervical radiculopathies are described following here.

C3 Radiculopathy

Because the interspace at the C2–C3 level is minimally involved in neck flexion and extension, clinically significant disk disease at the C2–C3 level (and thus C3 radiculopathy) is rare. When it occurs, the patient may complain of posterior neck and suboccipital pain, sometimes affecting the ear. There is no motor deficit, and numbness is rarely noticed by the patient.

C4 Radiculopathy

A C4 radiculopathy is clinically expressed as paraspinous pain extending from the root of the neck to the midshoulder and posteriorly to the level of the scapula. As with other radiculopathies, the pain may be aggravated by neck extension. Numbness is rare, and there is no motor deficit. Although the C4 nerve root innervates the diaphragm, diaphragmatic abnormalities due to C4 radiculopathy are rare.

C5 Radiculopathy

Pain in the top of the shoulder to a point midway on the lateral aspect of the upper arm is the cardinal manifestation of a C5 radiculopathy. Local shoulder pain and numbness can be confused with mechanical or inflammatory shoulder pathology, but there are no physical signs to corroborate this, such as pain with manual rotation of the shoulder. The principal motor deficit is deltoid weakness, which may be disabling. Loss of the biceps reflex occurs inconsistently.

C6 Radiculopathy

C6 radiculopathy, due to herniation of the C5–C6 disk, is the second most common cervical radiculopathy following herniation at the C6–C7 level. Pain and paresthesias radiate from the neck through the biceps, the lateral forearm, the lateral dorsum of the hand, and into the thumb and index finger. Weakness may involve the radial wrist extensor group and the biceps muscle. Such weakness may be detected on physical examination before the patient is aware that it exists. The presence and pattern of numbness are variable, although they typically involve the lateral forearm and the first and second digits. The brachioradialis reflex (C6) is often reduced or absent, and the biceps reflex (C5, C6) may also be depressed.

C7 Radiculopathy

Disk herniations at the C6–C7 interspace are the most common in the cervical region, and thus C7 radiculopathy occurs frequently. Pain and paresthesias radiate across the back of the shoulder, through the triceps and the posterolateral forearm, and into the middle finger. The thumb and index finger, although predominantly C6 innervated, may also be involved. Weakness primarily affects the triceps muscle. The wrist flexors and finger extensor groups may also be involved. Despite its size, gravity can take over many of the functions of the triceps muscle; thus, the patient may be unaware of mild weakness in this muscle. Careful manual examination of the triceps is therefore important, the more so because sensory loss in this dermatome is unreliable. A reduced or absent triceps reflex is usually seen with a C7 radiculopathy.

C8 Radiculopathy

Pain is less frequently associated with C8 radiculopathy than any of the other cervical radiculopathies. When present, pain and numbness may involve the little and ring fingers, and less often the distal half of the medial aspect of the forearm. Confusion of this syndrome with the symptoms of ulnar neuropathy is not unusual. As with ulnar neuropathy, weakness due to C8 radiculopathy may be noticed early by the patient. Typically, this involves the intrinsic muscles of the hand (finger flexors), causing loss of strength of grip or other fine motor activities of the hand.

Fig. 4.13 **Cervical disk disease.**

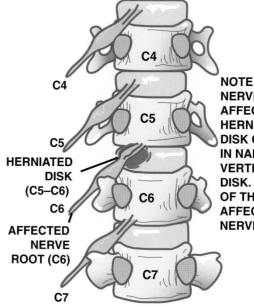

CARDINAL FEATURES

- NECK AND RADICULAR ARM PAIN ARE MOST COMMON SYMPTOMS
- DISTAL PARESTHESIAS AND MYOTOMAL WEAKNESS MAY DEVELOP
- SYMPTOMS ARE UNILATERAL AND MONORADICULAR
- PRESENTATION IS TYPICALLY ACUTE, ALTHOUGH SYMPTOMS MAY BECOME CHRONIC

NOTE THAT THE NERVE ROOT AFFECTED BY A HERNIATED CERVICAL DISK CORRESPONDS IN NAME TO THE VERTEBRA BELOW THE DISK. THUS, HERNIATION OF THE C5–C6 DISK AFFECTS THE C6 NERVE ROOT.

C4

C4

C5

C5

HERNIATED DISK (C5–C6)

C6

C6

AFFECTED NERVE ROOT (C6)

C7

C7

Cervical Spondylosis

See **Fig. 4.14**.

Cervical spondylosis is a form of osteophytosis due to degenerative disk disease. It may result in encroachment of the cervical neural foramen by the degenerative uncinate process, causing compression of the exiting nerve root.

The *uncinate process* is a ridge of bone that extends from the superior lateral aspect of each cervical vertebra. It serves to stabilize the spine and helps form the inferior medial wall of the neural foramina. Compression of a cervical nerve root due to enlargement of an uncinate process results in the same radicular syndromes that have been described for cervical disk disease. The hallmark of these syndromes is neck and radicular arm pain. Cervical pain may be more prominent due to the spondylotic process, a degenerative condition that tends to be diffuse.

Like cervical disk disease, the symptoms are unilateral and are aggravated by neck extension, which further narrows the lumen of the neural foramen.

Two clinical clues differentiate cervical disk disease from cervical spondylosis. First, although bilateral symptoms are uncommon in spondylosis, more than one cervical segment may be affected, and thus the symptoms may be more diffuse than those associated with cervical disk disease. Second, whereas cervical disk disease tends to present acutely, cervical spondylosis is classically a chronic and episodic disorder. As a result, muscle atrophy and fasciculations are more commonly observed in spondylosis than in disk disease. As mentioned earlier, neck pain may be more prominent in spondylosis.

Fig. 4.14 **Cervical spondylosis.**

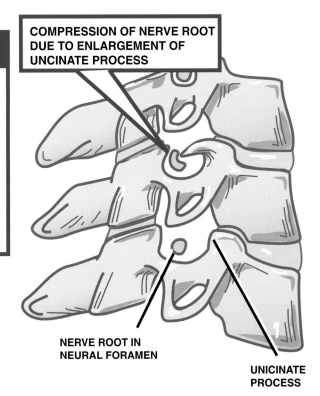

CARDINAL FEATURES

- **TEMPORAL PROFILE IS TYPICALLY CHRONIC AND EPISODIC**
- **NECK PAIN AND RADICULAR ARM PAIN ARE MOST COMMON SYMPTOMS**
- **PARESTHESIAS, SENSORY LOSS, AND WEAKNESS MAY DEVELOP**
- **MYOTOMAL ATROPHY AND FASCICULATIONS MAY BE PROMINENT**
- **SYMPTOMS ARE USUALLY UNILATERAL BUT MAY INVOLVE MULTIPLE LEVELS**

COMPRESSION OF NERVE ROOT DUE TO ENLARGEMENT OF UNCINATE PROCESS

NERVE ROOT IN NEURAL FORAMEN

UNICINATE PROCESS

Thoracic Disk Disease

See **Fig. 4.15**.

Although there is no typical clinical syndrome associated with thoracic disk herniation, radicular-type pain may predominate in cases where the disk protrusion occurs laterally. It typically causes cardiac-like pain across the chest wall, although the pain does not cross midline. Because thoracic radiculopathy involves the chest or abdominal walls, radicular-type pain due to thoracic disk herniation may be confused for cardiac or gastrointestinal disease. Frequently, thoracic disk herniations are centrally located. In those patients who present with myelopathic features—for example, spastic weakness of the lower extremities—it is important to determine whether the lesion is cervical or thoracic in origin. Obviously, neck pain and upper extremity involvement point to a cervical lesion, whereas the absence of these findings, in combination with the presence of a thoracic radiculopathy, midback pain, or a thoracic sensory level, point to a thoracic lesion.

Fig. 4.15 **Thoracic disk disease.**

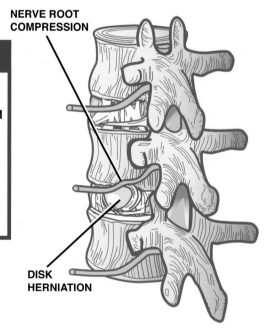

CARDINAL FEATURES

- LATERAL THORACIC DISK HERNIATION CAUSES COMPRESSION OF NERVE ROOT JUST PROXIMAL TO ITS SITE OF EXIT FROM THE CANAL
- RADICULAR-TYPE PAIN IN CHEST OR ABDOMINAL WALL IS MAJOR CLINICAL FEATURE
- IF DISK HERNIATION IS CENTRALLY LOCATED, SYNDROME MAY PRESENT AS MYELOPATHY

NERVE ROOT COMPRESSION

DISK HERNIATION

Lumbar Disk Disease

See **Fig. 4.16**.

Lumbar disk disease is predominantly a disease of young adulthood. Typically, it presents over a time course of weeks to months with an acute, persistent, unilateral monoradiculopathy that is aggravated by sitting, sneezing, or coughing and is relieved by standing or bed rest. The straight leg raise test is frequently positive, and there may be an associated motor or sensory deficit. Typically, this occurs in the L5 or S1 distribution, and in the latter case there is an associated decreased ankle jerk reflex.

In paracentral lumbar disk herniations, which are the most common kind, the affected nerve root corresponds in name to the vertebra below the herniated disk. Thus, an L4–L5 disk herniation is associated with an L5 radiculopathy. By contrast, the more unusual far lateral disk herniation affects the nerve that corresponds in name to the vertebra above the disk. Thus, a far lateral L4–L5 disk herniation is associated with an L4 radiculopathy. The rare central lumbar disk herniation may compress the entire thecal sac, causing symptoms of a cauda equina syndrome.

Fig. 4.16 **Lumbar disk disease.**

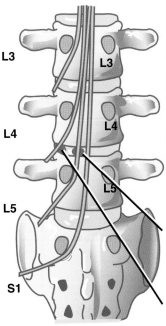

CARDINAL FEATURES

- BACK AND RADICULAR LEG PAIN ARE MOST COMMON SYMPTOMS
- YOUNG ADULTS ARE MOST FREQUENTLY AFFECTED
- PAIN IS EXACERBATED BY SITTING, SNEEZING, OR COUGHING, AND MAY BE RELIEVED BY STANDING OR BED REST
- STRAIGHT LEG RAISE TEST IS POSITIVE
- MOTOR OR SENSORY DEFICIT MAY DEVELOP
- L4–L5 IS MOST COMMONLY AFFECTED LEVEL; L5–S1 IS NEXT MOST COMMON
- SYMPTOMS ARE UNILATERAL AND MONORADICULAR

NOTE THAT THE NERVE ROOT AFFECTED BY A PARACENTRAL LUMBAR DISK HERNIATION CORRESPONDS IN NAME TO THE VERTEBRA BELOW THE DISK. THUS, AN L4–L5 DISK HERNIATION AFFECTS THE L5 NERVE ROOT.

NOTE THAT A FAR LATERAL DISK HERNIATION AFFECTS THE NERVE ROOT ABOVE THE DISK (i.e., L4).

PARACENTRAL DISK HERNIATION AFFECTS L5 NERVE ROOT (COMMON)

FAR LATERAL DISK HERNIATION AFFECTS L4 NERVE ROOT (UNCOMMON)

Lumbar Stenosis

See **Fig. 4.17**.

Lumbar stenosis classically presents in an elderly individual who complains of symptoms, progressive over years, consisting of chronic, intermittent bilateral posterior leg pain (neurogenic claudication). The pain typically begins in the buttocks and radiates downward in a nonradicular distribution. It is commonly described as a burning, cramping, or heavy feeling and is frequently associated with numbness or paresthesias. Classically, the pain is precipitated by prolonged standing or walking (spinal extension) and is improved by forward bending, sitting, or bed rest (spinal flexion). Typically, the patients are unable to ambulate for long distances. Surprisingly, they are able to ambulate for quite a distance in the grocery store while stooping forward when pushing a shopping cart (positive shopping cart sign). Characteristically, it is accompanied by minimal or no back pain, and motor deficits and sphincter dysfunction are a late and inconstant feature. The straight leg raise test is usually negative, and in general the disease is remarkable for its paucity of associated neurologic findings.

Fig. 4.17 **Lumbar stenosis.**

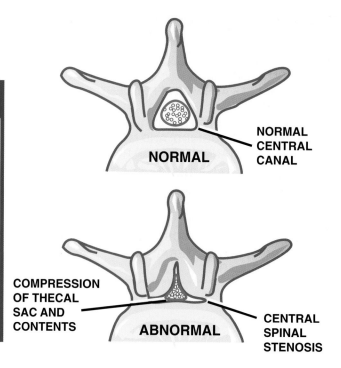

CARDINAL FEATURES

- **PREDOMINANTLY AFFLICTS THE ELDERLY**
- **PRESENTS AS NEUROGENIC CLAUDICATION**
- **WORSENED BY STANDING OR WALKING (spinal extension)**
- **IMPROVED BY FORWARD BENDING, SITTING, OR BED REST (spinal flexion)**
- **MINIMAL OR NO BACK PAIN**
- **MINIMAL OR NO NEUROLOGIC FINDINGS**
- **NEGATIVE STRAIGHT LEG RAISE TEST**

NORMAL CENTRAL CANAL

NORMAL

COMPRESSION OF THECAL SAC AND CONTENTS

ABNORMAL

CENTRAL SPINAL STENOSIS

Lateral Recess Stenosis

See **Fig. 4.18**.

Lateral recess stenosis is stenosis in the so-called lateral recess, a space that is bordered ventrally by the posterior vertebral body, laterally by the pedicle, and dorsally by the superior articular facet. Clinically, these patients complain of bilateral radicular pain, frequently associated with numbness and paresthesias, and mild or no low back pain. As in stenosis of the central spinal canal, the pain tends to worsen with standing or walking and improve with sitting or bed rest. Characteristically, the straight leg raise test is negative. Neurologic findings are usually minimal, although these patients tend to have weakness or atrophy more often than those with central stenosis only.

Fig. 4.18 **Lateral recess stenosis.**

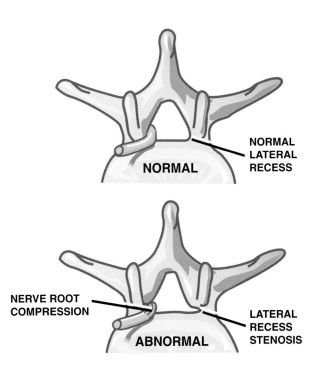

CARDINAL FEATURES

- **PRESENTS AS BILATERAL RADICULAR LEG PAIN**
- **WORSENED BY STANDING OR WALKING (spinal extension)**
- **IMPROVED BY FOWARD BENDING, SITTING, OR BED REST (spinal flexion)**
- **MILD OR NO BACK PAIN**
- **NEUROLOGIC FINDINGS ARE MINIMAL (although weakness and atrophy are more common than in central stenosis)**
- **NEGATIVE STRAIGHT LEG RAISE TEST**

Lumbar Spondylolisthesis

See **Fig. 4.19**.

Lumbar spondylolisthesis consists of forward displacement of one lumbar vertebral body on another. The most common clinical presentation of lumbar spondylolisthesis is mechanical low back pain, a deep, diffuse type of low back pain that is aggravated by activity and improved with rest. Spondylolisthesis may also produce radicular symptoms via traction or compression on the lumbar nerve roots. Neurologic findings are uncommon. Etiologies include degenerative facet joint disease (degenerative spondylolisthesis), spondylolysis (isthmic spondylolisthesis, a defect or fracture of the pars interarticularis), trauma (traumatic spondylolisthesis), and congenital abnormalities of the upper sacrum or arch of L5 (dysplastic spondylolisthesis). The most common cause is degenerative spondylolisthesis, which typically occurs at the L4–L5 level. Traumatic and dysplastic spondylolisthesis most commonly involves the L5–S1 level.

Fig. 4.19 **Lumbar spondylolisthesis.**

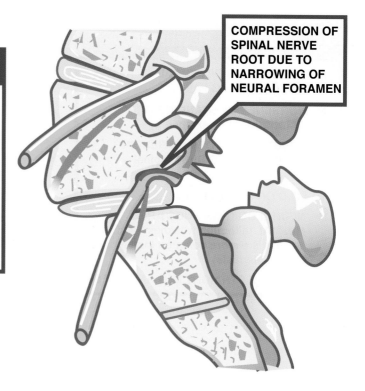

CARDINAL FEATURES

- **FORWARD DISPLACEMENT OF ONE VERTEBRAL BODY ON ANOTHER (spondylolisthesis)**
- **PRESENTS AS MECHANICAL LOW BACK PAIN**
- **RADICULOPATHY MAY BE PRESENT**
- **MINIMAL OR NO NEUROLOGIC FINDINGS**

COMPRESSION OF SPINAL NERVE ROOT DUE TO NARROWING OF NEURAL FORAMEN

Arachnoiditis

Arachnoiditis is a chronic inflammatory condition of the meninges, which most commonly occurs at the level of the lumbar spine. Causative factors include spinal surgery, myelography, and the introduction of other agents (e.g., antibiotics, anesthetics, or corticosteroids) into or around the thecal sac.

The clinical picture of arachnoiditis is usually a combination of back pain and radicular leg pain with or without neurologic deficits. The pain is characteristically constant and burning or tingling in quality. It is aggravated with activity but is not usually relieved with rest. The symptoms may be unilateral or bilateral and may involve one or up to all of the nerve roots of the cauda equina.

Cervical Nerve Root Avulsion

See **Fig. 4.20**.

Traumatic shoulder injuries, particularly traction injuries, are often associated with injury to the brachial plexus. Such plexus injuries may also be accompanied by avulsion of one or two cervical nerve roots. Clinically, cervical nerve root avulsion is expressed as radicular-type pain associated with severe motor and sensory loss in a radicular distribution. These lesions differ from the typical compressive radiculopathy, mainly in the degree of axon loss present.

The clinical diagnosis of nerve root avulsion is often masked by an associated brachial plexus injury. Fortunately, the electromyographic and nerve conduction velocity (NCV) findings of a cervical nerve root avulsion are typical: there is a severe reduction or absence in the compound motor action potentials (CMAPs), a remarkable increase in pathological fibrillation potentials, and yet completely normal sensory nerve action potentials (SNAPs). The presence of normal SNAPs (in the face of highly abnormal CMAPs) is explained by the anatomy of sensory root avulsion, which occurs proximal to the dorsal root ganglion.

Fig. 4.20 **Cervical nerve root avulsion.**

CARDINAL FEATURES

● MAJOR SYMPTOMS ARE RADICULAR ARM PAIN, ASSOCIATED WITH SEVERE RADICULAR MOTOR AND SENSORY LOSS

● MECHANISM OF INJURY OFTEN LEADS TO CONCURRENT BRACHIAL PLEXUS INJURY, MAKING CLINICAL DIAGNOSIS OF NERVE ROOT AVULSION DIFFICULT

● ELECTRICAL STUDIES DEMONSTRATE HIGHLY ABNORMAL MOTOR FINDINGS IN SETTING OF COMPLETELY NORMAL SENSORY FINDINGS DUE TO LOCATION OF INJURY PROXIMAL TO THE DORSAL ROOT GANGLION (DRG)

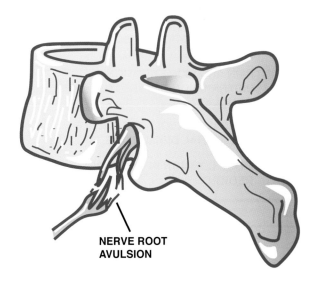

NERVE ROOT AVULSION

Herpes Zoster

See **Fig. 4.21**.

Herpes zoster (shingles) is a viral disease that is associated with inflammatory changes in an infected dorsal root ganglion. The virus typically lies dormant in the dorsal root ganglia and is activated when the body is stressed, such as during an acute illness. Clinically, it is characterized by pain and skin eruption in the distribution of the infected ganglion, the former usually preceding the latter. Typically, the lesion involves a single, unilateral dermatome, most commonly in the thoracic region. Tricyclic antidepressants and/or anticonvulsants may be used for the pain, although it is usually refractory.

Fig. 4.21 **Herpes zoster.**

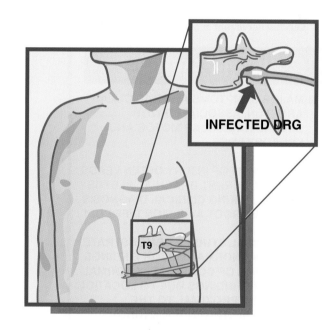

CARDINAL FEATURES

- VIRAL INFECTION OF DORSAL ROOT GANGLION (DRG)
- PAIN AND SKIN ERUPTION IN DISTRIBUTION OF INFECTED GANGLION
- TYPICALLY INVOLVES A SINGLE UNILATERAL DERMATOME
- MOST COMMON IN THORACIC REGION

INFECTED DRG

T9

Poliomyelitis

See **Fig. 4.22**.

Poliomyelitis is an acute viral infection of the spinal cord associated with destruction of the anterior horn cells. Fortunately, the viral infection typically presents with gastrointestinal and not neurologic symptoms. Only rarely are the anterior horn cells affected. Because the cells of the nerve roots are destroyed at affected levels, the clinical appearance of polio may be similar to that of a nerve root lesion. Muscle weakness may develop rapidly, reaching its maximal extent within 48 hours, or it may develop slowly or in a stuttering fashion, over a period of a week or more.

Like the temporal pattern, the anatomic pattern of polio is variable and may be related to the age of the patient. Thus, in children under 5 years of age, the most common clinical appearance is weakness of one leg; in older children, the most common presentation is weakness of an arm or both legs; and in adults, the most common form is an asymmetric weakness of all four limbs.

Finally, the degree of weakness varies among patients and may be determined by the presence and extent of redundant innervation of an affected muscle. Thus, the quadriceps muscle (L2–L4), which receives innervation from several lumbar nerve roots, may exhibit no or mild weakness, whereas the tibialis anterior muscle (L4), which is predominantly innervated by a single nerve root, may present with a more severe form of weakness (i.e., foot drop). This principle explains the relatively common finding of foot drop among polio patients.

Fig. 4.22 Polio.

CARDINAL FEATURES

- ACUTE VIRAL INFECTION INVOLVING ANTERIOR HORN CELLS
- MAY PRESENT WITH MYOTOMAL WEAKNESS
- TEMPORAL COURSE AND ANATOMIC PATTERN OF WEAKNESS ARE VARIABLE

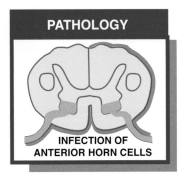

PATHOLOGY

INFECTION OF ANTERIOR HORN CELLS

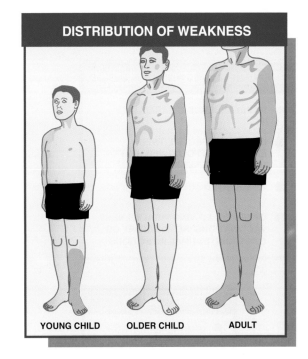

DISTRIBUTION OF WEAKNESS

YOUNG CHILD   OLDER CHILD   ADULT

Nerve Sheath Tumors

Nerve sheath tumors, neurofibromas, and schwannomas are derived from the dorsal roots at various segmental levels. These tumors are often associated with neurofibromatosis. The frequency of these lesions is distributed evenly among the cervical, thoracic, and lumbar regions. In neurofibromas, nerve fibers typically transverse the tumor, thus making the complete surgical removal difficult. In schwannomas, the nerve fibers are typically sprayed over the tumor capsule, making complete surgical resection possible. Occasionally, a neurofibroma may straddle the spinal canal, producing the so-called dumbbell configuration, with part of the tumor outside the canal, part inside, and the narrowest part of the tumor at the intervertebral foramen. Clinically, these lesions cause radicular-type pain that is typically worse at night. Associated findings may include signs and symptoms of a myelopathy, such as gait difficulties, bladder disturbances, and long tract signs, as a result of extrinsic compression of the spinal cord.

Guillain-Barré Syndrome

See **Fig. 4.23**.

This acute idiopathic inflammatory polyradiculitis often follows, by 1 to 3 weeks, a mild respiratory or gastrointestinal infection. It may also occur after a preceding viral illness or vaccination. The major clinical manifestation is ascending weakness, which evolves over a period of days to weeks. Pathologically, there is an immune-mediated segmental degeneration of the involved nerves. Typically, the proximal as well as distal limb muscles are equally involved, and the lower extremities are affected before the upper. Although objective sensory loss is usually negligible or absent, patients often complain of pain and aching in the muscles. As the disease progresses, trunk, intercostal, neck, and cranial muscles may all become involved. In the most severe cases, the patient succumbs from respiratory failure within a few days. Autonomic mobility is not common, which may consist of sinus tachycardia, bradycardia, or orthostatic hypotension. Treatment consists of supportive care and plasmapheresis in extreme cases. The majority of patients demonstrate complete recovery, whereas around one third have permanent residual deficits.

Fig. 4.23 **Guillain-Barré syndrome.**

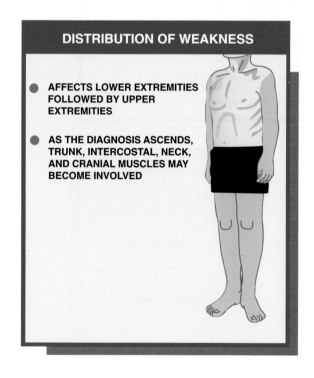

CARDINAL FEATURES

- RAPID ASCENDING PARALYSIS
- USUALLY AFFECTS LOWER EXTREMITIES FOLLOWED BY UPPER EXTREMITIES
- ASSOCIATED AREFLEXIA
- OFTEN FOLLOWING VIRAL ILLNESS, VACCINATIONS, RESPIRATORY OR GASTROINTESTINAL INFECTIONS

PATHOLOGY

- IMMUNE-MEDIATED SEGMENTAL DEGENERATION

DISTRIBUTION OF WEAKNESS

- AFFECTS LOWER EXTREMITIES FOLLOWED BY UPPER EXTREMITIES
- AS THE DIAGNOSIS ASCENDS, TRUNK, INTERCOSTAL, NECK, AND CRANIAL MUSCLES MAY BECOME INVOLVED

Diabetic Radiculopathy

See **Fig. 4.24**.

The most common peripheral nervous system manifestation of diabetes is a distal polyneuropathy. However, involvement of spinal nerve roots may also occur, presumably as a result of the same pathophysiological mechanism: microcirculation disease (i.e., ischemia). These patients usually complain of painful paresthesias in the feet. There is also an associated loss of sensation in stocking distribution on the lower extremities, often leading to skin ulcers, neuropathic joints, and/or loss of ankle jerk reflexes. The sensory loss may involve the myelinated fibers of the dorsal column, leading to the ataxia. Motor nerves may be involved, leading to either or both weakness and atrophy, especially involving the femoral and sciatic nerves. The autonomic system may also be adversely affected (e.g., bladder dysfunction or postural hypotension). Treatment usually consists of good blood glucose control and meticulous foot care. Tricyclic antidepressants may be used for burning pain; antiepileptic medications may be used for stabbing pain.

Fig. 4.24 **Diabetic radiculopathy.**

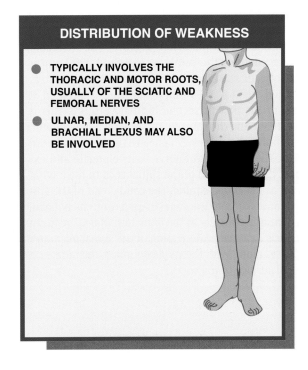

CARDINAL FEATURES

- PAINFUL PARESTHESIAS IN THE FEET

- WEAKNESS ATROPHY, TYPICALLY OF FEMORAL OR SCIATIC NERVES

- OFTEN SKIN ULCERS AND LOSS OF ACHILLES REFLEX

- AUTONOMIC SYMPTOMS OCCUR (e.g., bladder dysfunction and hypotension)

DISTRIBUTION OF WEAKNESS

- TYPICALLY INVOLVES THE THORACIC AND MOTOR ROOTS, USUALLY OF THE SCIATIC AND FEMORAL NERVES

- ULNAR, MEDIAN, AND BRACHIAL PLEXUS MAY ALSO BE INVOLVED

5 Spinal Cord

Fig. 5.1 **Spinal cord, nerve roots, and meninges.** ⟶

This chapter briefly describes the general gross and microscopic anatomy of the spinal cord. This is followed by a more lengthy discussion of clinical topics, including:
- Blood supply to the spinal cord
- Vascular syndromes of the spinal cord
- Spinal tumors
- Autonomic disturbances in spinal cord lesions
- Localization of spinal cord lesions according to level
- Clinical evaluation of the spinal cord patient
- Spinal cord syndromes

Gross Anatomy

General Features

The spinal cord forms a nearly cylindrical column that is situated within the spinal canal of the vertebral column. Three meningeal coverings surround the spinal cord: (1) the dura mater, which is attached to the lateral surface of the spinal cord by the denticulate ligament, (2) the arachnoid, and (3) the pia mater (**Fig. 5.1**). The subarachnoid space contains the cerebrospinal fluid (CSF) and is located between the arachnoid mater and the pia mater.

The caudal end of the adult spinal cord is situated at the level of the first or second lumbar vertebra. This is because, following the third month of fetal development, the vertebral column grows faster than the spinal cord (**Fig. 5.2**). The lumbosacral nerve roots elongate and extend past the caudal end of the spinal cord to form what is known as the *cauda equina*. The caudal end of the spinal cord tapers off into the cone-shaped *conus medullaris*, which continues distally as the *filum terminale*. The filum terminale is a caudal prolongation of the spinal *pia mater* that courses along with the cauda equina to terminate on the dorsal surface of the coccyx.

Fig. 5.2 **Differential rate of spinal growth.** ⟶

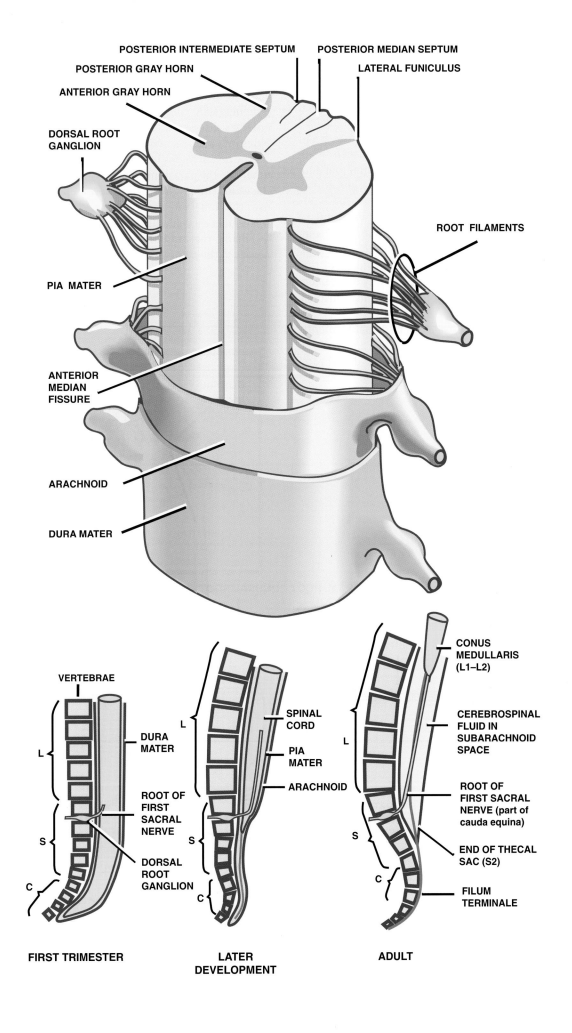

POSTERIOR INTERMEDIATE SEPTUM

POSTERIOR MEDIAN SEPTUM

POSTERIOR GRAY HORN

LATERAL FUNICULUS

ANTERIOR GRAY HORN

DORSAL ROOT GANGLION

ROOT FILAMENTS

PIA MATER

ANTERIOR MEDIAN FISSURE

ARACHNOID

DURA MATER

VERTEBRAE

DURA MATER

ROOT OF FIRST SACRAL NERVE

DORSAL ROOT GANGLION

SPINAL CORD

PIA MATER

ARACHNOID

CONUS MEDULLARIS (L1–L2)

CEREBROSPINAL FLUID IN SUBARACHNOID SPACE

ROOT OF FIRST SACRAL NERVE (part of cauda equina)

END OF THECAL SAC (S2)

FILUM TERMINALE

L

S

C

L

S

C

L

S

C

FIRST TRIMESTER

LATER DEVELOPMENT

ADULT

Spinal Nerves

See **Fig. 5.3**.

Thirty-one pairs of spinal nerves emerge from the human spinal cord: 8 cervical, 12 thoracic, 5 lumbar, 5 sacral, and 1 coccygeal. Each spinal nerve is formed in an intervertebral foramen by the union of a ventral root and dorsal root, and each one gives rise to a ventral and dorsal ramus.

A *ventral root* is composed of a series of ventral filaments that carry general somatic efferent (GSE) and general visceral efferent (GVE) fibers. The cell bodies of origin of these axons constitute the motor nuclei of the ventral horn of the spinal cord. More recently it has been shown that the ventral roots contain afferent (sensory) fibers as well.

The *dorsal roots* comprise a series of dorsal filaments that carry general somatic afferents (GSA) and general visceral afferents (GVA) that originate in the dorsal root ganglion (spinal ganglion).

Distally, the ventral and dorsal roots converge to form a *spinal nerve*, which contains all four functional components (GSA, GVA, GSE, and GVE). As the spinal nerve emerges distally from the intervertebral foramen, it divides into a dorsal and ventral ramus.

The *dorsal ramus* branches into peripheral nerves that innervate the paraspinal muscles and the skin of the back; the *ventral ramus* divides into peripheral nerves and plexuses that innervate the muscles and the skin of the anterolateral body wall, the limbs, and the perineum.

Finally, the *gray and white rami* connect the spinal nerves to the sympathetic trunk.

Fig. 5.3 **Spinal nerve.**

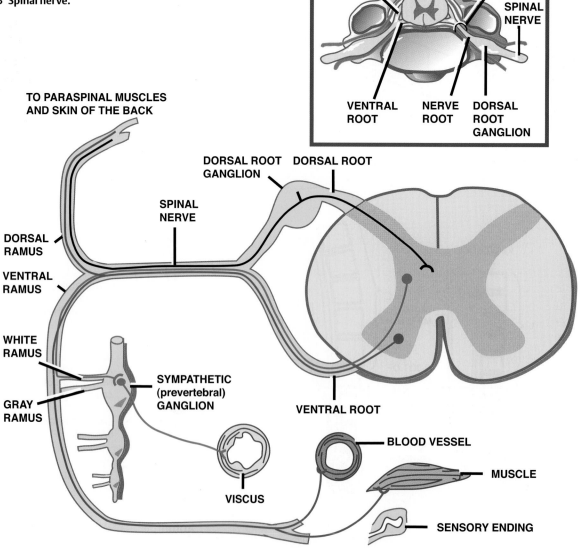

Segmental Innervation of the Body

See **Fig. 5.4**.

Skin

A dermatome comprises that area of skin that is innervated by the sensory fibers of an individual spinal nerve. However, the distribution of a single dermatome overlaps adjacent dermatomes, and thus destruction of a single spinal nerve does not produce clinically evident anesthesia. A dermatomal map is shown in **Fig. 5.4**. Key dermatomes include the following:

C3: Neck
C5: Deltoid region
C6: Radial forearm and thumb
C8: Ulnar aspect of hand and little finger
T4–T5: Nipple
T10: Umbilicus
L1: Groin
L3: Knee
L5: Dorsal surface of foot and great toe
S1: Lateral surface of foot and little toe
S3–S5: Genitoanal area

Muscle

Although their pattern of innervation is less obvious than in the case of sensory fibers, the motor fibers of a spinal nerve generally innervate those muscles that lie beneath the corresponding dermatome. Each spinal nerve supplies several voluntary muscles; likewise, each muscle is innervated by several spinal nerves.

Some of the more clinically relevant muscles and their innervation include the following:

Biceps brachii: C5–C6
Triceps: C6–C8
Brachioradialis: C5–C7
Intrinsic muscles of the hand:
    C8–T1
Thoracic musculature: T1–T8
Abdominal musculature: T6–T12
Quadriceps femoris: L2–L4
Gastrocnemius: S1–S2
Muscles of the perineum, bladder, and genitals: S3–S5

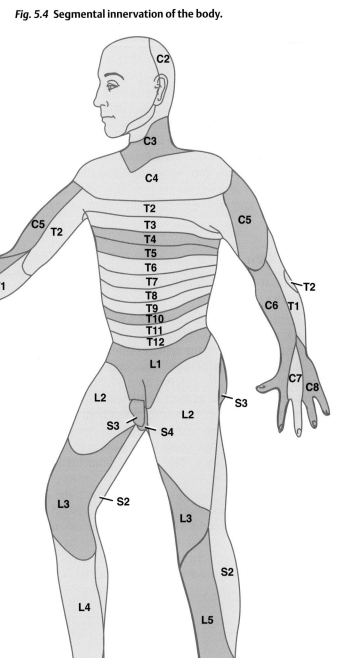

Fig. 5.4 Segmental innervation of the body.

Internal Structure

The internal structure of the spinal cord is organized into two discrete areas: (1) an inner core of gray matter containing cell bodies and mostly unmyelinated fibers and (2) an outer coat of white matter carrying both myelinated and unmyelinated fibers.

The distribution of gray and white matter in the spinal cord varies with the level of the spinal cord. For example, at cervical and lumbar levels that correspond to the innervation of the limbs, there is an increased proportion of gray matter. Furthermore, there is a decreased amount of white matter present at lower levels of the cord because the descending fibers exit the cord caudally, whereas ascending fibers enter rostrally.

Gray Matter

See **Fig. 5.5**.

The centrally located **H**-shaped gray matter is composed of nerve cells and their processes, neuroglia, and blood vessels . A small central canal, obliterated in places, is lined by ependymal epithelium. Each side of the gray matter is composed of (1) a *dorsal horn*, extending posterolaterally, (2) a *ventral horn*, extending anteriorly, and (3) an *intermediate gray*, which connects the dorsal and ventral horns. A small lateral horn is formed in the intermediate gray of the thoracic and upper lumbar segments.

Dorsal Horn

The dorsal horn is primarily composed of the following four cell groups:

1. *Posteromarginal nucleus*   This nucleus forms a cap on the dorsal horn. Many of the axons of the cells in this nucleus contribute to the spinothalamic tract.

2. *Substantia gelatinosa*   This cell group occupies most of the apex of the dorsal horn. It contains neurons and their processes, as well as afferent fibers from the dorsal nerve root and descending fibers from supraspinal levels. The functional significance of this cell group is in the modification of the sensation of pain.

3. *Nucleus proprius*   The nucleus proprius lies just anterior to the substantia gelatinosa. The axons of these cells are carried in the spinothalamic system, the spinocerebellar pathways, and the propriospinal system.

4. *Nucleus dorsalis* (*Clarke's column* or *nucleus thoracicus*)   This cell group is present at the base of the dorsal horn in segments C8–L3. It contains cell bodies whose axons form the dorsal spinocerebellar tract.

Intermediate Gray

Two cell groups contribute to the intermediate gray:

1. *Intermediolateral cell group*   This cell group forms the lateral horn in segments T1–L2. It gives rise to preganglionic sympathetic fibers. In segments S2–S4, an equivalent column of cells projects preganglionic parasympathetic fibers.

2. *Intermediomedial cell group*   The intermediomedial group lies just lateral to the central canal throughout the length of the spinal cord. It receives visceral afferent fibers from the dorsal roots.

Ventral Horn

The principal cells of the ventral horn are motor neurons. The motor activity of these neurons is subject to the influences of (1) interneurons, (2) dorsal root afferents (which act in spinal reflexes), and (3) the descending tracts of the brain.

Significantly, the neurons situated in the ventral horn are somatotopically organized in two ways. First, the neurons of the ventral horn that innervate the flexor muscles lie dorsal to those that innervate the extensor muscles; second, the neurons that innervate the muscles of the hand lie lateral to those that innervate the trunk. The logic of these relationships is made clear when one considers that the descending pathways associated mainly with the control of the flexor musculature, such as the corticospinal and rubrospinal tracts, are located dorsally in the lateral funiculus. On the other hand, the descending pathways associated mainly with the antigravity muscles (i.e., generally the extensor musculature) are situated in a more ventral position.

Two types of motor neurons are distinguished on the basis of the diameter of their axons. Large α motor neurons supply ordinary (extrafusal) muscle fibers of skeletal muscles; smaller γ motor neurons innervate intrafusal fibers of the neuromuscular spindles.

As mentioned, the ventral horn contains the following two groups of neurons:

1. *Medial group*   This group innervates the muscles of the axial skeleton and the abdominal and intercostal musculature.

2. *Lateral group*   The lateral group, present only in the cervical and lumbosacral enlargements, supplies the muscles of the limbs.

As an alternative classification, the gray matter of the spinal cord has also been divided into 10 layers of neurons, known as Rexed's laminae. Among the most important groups of laminae are the following (**Fig. 5.6**):

1. *Laminae I, II,* and *V* are important in the transmission of pain.

2. *Lamina VII* contains the nucleus dorsalis, the intermediolateral cell column, and the sacral autonomic nucleus.

3. *Lamina IX* contains the motor neurons that innervate the extremities. In addition, the phrenic nucleus and spinal accessory nucleus are located in this lamina, as is Onuf's nucleus. The nucleus of Onuf contributes axons to the pudendal nerve (roots S2–S4). These axons supply muscles in the pelvic floor, including the striated muscle sphincters that contribute to urinary and fecal continence.

Fig. 5.5 **Components of the gray matter of the spinal cord.**

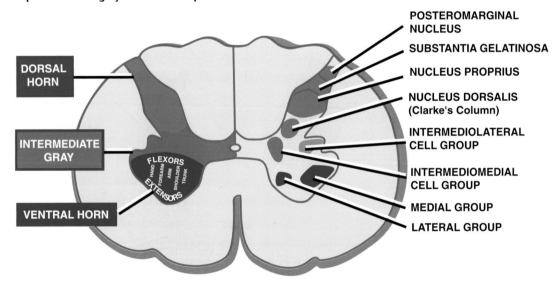

Fig. 5.6 **Organization of the gray matter of the spinal cord.**

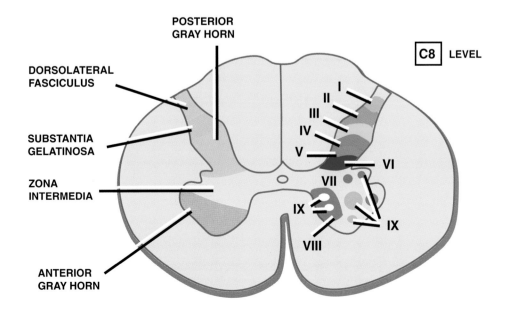

White Matter

See **Fig. 5.7**.

The white matter of the spinal cord may be divided into ventral, lateral, and dorsal funiculi. These funiculi contain the ascending and descending fiber bundles (fasciculi or tracts) that transmit signals both within the spinal cord and between the spinal cord and the brain. **Fig. 5.7** illustrates the relative position of the major tracts.

Fig. 5.7 **White matter of the spinal cord.**

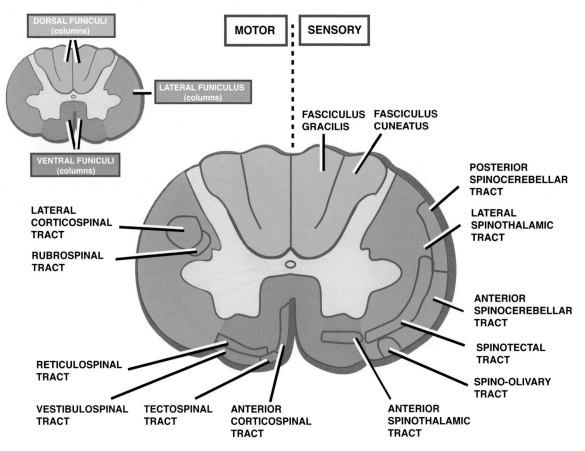

Ascending Tracts

See **Fig. 5.8**.

Dorsal Funiculi

Two dorsal or posterior white columns, the *fasciculus gracilis* and the *fasciculus cuneatus*, occupy the dorsal funiculi. The fasciculus cuneatus begins at T6, below which there is only the fasciculus gracilis. Separated from each other by a septum, these tracts mediate position sense, vibratory sense, and discriminative touch. The tracts are organized somatotopically. Those fibers that transmit sensation from the legs are located medially (fasciculus gracilis). Those fibers that transmit sensation from the arms are located laterally (fasciculus cuneatus).

Ventral Funiculi

The *anterior spinothalamic tract* lies anteromedial in relation to the lateral spinothalamic tract. It is concerned with light touch and pressure sensation.

Lateral Funiculi

1. The *posterior spinocerebellar tract* occupies the posterior part of the periphery of the lateral funiculi. It conveys position sense, touch, and pressure sense information to the cerebellum. It ascends uncrossed in the spinal cord.

2. The *anterior spinocerebellar tract* occupies the anterior part of the periphery of the lateral funiculi. The majority of ascending fibers in the anterior spinocerebellar tract are crossed.

3. Just medial to the anterior spinocerebellar tract is the *lateral spinothalamic tract*. This is the main ascending nerve, which mediates pain and temperature sensation. The lateral spinothalamic tract is somatotopically organized. Fibers that are located medially in the tract are concerned with sensation in the arms. Fibers that are located laterally in the tract are concerned with sensation in the legs.

4. The spinotectal tract, which is closely associated with the lateral and anterior spinothalamic tracts, conveys information to the superior colliculus of the midbrain. Its functional significance is unknown.

5. The posterolateral tract (Lissauer's tract) caps the dorsal gray horn. It carries fibers from two sources: (1) the dorsal nerve root and (2) gelatinosa cells that interconnect different levels of the substantia gelatinosa.

6. The spinoreticular tract travels in association with the lateral spinothalamic tract. It conveys information related to behavioral awareness.

7. The spino-olivary tract lies just anterior to the anterior spinocerebellar tract. It conveys sensory information to the cerebellum.

Fig. 5.8 Somatotopy of spinal tracts.

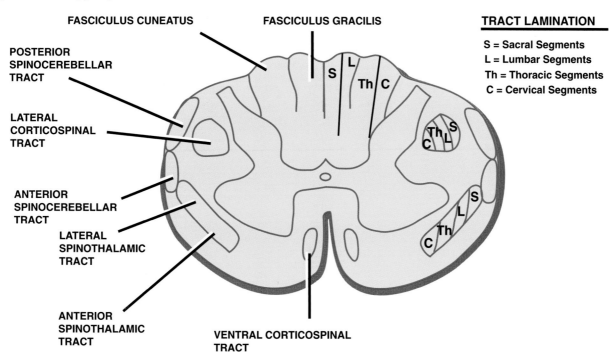

FASCICULUS CUNEATUS   FASCICULUS GRACILIS   **TRACT LAMINATION**

S = Sacral Segments
L = Lumbar Segments
Th = Thoracic Segments
C = Cervical Segments

POSTERIOR SPINOCEREBELLAR TRACT

LATERAL CORTICOSPINAL TRACT

ANTERIOR SPINOCEREBELLAR TRACT

LATERAL SPINOTHALAMIC TRACT

ANTERIOR SPINOTHALAMIC TRACT

VENTRAL CORTICOSPINAL TRACT

Descending Tracts

See **Fig. 5.9**.

Ventral Funiculi

1. The *anterior corticospinal tract*, present only in the cervical and upper thoracic segments, lies adjacent to the anterior median fissure. It conveys impulses related to voluntary movement.

2. The vestibulospinal tract occupies the periphery of the anterior funiculi. This tract descends uncrossed in the spinal cord. It facilitates extensor tone of muscles. It serves an important role in maintaining tone mainly in antigravity muscles.

3. The tectospinal tract is situated between the anterior corticospinal tract and the vestibulospinal tract. Fibers cross in the dorsal segmentation and are present only at cervical levels. It is thought to be concerned with reflex postural movements in response to visual and possibly auditory stimuli.

4. Scattered reticulospinal fibers concerned with motor control are contained in the anterior funiculi.

Lateral Funiculi

1. The *lateral corticospinal tract*, which lies lateral to the dorsal gray horn and medial to the spinocerebellar tract, mediates impulses concerned with voluntary movement, particularly fine motor movement. In the lower lumbar and sacral segments, where the posterior spinocerebellar tract is not present, the lateral corticospinal tract extends laterally to reach the dorsolateral surface of the spinal cord. The lateral corticospinal tract is somatotopically organized. Those fibers that are concerned with motor input to the arms are located medially. Those fibers that are concerned with motor input to the legs are located laterally.

2. The rubrospinal tract is situated anterior to the lateral corticospinal tract. This tract facilitates flexor muscle tone.

3. Descending autonomic fibers carrying impulses associated with the control of smooth muscle, cardiac muscle, glands, and body viscera are thought to be located in the lateral funiculi.

4. The lateral funiculi contain reticulospinal fibers concerned with motor control.

Fig. 5.9 Corticospinal tracts.

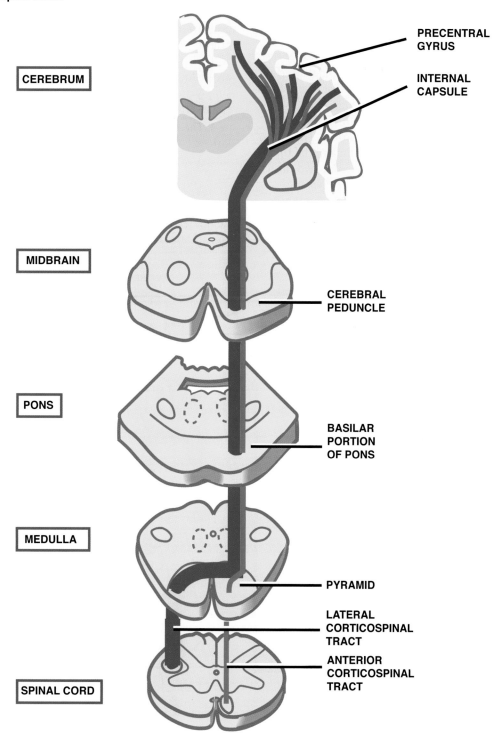

CEREBRUM

PRECENTRAL GYRUS

INTERNAL CAPSULE

MIDBRAIN

CEREBRAL PEDUNCLE

PONS

BASILAR PORTION OF PONS

MEDULLA

PYRAMID

LATERAL CORTICOSPINAL TRACT

ANTERIOR CORTICOSPINAL TRACT

SPINAL CORD

Blood Supply of the Spinal Cord

See **Fig. 5.10**.

The blood supply of the spinal cord is primarily derived from one anterior and two posterior spinal arteries. Both of these arteries are branches of the distal vertebral artery.

The *anterior spinal artery* arises from an anastomosis of two branches from the vertebral artery. The anterior spinal artery extends from the medulla to the tip of the conus medullaris. It supplies the anterior two thirds of the spinal cord. The *posterior spinal arteries* arise as paired branches from the intracranial vertebral artery, although they may also arise from the posteroinferior cerebellar arteries. They extend the length of the spinal cord and supply its dorsal third.

At the conus medullaris, the anterior and posterior spinal arteries anastomose. Throughout their course, both arteries receive supply from the radiculomedullary arteries, most of which are branches of the descending aorta. Three regions in the vertical axis of the spinal cord are distinguished by the relative richness of their arterial supply and are related to the distribution of the anterior spinal artery.

1. The cervicothoracic region (C1–T2) is richly vascularized.

2. The midthoracic region (T3–T8) is poorly vascularized.

3. The thoracolumbar region (T9 to conus) is richly vascularized. It receives the great radicular artery of Adamkiewicz, which most commonly (75%) enters the spinal canal at the T9–L2 segments on the left side.

Fig. 5.10 Blood supply of the spinal cord.

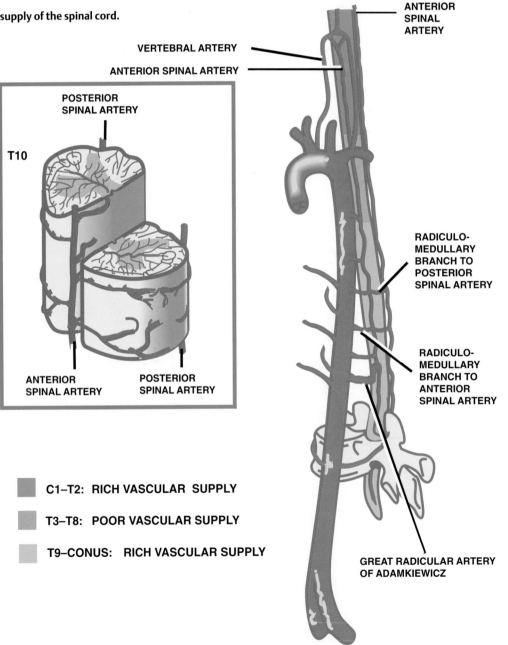

VERTEBRAL ARTERY

ANTERIOR SPINAL ARTERY

POSTERIOR SPINAL ARTERY

T10

ANTERIOR SPINAL ARTERY

POSTERIOR SPINAL ARTERY

ANTERIOR SPINAL ARTERY

RADICULO-MEDULLARY BRANCH TO POSTERIOR SPINAL ARTERY

RADICULO-MEDULLARY BRANCH TO ANTERIOR SPINAL ARTERY

GREAT RADICULAR ARTERY OF ADAMKIEWICZ

C1–T2: RICH VASCULAR SUPPLY

T3–T8: POOR VASCULAR SUPPLY

T9–CONUS: RICH VASCULAR SUPPLY

Vascular Syndromes of the Spinal Cord

Anterior Spinal Artery Syndrome

See **Fig. 5.11**.

Thrombotic occlusion of the anterior spinal artery is the most common vascular syndrome of the spinal cord. Most frequently it occurs in watershed or boundary zones, such as the midthoracic region (T3–T8). It has four essential features:

1. Quadriplegia or paraplegia (due to involvement of the *corticospinal tract*)

2. Impaired bowel and bladder control (due to involvement of the corticospinal tract)

3. Loss of pain and temperature sensation (due to involvement of the *lateral spinothalamic tract*)

4. Sparing of position sense, vibration, and light touch (due to preservation of the *dorsal columns*)

Posterior Spinal Artery Syndrome

This syndrome is rare. Manifestations may include loss of position, vibratory, and light touch sensation below the level of the lesion (due to involvement of the dorsal columns) with preservation of motor, pain, and temperature modalities.

Fig. 5.11 **Anterior spinal artery syndrome.**

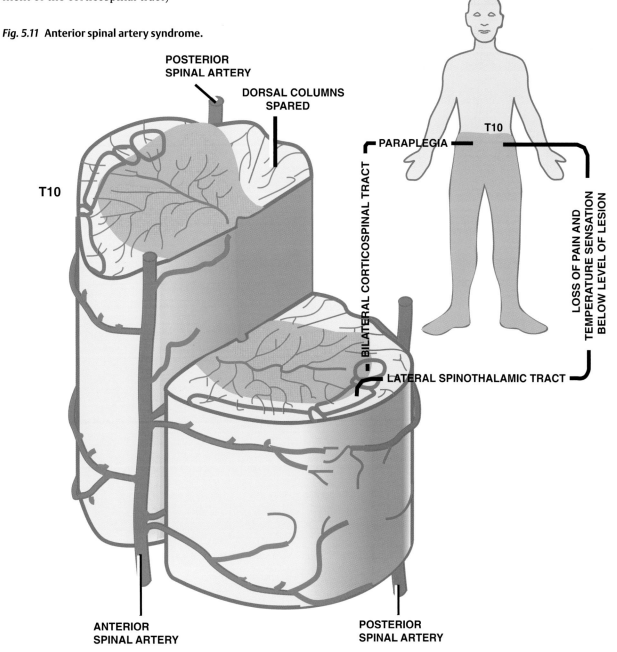

POSTERIOR SPINAL ARTERY

DORSAL COLUMNS SPARED

T10

PARAPLEGIA

T10

BILATERAL CORTICOSPINAL TRACT

LATERAL SPINOTHALAMIC TRACT

LOSS OF PAIN AND TEMPERATURE SENSATION BELOW LEVEL OF LESION

ANTERIOR SPINAL ARTERY

POSTERIOR SPINAL ARTERY

Spinal Tumors

See **Fig. 5.12**.

Spinal tumors fall into one of three categories: (1) extradural extramedullary, (2) intradural extramedullary, and (3) intradural intramedullary. Clinically, extradural and intradural extramedullary tumors are difficult to differentiate. The following discussion therefore describes both extradural and intradural extramedullary tumors together.

Extramedullary Tumors

Extramedullary tumors tend to produce pain in a radicular distribution. Frequently, this pain is associated with tenderness to palpation in the vertebral column. Ironically, this pain and tenderness are often accompanied by loss of normal pain and temperature sensation. The paraparesis associated with an extramedullary lesion tends to be spastic, and this spasticity persists even after paraplegia develops. There is little or no muscle atrophy associated with an extramedullary lesion. Muscle fasciculations are common. Trophic disturbances of the skin are usually absent. Bowel and bladder disturbances tend to occur late, unless the tumor is located in the sacral region.

Intramedullary Tumors

Radicular pain in intramedullary tumors is rare. Dysesthesias and paresthesias are common, as is dissociated sensory loss and sacral sparing (due to the somatotopic organization of the spinothalamic tract). Paraparesis is spastic in only 50% of cases and when present is less pronounced than in extramedullary tumors. Muscle atrophy is common, and muscle fasciculations are rare. Trophic disturbances of the skin are seen fairly frequently. Bowel and bladder disturbances tend to occur early.

Fig. 5.12 **Spinal tumors.**

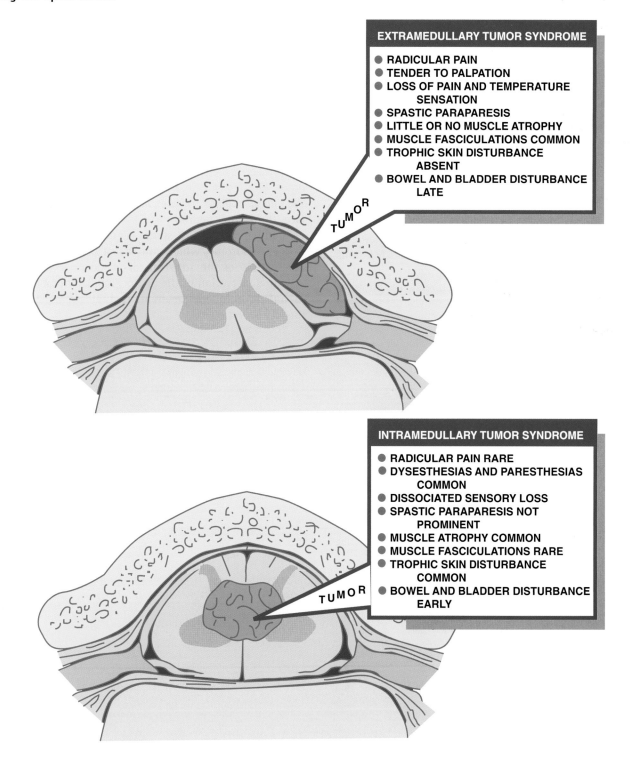

EXTRAMEDULLARY TUMOR SYNDROME

- RADICULAR PAIN
- TENDER TO PALPATION
- LOSS OF PAIN AND TEMPERATURE SENSATION
- SPASTIC PARAPARESIS
- LITTLE OR NO MUSCLE ATROPHY
- MUSCLE FASCICULATIONS COMMON
- TROPHIC SKIN DISTURBANCE ABSENT
- BOWEL AND BLADDER DISTURBANCE LATE

TUMOR

INTRAMEDULLARY TUMOR SYNDROME

- RADICULAR PAIN RARE
- DYSESTHESIAS AND PARESTHESIAS COMMON
- DISSOCIATED SENSORY LOSS
- SPASTIC PARAPARESIS NOT PROMINENT
- MUSCLE ATROPHY COMMON
- MUSCLE FASCICULATIONS RARE
- TROPHIC SKIN DISTURBANCE COMMON
- BOWEL AND BLADDER DISTURBANCE EARLY

TUMOR

Autonomic Disturbances in Spinal Cord Lesions

Respiratory Disturbances

Lesions at the level of C3–C5 may involve the phrenic nucleus, which innervates the diaphragm. Diaphragmatic paralysis causes limited lateral expansion of the lower rib cage during respiration, resulting in respiratory compromise.

Cardiovascular Disturbances

Upper cervical spinal cord lesions may be associated with bradycardia (due to interruption of fibers ascending to the cardiovascular center of the medulla). Such lesions may also be associated with hypotension (due to interruption of descending sympathetic fibers). The simultaneous presence of hypotension and bradycardia serves to distinguish hypotension due to loss of sympathetic tone from hypovolemic hypotension because the latter is typically associated with tachycardia. The former is seen during spinal shock following spinal cord injury.

Horner Syndrome

See **Fig. 5.13**.

Sympathetic fibers originate in the *hypothalamus* and descend through the brainstem to reach the *intermediolateral gray matter* of the C8–T2 spinal segments of the spinal cord (first-order neuron). Subsequent fibers are projected to the *superior cervical ganglion* (second-order neuron) and finally to the *superior tarsal muscle*, the *dilator pupillae* muscle, and the sweat glands of the face (third-order neuron).

Injury to the C8–T2 spinal segments may result in Horner syndrome, which consists of (1) *ptosis* (due to denervation of the superior tarsal muscle), (2) *miosis* (due to denervation of the dilator pupillae muscle), and (3) *anhidrosis* (due to denervation of the sweat glands of the face).

Fig. 5.13 Horner syndrome.

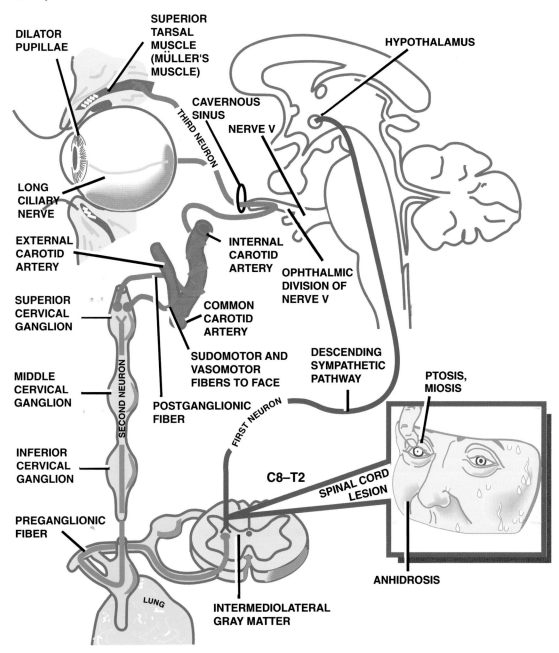

DILATOR
PUPILLAE

SUPERIOR
TARSAL
MUSCLE
(MÜLLER'S
MUSCLE)

HYPOTHALAMUS

CAVERNOUS
SINUS

NERVE V

THIRD NEURON

LONG
CILIARY
NERVE

EXTERNAL
CAROTID
ARTERY

INTERNAL
CAROTID
ARTERY

OPHTHALMIC
DIVISION OF
NERVE V

SUPERIOR
CERVICAL
GANGLION

COMMON
CAROTID
ARTERY

SUDOMOTOR AND
VASOMOTOR
FIBERS TO FACE

DESCENDING
SYMPATHETIC
PATHWAY

PTOSIS,
MIOSIS

MIDDLE
CERVICAL
GANGLION

SECOND NEURON

POSTGANGLIONIC
FIBER

INFERIOR
CERVICAL
GANGLION

FIRST NEURON

C8–T2

SPINAL CORD
LESION

PREGANGLIONIC
FIBER

LUNG

INTERMEDIOLATERAL
GRAY MATTER

ANHIDROSIS

Disturbances of Bladder Function

See **Figs. 5.14** and **5.15**.

The normal control of bladder function is mediated by two muscle groups. The *detrusor muscle* is composed of spiral, longitudinal, and circular smooth muscle bundles that surround the body of the bladder wall. Contraction of the detrusor muscle results in emptying of the bladder (micturition). The *external sphincter* is a skeletal muscle bundle that occurs on the distal segment of the urethra. Reflexive relaxation of this muscle is coordinated with contraction of the detrusor muscle during micturition. Voluntary contraction of this muscle stops micturition. (Separately, the *internal sphincter* is an extension of the detrusor muscle that consists of longitudinal muscle bundles that incompletely surround the proximal urethra. It plays a limited role in micturition, its major function apparently being to prevent semen from refluxing into the bladder during ejaculation.)

The nerve supply of the urinary bladder is derived mainly from two sources: the parasympathetic nervous system, which carries impulses of an involuntary nature to cause contraction of the detrusor muscle; and the cerebrospinopudendal pathway, which carries impulses related to voluntary control of the external sphincter muscle. Sensory afferents of the bladder are also carried in the *pelvic splanchnic* and *pudendal nerves*. Afferent impulses in these nerves continue in the ascending *lateral spinothalamic* and *dorsal column tracts*, relay in the *reticular formation*, and terminate in the *paracentral lobule* of the frontal lobe. The paracentral lobule, in turn, exerts voluntary control on the external sphincter via efferents that are carried in the corticospinal tract. The sympathetic nervous system also innervates the bladder, specifically the detrusor muscle and the base (output) of the bladder. The sympathetic output antagonizes the parasympathetic nervous system. Activation of the sympathetic system relaxes the detrusor muscle and contracts the base of the bladder, thus permitting bladder filling.

Fig. 5.14 Bladder innervation.

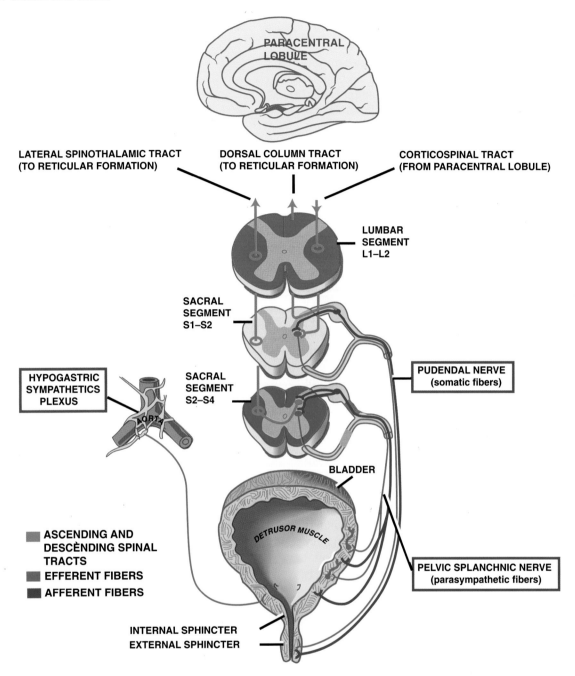

Reflecting the tiered system of bladder control, there are at least five distinct syndromes of bladder disturbance:

1. *Interruption of supraspinal control (uninhibited bladder)* This disorder is characterized by the sudden uncontrollable evacuation of urine due to a lack of supraspinal inhibition. **Bladder tone is normal, as is bladder capacity**. **Micturition occurs precipitously** at low bladder volumes (detrusor hyperreflexia). Frequently this occurs in inappropriate places and at inappropriate times. **Micturition is usually complete, with little or no residual urine**. **Bladder sensation is intact.** Clinical examples include frontal lobe tumors, parasagittal meningiomas, anterior communicating artery aneurysms, and normal pressure hydrocephalus.

2. *Spinal cord lesions above the sacral level (reflex bladder)* In spinal lesions above the S1 segment, bladder function is mediated solely by a reflex arc (reflex bladder). **Bladder tone is increased, and bladder capacity is decreased**. If the lesion is incomplete, there is urgency with little filling. Urgency is absent if the lesion is complete, in which case a rise in intravesical pressure may be manifest by sweating, pallor, flexor spasms, and systemic hypertension. Retention develops first, then overflow incontinence, and finally automaticity. A **small amount of residual urine** is present after voiding. **Bladder sensation is variably interrupted**, depending on the extent of the transverse lesion. Clinical examples include spinal cord trauma, spinal cord tumor, and multiple sclerosis.

3. *Spinal cord lesions involving the sacral level (autonomous bladder)* In lesions involving the sacral level, there is **denervation of both the afferent and the efferent supply to the bladder**. As a result, the bladder is autonomous (autonomous bladder). Clinically, this is manifest as overflow incontinence. **Bladder tone is flaccid. Urgency is absent. Bladder capacity is increased, as is residual urine. Bladder sensation is absent. Infection risk is high**.

4. *Lesions involving efferent motor neurons (motor paralytic bladder)* Lesions involving the efferent motor fibers to the detrusor muscle, or the detrusor motor neurons in the sacral spinal cord, produce a paralyzed bladder with intact sensation. **Bladder tone is flaccid, but urgency is present**. This results in **painful urinary retention or impaired bladder emptying. Bladder capacity and residual urine are markedly increased. Infection risk is high**.

5. *Lesions involving afferent sensory neurons (sensory paralytic bladder)* With lesions involving spinal or peripheral afferent pathways, voluntary micturition is possible, but **bladder sensation is impaired**. This results in **urinary retention or overflow incontinence**. As with an autonomous bladder, or a motor paralytic bladder, **infection risk is high**. Clinical examples include tabes dorsalis (dorsal column dysfunction) and diabetes mellitus (dorsal lumbar root dysfunction).

Fig. 5.15 **Disturbances of bladder function.**

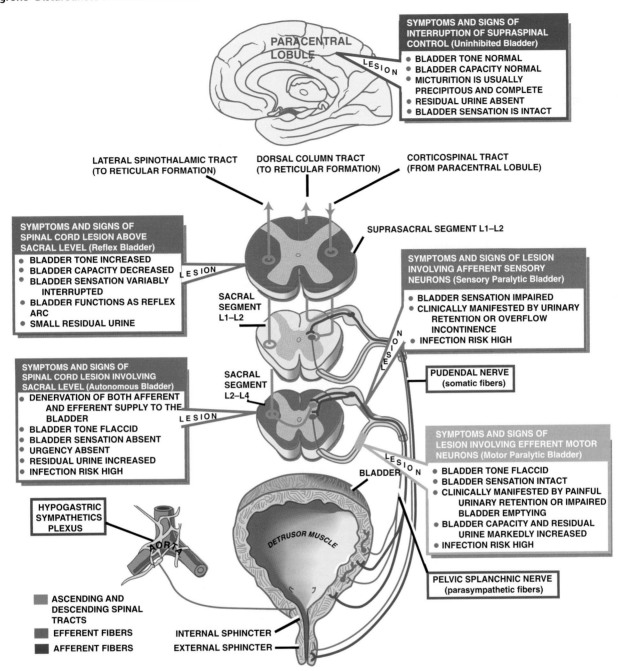

SYMPTOMS AND SIGNS OF INTERRUPTION OF SUPRASPINAL CONTROL (Uninhibited Bladder)
- BLADDER TONE NORMAL
- BLADDER CAPACITY NORMAL
- MICTURITION IS USUALLY PRECIPITOUS AND COMPLETE
- RESIDUAL URINE ABSENT
- BLADDER SENSATION IS INTACT

PARACENTRAL LOBULE

LESION

LATERAL SPINOTHALAMIC TRACT (TO RETICULAR FORMATION)

DORSAL COLUMN TRACT (TO RETICULAR FORMATION)

CORTICOSPINAL TRACT (FROM PARACENTRAL LOBULE)

SUPRASACRAL SEGMENT L1–L2

SYMPTOMS AND SIGNS OF SPINAL CORD LESION ABOVE SACRAL LEVEL (Reflex Bladder)
- BLADDER TONE INCREASED
- BLADDER CAPACITY DECREASED
- BLADDER SENSATION VARIABLY INTERRUPTED
- BLADDER FUNCTIONS AS REFLEX ARC
- SMALL RESIDUAL URINE

LESION

SACRAL SEGMENT L1–L2

SYMPTOMS AND SIGNS OF LESION INVOLVING AFFERENT SENSORY NEURONS (Sensory Paralytic Bladder)
- BLADDER SENSATION IMPAIRED
- CLINICALLY MANIFESTED BY URINARY RETENTION OR OVERFLOW INCONTINENCE
- INFECTION RISK HIGH

LESION

PUDENDAL NERVE (somatic fibers)

SYMPTOMS AND SIGNS OF SPINAL CORD LESION INVOLVING SACRAL LEVEL (Autonomous Bladder)
- DENERVATION OF BOTH AFFERENT AND EFFERENT SUPPLY TO THE BLADDER
- BLADDER TONE FLACCID
- BLADDER SENSATION ABSENT
- URGENCY ABSENT
- RESIDUAL URINE INCREASED
- INFECTION RISK HIGH

LESION

SACRAL SEGMENT L2–L4

BLADDER

LESION

SYMPTOMS AND SIGNS OF LESION INVOLVING EFFERENT MOTOR NEURONS (Motor Paralytic Bladder)
- BLADDER TONE FLACCID
- BLADDER SENSATION INTACT
- CLINICALLY MANIFESTED BY PAINFUL URINARY RETENTION OR IMPAIRED BLADDER EMPTYING
- BLADDER CAPACITY AND RESIDUAL URINE MARKEDLY INCREASED
- INFECTION RISK HIGH

HYPOGASTRIC SYMPATHETICS PLEXUS

AORTA

DETRUSOR MUSCLE

PELVIC SPLANCHNIC NERVE (parasympathetic fibers)

ASCENDING AND DESCENDING SPINAL TRACTS

EFFERENT FIBERS

AFFERENT FIBERS

INTERNAL SPHINCTER

EXTERNAL SPHINCTER

Disturbances of Rectal Function

See **Figs. 5.16** and **5.17**.

Innervation of the rectum is similar to that of the bladder. Parasympathetic neurons located in spinal segments S3–S5 are responsible for reciprocal contraction of the rectal muscles and relaxation of the internal sphincter muscle. Afferent impulses concerned with the sensation of rectal fullness are also carried in parasympathetic neurons.

Voluntary control of rectal emptying is facilitated by *somatic efferent neurons* that originate in the *paracentral lobule* of the frontal lobe and descend in the *corticospinal tracts*. These impulses synapse on ventral horn cells in the spinal *segments T6–T12*, which in turn innervate the abdominal muscles that are used in emptying the rectum.

Finally, sympathetic innervation of the rectum (not shown in the figure) impedes rectal emptying by inhibiting contraction of the rectal muscles.

Disturbances of rectal function may be divided into groups, based on the level of the offending lesion:

1. *Spinal cord lesions*　Lesions above the sacral level produce loss of voluntary sphincter control and loss of the sensation of rectal fullness. As a result, fecal retention occurs. Reflexive contraction of the sphincter usually persists, and the sphincter is usually spastic. High spinal lesions tend to produce less severe sphincter dysfunction, compared with lower-level lesions.

2. *Conus and cauda equina lesions*　Lesions involving the S3–S4 spinal segments produce paralysis of the sphincter muscle. As a result, fecal incontinence occurs.

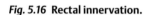

Fig. 5.16 **Rectal innervation.**

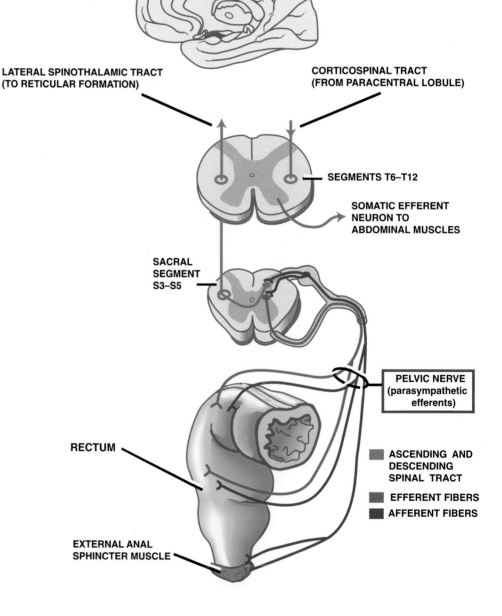

Fig. 5.17 **Disturbances of rectal function.**

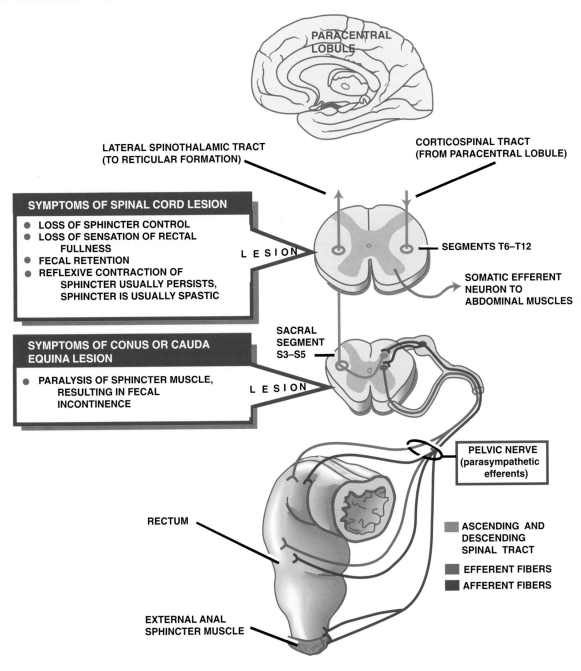

PARACENTRAL LOBULE

LATERAL SPINOTHALAMIC TRACT
(TO RETICULAR FORMATION)

CORTICOSPINAL TRACT
(FROM PARACENTRAL LOBULE)

SYMPTOMS OF SPINAL CORD LESION

- LOSS OF SPHINCTER CONTROL
- LOSS OF SENSATION OF RECTAL FULLNESS
- FECAL RETENTION
- REFLEXIVE CONTRACTION OF SPHINCTER USUALLY PERSISTS, SPHINCTER IS USUALLY SPASTIC

L E S I O N

SEGMENTS T6–T12

SOMATIC EFFERENT NEURON TO ABDOMINAL MUSCLES

SYMPTOMS OF CONUS OR CAUDA EQUINA LESION

- PARALYSIS OF SPHINCTER MUSCLE, RESULTING IN FECAL INCONTINENCE

L E S I O N

SACRAL SEGMENT S3–S5

PELVIC NERVE
(parasympathetic efferents)

RECTUM

ASCENDING AND DESCENDING SPINAL TRACT

EFFERENT FIBERS

AFFERENT FIBERS

EXTERNAL ANAL SPHINCTER MUSCLE

Disturbances of Sexual Function

See **Fig. 5.18**.

These disturbances can be divided into two distinct groups: disturbance in erection (including impotence and priapism) and disturbance in ejaculation.

Fig. 5.18 **Disturbances of sexual function.**

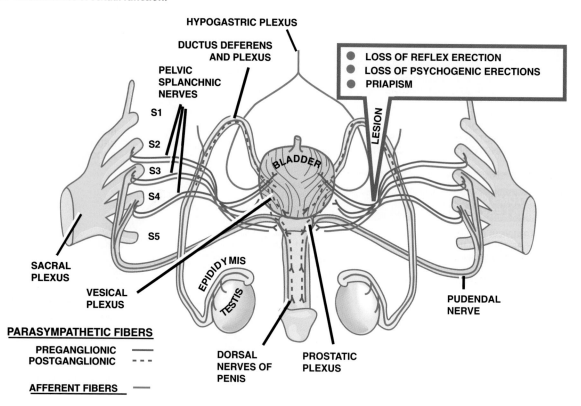

Erection

See **Fig. 5.19**.

The chief source of innervation in erection is the parasympathetic nervous system, which transmits impulses to the *corpus cavernosum* via the *pelvic splanchnic nerves*. Parasympathetic impulses facilitate erection by causing relaxation of the muscular cushions within the lumina of the cavernosus arteries, which normally obstruct the inflow of blood into the corpora cavernosa.

A complete lesion at the level of the S2–S4 segments results in loss of *reflex erection*, although *psychogenic erection* may still be possible. Psychogenic erection is due to hypothalamic impulses that are at least in part sympathetically mediated. Psychogenic erections are abolished by lesions above the T12 segment but are frequently preserved in lesions below this level.

Priapism, an abnormal persistent erection, commonly accompanies both traumatic and nontraumatic spinal cord lesions that occur above the lower thoracic levels. It is thought to be due, at least in part, to parasympathetically induced vasodilatation. Tonic contraction of the transverse perineal, bulbocavernosus, and ischiocavernosus muscles probably also contributes by preventing the escape of blood into the venous system.

Fig. 5.19 **Disturbances of erection.**

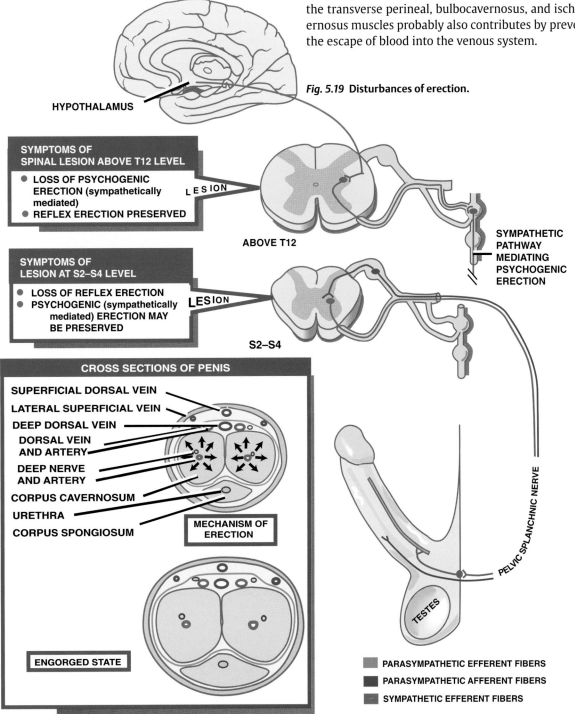

Ejaculation

See **Fig. 5.20**.

Ejaculation is a two-part process, which involves propulsion of semen into the urethra (emission) and propulsion of semen out of the urethra (ejaculation proper). Each of these parts is controlled by a reflex arc, as follows:

1. *Afferent limb*   Afferent limb impulses are carried from the *dorsal nerve of the penis* to the S3–S4 spinal segments via the *pudendal nerve.*

2. *Efferent limb*   From the S3–S4 spinal segments, afferent impulses reach two spinal centers. The first of these is a sympathetic center (T6–L3), which projects efferent fibers in the pelvic plexus and the *superior hypogastric plexus.* These fibers produce propulsion of semen into the urethra (emission) by inducing peristalsis of the *ampulla of the ductus vas deferens*, the *seminal vesicles*, and the *ejaculatory ducts.* The sympathetic ganglion at the L2 level plays an especially important role in this function. The second is a somatomotor center (S3–S4) that projects its efferent fibers in the pudendal nerve. These fibers produce ejaculation proper, the propulsion of semen out of the urethra, by inducing rhythmic contractions of the *bulbocavernosus and ischiocavernosus muscles.*

Spinal lesions above T6 may abolish normal ejaculation. However, ejaculatory reflex activity may be preserved and at times be so increased that the slightest stimulus may induce either an ejaculation or rhythmic contractions of the related pelvic musculature. In lesions involving segments S3–S5, ejaculation does not occur.

Fig. 5.20 **Disturbances of ejaculation.**

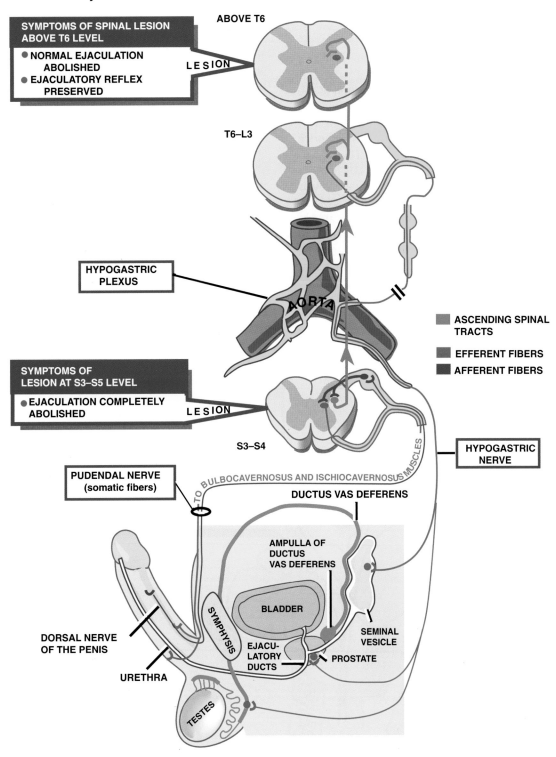

ABOVE T6

SYMPTOMS OF SPINAL LESION ABOVE T6 LEVEL
- **NORMAL EJACULATION ABOLISHED**
- **EJACULATORY REFLEX PRESERVED**

LESION

T6–L3

HYPOGASTRIC PLEXUS

AORTA

ASCENDING SPINAL TRACTS

EFFERENT FIBERS

AFFERENT FIBERS

SYMPTOMS OF LESION AT S3–S5 LEVEL
- **EJACULATION COMPLETELY ABOLISHED**

LESION

S3–S4

HYPOGASTRIC NERVE

PUDENDAL NERVE (somatic fibers)

TO BULBOCAVERNOSUS AND ISCHIOCAVERNOSUS MUSCLES

DUCTUS VAS DEFERENS

AMPULLA OF DUCTUS VAS DEFERENS

SYMPHYSIS

BLADDER

SEMINAL VESICLE

DORSAL NERVE OF THE PENIS

EJACU-LATORY DUCTS

PROSTATE

URETHRA

TESTES

Localization of Spinal Cord Lesions According to Level

Localization of the level of a lesion is one of the clinician's primary tasks in the care of a spinal-injured patient. If the patient is awake and cooperative, localization of the level of a lesion can almost invariably be ascertained by a focused neurologic examination. At a minimum, this should include an evaluation of motor strength, pinprick sensation, and deep tendon reflex activity. The following section illustrates a series of suggested tests in these three areas. For lesions that are located between levels C3 and T1, a negative test result is indicated by a blackened X or a blackened area. For lesions that are located at lumbosacral levels, only those tests that are expected to be abnormal are shown. For lesions between T2 and T12, a single illustration represents the various findings that may be observed.

Foramen Magnum

See **Fig. 5.21**.

The clinical presentation of foramen magnum lesions is variable. The most common presenting symptoms, in order of decreasing frequency, are suboccipital or neck pain, dysesthesias of the extremities (upper > lower), gait disturbance, and weakness (upper > lower). The weakness may involve first the arm, then the ipsilateral leg, then the contralateral leg. This is known as "around the clock" weakness. Other common early symptoms include clumsiness of the hands, bladder disturbance, dysphagia, nausea and vomiting, headache, "drop attacks," and dizziness.

An unusual feature of the weakness that develops is its occasional association with wasting of the intrinsic hand muscles. It has been proposed that this finding is caused by venous obstruction in the upper cervical spinal cord, leading to venous infarction in the lower cervical gray matter. Other less common but still frequent signs include downbeat nystagmus and accessory nerve palsy.

Fig. 5.21 **Foramen magnum lesion.**

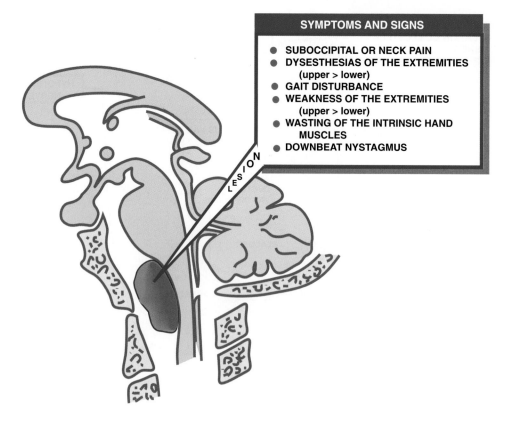

SYMPTOMS AND SIGNS

- SUBOCCIPITAL OR NECK PAIN
- DYSESTHESIAS OF THE EXTREMITIES (upper > lower)
- GAIT DISTURBANCE
- WEAKNESS OF THE EXTREMITIES (upper > lower)
- WASTING OF THE INTRINSIC HAND MUSCLES
- DOWNBEAT NYSTAGMUS

C3 Spinal Level (C3 Spared)

See **Fig. 5.22**.

Motor

Motor examination reveals quadriplegia.

Reflex

In the acute phase of a spinal injury, all deep tendon reflexes are absent. Later, all deep tendon reflexes may return and become exaggerated.

Sensory

Sensation is abolished below the base of the neck.

Respiration

Respiratory failure is also present because of denervation of the diaphragm.

Fig. 5.22 C3 spinal level lesion. Functions or responses marked with an "X" are impaired or absent.

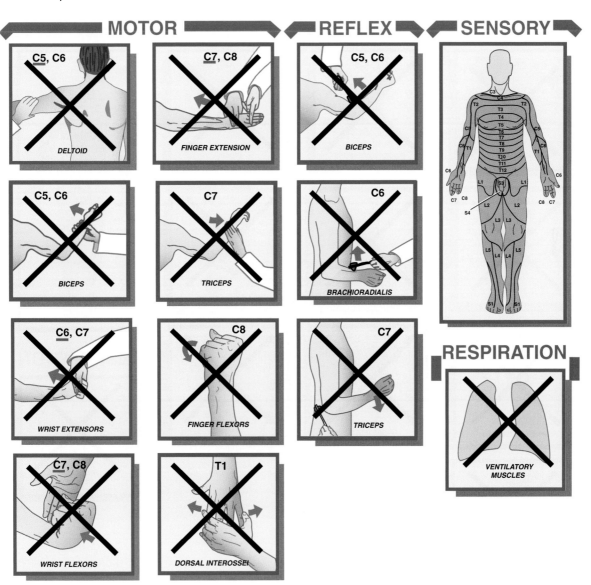

C4 Spinal Level (C4 Spared)

See **Fig. 5.23**.

Motor

Motor examination reveals quadriplegia.

Reflex

Initially, all deep tendon reflexes are absent. Recovery, and increased activity, may occur at a later time.

Sensory

Sensation is present in the upper anterior chest wall.

Respiration

Respiratory function (C3–C5) may be partially preserved, although paralysis of the intercostal and abdominal muscles further hampers spontaneous respiration.

Fig. 5.23 **C4 spinal level lesion.** Functions or responses marked with an "X" are impaired or absent.

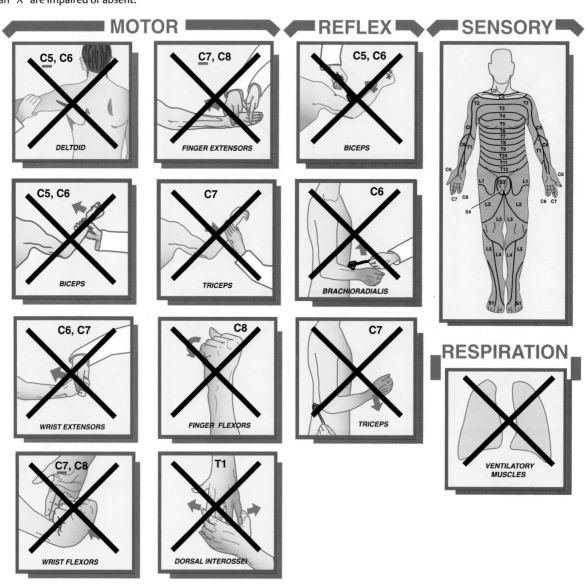

C5 Spinal Level (C5 Spared)

See **Fig. 5.24**.

Motor

Preserved muscles include the *deltoid* (C5) and, to a lesser degree, the *biceps* (C5–C6). Therefore, the patient is able to perform shoulder abduction and, to a lesser degree, elbow flexion.

Reflex

The biceps reflex (C5–C6) is normal or slightly decreased. As C6 returns, the reflex may become brisk.

Sensory

Sensation is preserved in the upper anterior chest and in the lateral aspect of the arm above the elbow.

Respiration

Respiratory reserve is compromised.

Fig. 5.24 **C5 spinal level lesion.** Functions or responses marked with an "X" are impaired or absent.

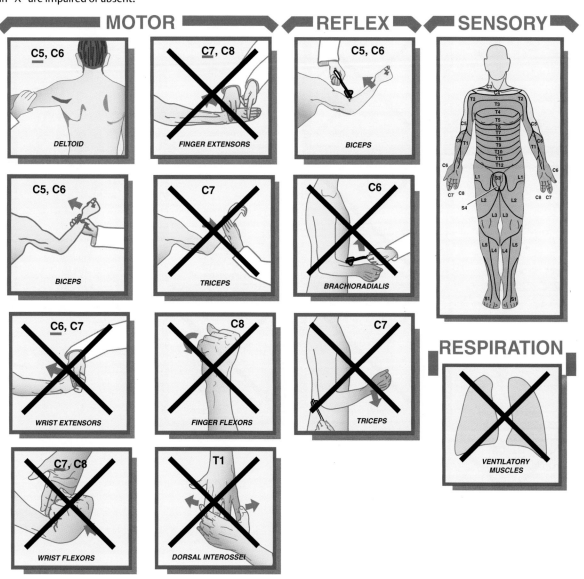

C6 Spinal Level (C6 Spared)

See **Fig. 5.25**.

Motor

The deltoid and biceps muscles are intact. Wrist extension is also present (extensor carpi radialis longus and brevis; C6), though slightly weakened (extensor carpi ulnaris; C7). Respiratory reserve is low.

Reflex

The biceps and brachioradialis reflexes are normal.

Sensory

Sensation is normal in the lateral upper extremity, including the thumb, the index finger, and half of the middle finger.

Fig. 5.25 **C6 spinal level lesion.** Functions or responses marked with an "X" are impaired or absent.

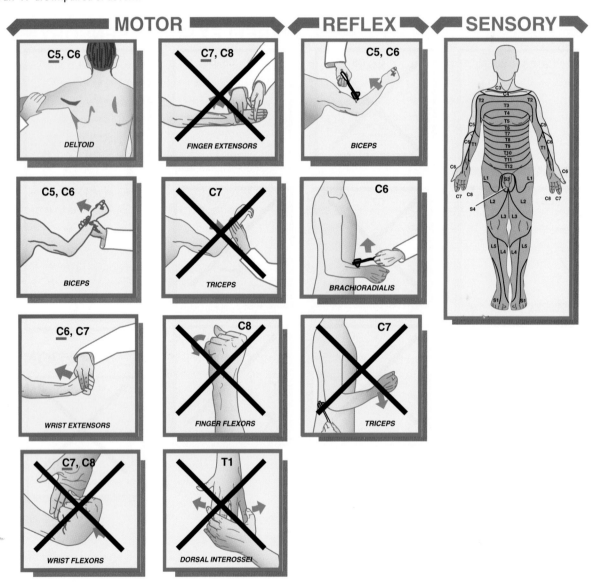

C7 Spinal Level (C7 Spared)

See **Fig. 5.26**.

Motor

The C7-innervated muscles, including the triceps, the wrist flexors, and the long finger extensors, are functional.

Reflex

The biceps (C5), the brachioradialis (C6), and the triceps (C7) reflexes are normal.

Sensory

The C7 innervation of the skin is limited. Therefore, sensation at this level is similar to the C6 level.

Fig. 5.26 **C7 spinal level lesion.** Functions or responses marked with an "X" are impaired or absent.

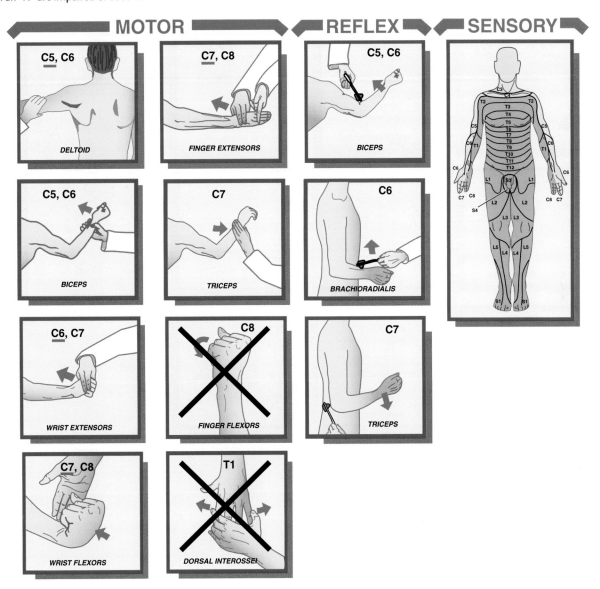

C8 Spinal Level (C8 Spared)

See **Fig. 5.27**.

Motor

Upper extremity motor function is normal with the exception of the hand intrinsics (dorsal interossei).

Reflex

The upper extremity deep tendon reflexes are normal.

Sensory

Sensation is normal in the lateral aspect of the arm and forearm, the hand, and the most distal portion of the medial aspect of the forearm.

Fig. 5.27 **C8 spinal level lesion.** Functions or responses marked with an "X" are impaired or absent.

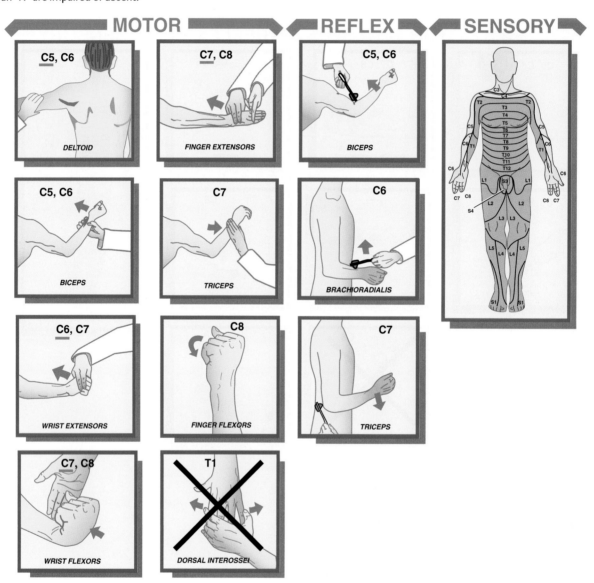

T1 Spinal Level (T1 Spared)

See **Fig. 5.28**.

Motor

Upper extremity strength is normal, leaving the patient paraplegic.

Reflex

The upper extremity reflexes are normal.

Sensory

Sensation is normal in the upper anterior chest and the entire upper extremity (except for the medial aspect of the most proximal part of the arm).

Fig. 5.28 T1 spinal level lesion.

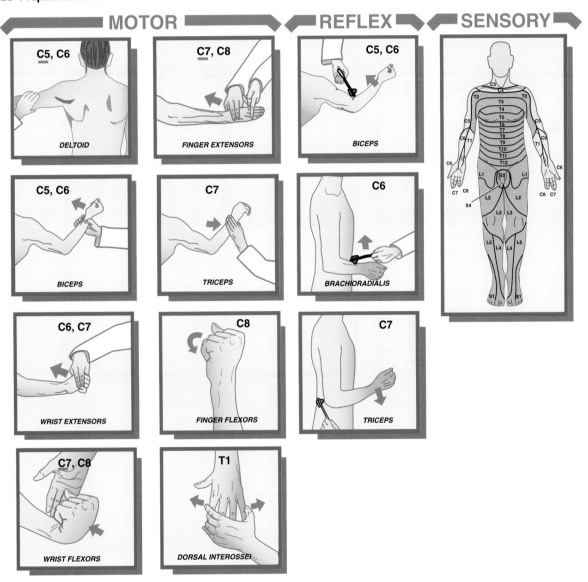

T2–T12 Spinal Levels

See **Fig. 5.29**.

Motor

The patient is paraplegic. Although an assessment of thoracic motor function is necessarily limited, some information about the intercostal and abdominal muscles may be obtained by attempting to elicit *Beevor's sign*. Beevor's sign is present when the umbilicus is pulled away from its normal location as the patient sits up from a supine position.

Reflex

Upper extremity reflexes are normal. Lower extremity reflexes are either absent (early) or increased (late).

Sensory

The level of the lesion determines the level of intact sensation.

Fig. 5.29 **T2–T12 spinal level lesion.**

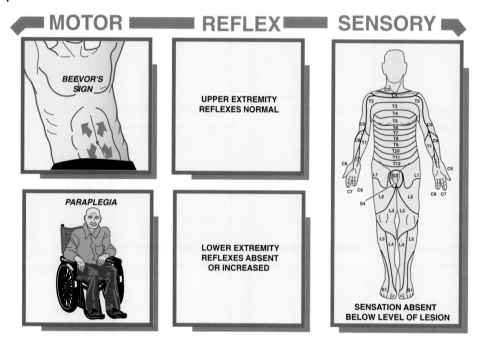

L1 Spinal Level (L1 Intact)

See **Fig. 5.30**.

Motor

Motor examination reveals paraplegia. The lower extremities are completely paralyzed, except for some hip flexion due to partial innervation of the iliopsoas (T12–L3).

Reflex

The patellar and Achilles reflexes are absent initially. Later, these reflexes may recover and become increased.

Sensory

Sensation is absent in the lower extremities except for the most proximal portion of the anterior thigh.

Bowel and Bladder

Bladder function is absent. Anal sphincter tone is decreased, and the superficial anal reflex is absent. With time, anal sphincter tone returns, and the anal reflex becomes hyperactive.

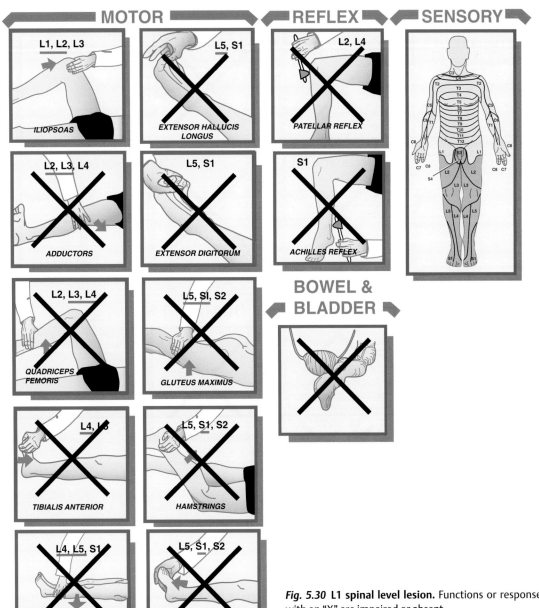

Fig. 5.30 **L1 spinal level lesion.** Functions or responses marked with an "X" are impaired or absent.

L2 Spinal Level (L2 Spared)

See **Fig. 5.31**.

Motor

Hip flexion is present, though diminished. The adductor muscles (L2–L4) are partially functional. Although the quadriceps (L2–L4) receive some innervation, it is not adequate for practical purposes. No other muscle activity is present. A flexion and adduction deformity may be present.

Sensory

Sensation is absent below the L2 dermatome, which is located halfway between the hip and the knee.

Reflex

The L2 contribution to the patellar reflex is small. Therefore, there is minimal or no reflex activity in the lower extremities.

Bowel and Bladder

Voluntary control of the bowel and bladder is absent.

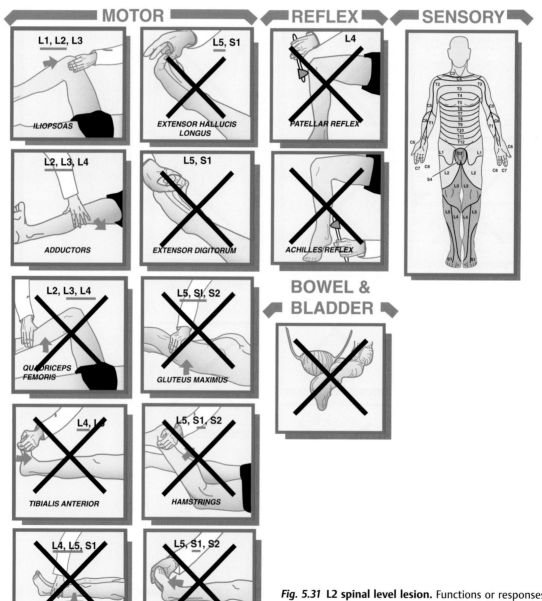

Fig. 5.31 L2 spinal level lesion. Functions or responses marked with an "X" are impaired or absent.

L3 Spinal Level (L3 Spared)

See **Fig. 5.32**.

Motor

The iliopsoas, the adductors, and the quadriceps muscles all show significant, if diminished, power. No other muscle activity is present.

Reflex

The patellar reflex, which is predominantly L4 innervated, is present but significantly decreased. The Achilles reflex is absent.

Sensory

Sensation of the entire thigh is normal but is absent below the knee (L3 dermatome).

Bowel and Bladder

There is no voluntary control of the bowel and bladder.

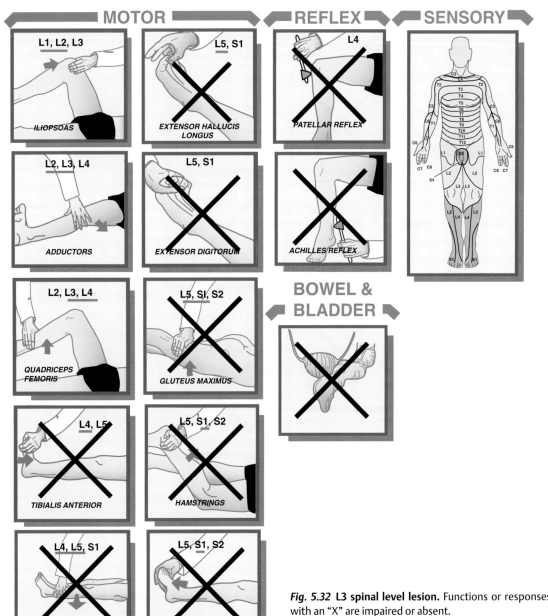

Fig. 5.32 **L3 spinal level lesion.** Functions or responses marked with an "X" are impaired or absent.

L4 Spinal Level (L4 Spared)

See **Fig. 5.33**.

Motor

Compared with the L3 level, the quadriceps are stronger, and in fact are normal. The tibialis anterior (L4) is the only functional muscle below the knee. It causes dorsiflexion and inversion of the foot. Although the gluteus medius (L4–S1) receives L4 innervation, it is significantly weakened.

Sensory

Sensation of the entire thigh is normal. It is also normal below the knee along the medial aspect of the tibia and the foot.

Reflex

The patellar reflex (predominantly L4) is present. The Achilles reflex is absent.

Bowel and Bladder

Voluntary control of the bowel and bladder is still absent.

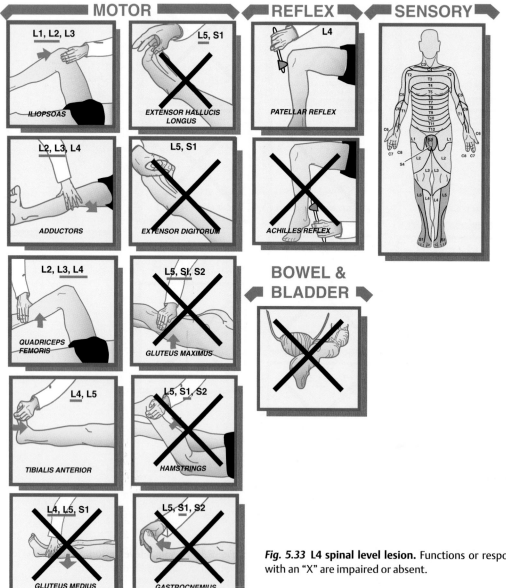

Fig. 5.33 L4 spinal level lesion. Functions or responses marked with an "X" are impaired or absent.

L5 Spinal Level (L5 Spared)

See **Fig. 5.34**.

Motor

Because the gluteus maximus (L5–S1) is not functional, the hip assumes a flexed posture. Adduction is opposed by the action of the gluteus medius (L4–S1), which is partially innervated. The quadriceps are intact. Knee flexion (hamstrings, L5–S2) is present but significantly weakened. The foot dorsiflexors and invertors are intact (tibialis anterior, L4; extensor hallucis and extensor digitorum, L5), but the plantar flexors and evertors are absent (gastrocnemius and peronei muscles, S1). Therefore, the foot is in dorsiflexion deformity.

Reflex

The patellar reflex is normal. The Achilles reflex is absent.

Sensory

Sensation is normal in the entire lower extremity, with the exception of the lateral and plantar aspects of the foot.

Bowel and Bladder

Voluntary control of the bowel and bladder is absent.

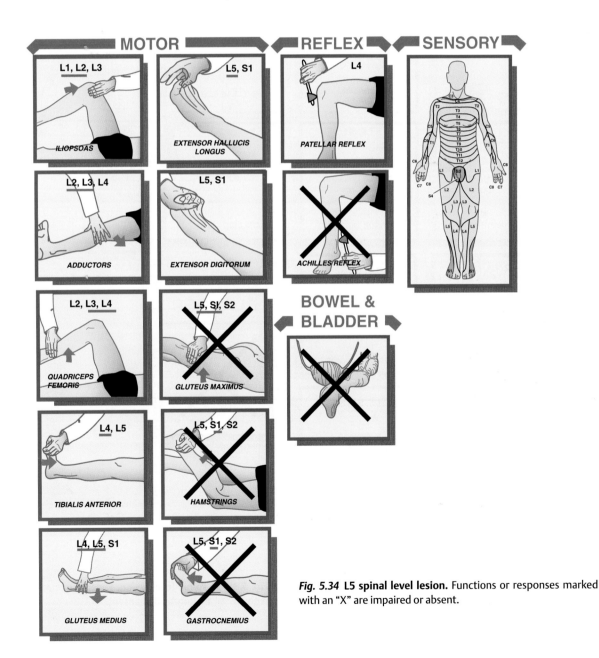

Fig. 5.34 L5 spinal level lesion. Functions or responses marked with an "X" are impaired or absent.

S1 Spinal Level (S1 Spared)

See **Fig. 5.35**.

Motor

Motor power in the lower extremity is essentially normal, with the exception of the intrinsic foot muscles (S2–S3), which are weak. As a result, the toes are in claw deformity.

Reflex

The lower extremity reflexes are normal

Sensory

Sensation in the lower extremity is normal, but saddle anesthesia persists.

Bowel and Bladder

There is loss of normal bowel and bladder function.

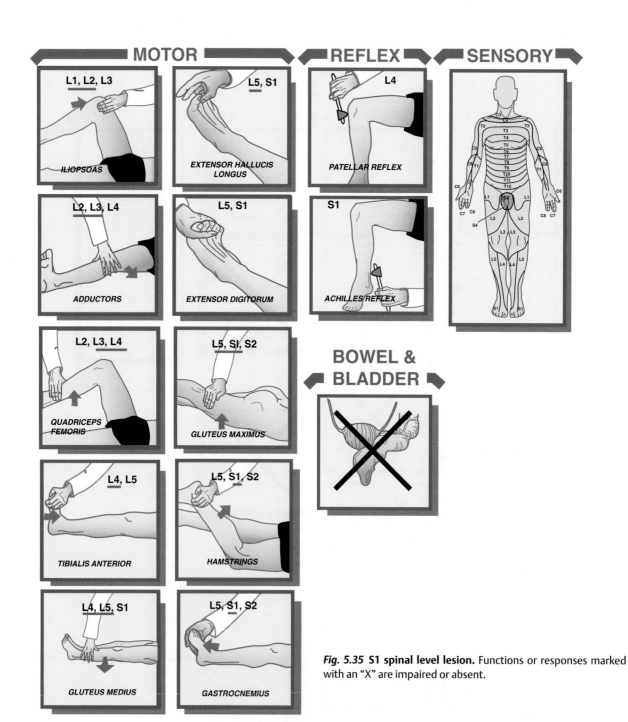

Fig. 5.35 S1 spinal level lesion. Functions or responses marked with an "X" are impaired or absent.

Conus Medullaris

See **Fig. 5.36**.

Lesions of the conus medullaris may result in any one or a combination of the following signs:

1. **An autonomous bladder**
2. **Fecal incontinence**
3. **Impotence**
4. **Saddle anesthesia**
5. **Absence of corticospinal tract signs or lower extremity weakness**

In reality this syndrome is often not present in its pure form. This is because lesions that involve the conus medullaris typically also involve the cauda equina. In contrast to a cauda equina lesion, in a lesion of the conus medullaris pain occurs late, sphincter disturbances occur early, saddle anesthesia is symmetrical, and motor disturbances in the lower extremities are absent.

Cauda Equina

See **Fig. 5.36**.

Lesions of the cauda equina may result in any one or a combination of the following signs:

1. **Radicular pain**
2. **Autonomous bladder**
3. **Fecal incontinence**
4. **Impotence**
5. **Asymmetric saddle anesthesia**
6. **Flaccid paraplegia**
7. **Absent deep tendon reflexes**

In contrast to conus medullaris lesions, pain occurs early, sphincter disturbances occur late, saddle anesthesia is asymmetrical, and weakness of the lower extremities is present.

Fig. 5.36 **Conus medullaris and cauda equina syndromes.**

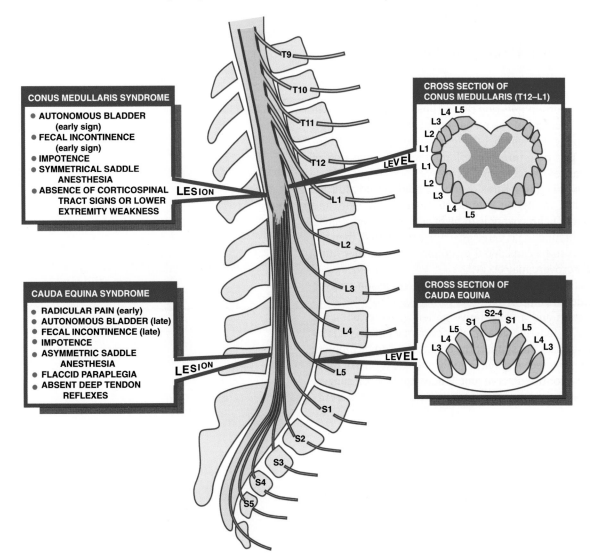

Clinical Evaluation of the Spinal Injured Patient

The Cardinal Manifestations of Spinal Cord Lesions

As a shortcut to establishing that a neurologic deficit has originated in the spinal cord, it is suggested that the clinician be in command of the most common signs and symptoms that are due to spinal cord lesions. Although each of these signs and symptoms will not occur in every instance, they should be sought in every case where a spinal cord lesion is suspected. The presence of a complete list of the findings given below almost invariably identifies a lesion as spinal in origin. There are four cardinal manifestations of spinal cord lesions:

1. **Spastic paraparesis** (or quadriparesis if cervical level)
2. **Bowel and bladder dysfunction**
3. **Sensory level** (dermatome below which no sensation is felt)
4. **Features of an upper motor neuron syndrome**

Complete or Incomplete Lesion

Prognostication is an important part of the overall management of the spinal-injured patient. Perhaps the single most important question that a clinician must answer in the early stages of the management of a spinal cord–injured patient is whether the lesion is complete or incomplete. This determination affords the best indication of the chances for functional recovery.

If no function returns over a 24-hour period after injury, then the lesion is to be considered complete, and no functional recovery is to be expected. If even a small return of function is detected in the early period, then the lesion is to be considered incomplete, and further functional recovery may occur.

It is important to emphasize that no lesion may be considered complete without a thorough neurologic examination and a cooperative patient. Furthermore, recovery of function at a single neurologic level is not by itself sufficient to support the diagnosis of an incomplete lesion. Such recovery may simply indicate return of function in a contused nerve root. It does not by itself suggest recovery below the nerve root.

Sacral Sparing

See **Fig. 5.37**.

Because the sacral fibers of the spinothalamic and corticospinal tracts are located peripherally in the spinal cord, preserved function in the sacral spinal segments is evidence of an incomplete spinal lesion. This is termed sacral sparing. Sacral sparing is evidence that a spinal lesion is incomplete. Because its presence suggests the possibility of functional recovery, sacral sparing should be routinely sought.

The identification of sacral sparing is based on the findings of three tests:

1. *Motor*   Flexion of the great toe (S1 innervation)
2. *Reflex*   Anal sphincter muscle (S2–S4)
3. *Sensory*   Perianal sensation (S2–S4)

Fig. 5.37 Sacral sparing.

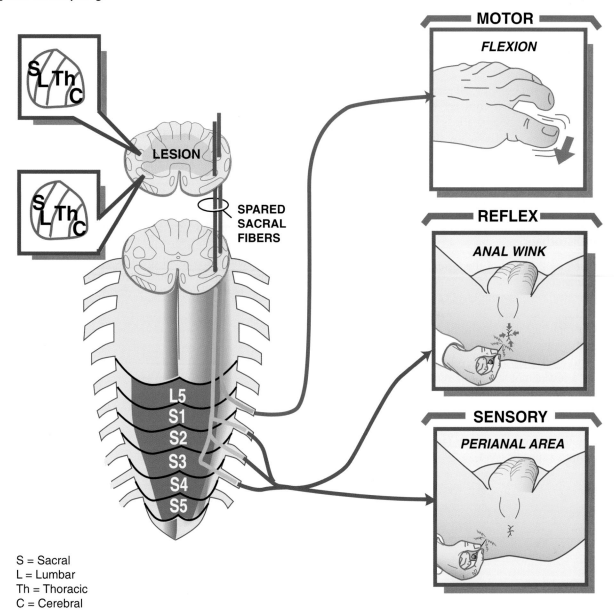

S = Sacral
L = Lumbar
Th = Thoracic
C = Cerebral

Spinal Cord Syndromes

Transverse Myelopathy

See **Fig. 5.38.**

In transverse myelopathy, all ascending and descending tracts of the spinal cord are disrupted (complete lesion). As a result, there is a loss of motor control and sensation to all modalities below the level of the lesion. Bowel and bladder control are also interrupted. Depending on whether the lesion is complete or incomplete, the loss of function may be complete and irreversible, or incomplete with a chance for functional recovery.

Motor Disturbances

Depending on the level of the lesion, interruption of the descending corticospinal tracts may result in paraplegia or quadriplegia. Below the level of the lesion, interruption of the corticospinal tracts eventually gives rise to an upper motor neuron syndrome (i.e., increased muscle tone and hyperreflexia), after an initial period of flaccidity and areflexia. At the level of the lesion there are signs of a lower motor neuron syndrome (i.e., atrophy, fasciculations, and loss of deep tendon reflexes) due to impairment of the anterior horn cells or their ventral roots. Identification of the segmental distribution of the lower motor neuron signs may facilitate localization of the lesion to a specific level.

Sensory Disturbances

Complete transverse myelopathies are associated with a loss of sensation in all sensory modalities below the level of the lesion. In practice, the sensory level that is evident clinically (usually by pinprick examination) may appear lower than the level of the actual lesion. This may be explained by the somatotopic organization of the lateral spinothalamic tract, in which the lower spinal segments are represented more superficially. Clinical evidence of segmental pain or paresthesias may identify the level of the lesion more precisely.

Autonomic Disturbances

Depending on the level and the completeness of the lesion, autonomic disturbances in transverse myelopathy may include any or all of the following: respiratory compromise, hypotension and bradycardia, Horner syndrome, bowel or bladder impairment, and sexual dysfunction.

Fig. 5.38 **Transverse myelopathy.**

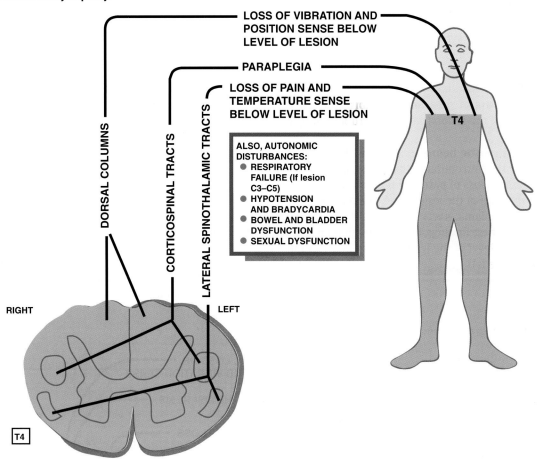

LOSS OF VIBRATION AND POSITION SENSE BELOW LEVEL OF LESION

PARAPLEGIA

LOSS OF PAIN AND TEMPERATURE SENSE BELOW LEVEL OF LESION

DORSAL COLUMNS

CORTICOSPINAL TRACTS

LATERAL SPINOTHALAMIC TRACTS

ALSO, AUTONOMIC DISTURBANCES:
- **RESPIRATORY FAILURE (If lesion C3–C5)**
- **HYPOTENSION AND BRADYCARDIA**
- **BOWEL AND BLADDER DYSFUNCTION**
- **SEXUAL DYSFUNCTION**

RIGHT

LEFT

T4

T4

Brown-Séquard Syndrome

See **Fig. 5.39**.

The Brown-Séquard syndrome is due to hemisection of the spinal cord, usually as a result of a penetrating spinal injury. The syndrome consists of the following three signs and symptoms:

1. **Ipsilateral loss of position and vibration sense** below the level of the lesion (due to interruption of the dorsal columns)

2. **Ipsilateral spastic hemiparesis** below the level of the lesion (due to interruption of the corticospinal tract)

3. **Contralateral loss of pain and temperature sensation** below the level of the lesion (due to interruption of the lateral spinothalamic tract)

In addition to these findings, lower motor neuron signs may occur at the level of the lesion (due to interruption of anterior horn cells).

Fig. 5.39 **Brown-Séquard syndrome.**

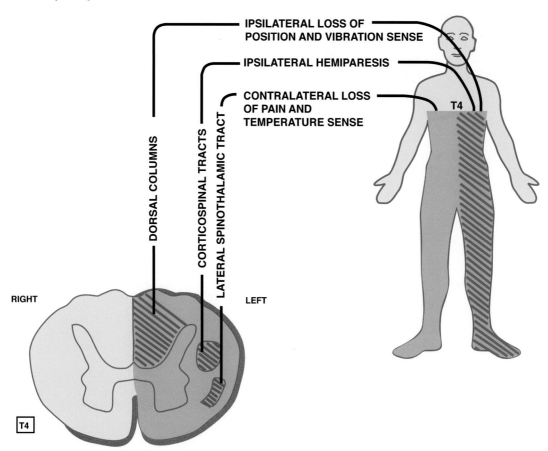

Anterior Spinal Cord Injury Syndrome

See **Fig. 5.40**.

This traumatic syndrome is clinically similar to the anterior spinal artery syndrome, and, indeed, the two syndromes may not be distinct (i.e., the mechanism of traumatic injury in the anterior spinal cord injury syndrome may be vascular). The syndrome is associated with damage to the anterior aspect of the cervical spinal cord. Its clinical findings include the following signs and symptoms:

1. **Spastic quadriparesis** (due to interruption of the corticospinal tract)

2. **Loss of the pain and temperature sensation** below the level of the lesion (due to interruption of the spino-thalamic tract)

3. **Preservation of position and vibration sense** (due to sparing of the dorsal columns)

Preservation of the dorsal columns, which also mediate crude touch, means that sensation below the level of the lesion is not completely abolished.

Fig. 5.40 **Anterior spinal cord injury syndrome.**

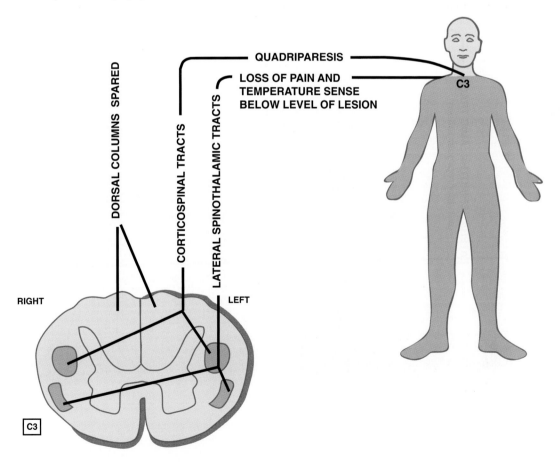

Central Spinal Cord Injury Syndrome

See **Fig. 5.41**.

Annular constriction of the spinal cord may lead to damage of the central portion of the spinal cord. Although the mechanism of injury in this syndrome is not entirely clear, it appears to represent the superimposition of a deforming insult on a stenotic spinal canal. Whether the direct mechanism of injury is ischemic or contusive is unknown.

The clinical findings of the syndrome are characteristic. They include weakness in the upper extremities out of proportion to weakness in the lower extremities. Furthermore, the upper extremity weakness is more severe distally than proximally. This characteristic pattern of weakness is explained by the somatotopy of the corticospinal tract, where the lower extremities are represented more superficially. Sensory loss in this syndrome is variable, but it also tends to involve the upper extremities disproportionately (again, due to somatotopy). Because the lesion is incomplete, at least partial functional recovery is the rule.

Fig. 5.41 **Central spinal cord injury syndrome.**

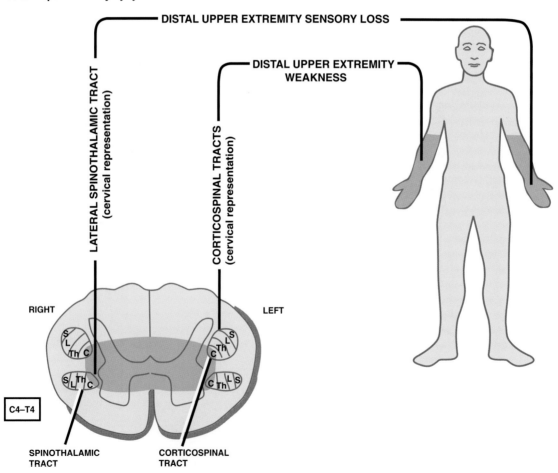

Anterior Horn Cell Syndrome

See **Fig. 5.42**.

Selective destruction of the anterior horn cells is classically associated with poliomyelitis and progressive spinal muscular atrophy. Motor involvement is characterized by flaccid paralysis of the muscles that are innervated by the affected anterior horn cells. Lower motor neuron signs are present in the involved muscles. Sensation is intact.

Fig. 5.42 Anterior horn cell syndrome.

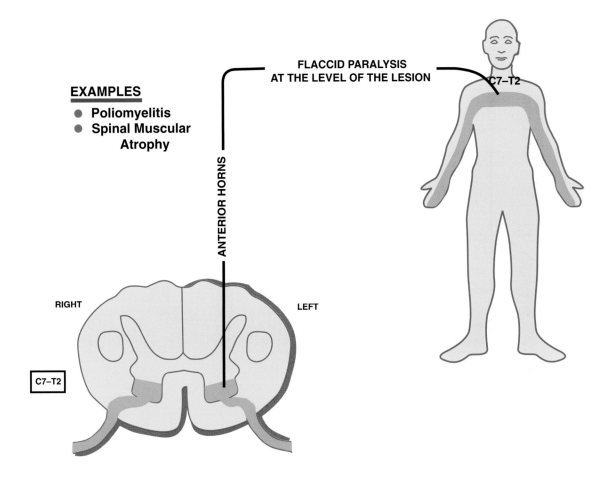

Lesions Affecting the Spinal Cord Centrally

See **Fig. 5.43**.

This syndrome is associated with syringomyelia and intramedullary spinal cord tumors. Characteristically, involvement of the decussating fibers of the spinothalamic tract results in a "suspended" sensory level. At cervical levels, the affected areas occur in a shawl-like distribution. Asymmetrical involvement of the more centrally located fibers in the corticospinal tract may result in an ipsilateral spastic monoparesis. Flaccid paralysis may occur at the level of the lesion due to involvement of the anterior horn cells. The dorsal columns are frequently spared.

The clinical presentation of this syndrome is variable. As the lesion enlarges and additional areas become involved, the nature and distribution of both the motor and the sensory disturbances change.

Fig. 5.43 **Lesions affecting the spinal cord centrally.**

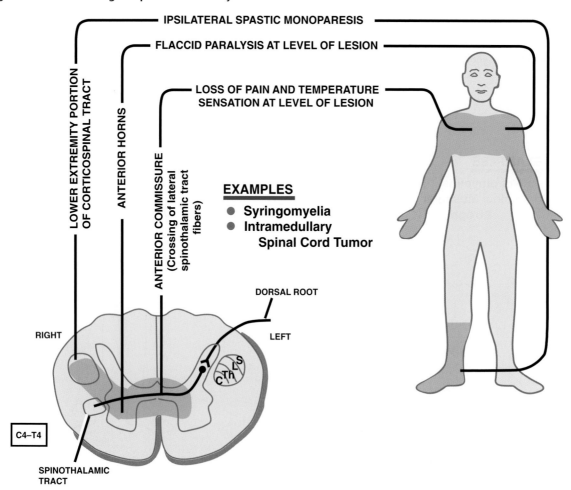

Amyotrophic Lateral Sclerosis

See **Fig. 5.44**.

Amyotrophic lateral sclerosis (ALS) is characterized by degeneration of the lateral corticospinal tracts and the anterior horn cells. Usually, it is unremitting and fatal. Clinically, it is marked by two manifestations:

1. **Flaccid paralysis at the level of the lesion** (due to degeneration of the anterior horn cells)

2. **Spastic paralysis below the level of the lesion** (due to degeneration of the corticospinal tracts)

Initially, the symptomatology is often focal or predominantly unilateral. Over time, however, the symptoms spread to involve a greater distribution, including the bulbar musculature. Bulbar impairment results in dysarthria and dysphagia. Frequently, there is also tongue atrophy and weakness, findings which should be routinely sought when this diagnosis is suspected.

The combination of upper and lower motor neuron findings is characteristic of ALS. As distinguished from the presentation of cervical spondylotic myelopathy (which is also associated with a combination of upper and lower motor neuron signs), sensation is entirely normal in ALS.

Fig. 5.44 **Amyotrophic lateral sclerosis (ALS).**

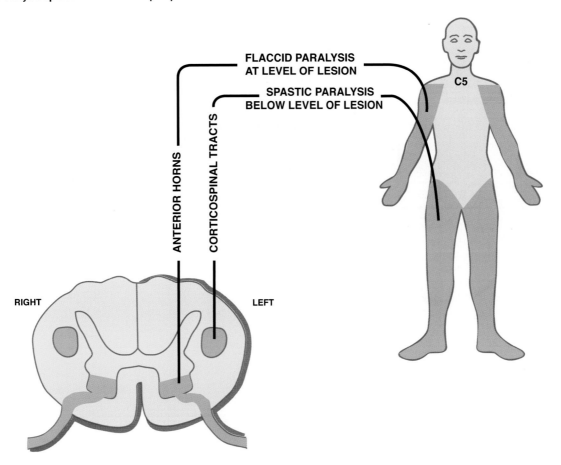

Tabes Dorsalis

See **Fig. 5.45.**

Tabes dorsalis is a neurologic sequela of neurosyphilis. Typically it develops 10 to 20 years after the onset of infection. Pathologically, it is characterized by selective destruction of the dorsal columns. Clinically, it is characterized by

1. **Loss of position and vibration sensation below the level of the lesion**. Usually, this is associated with **gait ataxia**, a **Romberg's sign**, and **decreased patellar and Achilles tendon reflexes**.

2. **Urinary incontinence**

3. **Lancinating (lightning-like) pains in the lower extremities**

Fig. 5.45 **Tabes dorsalis.**

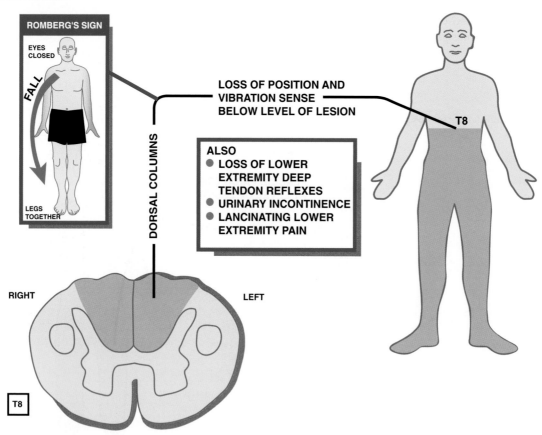

Friedreich's Ataxia

See **Fig. 5.46**.

Friedreich's ataxia is a syndrome consisting of degeneration in three tracts: the dorsal columns, the corticospinal tracts, and the spinocerebellar tracts. Clinically, it consists of the following findings:

1. **Loss of position and vibration sensation** (due to degeneration of the dorsal columns)

2. **Romberg's sign** (due to degeneration of the dorsal columns)

3. **Ataxia** (due to degeneration of the spinocerebellar tracts)

4. **Spastic paraparesis** (due to degeneration of the corticospinal tracts)

Additional findings that are frequently found in Friedreich's ataxia are a pes cavus foot deformity and spinal kyphosis or scoliosis.

Fig. 5.46 **Friedreich's ataxia.**

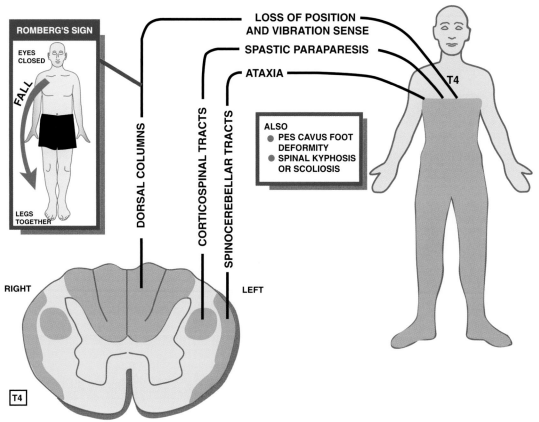

Subacute Combined Degeneration

See **Fig. 5.47**.

This syndrome is usually related to pernicious anemia, which is one of the causes of vitamin B12 deficiency. Pathologically, it is characterized by degeneration of the dorsal columns, and later the corticospinal tracts. Hence, it is referred to as a *combined* degeneration. Clinically, it is characterized by two major manifestations:

1. **Loss of position and vibration sensation** (due to degeneration of the dorsal columns)

2. **Spastic paraparesis** (due to degeneration of the corticospinal tracts)

As a result of the degeneration of the dorsal columns, there will be ataxia and a positive Romberg's sign.

Fig. 5.47 **Subacute combined degeneration.**

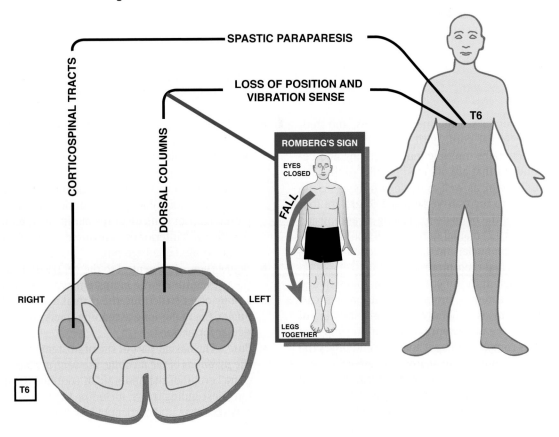

6 Brainstem

The brainstem comprises the medulla, pons, and midbrain. Like the spinal cord, with which it is caudally contiguous, it contains multiple long ascending and descending pathways that are oriented parallel to the long axis of the brainstem, as well as nuclei whose axons are oriented parallel to the transverse plane. There are four major elements of the brainstem: (1) long ascending and descending tracts, (2) cranial nerve nuclei and their fascicles, (3) cerebellar nuclei and their connections, and (4) reticular neurons and their processes.

Because brainstem dysfunction is both common and potentially life threatening, prompt recognition of its cardinal manifestations is imperative. An understanding of the principles of the brainstem's organization simplifies the study of its complex regional anatomy and offers the clinician a logical approach to anatomic diagnosis.

This chapter outlines the basic organization of the brainstem, then discusses the regional and functional anatomy of the cranial nerve nuclei, the long ascending and descending tracts, the cerebellar connections, and the reticular formation. A description of the blood supply of the brainstem is followed by a discussion of the localization of brainstem lesions, and finally by a description of classic brainstem syndromes.

The Brainstem Is Organized into Four Major Parts

Grossly, four major parts of the brainstem are contiguous throughout the length of the medulla, pons, and midbrain (**Fig. 6.1**):

- *Ventricular cavity*   The ventricular cavity of the brainstem is contiguous with the *central canal* of the spinal cord. It comprises the central canal (caudal medulla), the fourth ventricle (rostral medulla and pons), and the *cerebral aqueduct* of Sylvius (midbrain).

- *Roof*   Overlying the ventricular cavity is the roof of the brainstem, which comprises the choroid plexus and tela choroidea of the fourth ventricle (medulla), the cerebellum (pons), and the *tectum* (midbrain). The tectum consists of the rostral pretectum, the paired superior colliculi of the optic system, and the paired inferior colliculi of the auditory system. The superior and inferior colliculi are collectively known as the corpora quadrigemina.

- *Tegmentum*   Just ventral to the ventricular cavity is the tegmentum of the brainstem, which contains, among other structures, the cranial nerves and their nuclei, the major long ascending tracts, and the reticular formation.

- *Base*   The basilar part of the brainstem comprises the *pyramids of the medulla*, the *ventral pons*, and the crura cerebri of the midbrain. It contains the major long descending tracts, including the corticospinal, corticobulbar, and corticopontine tracts.

Fig. 6.1 **Brainstem.**

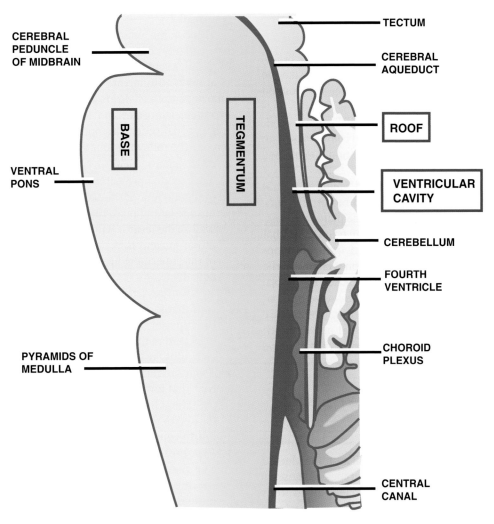

TECTUM

CEREBRAL
PEDUNCLE
OF MIDBRAIN

CEREBRAL
AQUEDUCT

BASE

ROOF

TEGMENTUM

VENTRICULAR
CAVITY

VENTRAL
PONS

CEREBELLUM

FOURTH
VENTRICLE

CHOROID
PLEXUS

PYRAMIDS OF
MEDULLA

CENTRAL
CANAL

Cranial Nerve Nuclei Are Organized into Longitudinal Columns

Ten of the 12 cranial nerves have their nuclei in the brainstem. (Cranial nerves I and II are the exceptions.) Like the spinal gray nuclei, the cranial nerve nuclei are grouped into longitudinal columns. These columns are both anatomically and functionally distinct: medial columns contain exclusively motor nuclei, and lateral columns contain exclusively sensory nuclei. This organization is explained by developmental events, as follows.

The alar and basal plates of the developing neural tube give rise to sensory afferents and motor efferents, respectively. Early in development, these plates are positioned in a dorsal/ventral orientation, an orientation that is maintained in the mature spinal cord. In the developing brainstem, however, this organization is changed: the lateral spread of the fourth ventricle causes the dorsal alar plate to rotate laterally in relation to the ventral basal plate. As a result, the lateral columns of the mature brainstem contain strictly sensory cranial nerve nuclei; the medial columns contain strictly motor cranial nerve nuclei.

Medial Columns Contain Three Types of Motor Nuclei

The medial columns are composed of somatic and visceral motor nuclei. Two types of visceral motor nuclei are distinguished on the basis of the two types of muscles their neurons innervate—striated muscle derived from primitive branchial arches and smooth muscle associated with viscera and glands. Three types of motor nuclei—one somatic, two visceral—thus comprise the three medial columns. The individual nuclei that form these columns, in medial to lateral order, are described in the following sections.

Column 1

See **Fig. 6.2**.

This column, which is not continuous longitudinally, is immediately adjacent to the midline, just below the floor of the ventricular system. It contains nuclei composed of neurons that innervate the striated muscles of the head and neck derived from embryonic myotomes (i.e., the extraocular muscles and the muscles of the tongue). In rostrocaudal order, the nuclei contained in this column include the following four structures:

- *Oculomotor nucleus* (III)   This nucleus contains neurons that project to the oculomotor nerve. They innervate four of the six extraocular muscles (i.e., all but the lateral rectus and the superior oblique) as well as the levator palpebrae superioris. The oculomotor nucleus is located in the midbrain at the level of the superior colliculus, just ventral to the cerebral aqueduct.
- *Trochlear nucleus* (IV)   This nucleus contains neurons that form the trochlear nerve. They innervate the superior oblique muscle. The trochlear nucleus is located in the midbrain at the level of the inferior colliculus, just ventral to the cerebral aqueduct.
- *Abducens nucleus* (VI)   This nucleus contains neurons that form the abducens nerve. They innervate the lateral rectus muscle. The abducens nucleus is located in the pons, just ventral to the floor of the fourth ventricle.
- *Hypoglossal nucleus* (XII)   This nucleus contains neurons that form the hypoglossal nerve. They innervate the muscles of the tongue. The hypoglossal nucleus is located in the medulla, just ventral to the floor of the fourth ventricle.

Fig. 6.2 **Somatic motor nuclei.**

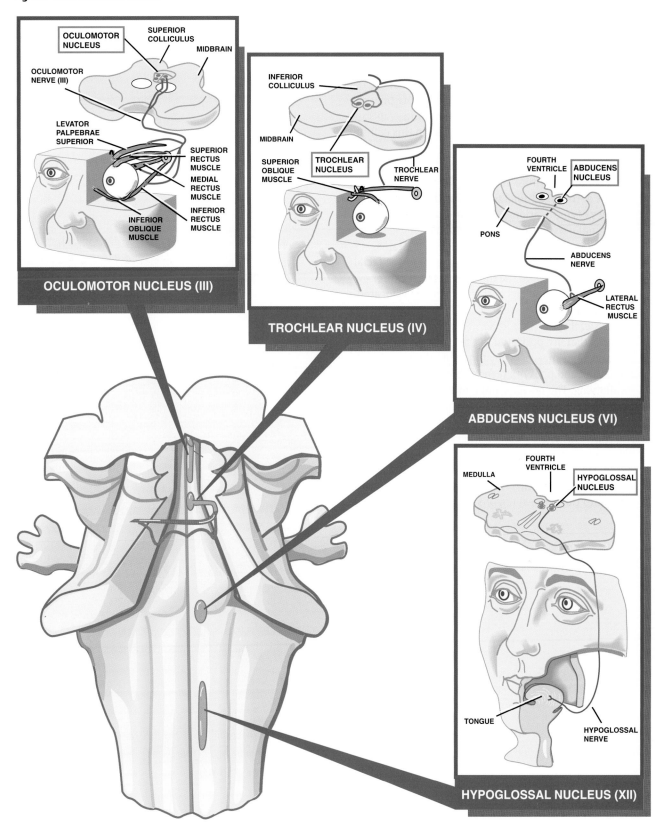

Column 2

See **Fig. 6.3**.

This column is located lateral and ventral to column 1. It contains nuclei composed of neurons that innervate the striated muscles of the head and neck derived from the branchial arches (i.e., the muscles of mastication, the muscles of facial expression, the muscles of the pharynx and larynx, and the sternocleidomastoid and trapezius muscles). In rostrocaudal order, the nuclei in this column include the following four structures:

- *Motor nucleus of the trigeminal nerve* (V)   This nucleus contains neurons that form the motor component of the trigeminal nerve. They innervate the muscles of mastication. The motor nucleus of the trigeminal nerve is located in the pons.
- *Facial motor nucleus* (VII)   This nucleus contains neurons that form the motor component of the facial nerve. They innervate the muscles of facial expression. The motor nucleus of the facial nerve is located in the pons.
- *Nucleus ambiguus* (IX and X)   This nucleus contains neurons that are projected in the glossopharyngeal (IX) and vagus nerves. They innervate the muscles of the larynx and pharynx responsible for speech and swallowing. The nucleus ambiguus, so-called because of its unclear borders in histological sections, is located in the medulla.
- *Nucleus of the spinal accessory nerve* (XI)   This nucleus contains neurons that form the spinal accessory nerve. They innervate the sternocleidomastoid and trapezius muscles. This nucleus extends from the medulla into the cervical regions of the spinal cord.

Fig. 6.3 **Visceral motor nuclei (striated muscle).**

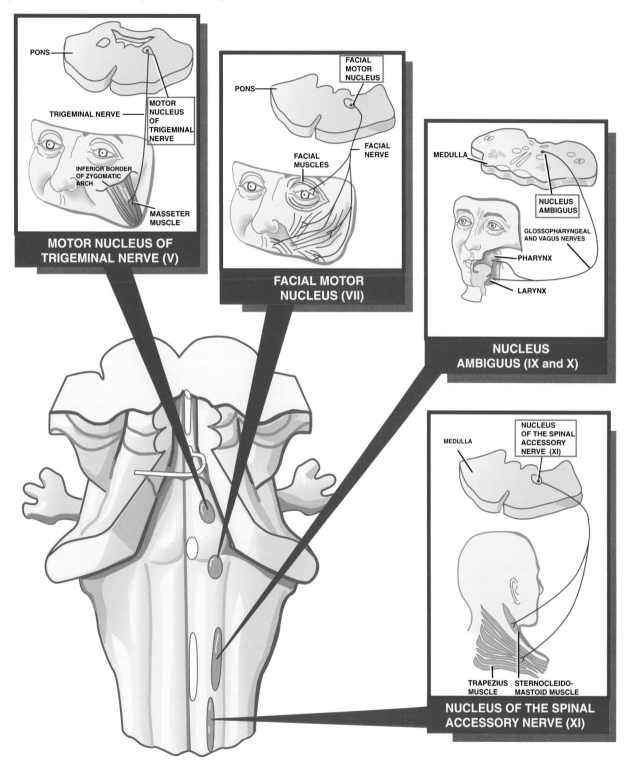

Column 3

See **Fig. 6.4**.

This column is located immediately lateral to column 1. It contains nuclei of preganglionic parasympathetic neurons that innervate the smooth muscles and glands of the head and neck, as well as the thoracic and parts of the abdominal viscera. (Preganglionic parasympathetics originating in sacral segments of the spinal cord supply the rest of the abdominal and pelvic viscera.) In rostro-caudal order, these parasympathetic nuclei include the following three structures:

- *Edinger-Westphal nucleus* (III)   This nucleus contains preganglionic parasympathetic neurons that are projected in the oculomotor nerve (III) to terminate in the ciliary ganglion. The ciliary ganglion contains postganglionic neurons that travel in the short ciliary nerve to innervate the pupillary constrictor and ciliary muscles of the eye. The Edinger-Westphal nucleus is located in the midbrain.
- *Superior and inferior salivatory nuclei* (VII and IX, respectively)   The superior salivatory nucleus contains preganglionic parasympathetic neurons that are projected in the facial nerve (VII) to terminate in the submandibular and pterygopalatine (sphenopalatine) ganglia. The submandibular ganglion contains postganglionic neurons that innervate the sublingual and submandibular glands, and the pterygopalatine ganglion contains postganglionic neurons that innervate the lacrimal gland. The inferior salivatory nucleus contains preganglionic parasympathetic neurons that are projected in the glossopharyngeal nerve (IX) to terminate in the otic ganglion. The otic ganglion contains postganglionic neurons that innervate the parotid gland. The superior and inferior salivatory nuclei are located in the medulla.
- *Dorsal motor nucleus of the vagus* (X)   This nucleus projects fibers carried in the vagus nerve that innervate the heart, lungs, and gastrointestinal tract. It is located in the medulla.

Fig. 6.4 **Visceral motor nuclei (smooth muscle).**

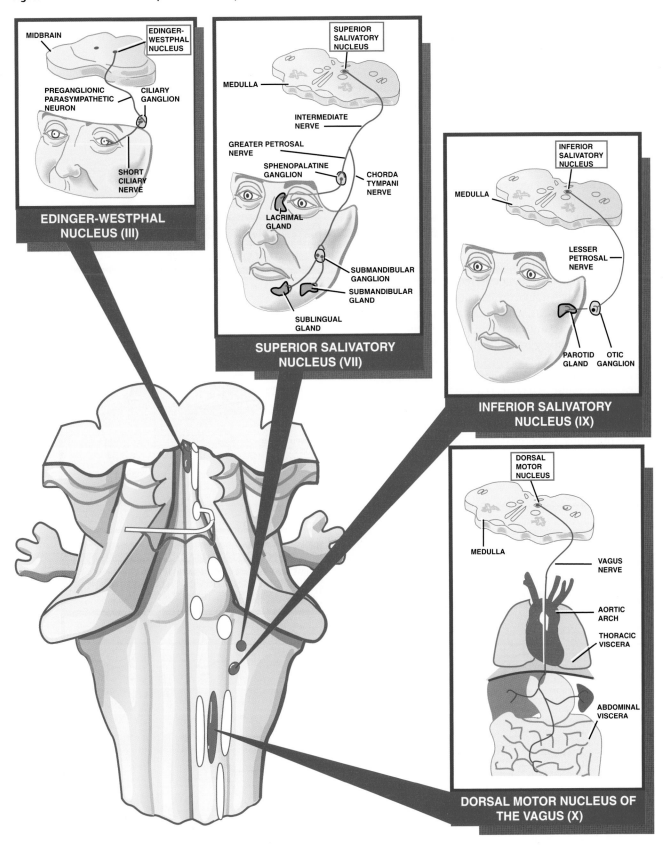

Lateral Columns Contain Three Sensory Nuclei

The lateral columns are composed of sensory nuclei. Unlike most motor nuclei, whose axons are carried in a single corresponding cranial nerve, each sensory nucleus receives input from several different cranial nerves. There are three major sensory nuclei in the brainstem (**Fig. 6.5**):

- The *trigeminal sensory nucleus* comprises three distinct nuclei: the *mesencephalic nucleus*, the *main sensory nucleus*, and the *spinal trigeminal tract nucleus*. These nuclei receive input from the trigeminal (V), facial (VII), glossopharyngeal (IX), and vagus (X) nerves, mediating proprioceptive (mesencephalic), light touch (main sensory), and pain and temperature (spinal trigeminal) sensation.
- The *vestibular* and *cochlear nuclei* extend from the rostral medulla into the pons, receiving input from fibers of the vestibulocochlear nerve (VIII).
- The *solitary nucleus*, which is located in the medulla, receives general and special visceral afferents carried in the facial (VII), glossopharyngeal (IX), and vagus (X) nerves. These nerves mediate taste sensation as well as general visceral sensations of the heart, lungs, and gastrointestinal tract. The cell bodies of these visceral afferents are located in sensory ganglia outside the brainstem; they possess central connections with the thalamus (taste sensation), the reticular formation, and the limbic system of the forebrain.

Fig. 6.5 **Sensory nuclei.**

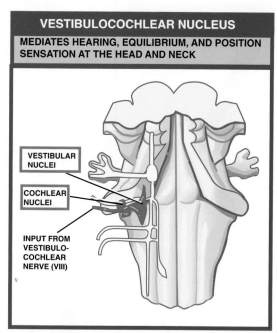

VESTIBULOCOCHLEAR NUCLEUS

MEDIATES HEARING, EQUILIBRIUM, AND POSITION SENSATION AT THE HEAD AND NECK

VESTIBULAR NUCLEI

COCHLEAR NUCLEI

INPUT FROM VESTIBULO-COCHLEAR NERVE (VIII)

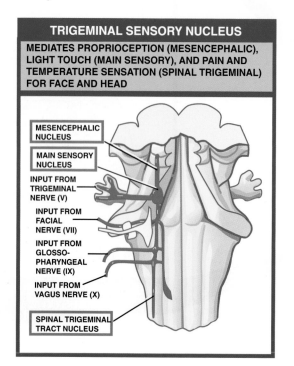

TRIGEMINAL SENSORY NUCLEUS

MEDIATES PROPRIOCEPTION (MESENCEPHALIC), LIGHT TOUCH (MAIN SENSORY), AND PAIN AND TEMPERATURE SENSATION (SPINAL TRIGEMINAL) FOR FACE AND HEAD

MESENCEPHALIC NUCLEUS

MAIN SENSORY NUCLEUS

INPUT FROM TRIGEMINAL NERVE (V)

INPUT FROM FACIAL NERVE (VII)

INPUT FROM GLOSSO-PHARYNGEAL NERVE (IX)

INPUT FROM VAGUS NERVE (X)

SPINAL TRIGEMINAL TRACT NUCLEUS

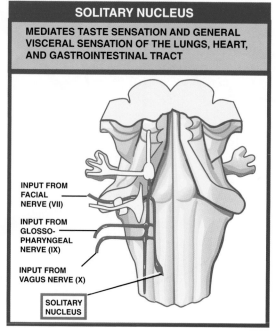

SOLITARY NUCLEUS

MEDIATES TASTE SENSATION AND GENERAL VISCERAL SENSATION OF THE LUNGS, HEART, AND GASTROINTESTINAL TRACT

INPUT FROM FACIAL NERVE (VII)

INPUT FROM GLOSSO-PHARYNGEAL NERVE (IX)

INPUT FROM VAGUS NERVE (X)

SOLITARY NUCLEUS

Long Ascending and Descending Tracts Traverse the Brainstem

Four long tracts, two ascending, two descending, provide landmarks along the transverse axis of the brainstem. The spinothalamic tract lies laterally in the brainstem, whereas the medial lemniscus, the corticospinal tract, and the corticobulbar tract lie medially.

Two Ascending Tracts Occur Laterally and Medially

Spinothalamic Tract

See **Fig. 6.6**.

The lateral and anterior spinothalamic tracts are responsible for pain, temperature, and light touch sensation. They are located in the lateral aspect of the tegmentum throughout the brainstem, adjacent to the descending sympathetic tract. They occur in essentially the same position they occupy in the spinal cord. The spinothalamic tract consists of second-order neurons that originate in the *dorsal gray horn* of the spinal cord, cross the midline in the *anterior white commissure*, and project to the *ventral posterolateral (VPL) nucleus of the thalamus*. Third-order neurons in the VPL thalamus send axons to the *postcentral gyrus*. Because of the close proximity of the spinothalamic tract to the descending sympathetic fibers, both systems are typically impaired as a result of damage to the lateral tegmentum, where they represent important landmarks. An ipsilateral Horner syndrome (descending sympathetic lesion) is thus often associated with a contralateral hemisensory loss (spinothalamic lesion), which may be caused by a lesion in the lateral medulla or pons.

Fig. 6.6 Spinothalamic tract.

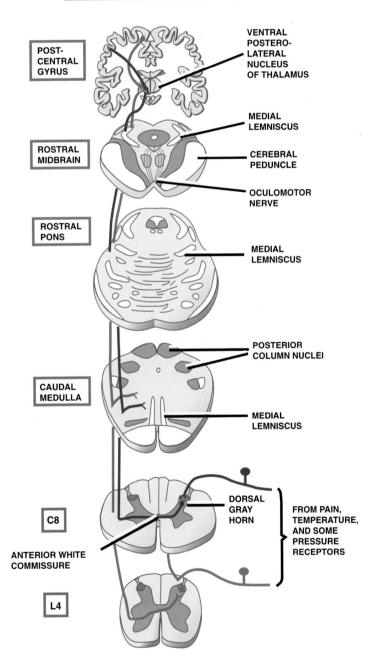

Medial Lemniscus

See **Fig. 6.7**.

The medial lemniscus, which is the rostral continuation of the dorsal columns of the spinal cord, mediates position sense and discriminative touch. It consists of second-order neurons that originate in the *nucleus cuneatus* and *nucleus gracilis*. These nuclei receive input from the spinal cord via the cuneate and gracile fasciculi (dorsal columns), which carry impulses from the upper and lower extremities, respectively. After synapse in the ipsilateral cuneate and gracile nuclei, these axons act as the internal arcuate fibers and ascend to the contralateral VPL thalamus. From here they ascend to the sensory cortex. The medial lemniscus is situated in the medulla close to the midline between the posteriorly situated medial longitudinal fasciculus (MLF) and the anteriorly situated corticospinal and corticopontine tracts. In its rostral ascent, the medial lemniscus moves laterally but remains an important landmark of the medial aspect of the medulla and pons.

Fig. 6.7 **Medial lemniscus.**

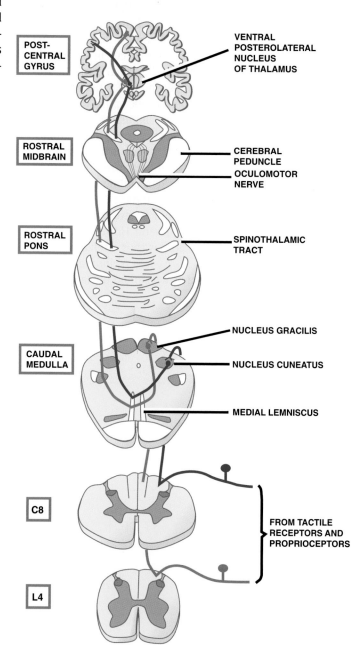

FUNCTION

MEDIATES POSITION, SENSATION, AND DISCRIMINATIVE TOUCH

POST-CENTRAL GYRUS

VENTRAL POSTEROLATERAL NUCLEUS OF THALAMUS

ROSTRAL MIDBRAIN

CEREBRAL PEDUNCLE

OCULOMOTOR NERVE

ROSTRAL PONS

SPINOTHALAMIC TRACT

NUCLEUS GRACILIS

CAUDAL MEDULLA

NUCLEUS CUNEATUS

MEDIAL LEMNISCUS

C8

FROM TACTILE RECEPTORS AND PROPRIOCEPTORS

L4

Two Descending Tracts Occur Medially

Corticospinal Tract

See **Fig. 6.8**.

The corticospinal tract transmits motor-related impulses from the cerebral cortex to laminae IV through IX (few fibers synapse directly with IX motor neurons in laminae IX) of the spinal gray matter. The fibers of this tract traverse the *corona radiata* and the *posterior limb of the internal capsule* and continue in the middle of the midbrain crura cerebri, flanked by more numerous corticopontine fibers on each side. At the level of the pons, the corticospinal tract is broken up into small bundles by transverse pontocerebellar fibers, which cross the midline to reach the contralateral cerebellar hemisphere via the middle cerebellar peduncle. At lower pontine levels, the corticospinal fibers come together again and form the medullary *pyramids*. As they reach the *caudal medulla*, approximately 85% of corticospinal fibers cross the midline in the decussation of the pyramids to form the *lateral corticospinal tract* (the other 15% of fibers continue in the uncrossed *anterior corticospinal tract*, which later decussates in the anterior commissure at cervical and upper thoracic levels). Separate from direct corticopontine fibers, numerous collateral branches of the corticospinal fibers innervate the pontine nuclei, including those of the reticular formation. Like the medial lemniscus, the corticospinal tract courses close to the midline throughout the pons and medulla, providing an important medial brainstem landmark.

Fig. 6.8 Corticospinal tract.

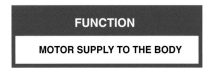

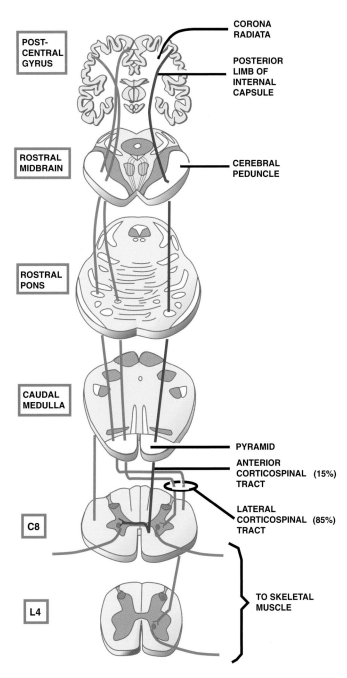

Corticobulbar Tract

See **Fig. 6.9**.

The corticobulbar tract comprises fibers projecting from the cerebral cortex to the lower brainstem. Among the neurons that receive these projections are several motor cranial nerve nuclei, including the trigeminal, facial, and hypoglossal nuclei. Except for part of the facial motor nucleus, the cortical input to these nuclei is more or less symmetrically bilateral. The muscles that receive their supply from these nuclei include the laryngeal, pharyngeal, palatal, upper facial, extraocular, and muscles of mastication. Because of their bilateral innervation, unilateral lesions interrupting the corticobulbar supply of these muscles cause only mild signs of paresis, whereas bilateral lesions are usually significant (pseudobulbar palsy). The clinically familiar contralateral paralysis of lower facial muscles (sparing the forehead) is evidence of predominantly crossed corticobulbar innervation of part of the facial motor nucleus. In addition to this direct corticobulbar pathway, corticoreticular fibers innervate neurons of the reticular formation, which serve to relay impulses indirectly from the cortex to the motor cranial nerve nuclei. As a landmark of the medial brainstem, the corticobulbar tract is associated with the medial lemniscus and the corticospinal tract.

Fig. 6.9 Corticobulbar tract.

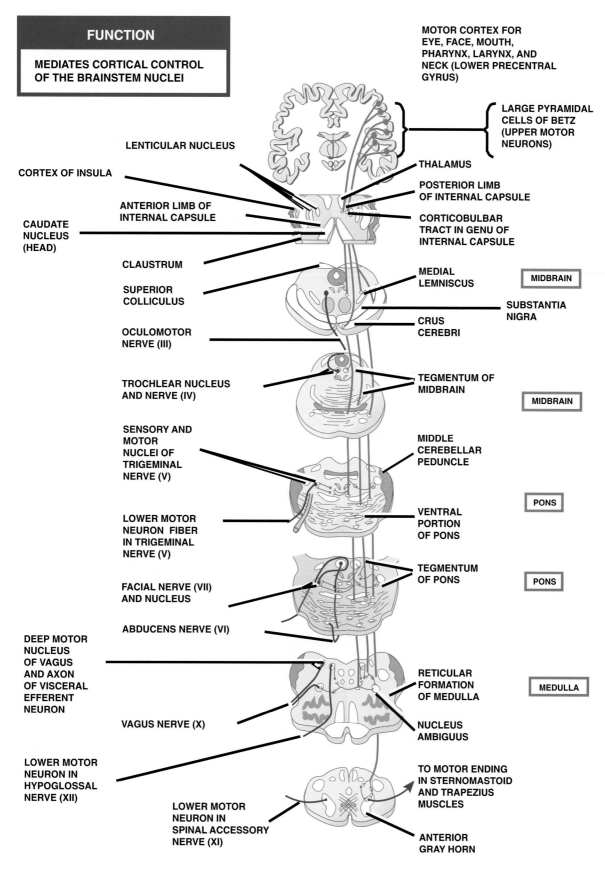

FUNCTION

MEDIATES CORTICAL CONTROL
OF THE BRAINSTEM NUCLEI

MOTOR CORTEX FOR
EYE, FACE, MOUTH,
PHARYNX, LARYNX, AND
NECK (LOWER PRECENTRAL
GYRUS)

LARGE PYRAMIDAL
CELLS OF BETZ
(UPPER MOTOR
NEURONS)

LENTICULAR NUCLEUS

CORTEX OF INSULA

ANTERIOR LIMB OF
INTERNAL CAPSULE

CAUDATE
NUCLEUS
(HEAD)

CLAUSTRUM

SUPERIOR
COLLICULUS

OCULOMOTOR
NERVE (III)

THALAMUS

POSTERIOR LIMB
OF INTERNAL CAPSULE

CORTICOBULBAR
TRACT IN GENU OF
INTERNAL CAPSULE

MEDIAL
LEMNISCUS

SUBSTANTIA
NIGRA

CRUS
CEREBRI

MIDBRAIN

TROCHLEAR NUCLEUS
AND NERVE (IV)

TEGMENTUM OF
MIDBRAIN

MIDBRAIN

SENSORY AND
MOTOR
NUCLEI OF
TRIGEMINAL
NERVE (V)

MIDDLE
CEREBELLAR
PEDUNCLE

LOWER MOTOR
NEURON FIBER
IN TRIGEMINAL
NERVE (V)

VENTRAL
PORTION
OF PONS

PONS

FACIAL NERVE (VII)
AND NUCLEUS

TEGMENTUM
OF PONS

PONS

ABDUCENS NERVE (VI)

DEEP MOTOR
NUCLEUS
OF VAGUS
AND AXON
OF VISCERAL
EFFERENT
NEURON

RETICULAR
FORMATION
OF MEDULLA

MEDULLA

VAGUS NERVE (X)

NUCLEUS
AMBIGUUS

LOWER MOTOR
NEURON IN
HYPOGLOSSAL
NERVE (XII)

TO MOTOR ENDING
IN STERNOMASTOID
AND TRAPEZIUS
MUSCLES

LOWER MOTOR
NEURON IN
SPINAL ACCESSORY
NERVE (XI)

ANTERIOR
GRAY HORN

Reciprocal Fibers Connect the Brainstem and Cerebellum

Three large fiber bundles, or cerebellar peduncles, connect the cerebellum to the brainstem. The superior, middle, and inferior cerebellar peduncles contain afferent and efferent fibers that pass between the cerebellum and the midbrain, pons, and medulla, respectively. The following brainstem nuclei are divided into those that send afferents to the cerebellum and those that receive cerebellar efferents.

Afferent Cerebellar Connections

The brainstem nuclei that send afferents to the cerebellum include the following (**Fig. 6.10**):

- *Pontine nuclei*   Corticopontine fibers originating in widespread areas throughout the cerebral cortex descend through the *internal capsule* and the *cerebral peduncles* to terminate in the *pontine nuclei*. These nuclei project crossed fibers that proceed through the *middle cerebellar peduncles* to reach the contralateral cerebellar hemisphere. Impulses from the cerebral cortex are concerned with the initiation and planning of movements. The pontine nuclei also relay information from the lateral geniculate body, the superior colliculus, and the striate cortex concerning vision.

- *Inferior olivary nucleus*   This nucleus is located in the rostral medulla. It receives input from widespread areas of the central nervous system, including the spinal cord, the brainstem, and the cerebral cortex. This input involves multiple sensory and motor impulses that cross the midline through the *inferior cerebellar peduncle* to reach the contralateral cerebellar hemisphere.

- *Vestibular nuclei*   These nuclei are located in the rostral medulla. Vestibular projections traverse the inferior cerebellar peduncle to terminate in the ipsilateral cerebellar hemisphere, providing information about eye movements, head movements, and changes in the position of the head.

- *Reticular formation*   Reticulocerebellar fibers originating in the medulla and pons project through the inferior cerebellar peduncles to both the ipsilateral and contralateral cerebellar hemispheres. They serve to integrate and relay information received from widespread parts of the central nervous system, including the spinal cord and higher regions of the brain.

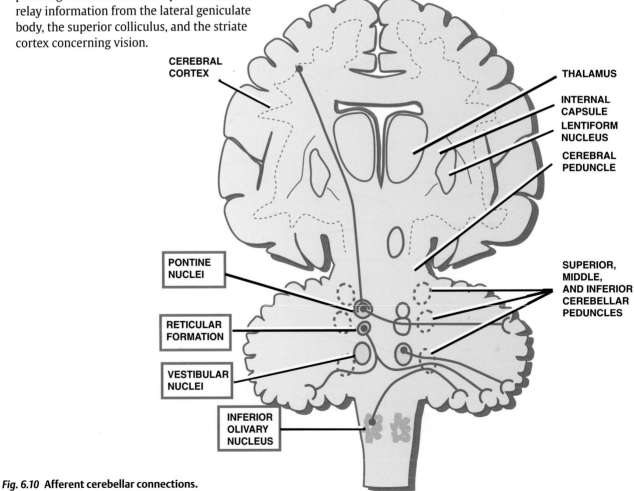

Fig. 6.10 **Afferent cerebellar connections.**

Efferent Cerebellar Connections

The following brainstem nuclei receive cerebellar efferents (**Fig. 6.11**):

- *Red nucleus*   This nucleus is located in the tegmentum of the midbrain just dorsal to the substantia nigra. It receives cerebellar fibers from the contralateral cerebellar hemisphere that cross the midline in the decussation of the *superior cerebellar peduncles*. The efferent fibers of the red nucleus descend in the crossed *rubrospinal tract* so that the red nucleus relays cerebellar impulses that influence flexor muscle tone on the ipsilateral side of the body.

- *Vestibular nuclei*   These nuclei receive input from the ipsilateral cerebellar hemisphere via the inferior cerebellar peduncle. They influence, in turn, (1) equilibrium and control of axial musculature (extensive muscle tone) via the uncrossed *vestibulospinal tract*, and (2) the coordination of eye movements via the uncrossed medial longitudinal fasciculus.

- *Reticular formation*   Cerebelloreticular fibers reach the ipsilateral reticular formation in the pons and medulla via the inferior cerebellar peduncle. The reticular formation, in turn, influences extensor muscle tone via the uncrossed pontine and medullary *reticulospinal tract*.

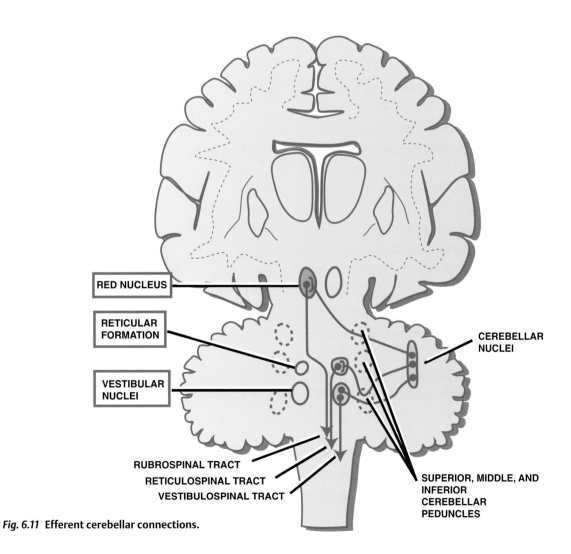

Fig. 6.11 **Efferent cerebellar connections.**

The Reticular Formation Is a Diffuse Aggregation of Cells in the Central Brainstem that Possesses an Unusually Wide Range of Neural Connections and Functions

Reticular neurons may be viewed as the rostral extension of spinal interneurons. Their widespread network of axonal projections from the brainstem are distributed rostrally as far as higher regions of the brain, and caudally as far as the spinal cord (**Fig. 6.12**).

- The *magnocellular zone*, which contains large cells that give rise to long ascending and descending pathways, is located in the medial two thirds of the reticular formation.
- The *parvocellular zone* contains predominantly small cells that send axons to the medial central nuclei.

The Reticular Formation Influences Several Functional Systems

Reticular formation (RF) function includes the following:

- *Motor control*   Reticular neurons influence muscle tone by innervating alpha and gamma spinal motor neurons via the descending reticulospinal tracts. These tracts originate in the medial portion of the medulla and pons and exert both facilitatory and inhibitory effects on extensor muscle tone. Because they receive ascending spinal impulses as well as descending impulses from the cerebellum and cerebral cortex, reticular neurons integrate and exercise a wide array of influences on motor control. The pontine reticular spinal tract is facilitating to extensive tone but is held in check by the medullary reticular spinal tract, which acts to inhibit this facilitatory action. The medullary reticular spinal tract is under facilitatory control of the cerebral cortex. An injury to the brainstem caudal to the red nucleus but rostral to the vestibular and reticular spinal nuclei results in extensor posturing. This occurs because the red nuclei projections (reticular spinal tract, flexor facilitator) are severed, and the cortical input to the medullary reticular spinal tract is also severed. This results in unapposed extensor tone initiated by the lateral vestibulospinal and pontine reticulospinal tracts.

- *Control of respiratory and cardiovascular systems* Respiratory-related reticular neurons are spread throughout the brainstem. The dorsal respiratory center is located in the dorsal medulla and controls inspiration. It is the main respiratory center. The ventral respiratory center is located in the ventrolateral medulla. It controls both inspiration and expiration but only during significant respiratory effects. The pneumotaxic center controls the rate and pattern of breathing and is located in the dorsal rostral pons. Reticular neurons receive afferent impulses from many sources and are directly influenced as well by the carbon dioxide content of the blood (more accurately the H^+ content of the blood). They send efferent impulses via reticulospinal pathways to end on spinal motor neurons that innervate the respiratory muscles. Cardiovascular–related reticular neurons are also involved in complex polysynaptic pathways. They receive afferent impulses from many sources, including peripheral sensory receptors such as the carotid sinus and higher regions of the brain such as the hypothalamus. They send efferent impulses via the reticulospinal tracts to end on spinal neurons that innervate both the heart and the peripheral circulation.

- *Sensory control*   Reticulospinal pathways modulate the sense of pain at the level of the dorsal horn of the spinal cord.

- *Consciousness*   The ascending reticular formation activating system (ARAS) modulates wakefulness and arousal. It receives collaterals from the long ascending sensory pathways, including the medial lemniscal and spinothalamic tracts. Efferent impulses are conducted via thalamic nuclei to widespread areas of the cerebral cortex. Stimulation of the reticular neurons of the ARAS induces wakefulness. These changes are reflected in the electroencephalogram (EEG), which records electrical activity in the cerebral cortex. The low voltage–high frequency activity of arousal replaces the high voltage–slow wave activity of somnolence. Brainstem lesions affecting the ARAS typically result in the impairment of consciousness—in the most extreme cases, causing coma.

Fig. 6.12 Reticular formation (RF).

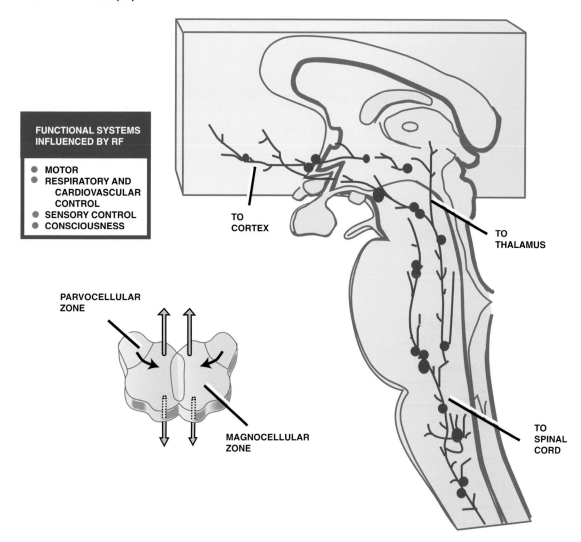

FUNCTIONAL SYSTEMS
INFLUENCED BY RF

- MOTOR
- RESPIRATORY AND
  CARDIOVASCULAR
  CONTROL
- SENSORY CONTROL
- CONSCIOUSNESS

TO
CORTEX

TO
THALAMUS

PARVOCELLULAR
ZONE

MAGNOCELLULAR
ZONE

TO
SPINAL
CORD

The Blood Supply of the Brainstem Is Derived from Branches of the Vertebral and Basilar Arteries

See **Fig. 6.13**.

Branches of the vertebral and basilar arteries may be conceptually subdivided into paramedian, short circumferential, and long circumferential branches. They supply the medial, anterolateral, and posterolateral brainstem, respectively.

Intracranially, each vertebral artery, which takes origin in the subclavian artery on the same side of the body, gives rise to (1) a posterior spinal artery (not shown in figure), (2) an *anterior spinal artery*, and (3) a *posteroinferior cerebellar artery*.

At the level of the pontomedullary junction, the two vertebral arteries come together to form the basilar artery, which gives rise to (1) the *anteroinferior cerebellar arteries*, (2) the *superior cerebellar arteries*, and (3) the *posterior cerebral arteries*. Numerous small paramedian and circumferential pontine branches also arise from the basilar artery.

Fig. 6.13 **Arterial supply.**

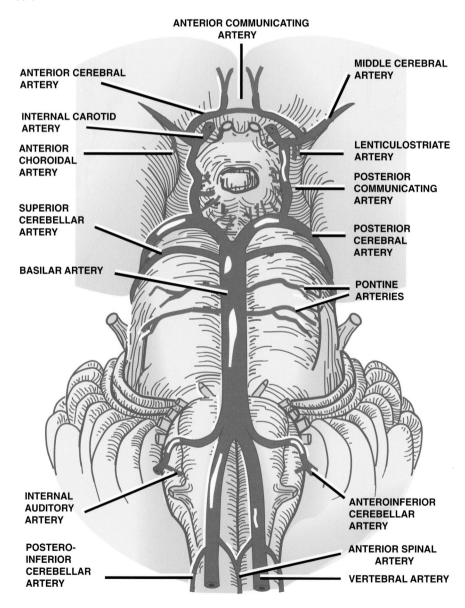

Most of the Midbrain Is Supplied by Branches of the Basilar Artery

See **Fig. 6.14**.

The predominant branch of the basilar artery that supplies the midbrain, the *posterior cerebral artery*, contributes *paramedian*, *short circumferential*, and *long circumferential branches*. The *superior cerebellar artery*, which takes off from the basilar artery just proximal to its bifurcation as the paired posterior cerebral arteries, also contributes short and long circumferential branches. As an exception to the otherwise exclusive supply of the brainstem by the vertebrobasilar system, the rostralmost midbrain receives supply from the internal carotid artery system via the posterior communicating artery.

Fig. 6.14 Arterial supply of the midbrain.

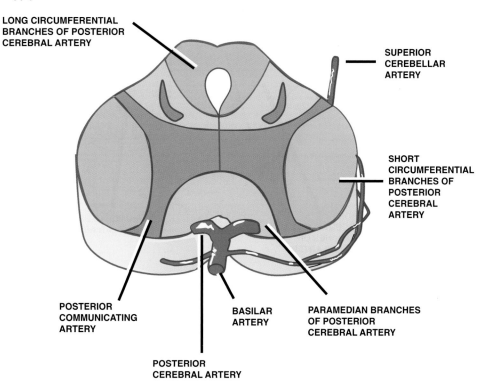

LONG CIRCUMFERENTIAL
BRANCHES OF POSTERIOR
CEREBRAL ARTERY

SUPERIOR
CEREBELLAR
ARTERY

SHORT
CIRCUMFERENTIAL
BRANCHES OF
POSTERIOR
CEREBRAL
ARTERY

POSTERIOR
COMMUNICATING
ARTERY

BASILAR
ARTERY

PARAMEDIAN BRANCHES
OF POSTERIOR
CEREBRAL ARTERY

POSTERIOR
CEREBRAL ARTERY

The Pons Is Supplied by Branches of the Basilar Artery

See **Fig. 6.15**.

The medial basal pons, including the corticospinal tract and the medial lemniscus, is supplied by *paramedian branches of the basilar artery*.

The lateral pons, including the spinothalamic tract, the descending sympathetic fibers, and the spinal tract and nucleus of the trigeminal nerve, is supplied by the superior cerebellar artery rostrally and the anteroinferior cerebellar artery caudally. Like the paramedian vessels, both of these arteries arise from the basilar artery.

Fig. 6.15 Arterial supply of the pons.

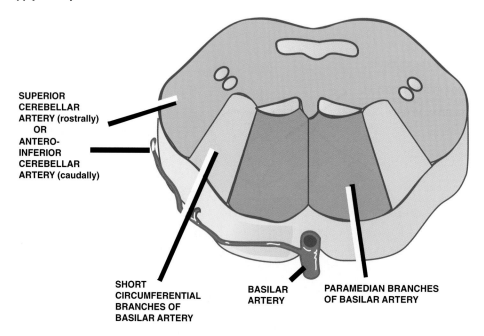

The Medulla Is Supplied by Branches of the Vertebral Artery

See **Fig. 6.16.**

The medial portion of the medulla, including the corticospinal tract and the medial lemniscus, is supplied by the vertebral artery or, at lower medullary levels, the anterior spinal artery.

The lateral portion of the medulla, including the spinothalamic tract, the descending sympathetic fibers, and the spinal tract and nucleus of the trigeminal nerve, is supplied by the vertebral artery or the posterior inferior cerebellar artery.

Fig. 6.16 Arterial supply of the medulla.

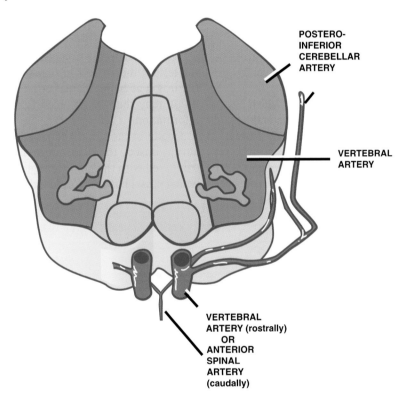

POSTERO-INFERIOR CEREBELLAR ARTERY

VERTEBRAL ARTERY

VERTEBRAL ARTERY (rostrally) OR ANTERIOR SPINAL ARTERY (caudally)

Constellations of Cranial Nerve and Long Tract Signs Provide Clues to the Localization of Brainstem Lesions

See **Fig. 6.17**.

Brainstem lesions are a common cause of neurologic dysfunction. Because both ascending and descending tracts and brainstem nuclei are located in the brainstem in close relation to one another, brainstem lesions typically damage several structures simultaneously.

A logical approach to the localization of brainstem lesions rests on four organizational principles: (1) functionally distinct ascending and descending tracts are spread along the transverse axis, (2) functionally distinct cranial nerve nuclei are spread along the rostrocaudal axis, (3) long tract signs occur contralateral to the lesion, and (4) cranial nerve signs occur ipsilateral to the lesion.

Three groups of cranial nerve nuclei aid in localizing the level of a brainstem lesion:

- The *oculomotor* and *trochlear nuclei*, which produce diplopia and ipsilateral pupillary disturbances with ptosis (oculomotor nerve), are located at the level of the midbrain.
- The *abducens nucleus* and the *facial nucleus*, which produce diplopia (abducens nerve) and ipsilateral facial weakness (facial nerve), are located at the level of the *pons*.
- The *nucleus ambiguus* (IX, X, and XI), the *dorsal motor nucleus* of the vagus, and the *hypoglossal nucleus*, which produce disturbances of speech and swallowing, are located at the level of the *medulla*.

Localizing long tracts include the following:

- The *corticospinal tract* and the *medial lemniscus*, which produce hemiplegia (corticospinal tract) and loss of vibratory and position sensation (medial lemniscus) on the side opposite the lesion, are located medial in the brainstem.
- The *lateral spinothalamic tract* and the descending sympathetic fibers, which produce contralateral loss of pain and temperature sensation (spinothalamic tract) and an ipsilateral Horner syndrome (descending sympathetic fibers), are located lateral in the brainstem.

The sine qua non of a lesion in the brainstem is thus the "crossed motor/sensory syndrome": motor/sensory loss affecting one side of the face and the opposite side of the body. This results because cranial nerve nuclei and long ascending and descending tracts produce ipsilateral and contralateral signs, respectively.

Two questions should arise regarding the patient with a crossed motor/sensory syndrome:

- What cranial nerves are involved?
- What long tracts are involved?

The answer to the first question identifies the level of the lesion; the answer to the second question identifies the lesion as being medial or lateral. Localization of the lesion may then be deduced from these two pieces of information.

Finally, in the clinical context of a vascular lesion (i.e., abrupt onset), the distribution of the lesion should be compared with the brainstem blood supply to determine which vessel has been occluded.

There Are Seven Major Vascular Brainstem Syndromes

See **Fig. 6.17**.

Identifying syndromes is an integral part of neurologic diagnosis. This is particularly true in the localization of brainstem lesions, which rarely result in only a single symptom.

Prompt syndrome identification lends efficiency to accurate anatomic diagnosis, and this is best accomplished by the application of the principles already outlined, in addition to familiarity with common brainstem syndromes. Two medullary, two pontine, and three midbrain syndromes are described following here. In most cases, these syndromes are manifestations of ischemia or infarction, and where appropriate the responsible artery is identified.

A word of caution: syndromes rarely occur in textbook form. A flexible mind is needed to correctly analyze and interpret the constellation of signs and symptoms with which patients, in the real world, present.

Fig. 6.17 **Brainstem localization.**

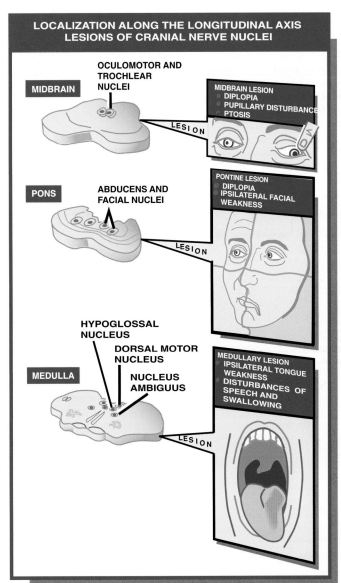

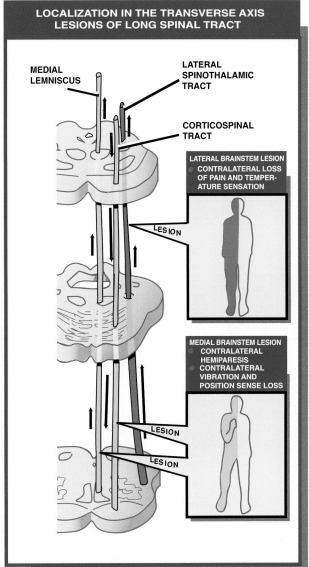

Lateral Medullary Syndrome (Wallenberg Syndrome)

See **Fig. 6.18**.

The lateral medulla is supplied by the vertebral artery or the posteroinferior cerebellar artery. Occlusion of these arteries produces the following signs and symptoms:

- **Ipsilateral impairment of facial pain and temperature sensation** (due to involvement of the *spinal tract and nucleus of the trigeminal nerve*)
- **Contralateral impairment of body pain and temperature sensation** (due to involvement of the *spinothalamic tract*)
- **Ipsilateral limb and gait ataxia** (due to involvement of *cerebellar connections*)
- **Ipsilateral Horner syndrome: ptosis, miosis, anhydrosis** (due to involvement of the *descending sympathetic fibers*)
- **Nausea, vomiting, vertigo, and nystagmus** (due to involvement of the *vestibular nuclei and connections*)
- **Dysphagia and dysarthria** (due to involvement of the *nucleus ambiguus*)

Fig. 6.18 Lateral medullary syndrome (Wallenberg syndrome).

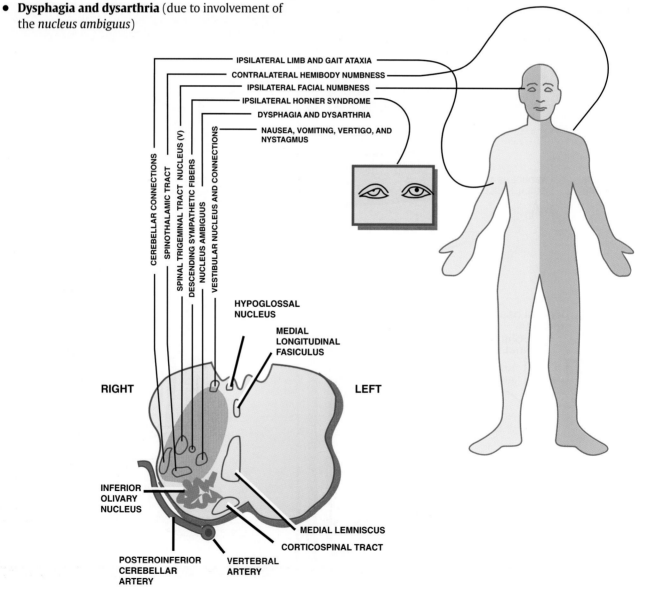

Medial Medullary Syndrome (Dejerine's Syndrome)

See **Fig. 6.19**.

The medial medulla contains the corticospinal tract, the medial lemniscus, and the hypoglossal nucleus. It is supplied by the vertebral artery or the anterior spinal artery. Occlusion of these arteries produces the following signs and symptoms:

- **Contralateral hemiparesis** (due to involvement of the *corticospinal tract*)
- **Contralateral loss of vibratory and position sense** (due to involvement of the *medial lemniscus*)
- **Ipsilateral paralysis of the tongue** (tongue deviates to side of lesion due to involvement of the *hypoglossal nucleus*)

Note that the dorsolateral spinothalamic tract is not affected. Therefore, pain and temperature sensation is spared. Bilateral lesions of the medial medulla result in quadriplegia (with facial sparing), complete paralysis of the tongue, and complete loss of vibratory and position sensation below the head.

Fig. 6.19 **Medial medullary syndrome (Dejerine's syndrome).**

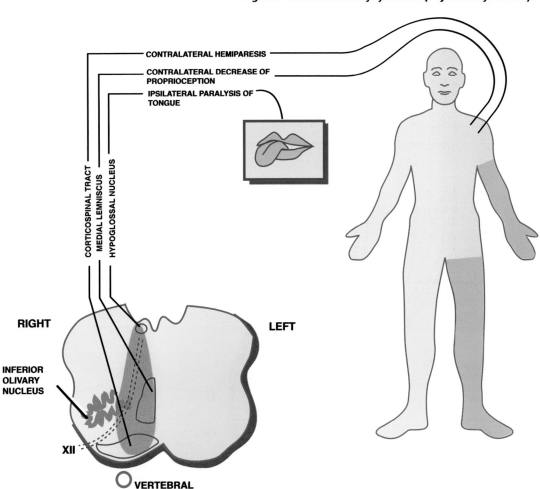

Lateral Pontine Syndrome (Millard-Gubler Syndrome)

See **Fig. 6.20**.

The lateral pons is supplied by the anteroinferior cerebellar artery caudally and the superior cerebellar artery rostrally. Occlusion of one or the other of these arteries causes the following signs and symptoms:

- **Ipsilateral impairment of facial pain and temperature sensation** (due to involvement of the *spinal tract and nucleus of the trigeminal nerve*)
- **Contralateral impairment of body pain and temperature sensation** (due to involvement of the *spinothalamic tract*)

- **Ipsilateral Horner syndrome** (due to involvement of *descending sympathetic fibers*)
- **Nausea, vomiting, vertigo, and nystagmus** (due to involvement of *vestibular nuclei and connections*)
- **Ipsilateral limb and gait ataxia** (due to involvement of *inferior cerebellar peduncle*)
- **Ipsilateral facial paralysis** (due to involvement of the *facial nerve*)
- **Paralysis of gaze to the side of the lesion** (due to involvement of the *paramedian pontine reticular formation*)
- **Deafness and tinnitus** (due to involvement of the *cochlear nerve or nucleus*)

Fig. 6.20 **Lateral pontine syndrome (Millard-Gubler syndrome).**

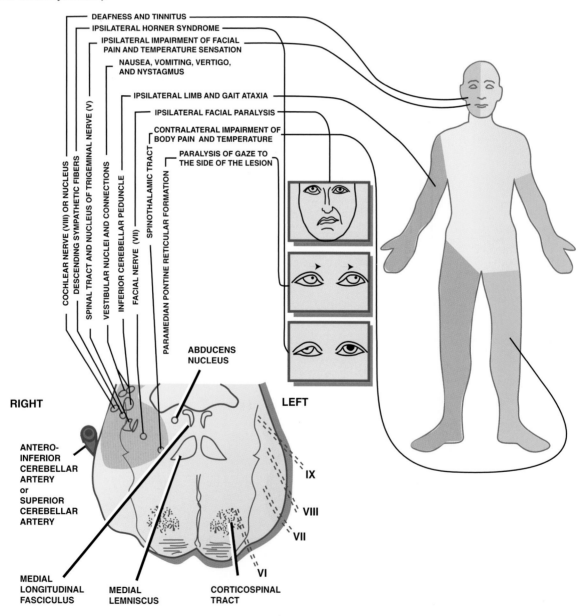

Medial Pontine Syndrome

See **Fig. 6.21**.

The medial pons is supplied by paramedian branches of the basilar artery. Occlusion of these arteries produces the following signs and symptoms:

- **Contralateral hemiparesis** (due to involvement of the *corticospinal tract*)
- **Contralateral loss of vibratory and position sense** (due to involvement of the *medial lemniscus*)
- **Ipsilateral limb and gait ataxia** (due to involvement of *cerebellar connections*)
- **Paralysis of the ipsilateral lateral rectus muscle** (due to involvement of the *abducens nerve*)

- **Internuclear ophthalmoplegia** (due to involvement of the *medial longitudinal fasciculus*)
- **Paralysis of gaze to the side of the lesion** (due to involvement of the *paramedian pontine reticular formation*)

Bilateral ventral pontine lesions (secondary to thrombosis of the basilar artery) result in the dramatic "locked-in syndrome." This consists of quadriplegia and complete aphonia due to interruption of the corticospinal and corticopontine pathways. The patient remains alert but is rendered immobile (with sparing of the oculomotor system) and noncommunicative.

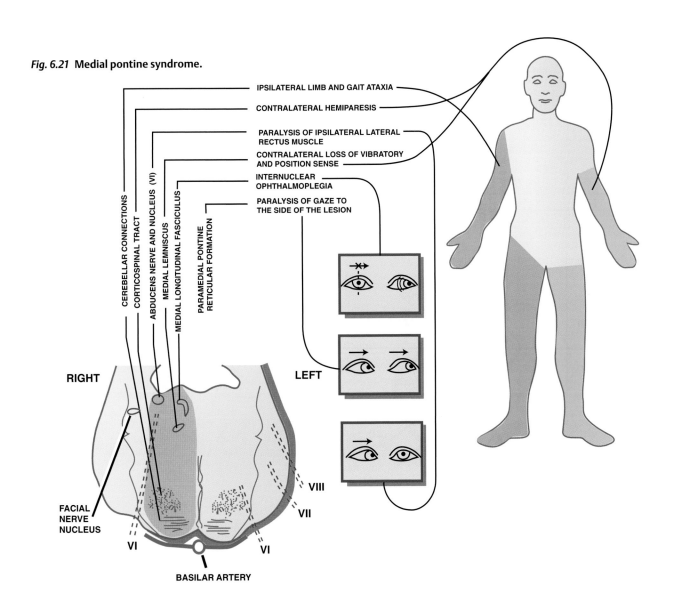

Fig. 6.21 **Medial pontine syndrome.**

IPSILATERAL LIMB AND GAIT ATAXIA

CONTRALATERAL HEMIPARESIS

PARALYSIS OF IPSILATERAL LATERAL RECTUS MUSCLE

CONTRALATERAL LOSS OF VIBRATORY AND POSITION SENSE

INTERNUCLEAR OPHTHALMOPLEGIA

PARALYSIS OF GAZE TO THE SIDE OF THE LESION

CEREBELLAR CONNECTIONS

CORTICOSPINAL TRACT

ABDUCENS NERVE AND NUCLEUS (VI)

MEDIAL LEMNISCUS

MEDIAL LONGITUDINAL FASCICULUS

PARAMEDIAL PONTINE RETICULAR FORMATION

RIGHT

LEFT

FACIAL NERVE NUCLEUS

VI

VIII

VII

VI

BASILAR ARTERY

Ventral Midbrain Syndrome (Weber's Syndrome)

See **Fig. 6.22.**

A lesion of the cerebral peduncle affects the corticospinal tract and fibers of the oculomotor nerve. This results in the following signs and symptoms:

- **Contralateral hemiparesis** (due to involvement of the *corticospinal tract*)
- **Ipsilateral third nerve palsy** (due to involvement of the oculomotor nucleus and nerve, including its parasympathetic fibers)

Fig. 6.22 **Ventral midbrain syndrome (Weber's syndrome).**

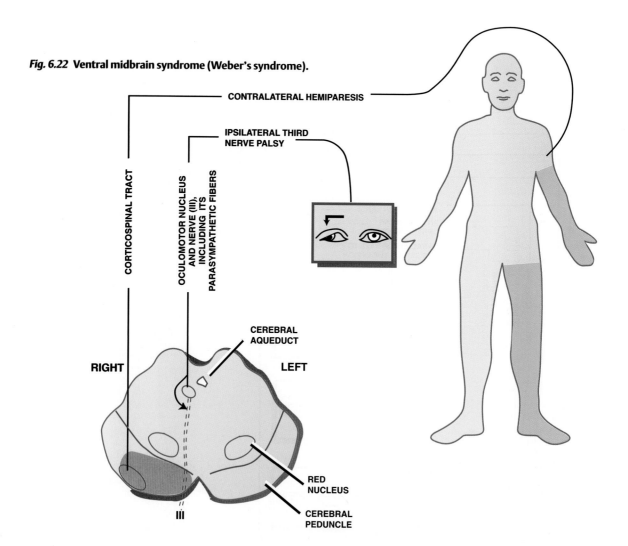

Central (Tegmental) Midbrain Syndrome (Benedikt's Syndrome)

See **Fig. 6.23**.

A lesion of the tegmentum of the midbrain affects the oculomotor nerve, the red nucleus, and the medial lemniscus. This results in the following signs and symptoms:

- **Ipsilateral third nerve palsy** (due to involvement of the oculomotor nucleus and nerve, including its parasympathetic fibers)
- **Tremor or involuntary movements of the contralateral limbs** (due to involvement of the *red nucleus*)
- **Impairment of contralateral vibratory and position sensation** (due to involvement of the *medial lemniscus*)

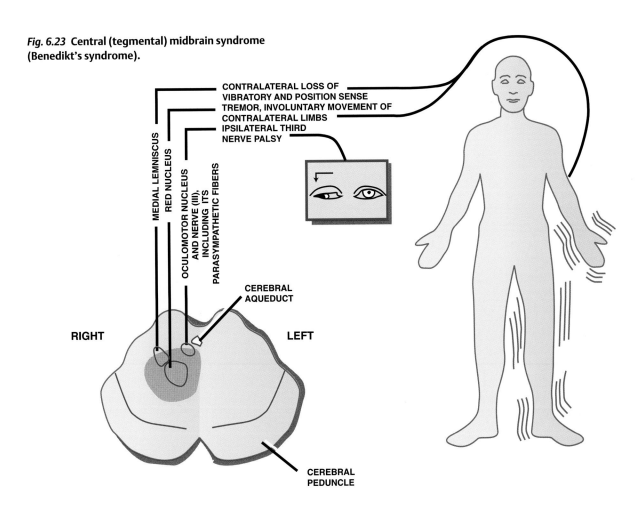

Fig. 6.23 **Central (tegmental) midbrain syndrome (Benedikt's syndrome).**

Dorsal Midbrain Syndrome (Parinaud's Syndrome)

See **Fig. 6.24**.

The responsible lesion, usually a tumor in the pineal region or hydrocephalus, results in compression of the *superior colliculi and tectum*, causing **isolated paralysis of upward gaze**, **pupillary dilation**, **lid retraction**, **convergence-retraction nystagmus**, and **dissociated near-light response** (near objects cause pupil to respond—accommodation—but there is no pupillary response to light).

Fig. 6.24 Dorsal midbrain syndrome (Parinaud's syndrome).

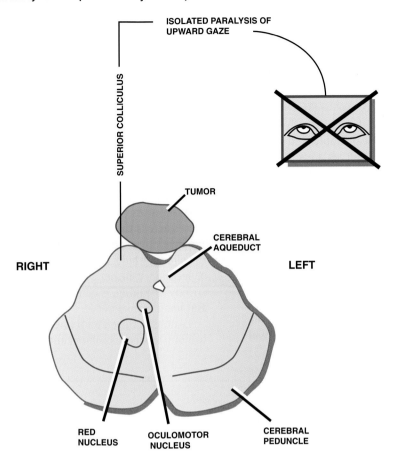

ISOLATED PARALYSIS OF UPWARD GAZE

SUPERIOR COLLICULUS

TUMOR

CEREBRAL AQUEDUCT

RIGHT

LEFT

RED NUCLEUS

OCULOMOTOR NUCLEUS

CEREBRAL PEDUNCLE

SIGNS AND SYMPTOMS

- IMPAIRED UPWARD GAZE
- PUPILLARY DILATATION
- LID RETRACTION
- CONVERGENCE-RETRACTION NYSTAGMUS
- DISSOCIATED NEAR-LIGHT RESPONSE

7 Cranial Nerves

Because of the density of their distribution throughout the brainstem, their heavy cortical supply, and their extracranial extension, the cranial nerves are sensitive indicators of both central and peripheral nervous system dysfunction. As such, an assessment of their integrity based on a knowledge of their anatomy is an important aspect of even a brief neurologic examination.

Collectively, the cranial nerves serve three functions:

- They supply motor and sensory input to the head and neck.
- They innervate the special sense organs.
- They carry parasympathetic nerve fibers responsible for visceral functions, such as pupillary constriction, gland secretion, breathing, blood pressure, and swallowing.

Cranial nerves are identified by their functional components, which indicate their function (sensory or motor) and the embryological origin of the target organ they innervate (visceral or somatic). Five functional components are distinguished: somatic sensory, somatic motor, visceral sensory, visceral motor, and special sense, the latter of which includes vision (II), hearing (VIII), taste (VII, IX, X), and smell (I). On the basis of their functional components, cranial nerves are classified as purely sensory (I, II, and VIII), purely motor (III, IV, VI, XI, and XII), or mixed (V, VII, IX, and X).

This chapter describes (1) the structure and function of the 12 cranial nerves, (2) the common signs and symptoms of cranial nerve dysfunction, and (3) the methods of cranial nerve testing. Subsequent chapters provide further discussion of the special senses, the somatic sensation of the face and head, and the autonomic nervous system.

The Olfactory Nerve

See **Fig. 7.1**.

The *first-order sensory neurons* of the olfactory system reside in the nasal cavity. They transduce chemical stimuli into impulses that travel via unmyelinated central processes across the *cribriform plate* of the ethmoid bone to synapse on *second-order sensory neurons* that make up the *olfactory bulb*. Because the olfactory bulb is composed of secondary, rather than primary, sensory neurons, it is, strictly speaking, a central nervous system (CNS) tract and not a cranial nerve.

Lesions of the olfactory nerve result from head trauma, tumors, tobacco smoking, and the common cold.

Fig. 7.1 **Olfactory nerve.**

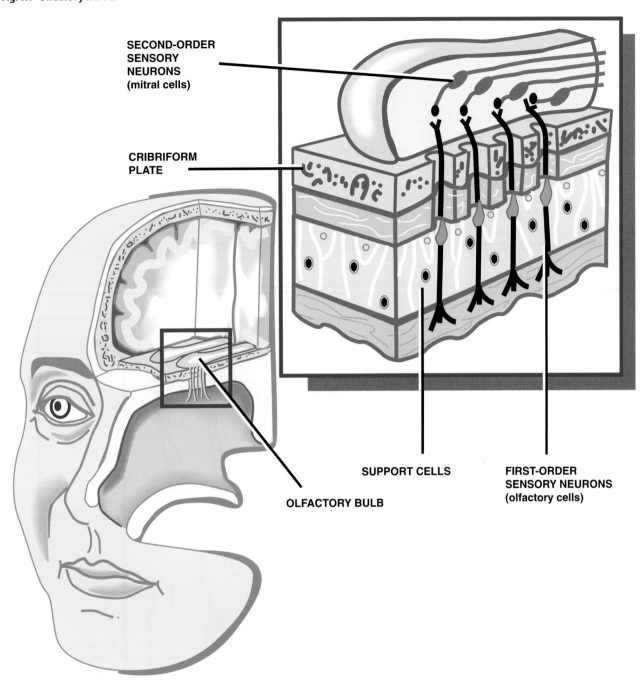

SECOND-ORDER
SENSORY
NEURONS
(mitral cells)

CRIBRIFORM
PLATE

OLFACTORY BULB

SUPPORT CELLS

FIRST-ORDER
SENSORY NEURONS
(olfactory cells)

The Optic Nerve and the Retina

See **Fig. 7.2**.

Like the olfactory nerve, the optic nerve is not composed of primary sensory neurons and is therefore, strictly speaking, not a peripheral nerve but a CNS tract. Axons in this tract originate in retinal *ganglion cells*, which carry impulses generated in the photoreceptor cell layer (*rods* and *cones*) that are relayed by the intermediary bipolar cells. Projected ganglion cell fibers converge on the *optic disc*, turn dorsally, penetrate the sclera, and form the optic nerve.

From the eyeball, the optic nerve exits the orbit through the optic canal to enter the middle cranial fossa, where it joins the contralateral optic nerve to form the optic chiasm. Central connections of the optic chiasm are described in Chapter 15.

Fig. 7.2 **Retina.**

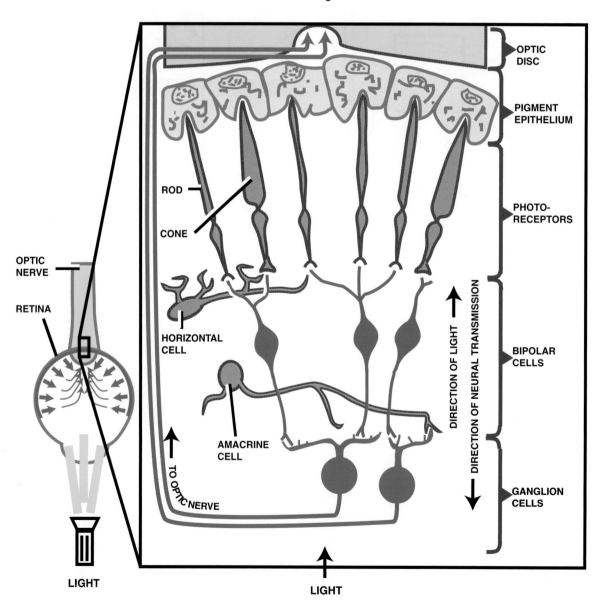

Papilledema

See **Fig. 7.3**.

The central retinal artery and vein pass through the ventral aspect of the optic nerve, which is surrounded by the three meningeal layers and bathed within the cerebrospinal fluid (CSF)–containing subarachnoid space. Because the optic nerve is confluent with the CSF, elevated CSF pressure secondary to elevated intracranial pressure is transmitted to the *optic nerve* and *disc*. The funduscopic picture that develops in this setting of increased intracranial pressure, known as papilledema, consists of (1) retinal vein engorgement and (2) blurring of the margins of the optic discs.

In addition to increased intracranial pressure, the optic nerve is subject to a variety of pathological processes, including tumors and infections, as well as toxins such as methyl alcohol. Optic neuritis, a remitting relapsing inflammatory process causing visual loss and pain, is a common complication of multiple sclerosis.

Fig. 7.3 Pathophysiology of papilledema.

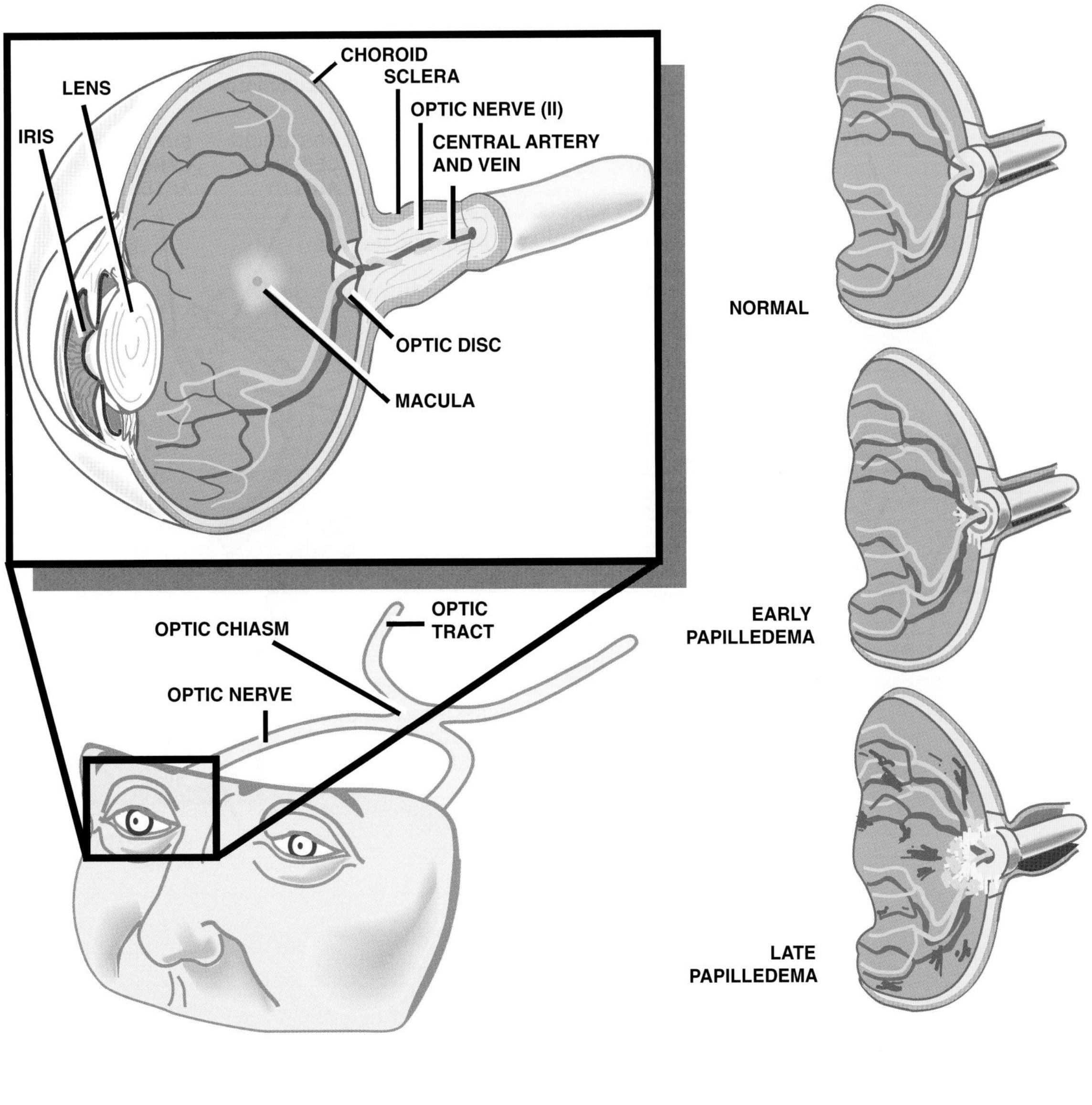

The Oculomotor Nerve

See **Fig. 7.4**.

The oculomotor nucleus is located in the midbrain at the level of the *superior colliculus*. Peripheral axons pass ventrally in the tegmentum of the midbrain. They penetrate the *red nucleus* and the *cerebral peduncles* to emerge between the *posterior cerebral* and *superior cerebellar arteries* in the interpeduncular fossa at the junction of the midbrain and the pons. After penetrating the dura, the oculomotor nerve courses laterally along the wall of the *cavernous sinus* and enters the orbit through the *superior orbital fissure*. At the orbital apex, the oculomotor nerve passes through the *anulus of Zinn*, which is the common tendinous origin of the extraocular muscles.

Somatic motor components of the oculomotor nerve innervate the *levator palpebrae superioris*, which is responsible for the elevation of the upper eyelid, and four of the six extraocular muscles: the medial, superior, and inferior recti and the inferior oblique (the abducens nerve supplies the lateral rectus, and the trochlear nerve supplies the superior oblique).

Fig. 7.4 **Anatomy of oculomotor nerve (III).**

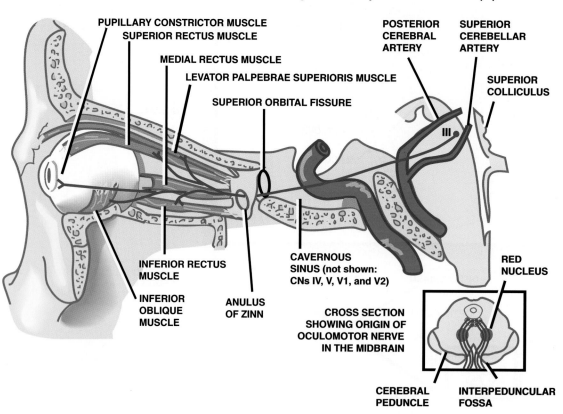

Parasympathetic Components

See **Fig. 7.5**.

Visceral motor components, which originate in the Edinger-Westphal nucleus of the oculomotor complex, consist of *preganglionic parasympathetic fibers*. These fibers synapse in the *ciliary ganglion* on postganglionic neurons that form the *short ciliary nerves*. The short ciliary nerves supply the ciliary and constrictor pupillae muscles, which cause (1) curvature of the lens (accommodation) and (2) constriction of the pupils, respectively. Pupillary dilatation is induced by the sympathetic stimulation.

The major functional components of the oculomotor nerve are summarized in **Table 7.1**.

Fig. 7.5 **Parasympathetic components of oculomotor nerve.**

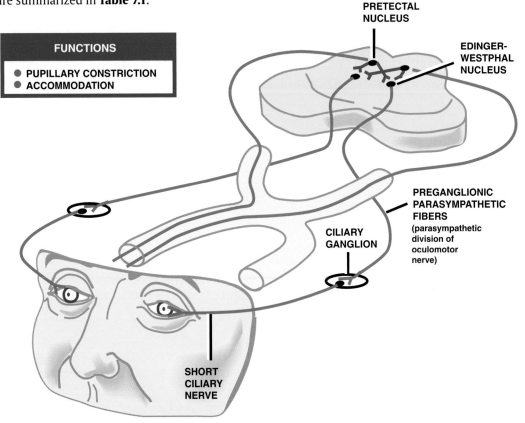

FUNCTIONS

- **PUPILLARY CONSTRICTION**
- **ACCOMMODATION**

Table 7.1 Functional Components of the Oculomotor Nerve (III)

Components	Ganglion	Nuclei	Exit through Skull	Target Organ	Function
Somatic motor		Oculomotor	Superior orbital fissure	Levator palpebrae superioris	Elevates upper eyelid
				Medial rectus muscle	Adducts eye
				Inferior oblique	Elevates, abducts, and externally rotates eye
				Superior rectus muscle	Depresses, abducts, and internally rotates eye
				Inferior rectus muscle	Elevates, abducts, and externally rotates eye
Visceral motor	Ciliary	Edinger-Westphal	Superior orbital fissure	Ciliary and constrictor pupillae muscles	Curvature of the lens and constriction of the pupils

Oculomotor Nerve Palsy

Oculomotor nerve palsy is relatively common in clinical practice. It usually presents with the following signs and symptoms (**Fig. 7.6**):

- **Inhibition of medial and vertical gaze with double vision (diplopia)** due to involvement of the extraocular muscles (the eye is therefore "down and out")
- **Drooping of the upper eyelid (ptosis)** due to paresis of the levator palpebrae superioris
- **Dilated pupil (mydriasis) and absent pupillary light reflex** due to involvement of the constrictor pupillae
- **Absent accommodation reflex** due to ciliary muscle involvement

Oculomotor nerve palsy is associated with four pathological processes (**Fig. 7.7**):

- *Aneurysms* of the posterior communicating artery, which compress the oculomotor nerve
- *Uncal herniation* due to increased intracranial pressure (tumor, abscess, hemorrhage), causing compression of the oculomotor nerve
- *Cavernous sinus thrombosis*, which may involve the oculomotor nerve
- *Midbrain infarction*, involving
  - The basal midbrain, which may cause ipsilateral ophthalmoplegia and contralateral hemiplegia (Weber's syndrome) following interruption of the oculomotor nerve and adjacent corticospinal fibers
  - The region of the red nucleus, which may cause ipsilateral ophthalmoplegia and contralateral intention tremor (Benedikt's syndrome) due to lesions in the oculomotor nerve and the red nucleus
  - Peripheral fibers of the oculomotor nerve as a complication of diabetes mellitus, which commonly causes paralysis of the extraocular muscles with sparing of pupillary constriction

Fig. 7.6 **Four clinical features of oculomotor nerve palsy.**

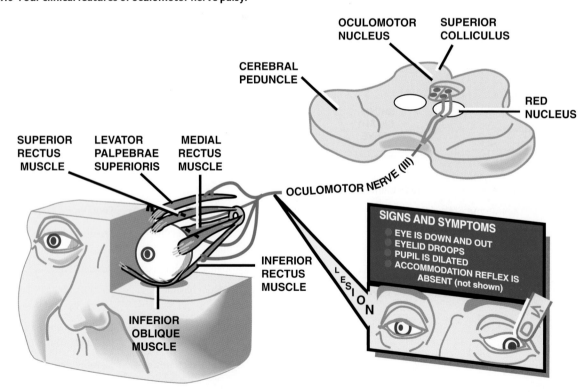

Fig. 7.7 Four common lesions of oculomotor nerve.

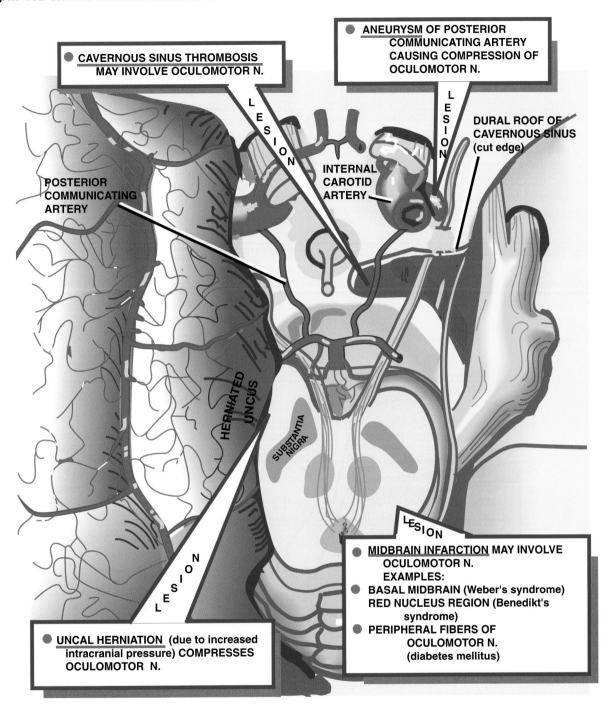

CAVERNOUS SINUS THROMBOSIS MAY INVOLVE OCULOMOTOR N.

ANEURYSM OF POSTERIOR COMMUNICATING ARTERY CAUSING COMPRESSION OF OCULOMOTOR N.

LESION

LESION

DURAL ROOF OF CAVERNOUS SINUS (cut edge)

INTERNAL CAROTID ARTERY

POSTERIOR COMMUNICATING ARTERY

HERNIATED UNCUS

SUBSTANTIA NIGRA

LESION

LESION

MIDBRAIN INFARCTION MAY INVOLVE OCULOMOTOR N.
EXAMPLES:
BASAL MIDBRAIN (Weber's syndrome)
RED NUCLEUS REGION (Benedikt's syndrome)
PERIPHERAL FIBERS OF OCULOMOTOR N. (diabetes mellitus)

UNCAL HERNIATION (due to increased intracranial pressure) **COMPRESSES OCULOMOTOR N.**

The Pupillary Light Reflex

The pupillary light reflex involves a reflex arc whereby a light stimulus elicits pupillary constriction. When light falls on the retina, impulses are generated that run along the optic nerve and tract to reach the ipsilateral pretectal nucleus. These impulses are passed on to the ipsilateral and contralateral Edinger-Westphal nuclei; from there they travel, via the ciliary ganglia, in preganglionic and postganglionic parasympathetic fibers to terminate in the constrictor pupillae. Impulses that cross the midline in their course from the pretectal region to the Edinger-Westphal nucleus constrict the contralateral pupil (indirect or consensual response); uncrossed impulses constrict the ipsilateral pupil (direct response).

Lesions of the Pupillary Light Reflex

See **Fig. 7.8**.
- A lesion of the *ipsilateral oculomotor nerve* results in a loss of the direct response.
- A lesion of the *contralateral oculomotor nerve* results in a loss of the consensual response.

- A lesion of the *ipsilateral optic nerve* results in a loss of both the direct and consensual responses.
- A lesion of the *contralateral optic nerve* does not affect the ipsilateral pupillary responses.

The Accommodation Reflex

The accommodation reflex occurs as a part of the adaptation of the eyes to near vision.

It involves a complex arc whose afferent limb terminates in the visual cortex and whose efferent limb terminates in the constrictor pupillae, medial rectus, and ciliary muscles by way of the pretectal region. Visual responses include pupillary constriction (constrictor pupillae), ocular convergence (pretectal nuclei, motor nuclei), and an increase in the curvature of the lens (contraction of the ciliary muscle), respectively.

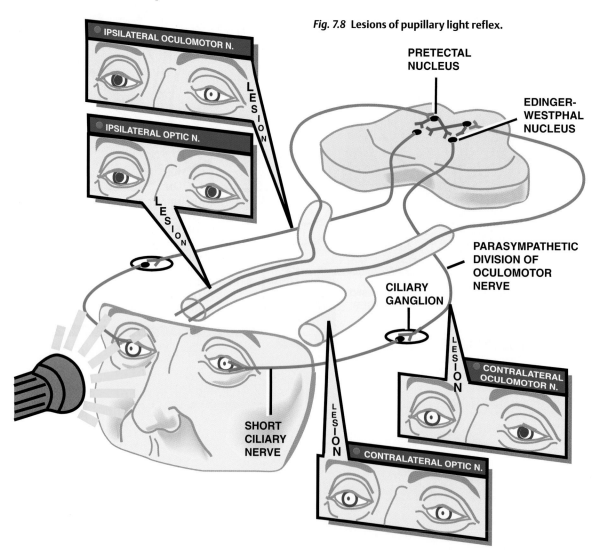

Fig. 7.8 **Lesions of pupillary light reflex.**

The Trochlear Nerve

See **Fig. 7.9**.

The trochlear nucleus is located in the midbrain just caudal to the oculomotor nucleus at the level of the *inferior colliculus*. After leaving the brainstem, the fibers of this nucleus pass through the *cavernous sinus* accompanying cranial nerves III, V1, V2, and VI and the internal carotid artery, to enter the orbit via the *superior orbital fissure*. The nerve then passes laterally to medially outside the *anulus of Zinn*, to innervate the *superior oblique muscle*. The superior oblique muscle causes inward rotation (intorsion) and downward movement of the adducted eye.

As compared with the other cranial nerves, two aspects of the anatomy of the trochlear nerve are exceptional: (1) it exits the dorsal (immediately caudal to the inferior colliculus), rather than the ventral, brainstem, and (2) its peripheral fibers decussate (in the superior medullary vellum) before they supply their target.

Table 7.2 summarizes the major functional components of the trochlear nerve.

Fig. 7.9 **Anatomy of trochlear nerve (IV).**

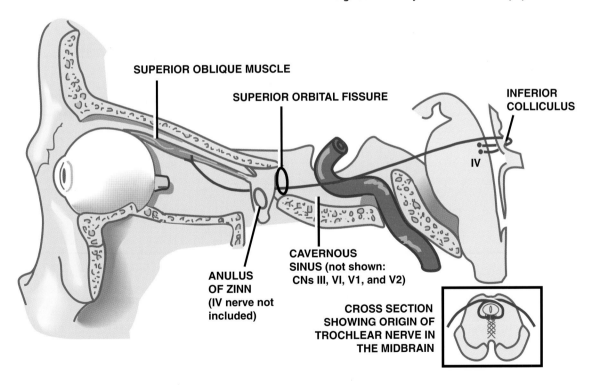

Table 7.2 Functional Components of the Trochlear Nerve (IV)

Component	Nucleus	Exit through Skull	Target Organ	Function
Somatic motor	Trochlear	Superior orbital fissure	Superior oblique muscle	Depresses, abducts, and internally rotates eye

Trochlear Nerve Palsy

See **Fig. 7.10**.

Isolated paralysis of the trochlear nerve, an uncommon event, forces the eye to rotate upward and inward. Clinically, this results in vertical diplopia, which is made worse when the eye is directed downward and inward. Classically, such patients complain of difficulty while walking downstairs, the head often tilted down and toward the contralateral shoulder.

Fig. 7.10 **Trochlear nerve palsy.**

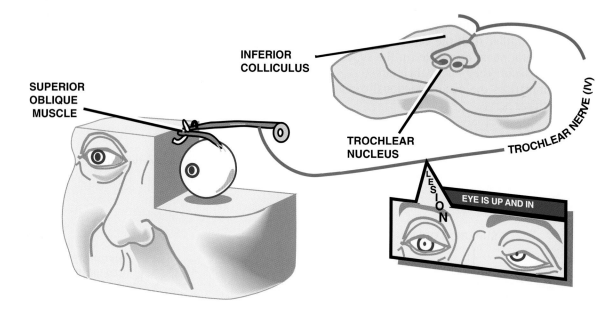

The Abducens Nerve

See **Fig. 7.11**.

The abducens nucleus is located in the pons just beneath the fourth ventricle. Dorsally, it is surrounded by the facial nerve, which drapes around the abducens nucleus, forming a bulge in the fourth ventricle called the facial colliculus.

After it emerges from the brainstem between the pons and the medullary pyramids, the abducens nerve courses through the *cavernous sinus* to enter the orbit via the *superior orbital fissure*. In the orbit, the abducens nerve passes through the *anulus of Zinn* to innervate the *lateral rectus muscle*. The lateral rectus muscle causes abduction of the eye.

Table 7.3 summarizes the major functional components of the abducens nerve.

Fig. 7.11 **Anatomy of abducens nerve (VI).**

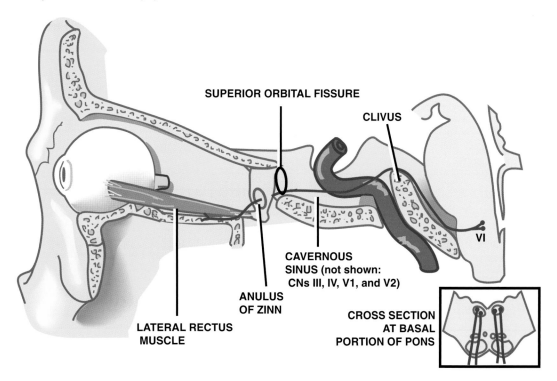

Table 7.3 Functional Components of the Abducens Nerve (VI)

Component	Nucleus	Exit through Skull	Target Organ	Function
Somatic motor	Abducens	Superior orbital fissure	Lateral rectus muscle	Abducts eye

Abducens Nerve Palsy

See **Fig. 7.12**.

Isolated paralysis of the abducens nerve causes horizontal diplopia, forcing the affected eye to orient inward, (i.e., medial deviation of the eye). The affected patient turns the head horizontally toward the ipsilateral shoulder for forward vision.

Fig. 7.12 **Abducens nerve palsy.**

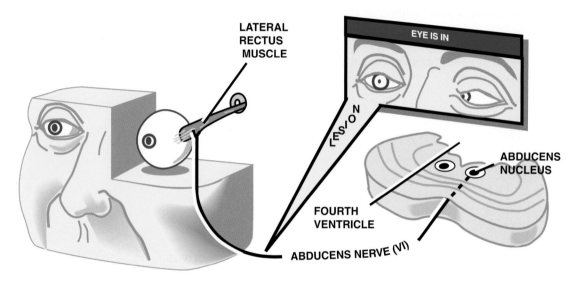

Conjugate Voluntary Horizontal Gaze

See **Fig. 7.13**.

A combination of voluntary and involuntary eye movements allows us to find, fixate on, and track visible objects in space. Conjugate voluntary eye movements are initiated in the frontal eye field, which lies anterior to the motor cortex in Brodmann's area 8 along the middle frontal gyrus. Frontal eye field fibers traverse the posterior limb of the internal capsule and the cerebral peduncle to terminate in the contralateral *paramedian pontine reticular formation* (PPRF), also known as the horizontal gaze center. PPRF neurons send axons in turn to the ipsilateral *abducens nucleus* and the contralateral *oculomotor nucleus*, the latter via the *medial longitudinal fasciculus* (MLF). The synchronous discharge that is produced in the ipsilateral *lateral rectus* and the contralateral *medial rectus* muscles results in voluntary conjugate horizontal gaze Activation of the left frontal eye fields results in conjugate horizontal gaze to the right. When rapid and precise, these voluntary conjugate eye movements are called saccades. Saccades permit the eyes to repeatedly sample the horizontal visual world to find and fixate on an object. A less characterized horizontal gaze center is located in the occipital lobe. This center permits voluntary smooth pursuit movements following objects moving in space.

Fig. 7.13 Pathway for conjugate horizontal gaze.

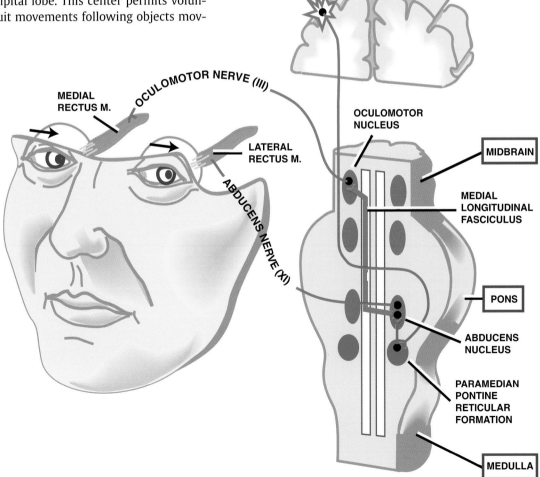

Supranuclear Palsies of Conjugate Horizontal Gaze

See **Fig. 7.14**.

The palsies of conjugate horizontal gaze are divided into three clinically distinct abnormalities in conjugate gaze, based on the site of the responsible lesion. Thus (1) a supranuclear palsy is produced by a lesion that is located "above" the oculomotor nuclear complex, (2) a nuclear palsy is produced by a lesion that is located within the oculomotor nuclear complex, and (3) an internuclear palsy is produced by a lesion that is located in the midline between the oculomotor complex on either side.

Supranuclear palsies involving the frontal eye field produce (1) ocular deviation in the direction of the lesion and (2) contralateral hemiplegia. Supranuclear ablation of right-sided cortical fibers in the frontal eye fields leads to unopposed action of left-sided fibers, which terminate on the right PPRF. These PPRF neurons project fibers, in turn, to the ipsilateral *abducens nucleus* as well as fibers that cross the midline in the MLF to reach the contralateral *oculomotor nucleus*. Activation of the left oculomotor nucleus and the right abducens nucleus evokes conjugate deviation of the eyes to the right, so that the patient "looks at his lesion." Because corticospinal fibers located near the frontal eye fields may also be involved, a contralateral hemiplegia often accompanies the ophthalmoplegia.

In contrast to an ablative lesion, irritative stimulation of area 8, as occurs during an epileptic seizure, produces ocular deviation away from the affected side so that the patient "looks away from his lesion."

Fig. 7.14 **Supranuclear palsies of conjugate horizontal gaze.**

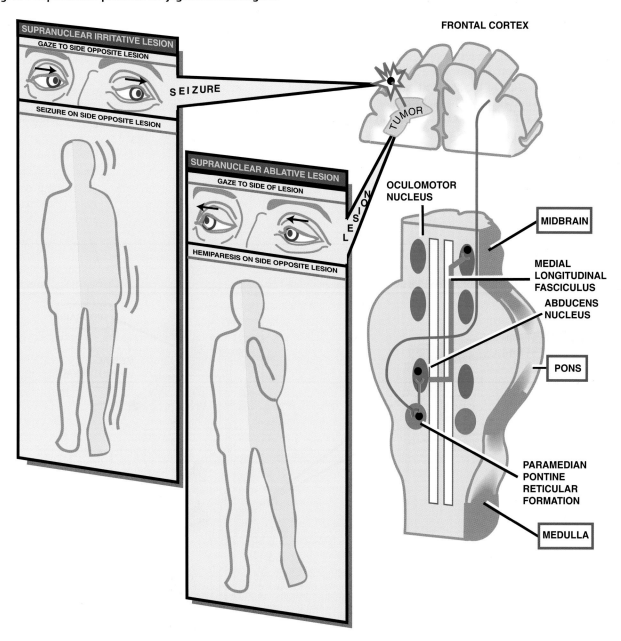

FRONTAL CORTEX

SUPRANUCLEAR IRRITATIVE LESION

GAZE TO SIDE OPPOSITE LESION

SEIZURE

SEIZURE ON SIDE OPPOSITE LESION

SUPRANUCLEAR ABLATIVE LESION

GAZE TO SIDE OF LESION

HEMIPARESIS ON SIDE OPPOSITE LESION

LESION

TUMOR

OCULOMOTOR NUCLEUS

MIDBRAIN

MEDIAL LONGITUDINAL FASCICULUS

ABDUCENS NUCLEUS

PONS

PARAMEDIAN PONTINE RETICULAR FORMATION

MEDULLA

Nuclear Palsy of Conjugate Horizontal Gaze

See **Fig. 7.15**.

A nuclear palsy involving the pons produces (1) ocular deviation away from the lesion and (2) contralateral hemiplegia. Interruption of right-sided PPRF fibers leads to unopposed activation of the left PPRF, which activates the left *abducens nucleus* and the right *oculomotor nucleus*, the latter via the crossed MLF. Activation of these nuclei results in conjugate deviation of the eyes to the left, so that the patient "looks away from his lesion." Because corticospinal fibers located in the pons may also be involved, contralateral hemiplegia frequently accompanies the ophthalmoplegia.

Fig. 7.15 **Nuclear palsy of conjugate horizontal gaze.**

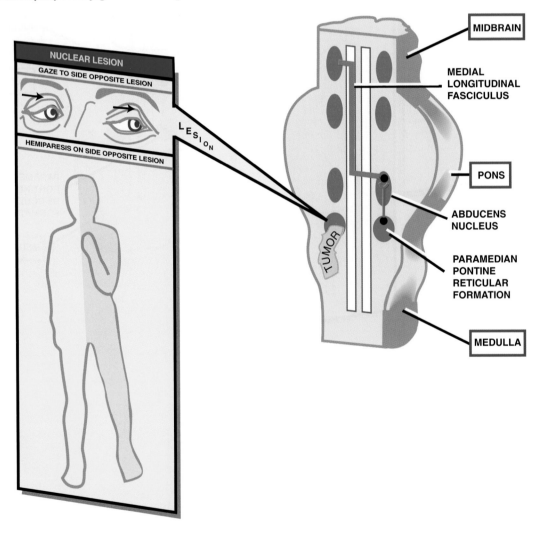

Internuclear Palsy of Conjugate Horizontal Gaze

See **Fig. 7.16**.

An internuclear palsy involving the MLF interrupts the oculomotor nucleus and results in loss of adduction of the ipsilateral eye. The contralateral eye often exhibits nystagmus (spontaneous rapid alternating movements). A lesion of the right MLF results in the left eye moving to the left (abduction), often with nystagmus, whereas the right eye cannot cross midline (i.e., cannot adduct). Bilateral MLF lesions are characteristically seen in patients with multiple sclerosis.

Fig. 7.16 **Internuclear palsy of conjugate horizontal gaze.**

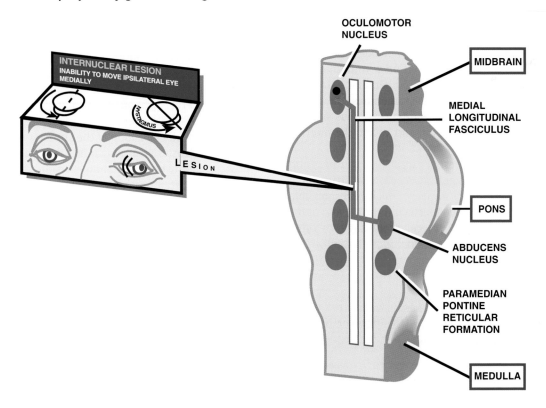

The Trigeminal Nerve

See **Fig. 7.17**.

The trigeminal nerve emerges from the brainstem at the level of the pons. It passes forward and laterally in the subarachnoid space from the posterior cranial fossa to the middle cranial fossa via Meckel's cave over the petrous portion of the temporal bone. Functionally, it contains somatic sensory fibers, proprioceptive fibers, and somatic motor fibers.

Somatic sensory fibers of cranial nerve V have their cell bodies in the trigeminal (gasserian) ganglion, which is situated in the middle cranial fossa. They innervate the skin of the face and forehead; the oral, nasal, and paranasal mucosa; and the teeth. In addition, they carry general sensory impulses from the anterior two thirds of the tongue (the posterior third is supplied by the glossopharyngeal nerve).

Peripheral processes of these fibers are distributed in three divisions: the ophthalmic (V1), maxillary (V2), and mandibular (V3) branches, which exit the skull via the superior orbital fissure, the foramen rotundum, and the foramen ovale, respectively (mnemonic: standing room only). The ophthalmic and (sometimes) the maxillary divisions reach the skull via the cavernous sinus in company with cranial nerves III and VI and the internal carotid artery.

Central processes of these sensory fibers continue into the brainstem, where they terminate on two trigeminal nuclei: the *main sensory nucleus*, which is responsible for light and discriminative touch, and the *nucleus of the spinal trigeminal tract*, which receives messages carrying pain and temperature information.

Proprioceptive fibers are carried in the mandibular division of the trigeminal nerve. They bypass the trigeminal ganglion and continue into the brainstem to synapse directly on the *mesencephalic nucleus*. This nucleus may be viewed as a sensory ganglion that has been displaced into the brainstem because the cell body of the nucleus actually lies within the brainstem.

Somatic motor fibers of cranial nerve V have their cell bodies in the motor trigeminal nucleus. Like the proprioceptive fibers, they are carried exclusively in the mandibular nerve. They innervate the muscles of mastication (the masseter, temporal, and pterygoids), the anterior digastric, the tensor tympani, and the tensor veli palatini muscles. As part of the jaw reflex (contraction of the muscles of mastication in response to a tap on the slightly relaxed jaw), the mesencephalic nucleus projects collaterals to the motor trigeminal nucleus, providing proprioceptive information on the muscles of mastication.

Table 7.4 summarizes the major functional components of the trigeminal nerve.

Clinically, several disease states may involve the trigeminal nerve. Trigeminal neuralgia (tic douloureux) refers to paroxysms of lancinating facial pain of unknown etiology in the territory of one or more branches of the trigeminal nerve, most often a combination of V2 and V3. The etiology is most often due to vascular compression of the nerve, usually by a loop of the superior cerebellar artery. Herpes zoster virus may infect the trigeminal nerve (most frequently the ophthalmic division). This results in shingles and often postherpetic neuralgia with trigeminal pain. A vasculitis may also occur and may result in blindness.

Table 7.4 Functional Components of the Trigeminal Nerve (V)

Components	Ganglion	Nuclei	Exit through Skull	Target Organ	Function
Somatic sensory	Trigeminal (gasserian)	Main sensory	Superior orbital fissure (V1); foramen rotundum (V2); foramen ovale (V3)	Skin of the face and forehead; oral, nasal, paranasal, mucosa; teeth	Light and discriminative touch sensation
		Spinal trigeminal tract			Pain and temperature sensation
		Mesencephalic	Foramen ovale (V3)	Mechanoreceptors in the muscles of mastication; collaterals to motor trigeminal nucleus	Proprioceptive sensation
Somatic motor		Motor trigeminal		Muscles of mastication, anterior digastric, tensor tympani, tensor veli palatini	Motor supply to masticators, temporomandibular joint, tympanic membrane, soft palate

Fig. 7.17 **Trigeminal nerve.**

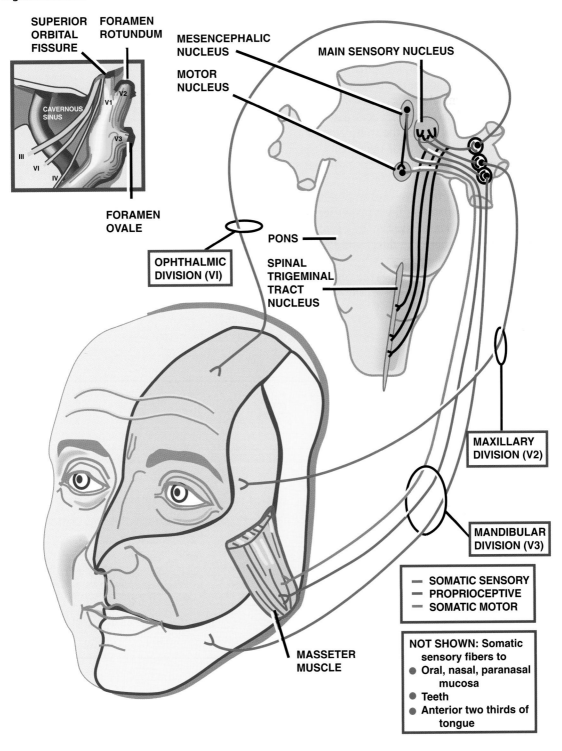

SUPERIOR ORBITAL FISSURE

FORAMEN ROTUNDUM

MESENCEPHALIC NUCLEUS

MAIN SENSORY NUCLEUS

MOTOR NUCLEUS

CAVERNOUS SINUS

V2
V1
V3
III
VI
IV

FORAMEN OVALE

OPHTHALMIC DIVISION (VI)

PONS

SPINAL TRIGEMINAL TRACT NUCLEUS

MAXILLARY DIVISION (V2)

MANDIBULAR DIVISION (V3)

— SOMATIC SENSORY
— PROPRIOCEPTIVE
— SOMATIC MOTOR

NOT SHOWN: Somatic sensory fibers to
- Oral, nasal, paranasal mucosa
- Teeth
- Anterior two thirds of tongue

MASSETER MUSCLE

The Corneal Reflex

See **Fig. 7.18**.

The corneal reflex consists of bilateral forced eye closure in response to stimulation of either cornea. The afferent limb of this reflex comprises somatic sensory fibers of the ophthalmic branch of the trigeminal nerve that synapse on the trigeminal sensory nucleus. The efferent limb comprises somatic motor fibers that begin in the trigeminal sensory nucleus of the stimulated side, project bilaterally on the facial motor nuclei, and continue in the facial nerves to terminate in the orbicularis oculi muscles.

Normally, stimulation of one eye causes simultaneous closure of both the ipsilateral (direct response) and contralateral (indirect response) eyes. A lesion of the trigeminal nerve abolishes both the direct and indirect responses when the ipsilateral eye is stimulated. By contrast, a lesion of the facial nerve abolishes the corneal reflex on the side of the affected facial nerve only (absence of direct *or* indirect response).

Fig. 7.18 **Corneal reflex.**

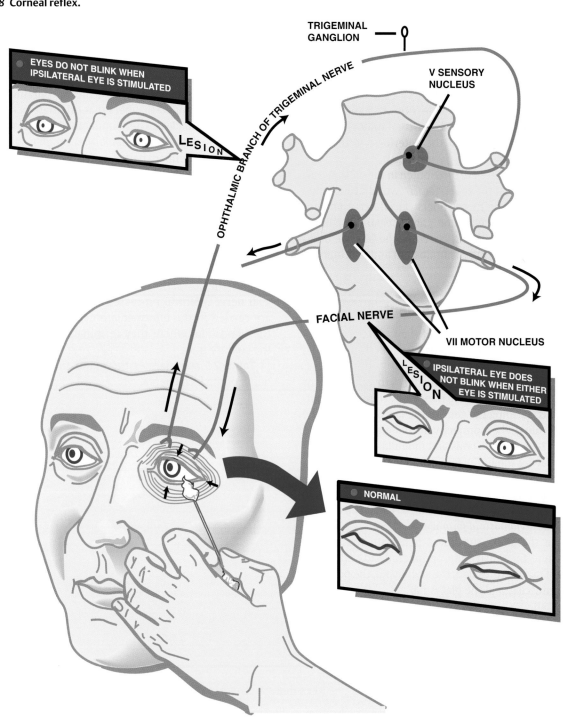

EYES DO NOT BLINK WHEN IPSILATERAL EYE IS STIMULATED

LESION

OPHTHALMIC BRANCH OF TRIGEMINAL NERVE

TRIGEMINAL GANGLION

V SENSORY NUCLEUS

FACIAL NERVE

VII MOTOR NUCLEUS

LESION

IPSILATERAL EYE DOES NOT BLINK WHEN EITHER EYE IS STIMULATED

NORMAL

The Facial Nerve

See **Fig. 7.19**.

Cranial nerve VII, the facial nerve, contributes mixed fibers to the face, comprising somatic motor, visceral motor, and special sensory components. These components supply the muscles of facial expression (somatic motor), the lacrimal and salivary glands (visceral motor), and the taste buds (special sense) of the anterior two thirds of the tongue.

Peripheral processes are distributed in the facial nerve, which emerges from the brainstem in two adjacent roots: one carrying somatic motor fibers (*facial nerve proper*), the other carrying visceral motor and special sense fibers (*intermediate nerve*). Both roots enter the *internal auditory meatus* upon exiting the brainstem and continue together in the *facial canal.*

The Somatic Motor Component

The somatic motor component of the facial nerve originates in the facial motor nucleus, situated in the caudal pontine tegmentum.

Efferent fibers project dorsomedially toward the floor of the fourth ventricle, where they loop around the *abducens nucleus* (forming the genu of the facial nerve and the facial colliculus), then project ventrolaterally to exit the brainstem between the pons and medulla.

After leaving the brainstem, these fibers enter the internal auditory meatus, accompanied by the intermediate nerve and the vestibulocochlear nerve (not shown in figure). They then continue in the facial canal and exit the skull via the *stylomastoid foramen.*

Outside the skull, the fibers penetrate the parotid gland, where they distribute peripherally to supply the muscles of facial expression, the stylohyoid, the posterior digastric muscles, and the platysma.

The Intermediate Nerve

During its course in the facial canal, the intermediate nerve carries fibers that distribute peripherally, in two branches: the *greater superficial petrosal nerve* and the *chorda tympani* nerve.

The greater superficial petrosal nerve contains preganglionic parasympathetic fibers that originate in the *superior salivatory nucleus*. They supply the lacrimal gland via the pterygopalatine (*sphenopalatine*) *ganglion.*

The chorda tympani nerve contains preganglionic parasympathetic fibers that originate in the superior salivatory nucleus. They supply the *sublingual* and *submandibular salivary glands* via the *submandibular ganglion.*

The chorda tympani also carries pseudounipolar gustatory neurons whose cell bodies are located in the geniculate ganglion. The peripheral processes of these neurons supply the taste buds in the anterior two thirds of the tongue (the dorsal third is supplied by the glossopharyngeal nerve). Central processes of the gustatory neurons are carried in the intermediate nerve and projected on the brainstem, where they terminate in the nucleus of the solitary tract.

Table 7.5 summarizes the major functional components of the facial nerve.

Table 7.5 Functional Components of the Facial Nerve (VII)

Components	Ganglia	Nuclei	Exit through Skull	Target Organ	Function
Somatic motor		Facial motor	Internal auditory meatus	Muscles of facial expression; stylohyoid, posterior digastric muscles; platysma	Multiple actions in the face and neck
Visceral motor	Pterygopalatine Submandibular	Superior salivatory		Lacrimal gland Submandibular and sublingual glands	Gland secretion
Special sense	Geniculate	Solitary tract		Taste buds in the anterior two thirds of the tongue	Taste

Fig. 7.19 **Facial nerve.**

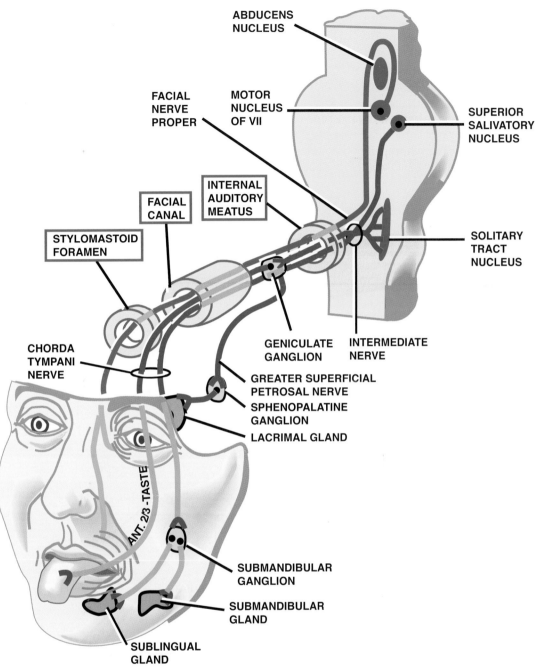

ABDUCENS
NUCLEUS

MOTOR
NUCLEUS
OF VII

SUPERIOR
SALIVATORY
NUCLEUS

FACIAL
NERVE
PROPER

INTERNAL
AUDITORY
MEATUS

FACIAL
CANAL

STYLOMASTOID
FORAMEN

SOLITARY
TRACT
NUCLEUS

GENICULATE
GANGLION

INTERMEDIATE
NERVE

CHORDA
TYMPANI
NERVE

GREATER SUPERFICIAL
PETROSAL NERVE

SPHENOPALATINE
GANGLION

LACRIMAL GLAND

ANT. 2/3 - TASTE

SUBMANDIBULAR
GANGLION

SUBMANDIBULAR
GLAND

SUBLINGUAL
GLAND

Facial Nerve Palsy Syndromes

See **Fig. 7.20**.

The following signs and symptoms of facial nerve palsies help localize the lesions that cause them:

- **Isolated unilateral facial paralysis** (somatic motor components), which results from lesions distal to the stylomastoid foramen
- **Unilateral facial paralysis and loss of taste sensation in the anterior two thirds of the tongue** (*chorda tympani*), which result from lesions within the facial canal proximal to the takeoff of the chorda tympani

- **Unilateral facial paralysis, loss of taste sensation in the anterior two thirds of the tongue, tinnitus, and deafness** (vestibulocochlear nerve) and **loss of tearing** (*greater petrosal nerve*), which result from lesions within the internal auditory meatus

Fig. 7.20 **Facial nerve palsy syndromes.**

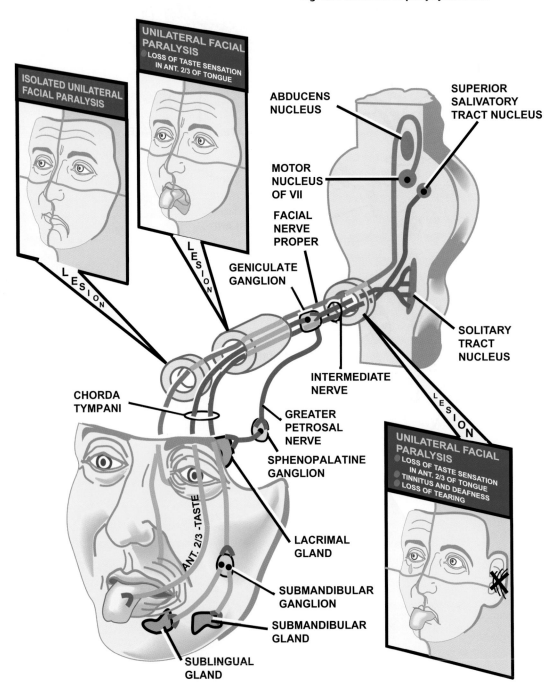

Upper and Lower Facial Palsies

See **Fig. 7.21**.

It is important to observe that the corticobulbar fibers that supply the face provide contralateral innervation of the lower face but bilateral innervation of the upper face. By contrast, the facial nerve supplies the ipsilateral upper and lower face. Thus, supranuclear palsies (interruption of the corticobulbar tract) result in lower facial paralysis on the side opposite the lesion ("central VII"), whereas nuclear or infranuclear palsies (interruption of the facial nucleus or nerve) result in ipsilateral involvement of both the upper and the lower face.

Clinical entities commonly associated with facial nerve palsies include fractures of the petrous bone, middle ear infections, tumors in the cerebellopontine angle (CPA) (e.g., the vestibular schwannoma), and inflammation of the parotid gland. Idiopathic Bell's palsy is the most frequently occurring lesion of the facial nerve.

Fig. 7.21 Upper and lower facial palsies.

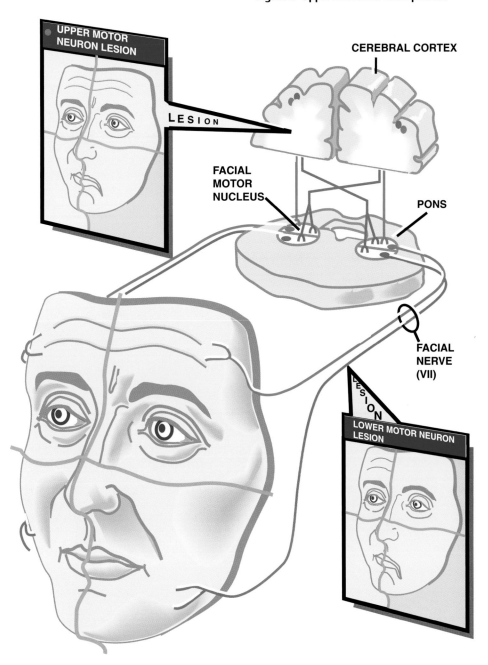

The Vestibulocochlear Nerve

See **Fig. 7.22**.

The vestibulocochlear nerve conducts auditory and vestibular-related impulses from the organ of Corti, the *semicircular ducts*, the utricle, and the saccule. *Vestibular* and *cochlear ganglia* contain the cell bodies of these neurons, the central processes of which traverse the internal auditory meatus, accompanied by the seventh cranial nerve. After exiting the *internal auditory meatus*, these neurons enter the pons, where they synapse in *vestibular* and *cochlear nuclei*.

Table 7.6 summarizes the major functional components of the vestibulocochlear nerve.

A variety of pathological processes, such as skull fractures, toxic drug effects, and infections in the ear, may produce symptoms of tinnitus, deafness, and vertigo secondary to involvement of the vestibulocochlear nerve; the most common tumor of the vestibulocochlear nerve, the vestibular schwannoma, frequently impairs the facial nerve as well.

Table 7.6 Functional Components of the Vestibulocochlear Nerve (VIII)

Components	Ganglia	Nuclei	Exit through Skull	Target Organ	Function
Special sense	Vestibular	Vestibular	Internal auditory meatus	Semicircular ducts; utricle and saccule	Equilibrium
	Cochlear	Cochlear		Organ of Corti	Hearing

Fig. 7.22 Vestibulocochlear nerve.

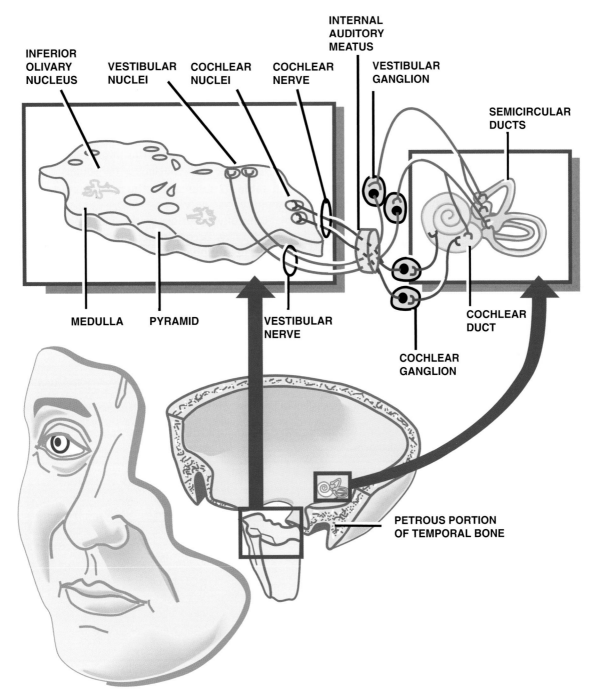

INTERNAL
AUDITORY
MEATUS

INFERIOR
OLIVARY
NUCLEUS

VESTIBULAR
NUCLEI

COCHLEAR
NUCLEI

COCHLEAR
NERVE

VESTIBULAR
GANGLION

SEMICIRCULAR
DUCTS

MEDULLA

PYRAMID

VESTIBULAR
NERVE

COCHLEAR
GANGLION

COCHLEAR
DUCT

PETROUS PORTION
OF TEMPORAL BONE

The Glossopharyngeal Nerve

See **Fig. 7.23**.

The glossopharyngeal nerve emerges from the medulla with the vagus and hypoglossal nerves and exits the skull via the *jugular foramen*, accompanied by the vagus and accessory nerves. Five functional components make up the glossopharyngeal nerve:

- *Somatic motor* fibers have their cell bodies in the *nucleus ambiguus*. They supply the stylopharyngeus muscle, which serves to elevate the pharynx.
- *Visceral motor* fibers have their cell bodies in the *inferior salivatory nucleus*. They supply the *parotid gland* via the *otic ganglion*.
- *Somatic sensory* fibers have their cell bodies in the *superior glossopharyngeal ganglion*. They supply the skin of the external ear and terminate in the nucleus of the spinal trigeminal tract.
- *Visceral sensory* fibers have their cell bodies in the *inferior glossopharyngeal ganglion*. They carry pain, temperature, and touch-related impulses from the posterior third of the tongue, the pharynx, and the eustachian tube, as well as chemo- and baroreceptive-related impulses from the *carotid sinus* and *carotid body*. The fibers that carry these impulses terminate in the *solitary tract nucleus*.
- *Special sensory* fibers have their cell bodies in the inferior glossopharyngeal ganglion. They supply the taste buds in the posterior third of the tongue and terminate in the nucleus of the solitary tract.

Table 7.7 summarizes the major features of the glossopharyngeal nerve.

Clinically, a lesion of the glossopharyngeal nerve, which rarely occurs in isolation, results in (1) a **hoarse voice**, (2) **dysphagia**, and (3) a **loss of the gag reflex**. Glossopharyngeal neuralgia, a syndrome of agonizing ear and throat pain, is similar in character to trigeminal neuralgia but less common.

Table 7.7 Functional Components of the Glossopharyngeal Nerve (IX)

Components	Ganglia	Nuclei	Exit through Skull	Target Organ	Function
Somatic motor		Nucleus ambiguus	Jugular foramen	Stylopharyngeus	Elevates pharynx
Visceral motor	Otic	Inferior salivatory		Parotid gland	Gland secretion
Somatic sensory	Superior glossopharyngeal	Spinal trigeminal tract		External ear	Somatic sensation
Visceral sensory	Inferior glossopharyngeal	Solitary tract		Carotid sinus and body; pharynx and posterior third of tongue	Baro- and chemoreceptor reflexes; pain, temperature, and touch sensation
Special sense				Taste buds in posterior third of tongue	Taste

Fig. 7.23 **Glossopharyngeal nerve.**

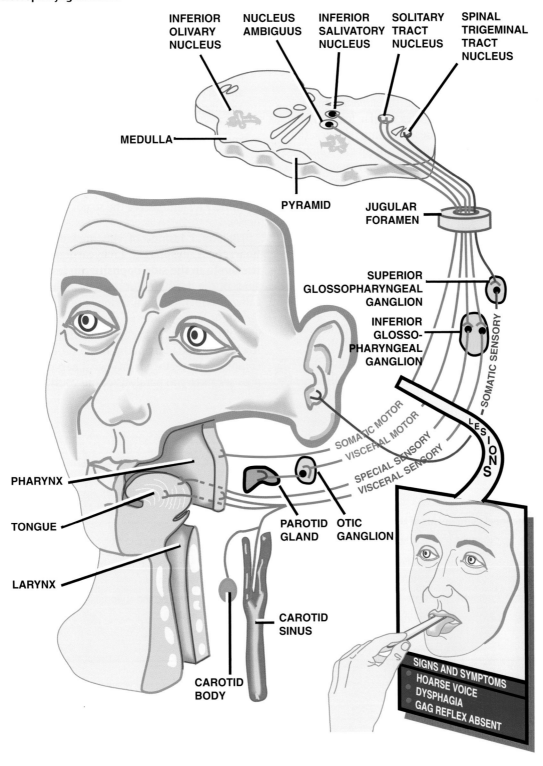

INFERIOR OLIVARY NUCLEUS

NUCLEUS AMBIGUUS

INFERIOR SALIVATORY NUCLEUS

SOLITARY TRACT NUCLEUS

SPINAL TRIGEMINAL TRACT NUCLEUS

MEDULLA

PYRAMID

JUGULAR FORAMEN

SUPERIOR GLOSSOPHARYNGEAL GANGLION

INFERIOR GLOSSO-PHARYNGEAL GANGLION

SOMATIC SENSORY

LESIONS

SOMATIC MOTOR

VISCERAL MOTOR

SPECIAL SENSORY

VISCERAL SENSORY

PHARYNX

TONGUE

LARYNX

PAROTID GLAND

OTIC GANGLION

CAROTID SINUS

CAROTID BODY

SIGNS AND SYMPTOMS
- HOARSE VOICE
- DYSPHAGIA
- GAG REFLEX ABSENT

The Vagus Nerve

See **Fig. 7.24**.

The vagus nerve emerges from the *medulla* to exit the skull through the *jugular foramen*, accompanied by the glossopharyngeal and accessory nerves. The cell bodies of its sensory fibers are located in the *superior* and *inferior ganglia*, which lie within the jugular fossa of the petrous (temporal) bone. As it descends into the neck, the vagus passes through the carotid sheath (dorsal), alongside the internal jugular vein (ventrolateral) and the internal carotid artery (ventromedial). The important role of the vagus nerve in the autonomic nervous system is discussed in Chapter 20.

Five functional components make up the vagus nerve:

- *Somatic motor* fibers have their cell bodies in the *nucleus ambiguus*. They supply the majority of the muscles of the *pharynx* and *larynx*, which are responsible for swallowing and the production of speech (exceptions: the glossopharyngeal nerve supplies the stylopharyngeus muscle, which elevates the pharynx but does not participate in swallowing; and the trigeminal nerve supplies the tensor veli palatini, which tenses the soft palate, thus opening the auditory tube, as occurs in the act of yawning).
- *Visceral motor* fibers have their cell bodies in the *dorsal motor nucleus* of the vagus. They supply the *viscera of the thoracic and abdominal cavities.*

- *Somatic sensory* fibers have their cell bodies in the *superior ganglion.* They carry pain, temperature, and touch-related impulses from the external ear to the nucleus of the *spinal trigeminal tract.*
- *Visceral sensory* fibers have their cell bodies in the *inferior ganglion.* They carry impulses from the pharynx and larynx, the *aortic arch* and body, and the thoracic and abdominal viscera. Central processes are projected to the *solitary tract nucleus.*
- *Special sensory* fibers have their cell bodies in the *inferior ganglion.* They carry taste-related impulses from the posterior pharynx that terminate in the nucleus of the solitary tract.

Table 7.8 summarizes the major features of the vagus nerve.

Unilateral lesions of the nucleus ambiguus cause **hoarseness, dysphagia, tachycardia,** and **deviation of the uvula to the side opposite the lesion**. Unilateral lesions of the dorsal motor nucleus are not manifest clinically, although bilateral lesions are life threatening. The recurrent laryngeal nerve supplies all the intrinsic muscles of the larynx except the cricothyroid muscle. Paratracheal lymphadenopathy or an aortic aneurysm may compress the recurrent laryngeal nerve, causing hoarseness secondary to paralysis of the vocal cords.

Table 7.8 Functional Components of the Vagus Nerve (X)

Components	Ganglia	Nuclei	Exit through Skull	Target Organ	Function
Somatic motor		Nucleus ambiguus	Jugular foramen	Muscles of the larynx and pharynx	Speech and swallowing
Visceral motor	Various	Dorsal motor nucleus of the vagus		Thoracic and abdominal viscera	Various autonomic (parasympathetic) effects on visceral organs
Somatic sensory	Superior	Spinal trigeminal tract		External ear	Somatic sensation
Visceral sensory	Inferior	Solitary tract		Pharynx, larynx, aortic arch and body, thoracic and abdominal viscera	Visceral sensation
Special sense				Pharynx	Taste

Fig. 7.24 **Vagus nerve.**

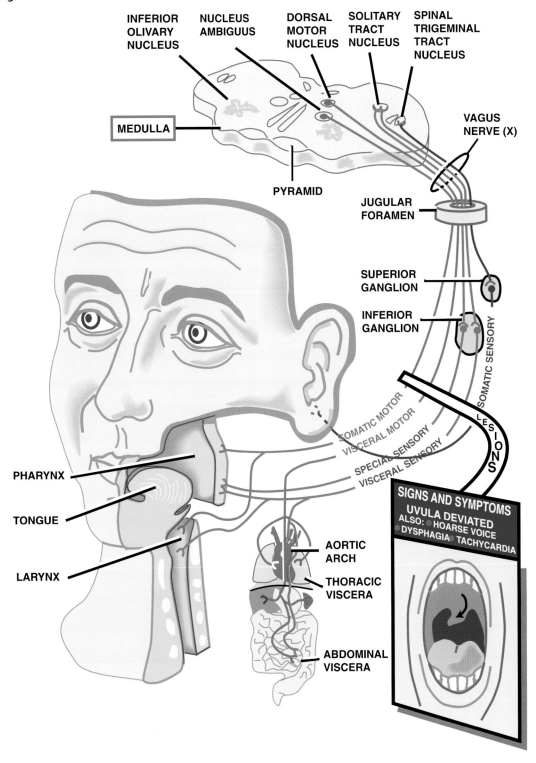

INFERIOR OLIVARY NUCLEUS

NUCLEUS AMBIGUUS

DORSAL MOTOR NUCLEUS

SOLITARY TRACT NUCLEUS

SPINAL TRIGEMINAL TRACT NUCLEUS

MEDULLA

PYRAMID

VAGUS NERVE (X)

JUGULAR FORAMEN

SUPERIOR GANGLION

INFERIOR GANGLION

SOMATIC SENSORY

SOMATIC MOTOR

VISCERAL MOTOR

SPECIAL SENSORY

VISCERAL SENSORY

LESIONS

PHARYNX

TONGUE

LARYNX

AORTIC ARCH

THORACIC VISCERA

ABDOMINAL VISCERA

SIGNS AND SYMPTOMS

UVULA DEVIATED

ALSO: HOARSE VOICE

DYSPHAGIA TACHYCARDIA

The Accessory Nerve

See **Fig. 7.25**.

The accessory nerve supplies the *sternocleidomastoid* and *trapezius muscles*. The cell bodies of the nerve are situated in the ventral horn of the upper five segments of the spinal cord. They send fibers through the *foramen magnum*, which then exit the skull with cranial nerves IX and X through the *jugular foramen*.

Table 7.9 summarizes the major functional components of the accessory nerve.

Paralysis of the accessory nerve results in **difficulty rotating the head to the side opposite the lesion** (sternocleidomastoid muscle) and **inability to shrug the ipsilateral shoulder** (trapezius muscle).

Table 7.9 Functional Components of the Accessory Nerve (XI)

Component	Nuclei	Exit through Skull	Target Organ	Function
Somatic motor	Anterior gray horn of spinal cord level C1–C5	Jugular foramen	Sternocleidomastoid; trapezius	Rotate head; elevate shoulder

Fig. 7.25 **Accessory nerve.**

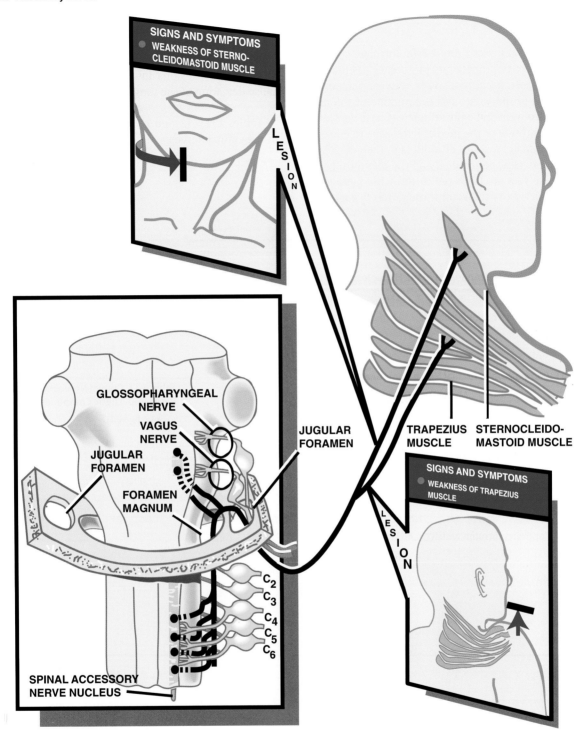

SIGNS AND SYMPTOMS
● WEAKNESS OF STERNO-CLEIDOMASTOID MUSCLE

GLOSSOPHARYNGEAL NERVE

VAGUS NERVE

JUGULAR FORAMEN

FORAMEN MAGNUM

JUGULAR FORAMEN

TRAPEZIUS MUSCLE

STERNOCLEIDO-MASTOID MUSCLE

C2
C3
C4
C5
C6

SPINAL ACCESSORY NERVE NUCLEUS

LESION

SIGNS AND SYMPTOMS
● WEAKNESS OF TRAPEZIUS MUSCLE

LESION

The Hypoglossal Nerve

See **Fig. 7.26**.

The hypoglossal nerve supplies the intrinsic and extrinsic muscles of the tongue. Its cell bodies are located in the *hypoglossal nucleus*, which lies between the dorsal motor nucleus of the vagus and the midline of the *medulla*. Fibers from the hypoglossal nucleus pass ventrally along the lateral side of the medial lemniscus to emerge from the medulla as a series of rootlets in the ventrolateral sulcus between the *pyramid* and the *inferior olivary nucleus*. These rootlets converge to form the hypoglossal nerve, which exits the skull through the *hypoglossal canal*.

Table 7.10 summarizes the major functional components of the hypoglossal nerve.

Upper motor neuron lesions involving the crossed corticobulbar supply of the hypoglossal nucleus cause deviation of the tongue to the side opposite the lesion; lower motor neuron lesions involving the hypoglossal nerve cause deviation of the tongue to the ipsilateral side.

Tables 7.11, **7.12**, and **7.13** present comparative features of the cranial nerves.

Table 7.10 Functional Components of the Hypoglossal Nerve (XII)

Components	Nucleus	Exit through Skull	Target Organ	Function
Somatic motor	Hypoglossal	Hypoglossal canal	Extrinsic and intrinsic muscles of the tongue	Movement of the tongue

Table 7.11 Comparison of Cranial Nerve Components

Sensory	Motor	Mixed Sensory/Motor
Olfactory (I)	Oculomotor (III)	Trigeminal (V)
Optic (II)	Trochlear (IV)	Facial (VII)
Vestibulocochlear (VIII)	Abducens (VI)	Glossopharyngeal (IX)
	Accessory (XI)	Vagus (X)
	Hypoglossal (XII)	

Table 7.12 Cranial Nerves with Parasympathetic Components

Cranial Nerves
Oculomotor (III)
Facial (VII)
Glossopharyngeal (IX)
Vagus (X)

Table 7.13 Foramina through which Cranial Nerves Exit Skull

Foramina	Cranial Nerves
Superior orbital fissure	Oculomotor (III)
	Trochlear (IV)
	Ophthalmic (V1)
	Abducens (VI)
Foramen rotundum	Maxillary (V2)
Foramen ovale	Mandibular (V3)
Internal auditory meatus	Facial (VII)
	Vestibulocochlear (VIII)
Jugular foramen	Glossopharyngeal (IX)
	Vagus (X)
	Accessory (XI)
Hypoglossal canal	Hypoglossal (XII)

Fig. 7.26 **Hypoglossal nerve.**

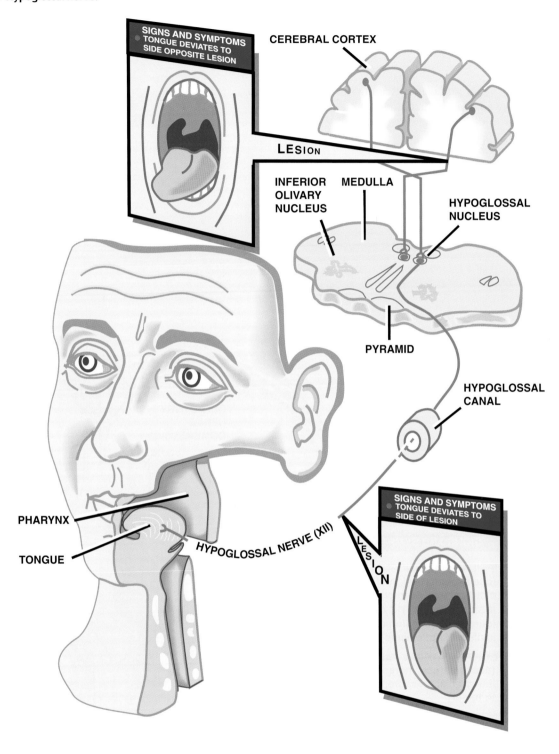

Cranial Nerve Syndromes

Foster Kennedy Syndrome

See **Fig. 7.27**.

Foster Kennedy syndrome is most commonly associated with olfactory groove or sphenoid ridge masses, often meningiomas. It has three signs and symptoms:

- **Ipsilateral anosmia** (due to compression of the olfactory bulb or tract)
- **Ipsilateral optic atrophy** (due to compression of the ipsilateral optic nerve)
- **Contralateral papilledema** (due to increased intracranial pressure)

Fig. 7.27 **Foster Kennedy syndrome.**

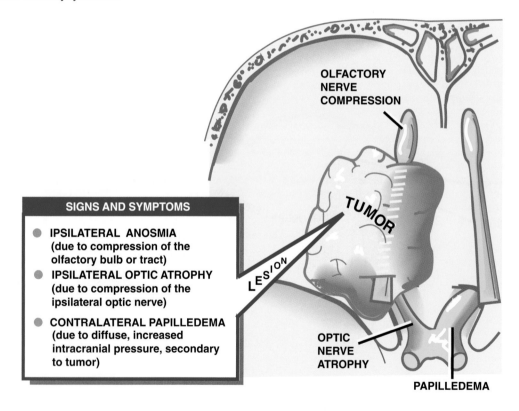

SIGNS AND SYMPTOMS

- IPSILATERAL ANOSMIA (due to compression of the olfactory bulb or tract)
- IPSILATERAL OPTIC ATROPHY (due to compression of the ipsilateral optic nerve)
- CONTRALATERAL PAPILLEDEMA (due to diffuse, increased intracranial pressure, secondary to tumor)

OLFACTORY NERVE COMPRESSION

TUMOR

LESION

OPTIC NERVE ATROPHY

PAPILLEDEMA

Raeder Paratrigeminal Syndrome

See **Fig. 7.28**.

Raeder paratrigeminal syndrome is usually due to lesions in the middle cranial fossa, most commonly between the *trigeminal ganglion* and the *internal carotid artery*. It has two signs and symptoms:

- **Pain in the distribution of V1 and V2**
- **Oculosympathetic paresis** (ptosis and miosis), but with preservation of sweating

Other less frequent symptoms include loss of sensation in a trigeminal nerve distribution and weakness of muscles innervated by the fifth nerve.

Fig. 7.28 **Raeder paratrigeminal syndrome.**

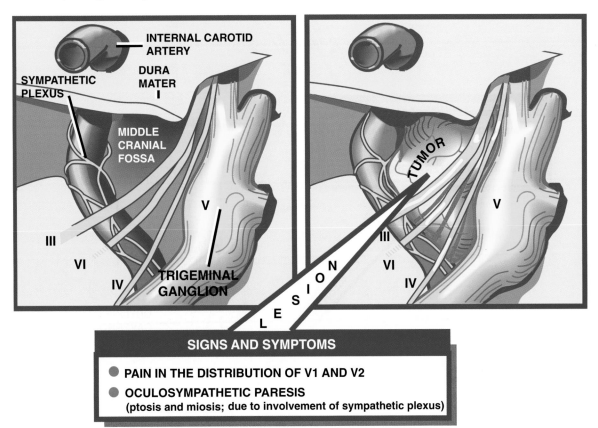

Gradenigo's Syndrome

See **Fig. 7.29**.

Gradenigo's syndrome is usually due to an inflammatory lesion at the apex of the petrous bone (petrous apicitis). It has two signs and symptoms:

- **Pain and sensory disturbance in the V1 distribution** (due to impairment of the ophthalmic nerve)
- **Ipsilateral lateral rectus palsy** (due to impairment of the abducens nerve)

Oculosympathetic paresis, with preservation of facial sweating, may also occur.

Fig. 7.29 **Gradenigo's syndrome.**

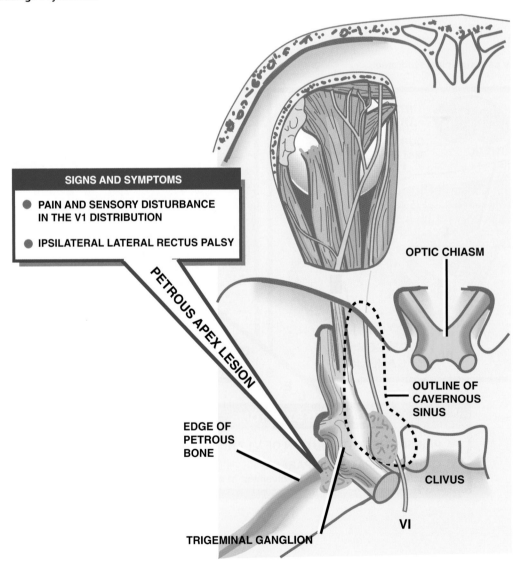

SIGNS AND SYMPTOMS

- PAIN AND SENSORY DISTURBANCE IN THE V1 DISTRIBUTION
- IPSILATERAL LATERAL RECTUS PALSY

PETROUS APEX LESION

OPTIC CHIASM

OUTLINE OF CAVERNOUS SINUS

EDGE OF PETROUS BONE

CLIVUS

TRIGEMINAL GANGLION

VI

Cavernous Sinus Syndrome

See **Fig. 7.30**.

Cavernous sinus syndrome is due to lesions involving the cavernous sinus. The syndrome has two signs and symptoms:

- **Pain and sensory disturbance in the V1 and (less often) V2 distribution**
- **Ipsilateral ophthalmoplegia** (due to impairment of the oculomotor, trochlear, and abducens nerves)

Oculosympathetic paresis, with preservation of facial sweating, may also occur. The eye may appear proptotic and injected.

Fig. 7.30 Cavernous sinus syndrome.

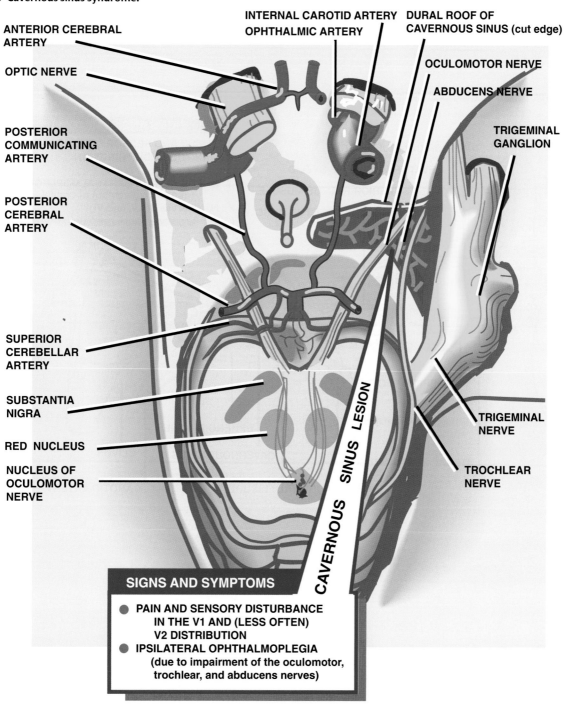

SIGNS AND SYMPTOMS

- PAIN AND SENSORY DISTURBANCE IN THE V1 AND (LESS OFTEN) V2 DISTRIBUTION
- IPSILATERAL OPHTHALMOPLEGIA (due to impairment of the oculomotor, trochlear, and abducens nerves)

Superior Orbital Fissure Syndrome

See **Fig. 7.31**.

Superior orbital fissure syndrome is due to a lesion in the superior orbital fissure. It has two symptoms that are clinically indistinguishable from the cavernous sinus syndrome:

- **Pain and sensory disturbance in the V1 distribution**
- **Ipsilateral ophthalmoplegia** (due to involvement of oculomotor, trochlear, and abducens nerve)

Oculosympathetic paresis, with preservation of facial sweating, may also occur.

Fig. 7.31 **Superior orbital fissure syndrome.**

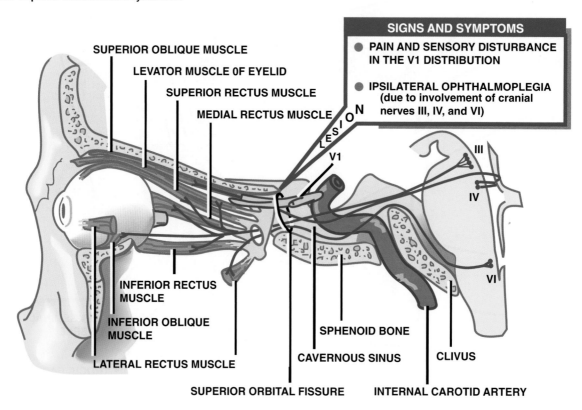

SUPERIOR OBLIQUE MUSCLE

LEVATOR MUSCLE 0F EYELID

SUPERIOR RECTUS MUSCLE

MEDIAL RECTUS MUSCLE

LESION

V1

SIGNS AND SYMPTOMS
- PAIN AND SENSORY DISTURBANCE IN THE V1 DISTRIBUTION
- IPSILATERAL OPHTHALMOPLEGIA (due to involvement of cranial nerves III, IV, and VI)

III

IV

VI

INFERIOR RECTUS MUSCLE

INFERIOR OBLIQUE MUSCLE

LATERAL RECTUS MUSCLE

SPHENOID BONE

CAVERNOUS SINUS

CLIVUS

SUPERIOR ORBITAL FISSURE

INTERNAL CAROTID ARTERY

Tolosa-Hunt Syndrome

See **Fig. 7.32**.

Tolosa-Hunt syndrome is due to a granulomatous lesion of the cavernous sinus or the superior orbital fissure. It has the following two signs and symptoms:

- **Retro-orbital pain and sensory loss in the V1 distribution**
- **Ipsilateral ophthalmoplegia**

Fig. 7.32 Tolosa-Hunt syndrome.

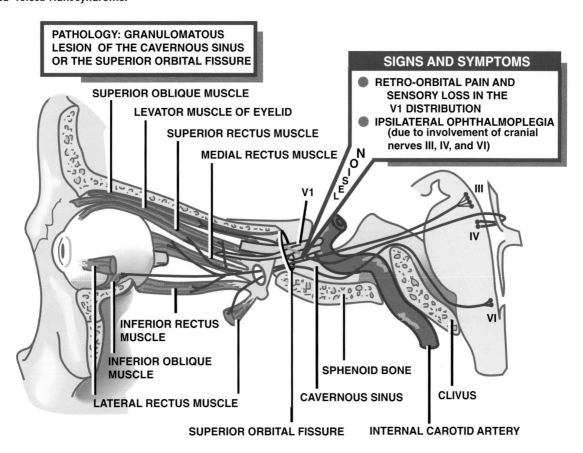

Millard-Gubler Syndrome

See **Fig. 7.33**.

Millard-Gubler syndrome is due to a lesion in the ventral pons. It has the following three signs and symptoms:

- **Ipsilateral facial paralysis** (due to interruption of the facial nerve)
- **Ipsilateral lateral rectus palsy** (due to interruption of the abducens nerve)
- **Contralateral hemiplegia** (due to interruption of the corticospinal tract)

Fig. 7.33 **Millard-Gubler syndrome.**

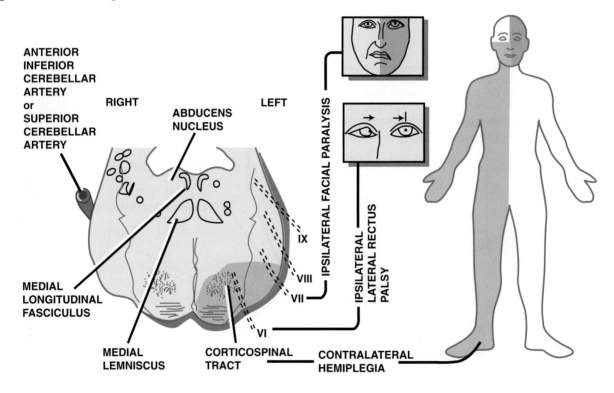

Foville's Syndrome

See **Fig. 7.34**.

Foville's syndrome is due to a lesion in the pontine tegmentum. It has the following three signs and symptoms:

- **Ipsilateral facial paralysis** (due to involvement of the facial nerve)
- **Paralysis of conjugate gaze to the side of the lesion** (due to involvement of the abducens nerve and the PPRF)
- **Contralateral hemiplegia** (due to involvement of the corticospinal tract)

Fig. 7.34 Foville's syndrome.

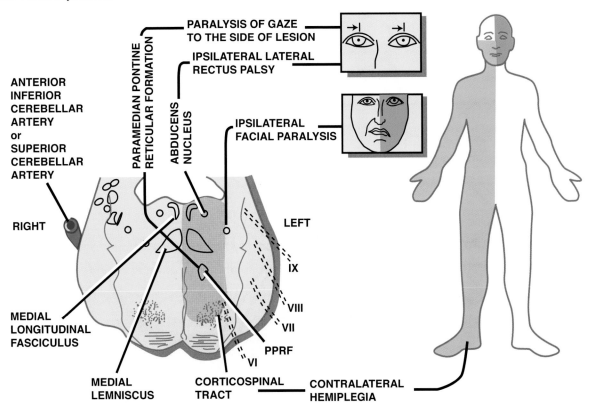

Cerebellopontine Angle Syndrome

See **Fig. 7.35**.

Cerebellopontine angle (CPA) syndrome is due to a mass in the CPA. This is most commonly a vestibular schwannoma (acoustic neuroma) and less commonly a meningioma. The syndrome has the following signs and symptoms:

- **Progressive sensorineural hearing loss**
- **Tinnitus**
- **Dizziness**
- **Unsteadiness**
- **Facial nerve palsy**
- **Facial pain and sensory loss and depressed corneal reflex**

Symptomatology in this syndrome is variable. In part, it is dependent on whether the lesion is a vestibular schwannoma or a meningioma. Vestibular schwannomas are associated with prominent early hearing loss, late facial nerve palsy, late trigeminal nerve involvement, and infrequent lower cranial nerve involvement. By contrast, meningiomas are associated with early facial nerve palsy, early trigeminal nerve involvement, late hearing loss, and, more commonly, involvement of the lower cranial nerves.

Fig. 7.35 **Cerebellopontine angle syndrome.**

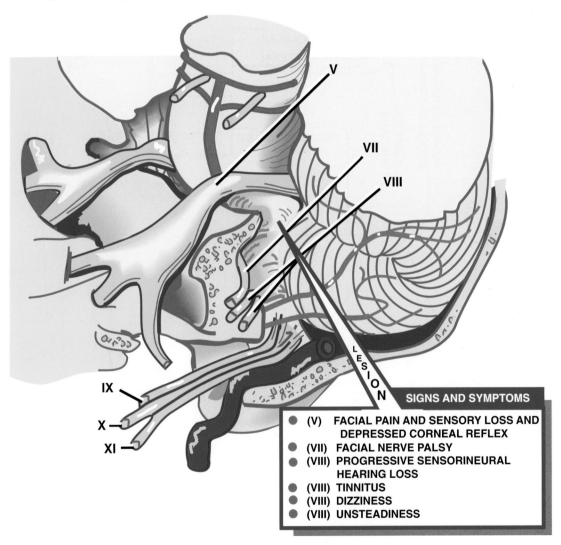

SIGNS AND SYMPTOMS

- (V) FACIAL PAIN AND SENSORY LOSS AND DEPRESSED CORNEAL REFLEX
- (VII) FACIAL NERVE PALSY
- (VIII) PROGRESSIVE SENSORINEURAL HEARING LOSS
- (VIII) TINNITUS
- (VIII) DIZZINESS
- (VIII) UNSTEADINESS

Topography of Cerebellopontine Angle Tumor

See **Fig. 7.36**.

The facial and the vestibulocochlear nerves are arranged within the internal auditory canal as follows. The *facial nerve* is located ventral and rostral; the *cochlear nerve* is located ventral and caudal; the *superior vestibular nerve* is located dorsal and superior; and the *inferior vestibular nerve* is located dorsal and caudal (remember: 7-Up, Coke down). Because acoustic neuromas most frequently arise in the dorsally situated vestibular nerves, they usually displace the facial and cochlear nerves ventrally. Variation in the direction of growth of these tumors may result in the displacement of the facial nerve anterosuperiorly or anteroinferiorly, rather than directly anteriorly.

Fig. 7.36 Topography of cerebellopontine angle tumor.

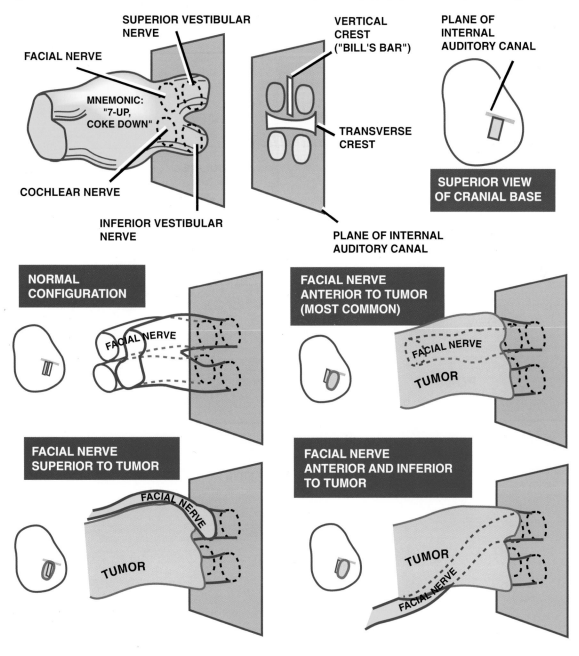

Ramsay Hunt Syndrome

See **Fig. 7.37**.

Ramsay Hunt syndrome is due to a viral infection of the geniculate ganglion by herpes zoster. It has the following four signs and symptoms:

- **Ipsilateral facial paralysis** (due to involvement of the motor division of the facial nerve)
- **Hyperacusis** (due to involvement of the stapedius branch of the facial nerve)
- **Loss of taste** (due to involvement of the geniculate ganglion)
- **Herpetic vesicles** on the eardrum, the external auditory canal, or palate

Fig. 7.37 **Ramsay Hunt syndrome.**

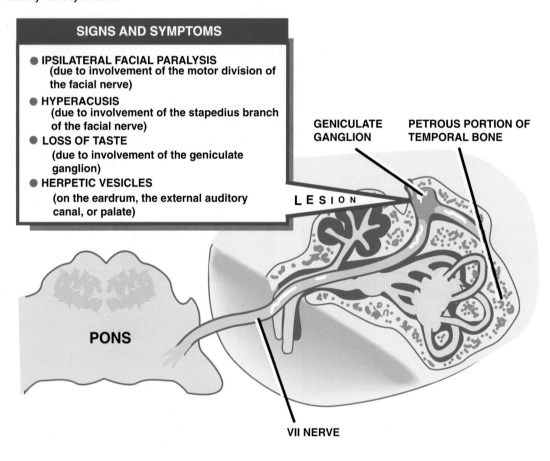

SIGNS AND SYMPTOMS

- IPSILATERAL FACIAL PARALYSIS
  (due to involvement of the motor division of the facial nerve)
- HYPERACUSIS
  (due to involvement of the stapedius branch of the facial nerve)
- LOSS OF TASTE
  (due to involvement of the geniculate ganglion)
- HERPETIC VESICLES
  (on the eardrum, the external auditory canal, or palate)

GENICULATE GANGLION

PETROUS PORTION OF TEMPORAL BONE

LESION

PONS

VII NERVE

Jugular Foramen Syndrome (Vernet's Syndrome)

See **Fig. 7.38**.

Vernet's syndrome is due to a lesion in the jugular foramen, most commonly a glomus jugulare tumor. It has the following signs and symptoms:

- **Loss of taste sensation in the posterior third of the tongue** (due to involvement of the glossopharyngeal nerve)
- **Paralysis of vocal cords and palate, anesthesia of larynx and pharynx** (due to involvement of the vagus nerve)
- **Ipsilateral trapezius and sternocleidomastoid muscle weakness and atrophy** (due to involvement of the accessory nerve)

Fig. 7.38 Jugular foramen syndrome (Vernet's syndrome).

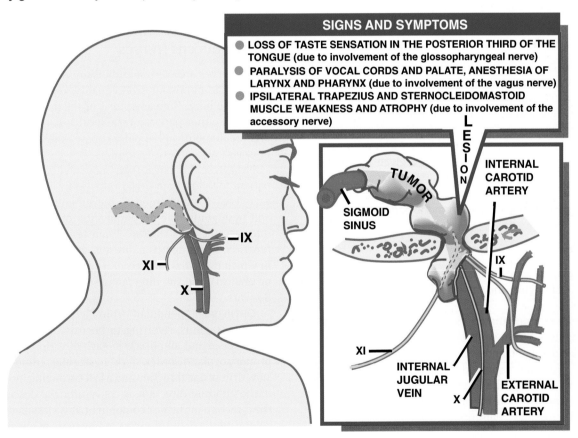

Cranial Nerve Testing

Cranial nerve testing constitutes an integral part of the traditional five-part neurologic examination. An orderly procedure, as described here, is suggested.

Olfactory Nerve

Ask the patient to close one nostril and use the other nostril to identify a common odor, such as coffee, cloves, or tobacco. Ensure the patency of each nostril by compressing them one at a time, asking the patient to sniff through the opposite nostril.

Avoid ammonia and other noxious substances, which test other functions as well. A normal response includes appreciation without identification of the odor.

Optic Nerve

Visual Acuity

Test distant vision with the Snellen eye chart. Have the patient, positioned 20 feet from the chart, read the smallest line of print possible, covering one eye at a time. In recording visual acuity, which is expressed as a fraction where the numerator represents the patient's distance from the chart and the denominator represents the normal distance required to read a given line, indicate whether vision was corrected with eyeglasses.

Near vision may be similarly tested using a handheld chart positioned 14 inches from the patient's face.

Fundus

To begin, examine the optic disc, noting its color, the clarity of its margins, and the size of its central physiological cup.

Next, examine the arterioles and veins. Arterioles are distinguished from veins by their lighter red color, their smaller diameter, and their central white stripe or light reflex. Note any narrowed segments or aneurysmal dilatations affecting the arterioles and any nicking of the veins (compression by thickened arterioles at arteriovenous crossings). Pulsations should be visualized.

Next, examine the macular area, which is located two to three disc diameters temporal to the optic disc, noting any hemorrhages or exudates.

Finally, note any hemorrhages, exudates, or abnormal pigmentation in the undifferentiated retina.

Visual Fields

Testing of visual fields by confrontation provides only a gross measure of peripheral vision but is valuable nevertheless in revealing a variety of cerebral lesions.

First, position the patient's face directly opposite yours and hold up both hands in the outer parts of opposite visual fields. Moving one hand, then the other, then both simultaneously, ask the patient to indicate which hand is moving. Patients with parietal lobe lesions may correctly identify movement in each hand individually but then preferentially neglect a field when both hands move simultaneously.

Next, ask the patient to cover the right eye and to fixate the left eye on your right. Moving a pencil or penlight from the periphery to the center of each of the four quadrants, use your right hand to test temporal and left hand to test nasal quadrants and ask the patient to indicate when the object comes into view. Then repeat with the other eye.

Examiners can use their own field of vision as a control by covering their own eye opposite the patient's covered eye and comparing the patient's visual fields with their own.

Oculomotor, Trochlear, and Abducens Nerves

These nerves are conveniently examined together. First, inspect the pupils for size, equality, regularity, and reactivity to light. Note any ptosis of the upper lids, which indicates either paresis of the levator palpebrae superioris (oculomotor nerve palsy) or weakness of the tarsal muscles (sympathetic lesion).

Next, test the extraocular movements by asking the patient to follow your finger into the six cardinal fields of gaze. Look for dysconjugate movements, saccadic jerks, and nystagmus. The decomposition of smooth pursuits into saccadic jerks suggests brainstem or cerebellar dysfunction. If nystagmus is present, note the field of gaze in which it occurs, the axis of its movements (horizontal or vertical), and the direction of the fast and slow components.

Distinguish "pendular" from "jerk" nystagmus. Pendular nystagmus, referring to horizontal oscillations of equal speed and amplitude in each direction, indicates a primary ocular disorder. "Jerk" nystagmus, composed of a slow drift in one direction and a fast correcting movement in the opposite direction, is conventionally described by the direction of the fast component. It is classified as horizontal, vertical, or rotary according to its plane of movement. Lesions in the labyrinth, the brainstem, and the cerebellum are most commonly responsible.

Trigeminal Nerve

Motor

With the patient's teeth clenched, palpate first the masseter and then the temporal muscles, observing their symmetry and strength of contraction.

Sensory

With the patient's eyes closed, test separately the forehead, cheeks, and jaw on each side, using a safety pin for pain sensation (nucleus of the spinal trigeminal tract) and a wisp of cotton for light touch (main sensory nucleus), asking the patient in each instance to describe the sensation.

Corneal Reflex

Ask the patient to look up and away from you. Carefully avoiding the eyelashes and conjunctiva, touch the cornea of the eye with a wisp of cotton and look for a reflexive blink *in both eyes*. The afferent limb of this reflex is carried in the ophthalmic division of the trigeminal nerve, the efferent limb in the facial nerve. Afferent lesions of the stimulated side result in loss of the ipsilateral and contralateral response, whereas efferent lesions result in loss of response in the affected side alone.

Facial Nerve

Motor

Inspect the face at rest for any weakness or asymmetry. Noting any signs of weakness or asymmetry, such as flattening of the nasolabial folds and drooping of the lower eyelid, ask the patient to smile, raise the eyebrows, puff out the cheeks, shut the eyes tightly, frown, and show some teeth. The distinction, described above, between an upper and lower motor neuron lesion here is critical.

Sensory

More difficult than the motor examination is testing the sense of taste on the anterior two thirds of the tongue. This is supplied by a branch of the facial nerve, proximal to the chorda tympani, which is tested by touching the lateral aspect of the tongue with sugar, salt, or vinegar, then asking the patient to identify the taste.

Vestibulocochlear Nerve

Cochlear

Test the sense of hearing by whispering a number into the patient's ears, noting the maximum distance at which the patient can accurately repeat the number. Next, determine whether air conduction is greater than bone conduction (Rinne test) and whether a tuning fork applied to the center of the forehead lateralizes (Weber test).

Vestibular

Vestibular testing is not a part of the routine neurological exam, although nystagmus (see earlier discussion) is a sign of vestibular dysfunction.

Glossopharyngeal and Vagus Nerves

As a test of the vagus nerve, observe the quality of the patient's voice: hoarseness is a sign of vocal cord paralysis; a nasal voice reflects paralysis of the palate.

Next, instruct the patient to say "ah" and observe the elevation of the palate. In bilateral lesions of the vagus nerve, the palate fails to rise, whereas in unilateral paralysis, both the palate and the uvula deviate to the normal side.

Finally, test the gag reflex. Stimulation of the dorsal wall of the pharynx with an applicator stick normally causes contraction of the pharyngeal muscles. Absence of the gag reflex suggests a lesion in the glossopharyngeal or vagus nerves, although it also occurs in normals.

Accessory Nerve

Estimate the strength of contraction of the sternocleidomastoid muscle as the patient turns his or her head against resistance. Estimate also the strength of contraction of the trapezii muscles as the patient shrugs the shoulders against resistance.

Hypoglossal Nerve

Ask the patient to protrude the tongue, noting any deviation from the midline, atrophy, or fibrillations. Atrophy and fibrillations are the hallmarks of the lower motor neuron lesion, which results in tongue deviation to the weakened side.

8 Cerebellum

External Appearance

See **Fig. 8.1**.

The cerebellum is composed of two cerebellar hemispheres joined by a median vermis. The *superior vermis* is confluent with the hemispheres, whereas the *inferior vermis* is a well-delineated structure that is located in a deep depression in the midline (the vallecula).

The cerebellum is divided into three lobes: the anterior lobe, the posterior lobe, and the flocculonodular lobe. The *anterior lobe* (paleocerebellum) constitutes the rostral portion of the rostral cerebellar surface; the *flocculonodular lobe* (archicerebellum) constitutes the rostral portion of the caudal cerebellar surface; and the *posterior lobe* (neocerebellum) makes up the remainder of the cerebellum on both surfaces.

Two major fissures of the cerebellum are identified: the *primary fissure* separates the anterior lobe from the posterior lobe on the superior surface, and the *dorsolateral fissure* separates the posterior lobe from the flocculonodular lobe on the inferior surface.

The rostral portion of the roof of the fourth ventricle is formed by the *superior cerebellar peduncles*. The caudal aspect of the roof of the fourth ventricle is formed by the *inferior medullary velum*, which frequently adheres to the inferior vermis. The foramen of Magendie is a median aperture, which constitutes an opening in the inferior medullary velum that connects the fourth ventricle with the cisterna magna. The three cerebellar peduncles are attached to the cerebellum in the interval between the anterior and the flocculonodular lobes.

Fig. 8.1 External appearance of cerebellum.

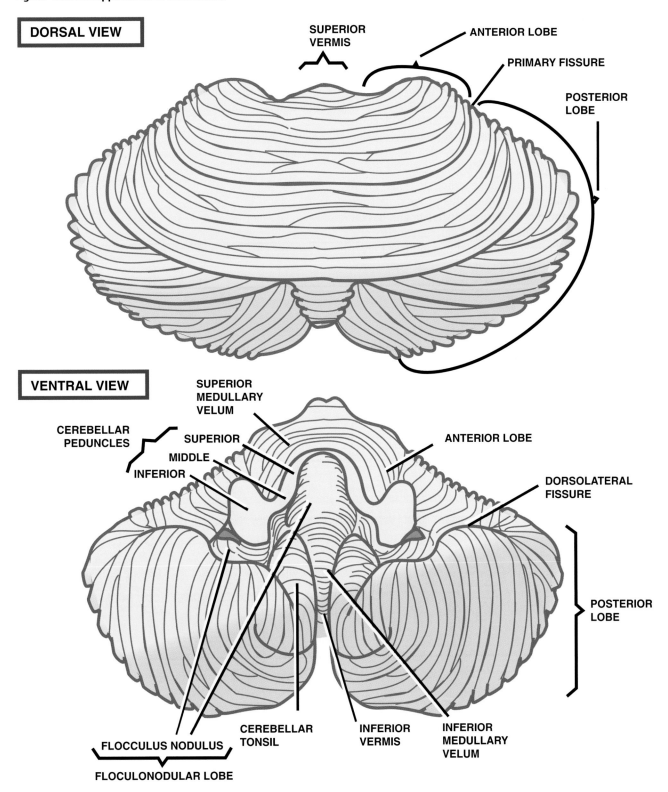

DORSAL VIEW

SUPERIOR VERMIS

ANTERIOR LOBE

PRIMARY FISSURE

POSTERIOR LOBE

VENTRAL VIEW

SUPERIOR MEDULLARY VELUM

CEREBELLAR PEDUNCLES

SUPERIOR

MIDDLE

INFERIOR

ANTERIOR LOBE

DORSOLATERAL FISSURE

POSTERIOR LOBE

FLOCCULUS NODULUS

FLOCULONODULAR LOBE

CEREBELLAR TONSIL

INFERIOR VERMIS

INFERIOR MEDULLARY VELUM

Cerebellar Cortex

Cortical Layers

See **Fig. 8.2**.

The cerebellar cortex is divided into three layers: a superficial *molecular layer*, a middle *Purkinje layer*, and a deep *granular layer*. These layers are collectively composed of five cell types: *stellate, basket, Purkinje, Golgi,* and *granule cells*.

The molecular layer is so-called because of its punctuated, sparsely populated appearance. It is largely a synaptic layer that contains dendrites of Purkinje cells and axons of granule cells. Scattered stellate and basket cells are also present. The Purkinje cell layer consists of a single row of Purkinje cell bodies; the granule cell layer consists of densely packed neurons that send axonal pro-jections into the molecular layer. The granule cell layer is composed of granule and Golgi cells.

An embryonic cerebellar layer, the external granule cell layer, is present during the prenatal and early post-natal periods but is completely gone by the first year of life. This layer is superficial to the molecular layer, and its cells are thought to be the cell of origin of medullo-blastomas.

Fig. 8.2 **Layers of the cerebellum.**

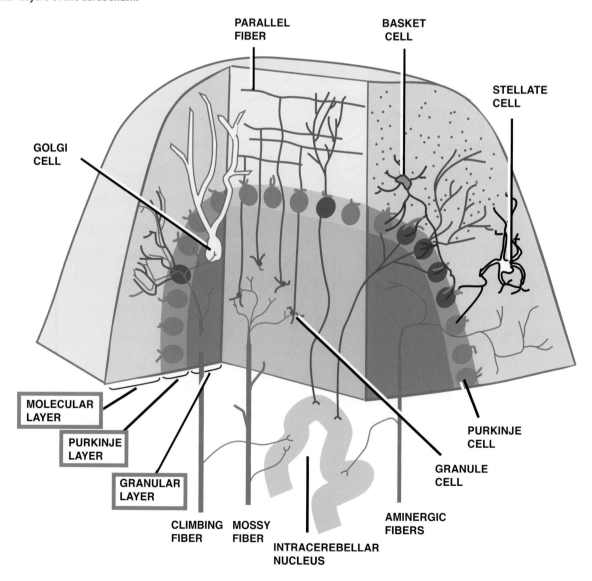

Intrinsic Circuitry

See **Fig. 8.3**.

The intrinsic circuitry of the cerebellar cortex is primarily composed of two interrelated circuits, which receive input from two afferent nerve fibers, the climbing fibers and the mossy fibers. The input from these fiber systems is received by the Purkinje cells (directly and indirectly), which in turn project to the neurons in the deep cerebellar nuclei.

Climbing fibers, most of which originate in the inferior olive, make direct contacts with the dendrites of a limited number of Purkinje cells. By contrast, *mossy fibers*, which are derived from a variety of sources, indirectly influence a large number of Purkinje cells. To accomplish this, the mossy fibers branch extensively in the granule cell layer, where they establish synaptic contacts with the granule cells. Rosettes are the sites of synapses between mossy fibers and the clawlike terminals of granule cell dendrites. Mossy fiber rosettes also establish synapses with Golgi type II cell bodies. The granule cells project superficially to the molecular layer, where they bifurcate in a **T**-shaped manner to form the so-called parallel fibers. Each parallel fiber establishes contacts with a large number of Purkinje cell dendrites.

Thus, the climbing fibers exert a powerful influence on a few specific Purkinje cells, whereas the mossy fibers modulate a large number of Purkinje cells through a relay in the granular layer. In other words, a single climbing fiber may stimulate a Purkinje cell in an all-or-none phenomenon, whereas many mossy fiber discharges are required to stimulate a Purkinje cell.

A third category of afferent axons, the aminergic fibers, are distinct both from climbing and mossy fibers in that they contain biogenic amines. These fibers, which show a widespread distribution in the cerebellar cortex, are divided into two different types: serotonin-containing axons that originate in the raphe nuclei of the brainstem, and norepinephrine-containing axons that originate in the locus ceruleus.

These circuits involving climbing fibers, mossy fibers, and aminergic fibers are modified by intracortical circuits formed by three types of interneurons that appear to function as modulators of Purkinje cell activity. These are the *Golgi, basket,* and *stellate cells*. Like the Purkinje cells, these interneurons are inhibitory in nature, and they contain the neurotransmitter gamma-aminobutyric acid (GABA). Thus, four out of the five cells in the cerebellar cortex are GABA-containing inhibitory neurons. Only the granule cells and the afferent fiber system are excitatory.

The overall circuit in the cerebellar cortex may be summarized as follows. Excitatory input to the cerebellar cortex is primarily derived from the mossy fibers and the climbing fibers. This excitatory input is received by the Purkinje cells (directly and indirectly), which are responsible, in turn, for the entire (inhibitory) output of the cerebellar cortex. The excitatory input to the Purkinje cells is further modified by the inhibitory influences of the modulating interneurons. The Purkinje cells project into the deep cerebellar nuclei.

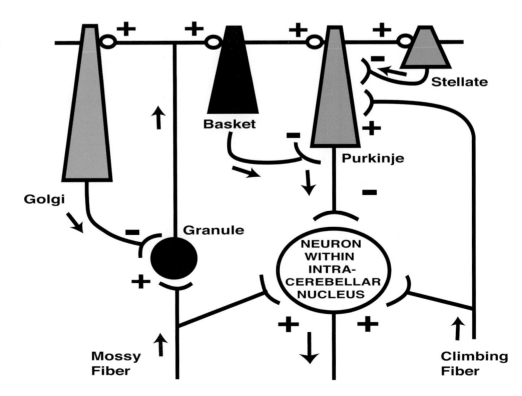

Fig. 8.3 **Intrinsic circuitry.**

Deep Cerebellar Nuclei

See **Fig. 8.4**.

Four pairs of nuclei are located in the white matter of the cerebellum. From medial to lateral on each side of the midline, they are the *fastigial, globose, emboliform,* and *dentate nuclei*. The globose and the emboliform nuclei are collectively known as the interposed nuclei because they are interposed between the fastigial and dentate nuclei.

The input to the cerebellar nuclei is derived from two sources: (1) excitatory input is derived from fibers that originate in cells that lie outside the cerebellum, and (2) inhibitory input is derived from fibers that arise from the Purkinje cells of the cortex. Cells outside the cerebellum that send afferents directly to the cerebellar nuclei include pontocerebellar, spinocerebellar, and olivocerebellar fibers, most of which give collaterals to the cerebellar nuclei, then continue on to the cerebellar cortex.

The cells that constitute the intracerebellar nuclei act to modify muscular activity through the motor control areas of the brainstem and cerebral cortex. Efferents from the fastigial nucleus project to the brainstem through the inferior cerebellar peduncle, whereas efferents from the other nuclei are projected to the brainstem and cerebral cortex (with relays in the thalamus) through the superior cerebellar peduncle.

Fig. 8.4 Deep cerebellar nuclei.

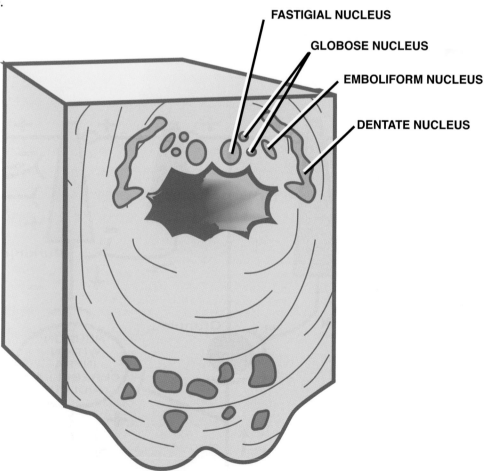

FASTIGIAL NUCLEUS

GLOBOSE NUCLEUS

EMBOLIFORM NUCLEUS

DENTATE NUCLEUS

Cerebellar Connections

Afferent Connections

See **Fig. 8.5**.

Cerebellar afferents are derived from three main sources: the cerebral cortex, the spinal cord, and the vestibular nerve. A small number of afferents originate in the red nucleus and the tectum.

Fig. 8.5 **Afferent cerebellar connections.**

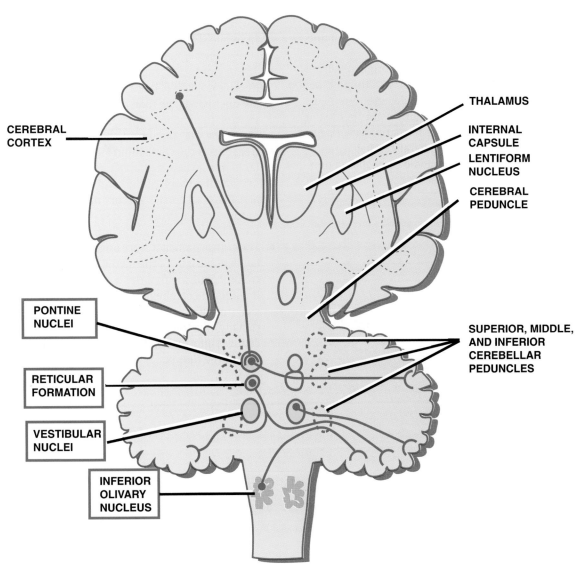

CEREBRAL CORTEX

THALAMUS

INTERNAL CAPSULE

LENTIFORM NUCLEUS

CEREBRAL PEDUNCLE

PONTINE NUCLEI

RETICULAR FORMATION

VESTIBULAR NUCLEI

INFERIOR OLIVARY NUCLEUS

SUPERIOR, MIDDLE, AND INFERIOR CEREBELLAR PEDUNCLES

Cerebral Cortex

See **Fig. 8.6**.

Before reaching the cerebellum, cortical projections establish synaptic contacts with three brainstem structures: (1) the *pontine nuclei*, (2) the *inferior olivary nucleus*, and (3) the *reticular formation.*

The *corticopontocerebellar pathway* originates from a large area of the cerebral cortex, descends through the corona radiata and the internal capsule, and terminates in the pontine nuclei. The cells of the pontine nuclei give rise to mossy fibers that cross the midline to reach the opposite cerebellar hemisphere via the middle cerebellar peduncle.

The *cortico-olivocerebellar pathway* also originates from a large area of the cerebral cortex, descends through the corona radiata and the internal capsule, and terminates bilaterally in the inferior olivary nuclei. The cells of the inferior olivary nuclei give rise to climbing fibers that cross the midline to enter the opposite cerebellar hemisphere via the inferior cerebellar peduncle.

The *corticoreticulocerebellar pathway* originates from a large area of the cerebral cortex, descends through the corona radiata and the internal capsule, and terminates bilaterally in the reticular formation of the pons and medulla. The cells of the reticular formation give rise to mossy fibers that enter the ipsilateral cerebellar hemisphere via the inferior and the middle cerebellar peduncles.

Spinal Cord

See **Fig. 8.7**, p. 288.

Spinal cord projections to the cerebellum are carried in three spinocerebellar pathways: (1) the *ventral spinocerebellar tract*, (2) the *dorsal spinocerebellar tract*, and (3) the *cuneocerebellar tract.*

- The ventral spinocerebellar tract originates in the ventral and intermediate gray matter of the spinal cord. Most of its fibers cross the midline to enter the ventral spinocerebellar tract on the opposite side, although a small number of fibers are uncrossed. The tract ascends bilaterally in the dorsolateral region of the lateral funiculus. After ascending the spinal cord, the ventral spinocerebellar tract enters the cerebellum via the superior cerebellar peduncle, crosses the midline for a second time, and terminates as mossy fibers in the cerebellar cortex. Functionally, this tract carries sensory information (mainly proprioceptive) from one side of the body (lower limbs) to the same side of the cerebellum.
- The dorsal spinocerebellar tract originates in the nucleus dorsalis (Clark's column). Most of its fibers are uncrossed. The tract ascends bilaterally in the ventrolateral region of the lateral funiculus. After ascending the spinal cord, the dorsal spinocerebellar tract enters the cerebellum via the inferior cerebellar peduncle and terminates as mossy fibers in the intermediate zone of the cerebellar cortex. Functionally, this tract carries sensory information (mainly proprioceptive) from one side of the body (trunk and lower limbs) to the cerebellum ipsilaterally.
- The cuneocerebellar tract originates in the accessory cuneate nucleus of the medulla. It is the upper extremity equivalent of the dorsal spinocerebellar tract. It enters the cerebellar hemisphere on the ipsilateral side through the inferior cerebellar peduncle. Functionally, this tract transmits sensory (mainly proprioceptive) information from the upper limb and upper part of the thorax.

Fig. 8.6 **Afferent cerebellar connections from cortex.**

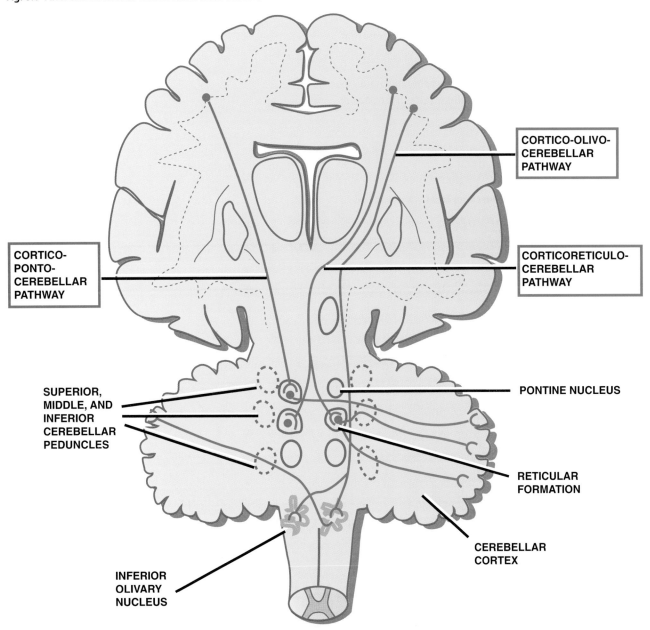

CORTICO-OLIVO-
CEREBELLAR
PATHWAY

CORTICO-
PONTO-
CEREBELLAR
PATHWAY

CORTICORETICULO-
CEREBELLAR
PATHWAY

SUPERIOR,
MIDDLE, AND
INFERIOR
CEREBELLAR
PEDUNCLES

PONTINE NUCLEUS

RETICULAR
FORMATION

CEREBELLAR
CORTEX

INFERIOR
OLIVARY
NUCLEUS

Vestibular Nerve

See **Fig. 8.7**.

The vestibular nerve gives rise to afferent fibers that terminate in the *vestibular nuclei* of the brainstem. The neurons of the vestibular nuclei in turn give rise to mossy fibers that pass through the inferior cerebellar peduncle to enter the ipsilateral flocculonodular lobe on the same side.

Fig. 8.7 **Afferent cerebellar connections from brainstem and spinal cord.**

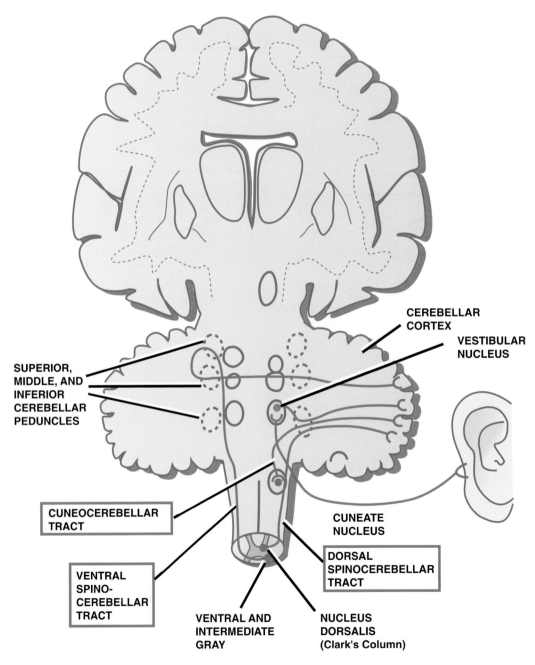

CEREBELLAR
CORTEX

VESTIBULAR
NUCLEUS

SUPERIOR,
MIDDLE, AND
INFERIOR
CEREBELLAR
PEDUNCLES

CUNEOCEREBELLAR
TRACT

CUNEATE
NUCLEUS

DORSAL
SPINOCEREBELLAR
TRACT

VENTRAL
SPINO-
CEREBELLAR
TRACT

VENTRAL AND
INTERMEDIATE
GRAY

NUCLEUS
DORSALIS
(Clark's Column)

Efferent Connections

The entire output of the cerebellar cortex is transmitted by the inhibitory Purkinje cells, most of which terminate on the deep cerebellar nuclei (a few Purkinje cell axons continue past the cerebellar nuclei to synapse on the lateral vestibular nucleus in the medulla). The cells of the cerebellar nuclei constitute the entire efferent outflow system of the cerebellum. These cells leave the cerebellum through the superior and inferior cerebellar peduncles to terminate in the following four destinations: (1) the red nucleus, (2) the thalamus, (3) the vestibular complex, and (4) the reticular formation.

The superior cerebellar peduncle transmits those fibers that ascend to the red nucleus and the thalamus. These constitute the majority of the fibers. The inferior cerebellar peduncle transmits those fibers that descend to the vestibular and the reticular formation.

Red Nucleus

See **Fig. 8.8**.

The axons of neurons in the *globose* and *emboliform nuclei* pass out of the cerebellum through the *superior cerebellar peduncle* and cross the midline. These axons ascend and synapse in the contralateral *red nucleus*, which in turn projects fibers in the crossed *rubrospinal tract*. Thus, projections from the globose and emboliform nuclei, which cross twice before reaching their final destination, influence motor body activity ipsilaterally. The rubrospinal tract influences flexor activity of the extremities. Therefore, the globose and emboliform nuclei are involved with tone.

Fig. 8.8 **Efferent cerebellar connections to red nucleus.**

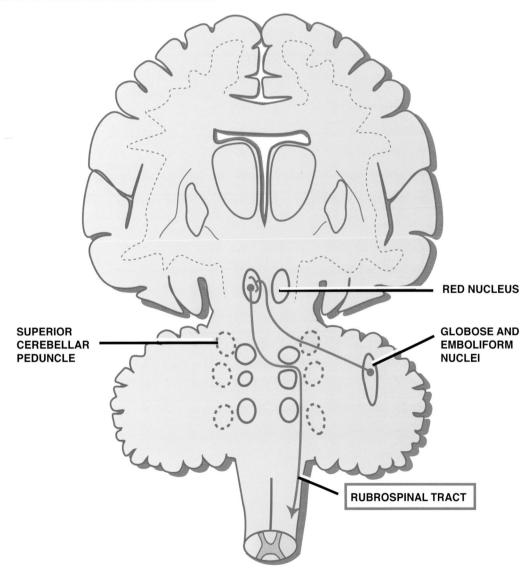

SUPERIOR CEREBELLAR PEDUNCLE

RED NUCLEUS

GLOBOSE AND EMBOLIFORM NUCLEI

RUBROSPINAL TRACT

Thalamus

See **Fig. 8.9**.

The axons of neurons in the *dentate nucleus* (and some from the globose and emboliform nuclei) exit the cerebellum through the *superior cerebellar peduncle* and cross the midline in the same decussation. These axons ascend to synapse in the contralateral ventrolateral, ventroposterolateral, and centrolateral nuclei of the thalamus, which in turn project axons through the internal capsule and the corona radiata to terminate in the primary motor cortex. The dentate nucleus thus influences the motor neurons of the cerebral cortex on the contralateral side. The motor cortex, however, projects descending fibers in the corticospinal tract, which cross the midline in the decussation of the pyramids. Thus, the neurons in the dentate nucleus influence motor activity on the same side of the body. Therefore, the dentate mainly influences coordination of the ipsilateral body.

Fig. 8.9 **Efferent cerebellar connections to thalamus.**

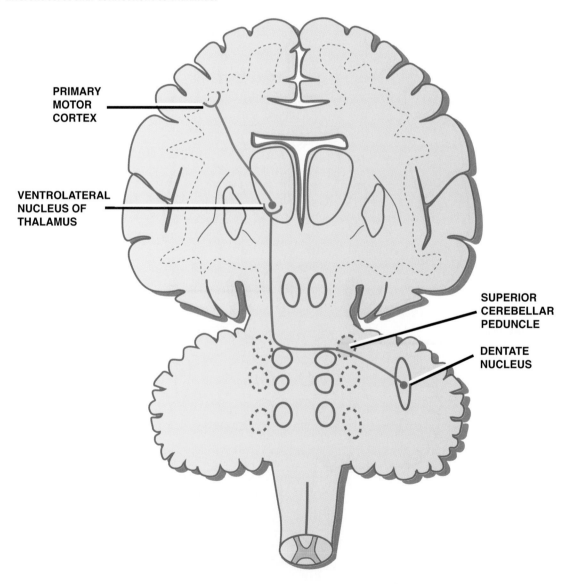

PRIMARY
MOTOR
CORTEX

VENTROLATERAL
NUCLEUS OF
THALAMUS

SUPERIOR
CEREBELLAR
PEDUNCLE

DENTATE
NUCLEUS

Vestibular Complex

See **Fig. 8.10**.

The axons of the neurons in the fastigial nucleus pass out of the cerebellum through the inferior cerebellar peduncle. These axons descend to terminate on the lateral vestibular nucleus on both sides. As already stated, a few Purkinje cell axons pass the deep cerebellar nuclei and project directly on the lateral vestibular nucleus. The neurons of the lateral vestibular nucleus form the uncrossed descending vestibulospinal tract. Thus, the neurons in the fastigial nucleus influence motor activity (facilitate extensor muscle tone) on the same side of the body. Fibers also synapse on the superior and medial vestibular nuclei. Therefore, the coordination of extensor muscles is also influenced by the cerebellum.

Reticular Formation

The axons of the neurons in the fastigial nucleus pass out of the cerebellum through the inferior cerebellar peduncle. Some of these axons descend to synapse with cells in the reticular formation on both sides. The reticular formation in turn gives rise to the descending reticulospinal tract, which projects both ipsilaterally and bilaterally to the spinal gray matter. The axons of the reticulospinal tract end on interneurons and influence motor neurons indirectly through synaptic relays within the spinal cord.

Fig. 8.10 **Efferent cerebellar connections to vestibular complex.**

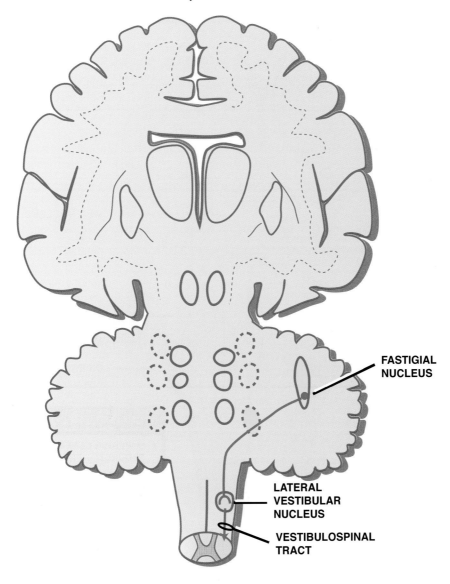

FASTIGIAL
NUCLEUS

LATERAL
VESTIBULAR
NUCLEUS

VESTIBULOSPINAL
TRACT

Cerebellar Peduncles

See **Fig. 8.11**.

All the efferent and afferent fibers of the cerebellum reside in the three cerebellar peduncles. The *superior cerebellar peduncle* consists primarily of efferent fibers to the globose, emboliform, and dentate nuclei. A smaller number of afferent fibers, including the ventral spinocerebellar tract, are also present.

The *middle cerebellar peduncle* is the largest of the three peduncles. It contains the afferent pontocerebellar fibers that arise from the contralateral side.

The *inferior cerebellar peduncle* consists primarily of afferent fibers, including (1) the dorsal spinocerebellar tract, (2) the cuneocerebellar tract, (3) the olivocerebellar tract, (4) the reticulocerebellar tract, and (5) the vestibulocerebellar tract. A smaller group of efferent fibers include those that originate in the flocculonodular lobe and the fastigial nucleus, to project on the vestibular nuclei and the central group of reticular nuclei of the medulla and the pons.

Fig. 8.11 **Cerebellar peduncles.**

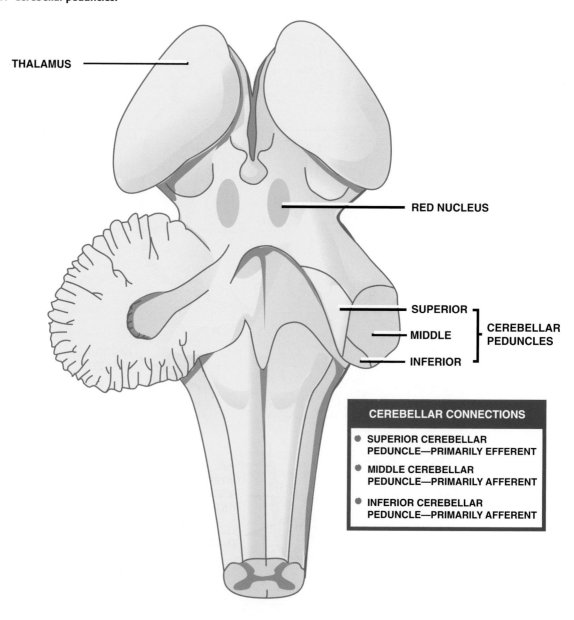

THALAMUS

RED NUCLEUS

SUPERIOR
MIDDLE · CEREBELLAR PEDUNCLES
INFERIOR

CEREBELLAR CONNECTIONS

- SUPERIOR CEREBELLAR PEDUNCLE—PRIMARILY EFFERENT
- MIDDLE CEREBELLAR PEDUNCLE—PRIMARILY AFFERENT
- INFERIOR CEREBELLAR PEDUNCLE—PRIMARILY AFFERENT

Cerebellar Function

See **Fig. 8.12**.

The cerebellum influences motor activity through its connections with the brainstem and cerebral cortex. It receives information on the activity of the muscles via proprioceptive input from the cerebral cortex, the muscles, the tendons, and the joints. It also receives input concerning equilibrium from the vestibular nuclei.

This afferent input is transmitted to the cerebellar cortex by the excitatory *climbing* and *mossy fibers*. These fibers establish direct or indirect synaptic contacts with the *Purkinje cells*, which in turn exert an inhibitory influence on the *deep cerebellar nuclei* and the lateral vestibular nuclei of the brainstem. Purkinje cell fibers located in the lateral cerebellar hemispheres project to the dentate nuclei; those located in the cerebellar vermis project to the fastigial nuclei; and those located in between project to the globose and emboliform nuclei.

Almost the entire cerebellar output is derived from the cells of the cerebellar nuclei. This output is directed to the sites of origin of the primary descending motor pathways, although it is interesting to note that no direct contacts are made between the cerebellar efferents and the alpha motor neurons. Instead, the cerebellum provides an ongoing comparison of the motor output of the cerebral cortex with the proprioceptive information received from the peripheral nervous system. This allows the cerebellum to continuously make minor motor output adjustments based on information regarding ongoing muscle activity.

Fig. 8.12 **Cerebellar function.**

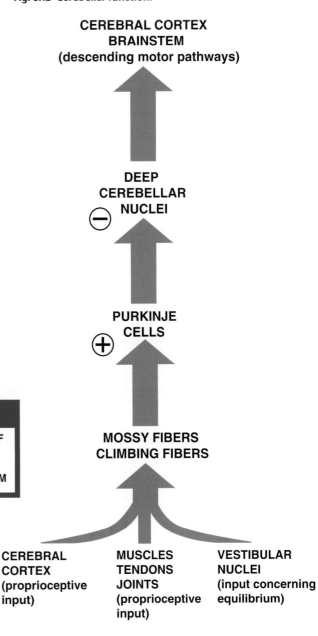

Functional Anatomic Organization of Cerebellum

The cerebellum may be loosely divided into three separate parts that are distinguished by their input and their major functional activities. These are the vestibulocerebellum, the spinocerebellum, and the pontocerebellum.

Vestibulocerebellum

See **Fig. 8.13**.

The vestibulocerebellum primarily consists of the flocculonodular lobe. It receives mossy fibers from the ipsilateral *vestibular nuclei* and the *vestibular ganglion* via the inferior cerebellar peduncles. It also receives visual information from the lateral geniculate nucleus, superior colliculi, and striate cortex.

Purkinje cell axons of the vestibulocerebellum primarily project to the *fastigial nucleus*. Axons of the cells in the fastigial nucleus leave the cerebellum via the inferior cerebellar peduncles to terminate in the vestibular nuclei.

The vestibulocerebellum influences primary motor activity through its contacts with the vestibulospinal tract. It is concerned with the adjustment of axial muscle tone and the maintenance of equilibrium. It also plays a role in eye movements, control, and the coordination of head and eye movements.

Fig. 8.13 Vestibulocerebellum.

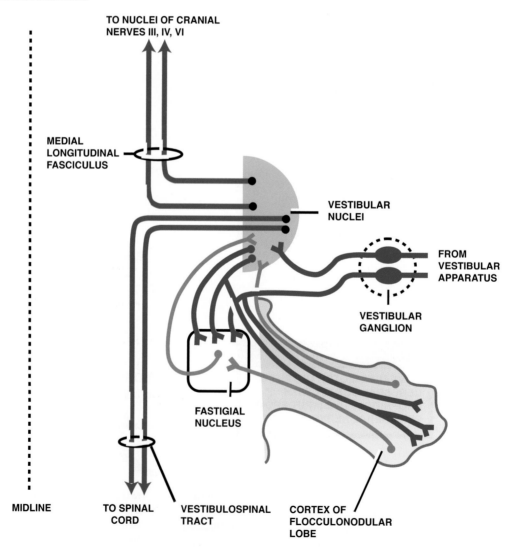

Spinocerebellum

See **Fig. 8.14**.

The spinocerebellum primarily consists of the vermis and the intermediate part of the cerebellar hemispheres. Its primary source of input is somatosensory information from the *dorsal* and *ventral spinocerebellar tracts* of the spinal cord. It also receives information from the auditory, visual, and vestibular systems.

The two parts of the spinocerebellum are composed of two separate output pathways. Purkinje cells in the vermis of the cerebellum send axons to the fastigial nucleus. Axons from this nucleus then project to the brainstem reticular formation, the lateral vestibular nuclei, and the primary motor cortex (via relays in the ventrolateral thalamus). This portion of the spinocerebellum is responsible for control of the medial descending systems, which regulate axial and proximal musculature.

By contrast, Purkinje cells in the intermediate part of the cerebellar hemispheres send axons to interposed nuclei, which in turn project to the rubrospinal and lateral corticospinal tracts. A smaller number of projections from the interposed nuclei relay in the ventrolateral thalamus and continue on to the primary motor cortex. The hemispheric part of the spinocerebellum is responsible for control of the lateral descending systems, which regulate the distal limb muscles.

Efferent fibers from the intermediate zone of the cerebellar hemispheres leave the cerebellum through the superior cerebellar peduncles to reach the rubrospinal and lateral corticospinal tracts. Along the way, these fibers cross in the decussation of the superior cerebellar peduncles. Because the rubrospinal and lateral corticospinal tract fibers also cross the midline before they terminate in the spinal cord, destructive lesions in the intermediate zone of the cerebellar hemispheres result in neurologic deficits on the ispilateral side of the body: the spinocerebellum influences the skeletal musculature on the ipsilateral side of the body.

The spinocerebellum controls the execution of movement and regulates muscle tone. It carries out these functions by continuously comparing information about the intended motor commands of the primary motor cortex with feedback about ongoing movement that is received from the spinal cord and periphery. This organization allows the spinocerebellum to correct for deviations in intended movement.

Fig. 8.14 **Spinocerebellum.**

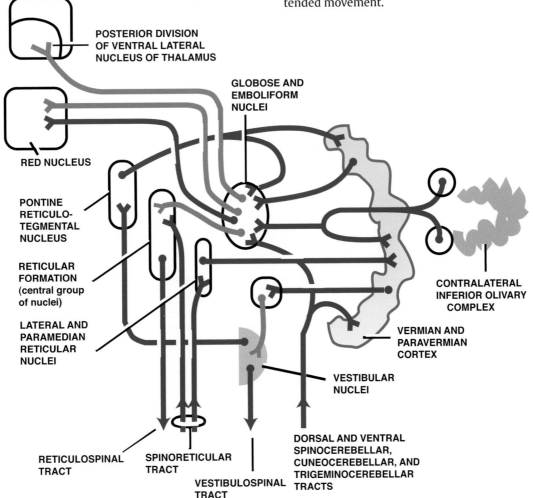

POSTERIOR DIVISION OF VENTRAL LATERAL NUCLEUS OF THALAMUS

GLOBOSE AND EMBOLIFORM NUCLEI

RED NUCLEUS

PONTINE RETICULO-TEGMENTAL NUCLEUS

RETICULAR FORMATION (central group of nuclei)

LATERAL AND PARAMEDIAN RETICULAR NUCLEI

CONTRALATERAL INFERIOR OLIVARY COMPLEX

VERMIAN AND PARAVERMIAN CORTEX

VESTIBULAR NUCLEI

RETICULOSPINAL TRACT

SPINORETICULAR TRACT

VESTIBULOSPINAL TRACT

DORSAL AND VENTRAL SPINOCEREBELLAR, CUNEOCEREBELLAR, AND TRIGEMINOCEREBELLAR TRACTS

Pontocerebellum

See **Fig. 8.15**.

The pontocerebellum primarily consists of the large lateral regions of the cerebellar hemispheres. Its primary source of input is from large areas of the contralateral *cerebral cortex* (especially that of the frontal and parietal lobes). These corticopontine fibers relay in the *pontine nuclei* and then enter the cerebellum through the middle cerebellar peduncles, of which they are the sole constituents. The information that is transmitted from the cerebral cortex to the cerebellum concerns volitional movements that are ongoing or are about to happen.

Purkinje cell axons of the pontocerebellar cortex project to the *dentate nucleus*, which in turn projects fibers via the superior cerebellar peduncles to the *ventrolateral nucleus of the thalamus*. Pontocerebellar afferents make up most of the fibers in the superior cerebellar peduncles. Axons from the nucleus of the ventrolateral thalamus project to the *primary motor cortex*, thus completing the corticopontine–thalamic–cortical loop.

Because of decussations in both the superior cerebellar peduncles and the corticospinal tract and other descending pathways, the pontocerebellum exerts its influence on the ipsilateral side of the body.

The pontocerebellum is concerned with precision in the control of rapid limb movements and with tasks requiring fine dexterity. It ensures a smooth and orderly sequence in muscle contractions and regulates the force, direction, and extent of volitional movement. It functions in these capacities by modulating activity in the primary motor cortex, a role that is also performed by the premotor cortical areas. Destructive lesions in the pontocerebellum may lead to various movement disorders, such as delays in the initiation or termination of movement, or involuntary tremor at the end of a movement.

Fig. 8.15 **Pontocerebellum.**

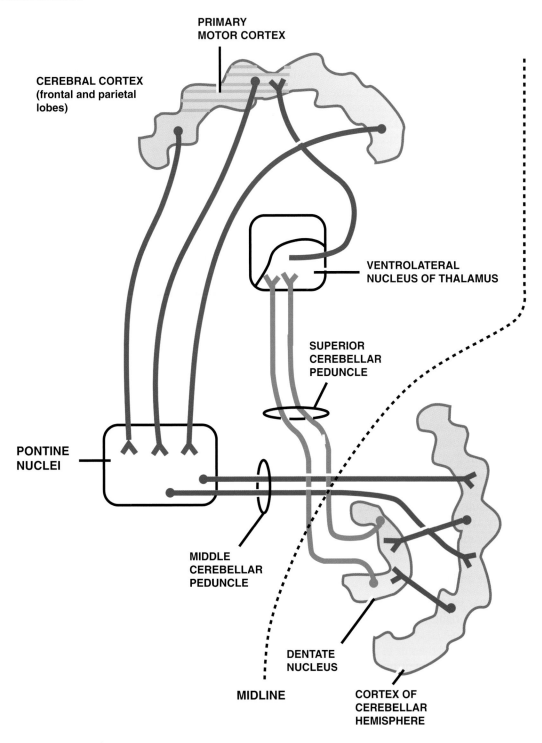

PRIMARY
MOTOR CORTEX

CEREBRAL CORTEX
(frontal and parietal
lobes)

VENTROLATERAL
NUCLEUS OF THALAMUS

SUPERIOR
CEREBELLAR
PEDUNCLE

PONTINE
NUCLEI

MIDDLE
CEREBELLAR
PEDUNCLE

DENTATE
NUCLEUS

MIDLINE

CORTEX OF
CEREBELLAR
HEMISPHERE

Clinical Manifestations of Cerebellar Disease

The clinical manifestations of cerebellar disease may be divided into three categories: (1) the symptoms of cerebellar disease, (2) the signs of midline cerebellar disease, and (3) the signs of lateral (hemispheric) cerebellar disease. Although the functional anatomy of the cerebellum comprises three separate zones—a midline, an intermediate, and a lateral (hemispheric) zone—only the midline and lateral zones are associated with distinct abnormalities; no abnormalities that are specifically associated with the intermediate zone have been identified. Furthermore, many of the signs that are observed with midline lesions may also be associated with lateral lesions, and vice versa.

Symptoms of Cerebellar Disease

The symptoms of cerebellar disease are nonspecific. They include **headache, nausea and vomiting, gait difficulty**, and **vertigo**.

Signs of Midline Cerebellar Disease

See **Fig. 8.16**.

The midline of the cerebellum comprises the anterior and posterior vermis, the flocculonodular lobe, and the fastigial nuclei. Functionally, this zone is responsible for equilibrium required during ambulation, the maintenance of truncal posture, the position of the head in relation to the trunk, and the control of extraocular eye movements. As a result, lesions in this area tend to produce **gait difficulty, truncal imbalance, abnormal head postures**, and **ocular motor dysfunction**.

Disorders of Stance and Gait

Truncal instability may be manifested during walking by a tendency to fall to the right, left, forward, or backward. While sitting, the patient may lean or fall to one side. These tendencies tend to be toward the side of the lesion.

Several abnormalities of gait, which are collectively described as gait ataxia, include a wider than normal base, unsteadiness and irregularity of steps, and lateral veering. The steps may be uncertain, some shorter and some longer than intended, and there may be a tendency to stagger or lurch to one side. There is little localizing value in cerebellar gait disorders to distinguish between midline and lateral cerebellar lesions, although lateral lesions tend to cause the patient to veer toward the side of the lesion.

Mild cerebellar gait disorders may be exacerbated by asking the patient to tandem walk. The Romberg's sign, in which the patient loses balance after closing the eyes, is a result of disordered position sensation secondary to posterior column disease and is not related to cerebellar dysfunction.

Abnormal Postures of the Head

Abnormal postures of the head may be due to midline or lateral cerebellar lesions. They may present as a head tilt (i.e., lateral deviation of the head) or a rotated posture of the head.

Ocular Motor Dysfunction

Like the clinical signs already described, ocular motor dysfunction may occur in association with midline cerebellar lesions but is also associated with lesions in other parts of the cerebellum.

The cerebellum and brainstem are involved in computing the location of targets in space, deriving temporal information from spatial information for appropriate muscle innervation, and adjusting the gain on saccadic eye movements to minimize target overshoot and undershoot. As a result, the primary disorders of extraocular movements in midline cerebellar disease are nystagmus and ocular dysmetria.

Nystagmus consists of rhythmic oscillatory movements of one or both eyes, occurring with the eyes in the primary position or with ocular deviation. The most common types of nystagmus observed in association with midline cerebellar lesions are (1) *gaze-evoked nystagmus*, (2) *rebound nystagmus*, and (3) *optokinetic nystagmus*.

Gaze-evoked nystagmus occurs when an individual cannot maintain conjugate eye deviation away from the midposition. Conjugate lateral gaze is accompanied by a slow, involuntary drift of the eyes back to midposition, followed by a rapid corrective return of the eyes to the laterally located target. The result is a to-and-fro oscillation of the eyes involving a fast component in the direction of gaze and a slow component away.

Rebound nystagmus is specific for cerebellar disease, although it is poorly localized within the cerebellum. It essentially represents a type of gaze-evoked nystagmus that changes direction after sustained lateral gaze or after refixation to the primary position.

Optokinetic nystagmus is a nonpathological nystagmus that develops normally when an individual attempts to count the stripes on a rotating drum or a moving cloth strip. In the presence of cerebellar disease, optokinetic nystagmus may become exaggerated, producing unusually large amplitudes of both the fast and the slow components.

Ocular dysmetria is defined as the conjugate overshoot of a target with voluntary saccades. The eyes appear to jerk back and forth because of repeated inaccuracies in saccadic movements intended to bring the target to the fovea.

Fig. 8.16 **Signs of midline cerebellar disease.**

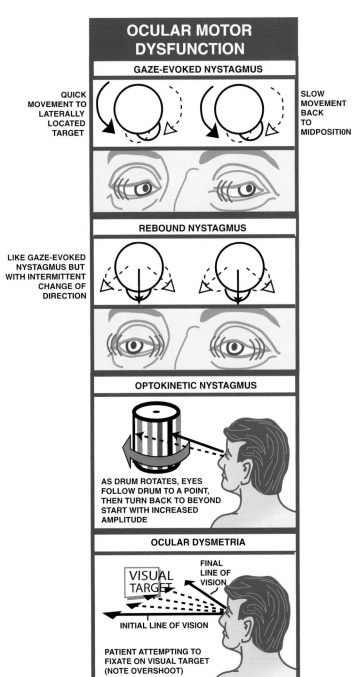

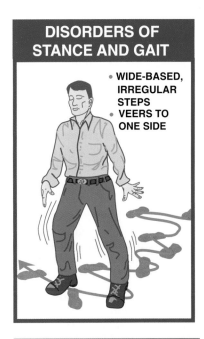

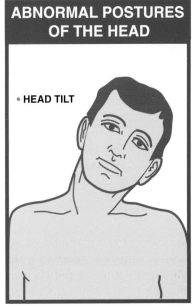

Signs of Lateral (Hemispheric) Cerebellar Disease

The lateral (hemispheric) zone of the cerebellum comprises the cerebellar hemisphere and the dentate and interposed nuclei of each side. The intermediate zone is also included here because it does not appear to be associated with distinct abnormalities. Compared with the midline zone, the lateral zone is involved in a greater variety of clinical disorders. These include (1) **hypotonia**, (2) **dysarthria**, (3) **limb ataxia**, (4) **intention tremor**, (5) **impaired check**, and (6) **oculomotor disorders**.

Hypotonia

Hypotonia, a decrease in resistance to passive movement of the limbs, is associated with lateral cerebellar lesions. It is best demonstrated by grasping the patient's forearms and shaking the relaxed wrists. Typically, the hypotonic limb is identified as the limb with more of a flail hand. In addition, examination of the patellar reflex in a hypotonic lower limb may demonstrate an increased duration and amplitude of swing. This pendular cerebellar reflex should be distinguished from clonus, due to corticospinal tract disease, which occurs at a more rapid rate than the pendular reflex.

Dysarthria

The dysarthria of cerebellar disease is characterized by slow, labored, slurred, or garbled speech that may be mistaken, like cerebellar ataxia, as a manifestation of alcohol intoxication. Comprehension and grammar remain intact.

Limb Ataxia

Limb ataxia, like gait ataxia, comprises a combination of disturbances in voluntary movement, the most important of which are dysmetria and the decomposition of movement.

Dysmetria consists of an error in trajectory and speed of movement. It is most easily demonstrated in the upper extremity, where it is tested by asking patients to touch the nose with the finger. Frequently, patients with lateral cerebellar disease undershoot or overshoot (past-pointing) the target. As the finger approaches the nose, it may oscillate around the nose and strike the cheek (overshoot) or stop short of touching the nose (undershoot). To test the lower extremity, ask the patient, in the supine position, to raise the heel of one foot over the knee of the other and to slide the heel smoothly down the shin. Frequent deviations to one side or the other are indicative of dysmetria in that limb.

Decomposition of movement involves errors in the sequence and speed of the component parts of a movement. An affected limb is unable to execute a movement, such as reaching out to grasp a glass of water, in a smooth and fluid manner. Instead, the movement is halting, imprecise, and jerky. Decomposition of movement may be tested by the same finger-to-nose test just described. Alternatively, decomposition of movement may be brought out in examination by asking the patient to perform a series of rapidly alternating or fine repetitive movements, such as a sequence of pronation and supination movements of the hand. The presence of decomposition of movement during this maneuver is referred to as dysdiadochokinesis.

Intention Tremor

Intention tremor is an irregular, more or less rhythmic, interruption of a voluntary movement that begins and increases as the patient approaches a target. It may be tested, like ataxia, by asking the patient to perform a finger-to-nose maneuver. Intention tremor is distinguished from the rest tremor of parkinsonism, which only occurs at rest, and the action tremor of familial or essential origin, which characteristically occurs during a sustained posture and from the beginning to the end of a movement.

Impaired Check

An impaired check response is characterized by the wide excursion of an affected limb following an involuntary displacement of the limb by an examiner. It may be tested by tapping the wrists of a patient with outstretched, pronated arms. With the patient's eyes closed, normally there is a small displacement of the arm that has been tapped, followed by a rapid, accurate return to the original position. In a patient with cerebellar disease, the displaced arm demonstrates an unusually wide excursion, followed by an overshoot of the original position. The original position is finally reached only after considerable oscillation about it.

Another method that may be used to test for an impaired check response is to provide resistance against a patient's flexed arm. On abrupt release of an affected arm, the arm will continue unchecked in the direction of its force and will strike the patient's chest.

Oculomotor Disorders

See **Fig. 8.17**.

Many oculomotor disturbances are associated with both lateral and midline cerebellar disorders but defy more specific localization. Several of these disturbances have already been described, such as gaze-evoked nystagmus, rebound nystagmus, ocular dysmetria, and optokinetic nystagmus. Other oculomotor disorders are frequently associated with widespread cerebellar disease or with disease involving both the cerebellum and the brainstem, including the following:

- *Opsoclonus* This disorder is characterized by constant, random, conjugate saccades of unequal amplitudes in all directions. Frequently, they are most marked immediately before and after a fixation.
- *Ocular flutter* Ocular flutter is defined as rapid to-and-fro oscillations of the eyes. These abnormal movements may develop abruptly, last for only seconds, and disturb vision for the duration of the episode.

- *Ocular bobbing* Ocular bobbing comprises intermittent (abrupt) downward displacement of the eyes, followed by a slow, synchronous return to the primary position. The relatively quick downward displacement is slower than the fast component of nystagmus; this disorder should therefore be distinguished from downbeat nystagmus, which is associated with lesions in the cervicomedullary junction. Horizontal eye movements are typically paralyzed.
- *Ocular myoclonus* Ocular myoclonus is defined as a rhythmic, pendular oscillation of the eyes that is associated with synchronous oscillation of the plate (palatal myoclonus).

Fig. 8.17 **Signs of lateral cerebellar disease (oculomotor disorders).**

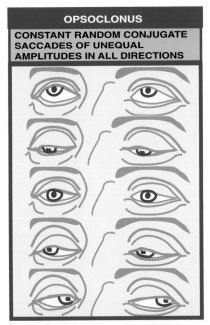
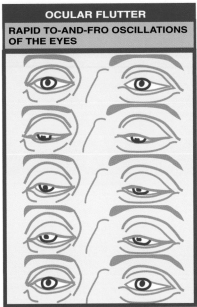
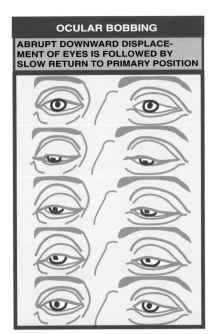
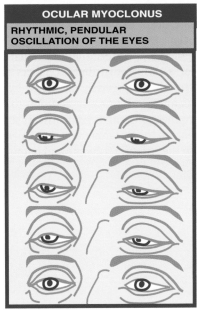

9 Thalamus

The cerebrum comprises a central core, or diencephalon, surrounded by the cerebral hemispheres, or telencephalon. The diencephalon contains the third ventricle and adjacent structures, including (1) the thalamus, (2) the subthalamus, (3) the epithalamus, and (4) the hypothalamus.

The boundaries of the diencephalon extend from the posterior commissure dorsally to the interventricular foramina ventrally. Dorsally it is bordered by the roof of the third ventricle; ventrally it is bordered, ventral to dorsal, by the optic chiasm, the infundibulum, and the mammillary bodies. The internal capsule comprises the lateral boundaries.

Thalamus

See **Figs. 9.1**, **9.2**, **9.3**, and **9.4**.

The thalamus is a large, ovoid mass of gray matter situated on either side of the third ventricle. The medial surfaces of the thalami often meet within the third ventricle to form the interthalamic connection (or *massa intermedia*).

The thalamus is the gateway to the cerebral cortex: all major sensory pathways, except olfactory, relay in the thalamus before ascending to the cortex. The thalamus also has important connections with the extrapyramidal motor system, the consciousness system, the visual system, and the limbic system. Therefore, lesions in the thalamus result in sensory and motor disturbances, as well as disturbances in alertness, vision, and behavior.

The reticular nucleus excepted, each thalamic nucleus sends axons to the cerebral cortex. These terminate in either a discrete or a diffuse distribution. Fibers that are distributed discretely are precisely paralleled by reciprocal corticothalamic projections. In addition to the two-way cortical connections, other (subcortical) structures project afferents to the thalamus, and the thalamus projects efferents to the striatum (caudate and putamen) and hypothalamus.

The reticular nucleus receives collaterals from both afferent and efferent thalamic axons and projects in turn to the other nuclei of the thalamus. No other thalamic nucleus projects to other thalamic nuclei, although each individual nucleus contains interneurons.

In what follows, we first describe the structural organization of the thalamus and its nuclei, then describe a second classification based on function. After a brief description of thalamic vascular supply, we summarize the clinical manifestations that result from thalamic dysfunction.

Fig. 9.1 Thalamus anatomy.

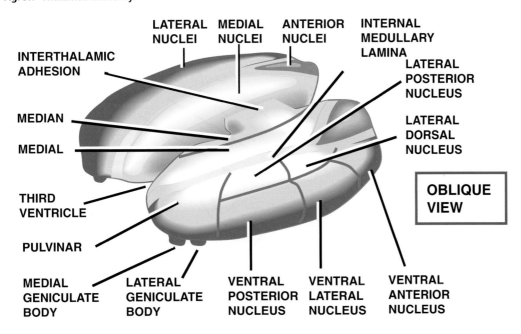

LATERAL NUCLEI

MEDIAL NUCLEI

ANTERIOR NUCLEI

INTERNAL MEDULLARY LAMINA

INTERTHALAMIC ADHESION

LATERAL POSTERIOR NUCLEUS

MEDIAN

LATERAL DORSAL NUCLEUS

MEDIAL

THIRD VENTRICLE

OBLIQUE VIEW

PULVINAR

MEDIAL GENICULATE BODY

LATERAL GENICULATE BODY

VENTRAL POSTERIOR NUCLEUS

VENTRAL LATERAL NUCLEUS

VENTRAL ANTERIOR NUCLEUS

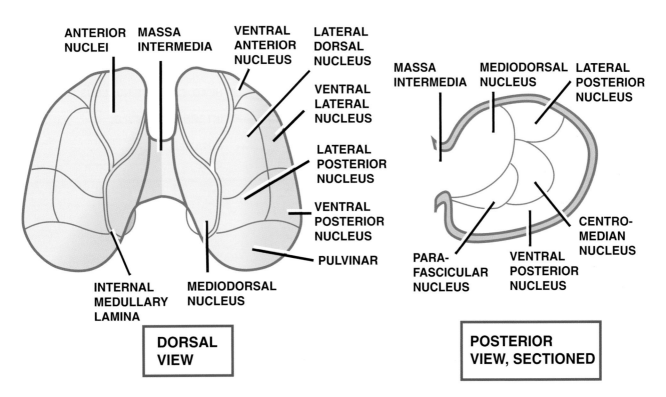

ANTERIOR NUCLEI

MASSA INTERMEDIA

VENTRAL ANTERIOR NUCLEUS

LATERAL DORSAL NUCLEUS

MASSA INTERMEDIA

MEDIODORSAL NUCLEUS

LATERAL POSTERIOR NUCLEUS

VENTRAL LATERAL NUCLEUS

LATERAL POSTERIOR NUCLEUS

VENTRAL POSTERIOR NUCLEUS

PULVINAR

CENTRO-MEDIAN NUCLEUS

INTERNAL MEDULLARY LAMINA

MEDIODORSAL NUCLEUS

PARA-FASCICULAR NUCLEUS

VENTRAL POSTERIOR NUCLEUS

DORSAL VIEW

POSTERIOR VIEW, SECTIONED

Fig. 9.2 **Coronal thalamus.**

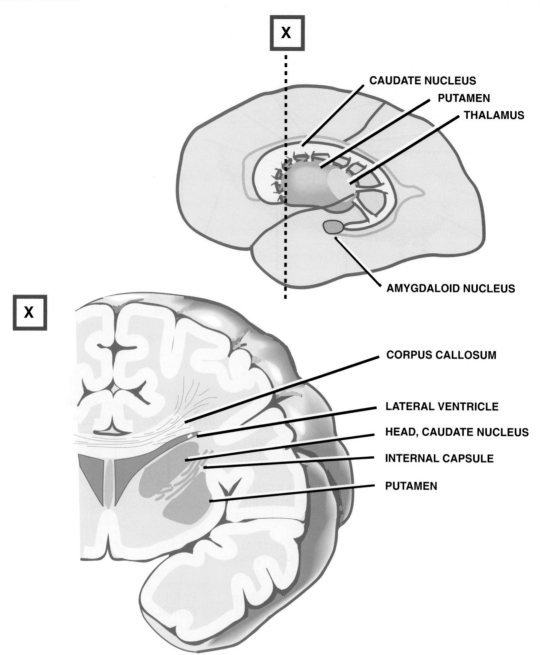

Fig. 9.3 Thalamic nuclei and their respective projections to the cortex.

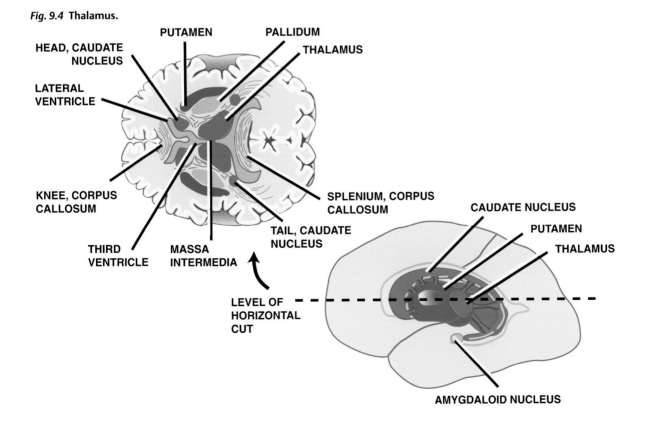

DORSAL VIEW

VENTRAL ANTERIOR NUCLEUS

LATERAL DORSAL NUCLEUS

VENTRAL LATERAL NUCLEUS

LATERAL POSTERIOR NUCLEUS

VENTRAL POSTERIOR NUCLEUS

PULVINAR

LATERAL GENICULATE BODY

DORSOMEDIAL NUCLEUS

MEDIAL GENICULATE BODY

LATERAL VIEW

PREFRONTAL CORTEX

PREMOTOR CORTEX

MOTOR CORTEX

SOMATOSENSORY CORTEX

PRIMARY AUDITORY CORTEX

PRIMARY VISUAL CORTEX

MEDIAL VIEW

CENTRAL SULCUS

CINGULATE GYRUS

CALCARINE SULCUS

Fig. 9.4 Thalamus.

PUTAMEN

PALLIDUM

THALAMUS

HEAD, CAUDATE NUCLEUS

LATERAL VENTRICLE

KNEE, CORPUS CALLOSUM

SPLENIUM, CORPUS CALLOSUM

THIRD VENTRICLE

MASSA INTERMEDIA

TAIL, CAUDATE NUCLEUS

LEVEL OF HORIZONTAL CUT

CAUDATE NUCLEUS

PUTAMEN

THALAMUS

AMYGDALOID NUCLEUS

Morphological Classification

See **Fig. 9.5**.

Rostrally, the thalamus is covered by a thin white matter layer termed the stratum zonale. Laterally, it is covered by another white matter layer termed the *external medullary lamina*. The thalamus is divided into three main parts by a **Y**-shaped white matter layer termed the *internal medullary lamina*. The internal medullary lamina divides the thalamus into anterior, medial, and lateral aspects, the anterior portion lying between the limbs of the **Y**, the medial and lateral parts lying on either side of its stem.

The lateral part of the thalamus is divided into two tiers: a dorsal tier that contains (1) the *lateral dorsal nucleus*, (2) the *lateral posterior nucleus*, and (3) the *pulvinar*; and a ventral tier that contains (1) the *ventral anterior nucleus*, (2) the *ventral lateral nucleus*, (3) the *ventral posterior nucleus*, and (4) the *medial and lateral geniculate nuclei*.

Other thalamic nuclei not included in the three-part scheme are (1) the *reticular nucleus*, which is located on the lateral surface of the thalamus between the external medullary lamina and the internal capsule; (2) the *intralaminar nuclei*, which are located within the internal medullary lamina; and (3) the *midline nuclei*, which are located on the medial surface of the thalamus in the interthalamic connection.

Fig. 9.5 **Morphological classification of thalamic nuclei.** ⟶

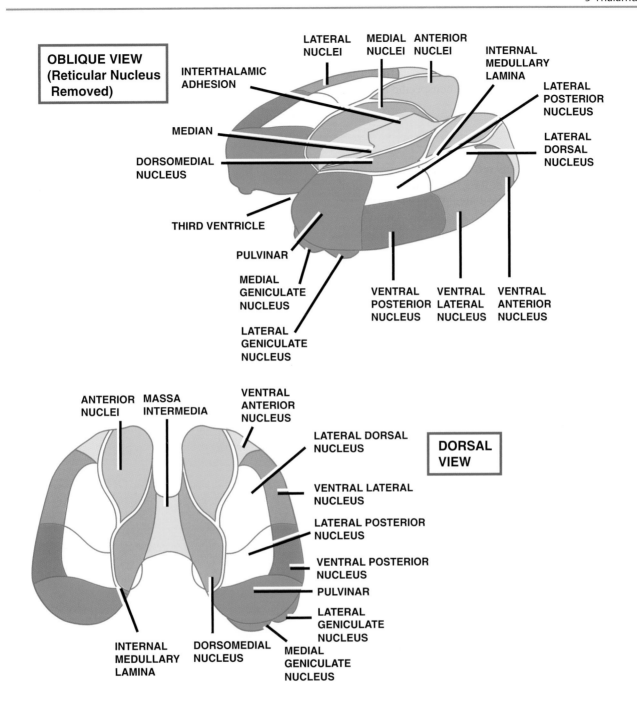

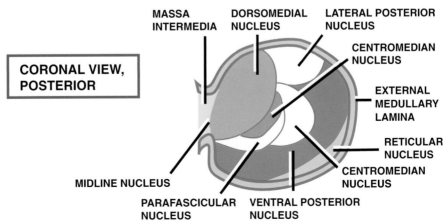

Functional Classification

See **Fig. 9.6**.

There are three groups of functionally distinct thalamic nuclei: specific relay nuclei, nonspecific thalamic nuclei, and association nuclei.

Specific Relay Nuclei

Each specific relay nucleus receives discrete input from a single sensory modality or a particular motor function and projects to a well-defined area of the primary sensory and motor cortex. Reciprocal corticothalamic connections faithfully copy each "specific" thalamocortical projection.

The specific nuclei include the *anterior nucleus* and the ventral tier of the lateral nuclear group (*ventral anterior, ventral lateral, ventral posterior, medial geniculate,* and *lateral geniculate nuclei*).

- The anterior nucleus receives input from the hypothalamus (mammillary bodies and the mammillothalamic tract) and projects to the cingulate gyrus. It is concerned with emotional states and memory.
- The ventral anterior and ventral lateral nuclei receive input from the basal ganglia and the cerebellum and project to the motor and premotor cortices. They provide the motor cortex with information received from the cerebellum and basal ganglia and other motor areas of the brain.
- The ventral posterior nucleus is subdivided into lateral and medial parts. The ventroposterolateral (VPL) nucleus receives somatosensory input (related to the body) from the medial lemniscal and spinothalamic tracts. The ventroposteromedial (VPM) nucleus receives somatosensory input (related to the face) from the sensory nuclei of the trigeminal nerve. Both the VPL and VPM nuclei project to the primary sensory cortex.
- The medial and lateral geniculate nuclei are concerned with hearing and vision, respectively. The lateral geniculate body receives input from retinal ganglion cells via the optic nerve and optic tract and projects to the visual cortex of the occipital lobe. The medial geniculate body receives input independently from the cholear nuclei (hearing). Projections then continue on to the primary superior temporal convolution (transverse gyrus of Heschl).

Fig. 9.6 Specific relay nuclei of thalamus.

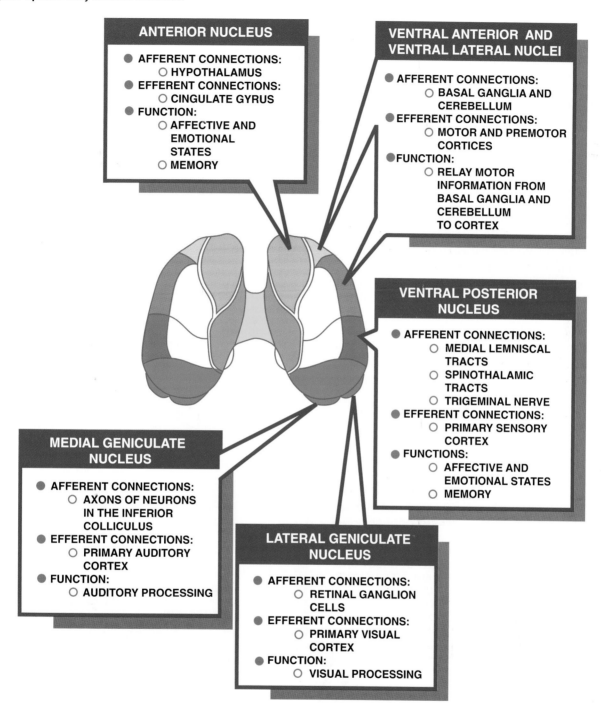

ANTERIOR NUCLEUS

- AFFERENT CONNECTIONS:
  - HYPOTHALAMUS
- EFFERENT CONNECTIONS:
  - CINGULATE GYRUS
- FUNCTION:
  - AFFECTIVE AND EMOTIONAL STATES
  - MEMORY

VENTRAL ANTERIOR AND VENTRAL LATERAL NUCLEI

- AFFERENT CONNECTIONS:
  - BASAL GANGLIA AND CEREBELLUM
- EFFERENT CONNECTIONS:
  - MOTOR AND PREMOTOR CORTICES
- FUNCTION:
  - RELAY MOTOR INFORMATION FROM BASAL GANGLIA AND CEREBELLUM TO CORTEX

VENTRAL POSTERIOR NUCLEUS

- AFFERENT CONNECTIONS:
  - MEDIAL LEMNISCAL TRACTS
  - SPINOTHALAMIC TRACTS
  - TRIGEMINAL NERVE
- EFFERENT CONNECTIONS:
  - PRIMARY SENSORY CORTEX
- FUNCTIONS:
  - AFFECTIVE AND EMOTIONAL STATES
  - MEMORY

MEDIAL GENICULATE NUCLEUS

- AFFERENT CONNECTIONS:
  - AXONS OF NEURONS IN THE INFERIOR COLLICULUS
- EFFERENT CONNECTIONS:
  - PRIMARY AUDITORY CORTEX
- FUNCTION:
  - AUDITORY PROCESSING

LATERAL GENICULATE NUCLEUS

- AFFERENT CONNECTIONS:
  - RETINAL GANGLION CELLS
- EFFERENT CONNECTIONS:
  - PRIMARY VISUAL CORTEX
- FUNCTION:
  - VISUAL PROCESSING

Nonspecific Thalamic Nuclei

See **Fig. 9.7**.

In contrast to specific nuclei, nonspecific thalamic nuclei receive input from diverse sources, then project diffusely to widespread areas of the brain.

The nonspecific nuclei include the intralaminar, reticular, and midline nuclei.

- The *centromedian nucleus* is the largest of the intralaminar nuclei. It receives input from the cerebral cortex and globus pallidus and projects to the caudate nucleus and putamen. Other intralaminar nuclei influence levels of arousal as part of the ascending reticular activating system. They receive input from the brainstem reticular formation and project diffusely to widespread areas of the cortex.

- As noted, the *reticular nucleus* receives input from collateral branches of thalamocortical and corticothalamic fibers and projects in turn on other thalamic nuclei. In this way, the reticular nucleus modulates the influence that the thalamus exerts on the cortex.

- The *midline nucleus* receives input from the brainstem reticular formation and projects to limbic structures, such as the amygdaloid nucleus and cingulate gyrus. The precise function of the midline nucleus is unknown.

Fig. 9.7 **Nonspecific nuclei of the thalamus.**

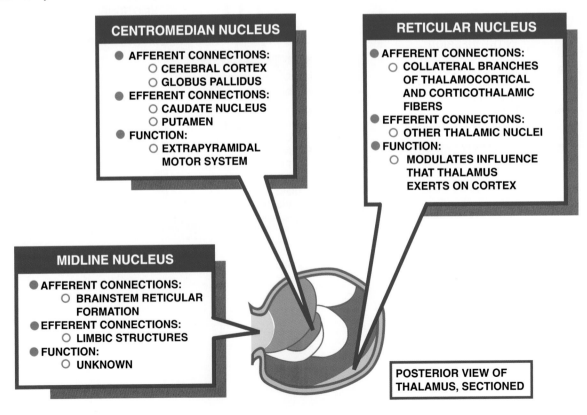

CENTROMEDIAN NUCLEUS
- AFFERENT CONNECTIONS:
  - CEREBRAL CORTEX
  - GLOBUS PALLIDUS
- EFFERENT CONNECTIONS:
  - CAUDATE NUCLEUS
  - PUTAMEN
- FUNCTION:
  - EXTRAPYRAMIDAL MOTOR SYSTEM

RETICULAR NUCLEUS
- AFFERENT CONNECTIONS:
  - COLLATERAL BRANCHES OF THALAMOCORTICAL AND CORTICOTHALAMIC FIBERS
- EFFERENT CONNECTIONS:
  - OTHER THALAMIC NUCLEI
- FUNCTION:
  - MODULATES INFLUENCE THAT THALAMUS EXERTS ON CORTEX

MIDLINE NUCLEUS
- AFFERENT CONNECTIONS:
  - BRAINSTEM RETICULAR FORMATION
- EFFERENT CONNECTIONS:
  - LIMBIC STRUCTURES
- FUNCTION:
  - UNKNOWN

POSTERIOR VIEW OF THALAMUS, SECTIONED

Association Nuclei

See **Fig. 9.8**.

Between the precise projections of the specific thalamic nuclei and the loosely organized projections of the nonspecific thalamic nuclei, the association nuclei receive input from several sources, then project to one of three areas of the association cortex. These are the parietal-temporal-occipital association cortex, the prefrontal association cortex, and the limbic association cortex.

The association nuclei include the medial nucleus (*dorsomedial nucleus*) and the dorsal tier of the lateral nuclei (*lateral dorsal nucleus*, *lateral posterior nucleus*, and *pulvinar*).

- The dorsomedial nucleus receives input from the olfactory cortex, the amygdaloid nucleus, and the hypothalamus. There are reciprocal connections between the dorsomedial nucleus and the association cortex of the frontal lobe (prefrontal cortex). Psychosurgical studies suggest that the dorsomedial nucleus and the prefrontal cortex are concerned with affective behavior. Further, visceral afferents coming from the hypothalamus appear to influence mood. Clinicopathologic correlation in the form of Korsakoff's syndrome, which is characterized by memory loss and damage to the dorsomedial nucleus, suggests yet another role in memory.

- The lateral dorsal nucleus, like the anterior thalamic nuclei, is part of the limbic system, related to emotional behavior. It receives input from the hippocampal formation and projects to the cingulate gyrus.
- The afferent connections of the lateral posterior nucleus are unknown. It projects to the somatosensory association cortex of the parietal lobe.
- The pulvinar receives input concerning vision from the superior colliculus of the midbrain. It also receives input from the sensory association areas of the parietal, temporal, and occipital lobes, and projects back to the same areas.

Fig. 9.8 Association nuclei of the thalamus.

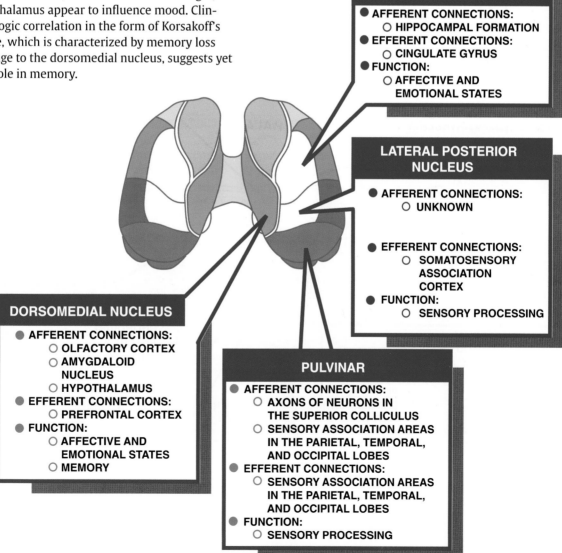

LATERAL DORSAL NUCLEUS
- AFFERENT CONNECTIONS:
  ○ HIPPOCAMPAL FORMATION
- EFFERENT CONNECTIONS:
  ○ CINGULATE GYRUS
- FUNCTION:
  ○ AFFECTIVE AND EMOTIONAL STATES

LATERAL POSTERIOR NUCLEUS
- AFFERENT CONNECTIONS:
  ○ UNKNOWN
- EFFERENT CONNECTIONS:
  ○ SOMATOSENSORY ASSOCIATION CORTEX
- FUNCTION:
  ○ SENSORY PROCESSING

DORSOMEDIAL NUCLEUS
- AFFERENT CONNECTIONS:
  ○ OLFACTORY CORTEX
  ○ AMYGDALOID NUCLEUS
  ○ HYPOTHALAMUS
- EFFERENT CONNECTIONS:
  ○ PREFRONTAL CORTEX
- FUNCTION:
  ○ AFFECTIVE AND EMOTIONAL STATES
  ○ MEMORY

PULVINAR
- AFFERENT CONNECTIONS:
  ○ AXONS OF NEURONS IN THE SUPERIOR COLLICULUS
  ○ SENSORY ASSOCIATION AREAS IN THE PARIETAL, TEMPORAL, AND OCCIPITAL LOBES
- EFFERENT CONNECTIONS:
  ○ SENSORY ASSOCIATION AREAS IN THE PARIETAL, TEMPORAL, AND OCCIPITAL LOBES
- FUNCTION:
  ○ SENSORY PROCESSING

Blood Supply of the Thalamus

See **Fig. 9.9**.

The predominant blood supply of the thalamus comes from the *posterior communicating artery* of the anterior circulation and, more abundantly, the *posterior cerebral artery* of the posterior circulation. Named branches of the latter artery include the *thalamoperforate artery* and the *thalamogeniculate artery*. Additional supply is provided by the *anterior* and *posterior choroidal arteries*.

Fig. 9.9 **Blood supply of the thalamus.**

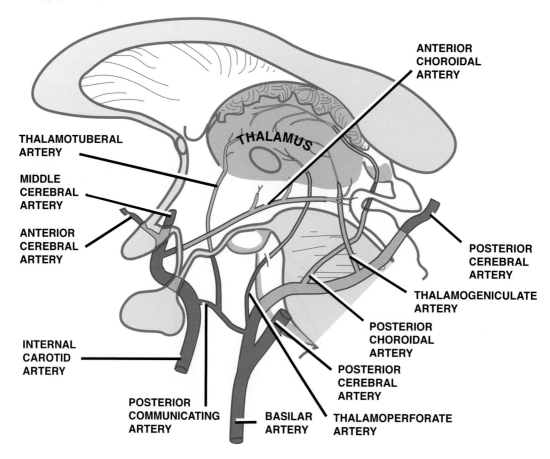

Clinical Manifestations of Thalamic Lesions

The interpretation of clinical signs and symptoms that result from thalamic lesions, which are predominantly caused by infarction, is complicated because these lesions often extend beyond the thalamus.

For example, an altered level of consciousness may reflect involvement of the midbrain, and motor and sensory disturbances may represent involvement of the internal capsule.

Further, thalamic lesions rarely respect the boundaries of individual thalamic nuclei; therefore, many thalamic functions may be impaired. The resulting thalamic syndromes are often complex, so we shall concentrate on the individual signs and symptoms.

Sensory Disturbances

See **Fig. 9.10**.

Sensory disturbances result from lesions in the *ventral posterior nucleus* (VPL and VPM).

The disturbances may be negative or positive phenomena; the former are marked by sensory loss, the latter include pain and paresthesias. Both types of sensory phenomena affect the contralateral side of the body.

Although all sensory modalities are represented in the thalamus, thalamic sensory loss most frequently affects position sense. Further, deep sensation is usually more severely affected than cutaneous sensation.

Clinically distinguishing cortical from thalamic causes of sensory loss may be difficult, but because vibratory sense is spared in lesions of the parietal somatosensory cortex, loss of vibratory sense localizes a lesion to the thalamus.

Pain associated with thalamic lesions assumes an especially peculiar form: it is often severely unpleasant, is primarily felt close to the skin, and may occur spontaneously or may linger long after a cutaneous stimulus is removed.

Thalamic paresthesias predominantly affect the circumoral region and the distal parts of the limbs. This is because these areas of the body possess the largest representation in the sensory thalamus.

Fig. 9.10 **Sensory disturbances.**

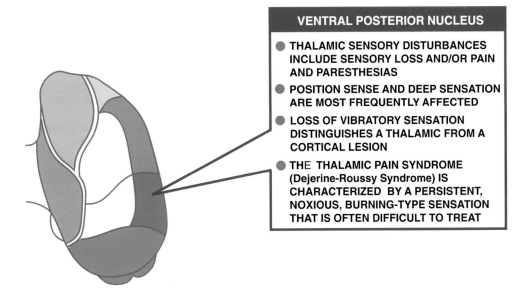

VENTRAL POSTERIOR NUCLEUS

- THALAMIC SENSORY DISTURBANCES INCLUDE SENSORY LOSS AND/OR PAIN AND PARESTHESIAS
- POSITION SENSE AND DEEP SENSATION ARE MOST FREQUENTLY AFFECTED
- LOSS OF VIBRATORY SENSATION DISTINGUISHES A THALAMIC FROM A CORTICAL LESION
- THE THALAMIC PAIN SYNDROME (Dejerine-Roussy Syndrome) IS CHARACTERIZED BY A PERSISTENT, NOXIOUS, BURNING-TYPE SENSATION THAT IS OFTEN DIFFICULT TO TREAT

Motor Disturbances

See **Fig. 9.11**.

Motor disturbances result from lesions in the ventral anterior and ventral lateral nuclei. These interrupt connections between the thalamus and the extrapyramidal motor system (basal ganglia and cerebellum).

Thalamic motor disturbances, which affect the opposite side of the body, include hemiataxia and abnormal involuntary movements. Such abnormal involuntary movements include a 3 to 5 Hz hand tremor, which worsens with use (action tremor), and choreoathetosis, which is the combination of writhing, sinuous, and rapid, jerky movements, particularly involving the distal part of the affected limb.

An affected hand may assume an abnormal posture of flexion at the wrist and metacarpophalangeal joints, with hyperextension at the interphalangeal joints (thalamic hand).

Transient hemiparesis on the opposite side of the body may occur with thalamic lesions, but this is thought to result from extension of the lesion into the internal capsule, rather than thalamic involvement per se.

Fig. 9.11 **Motor disturbances.**

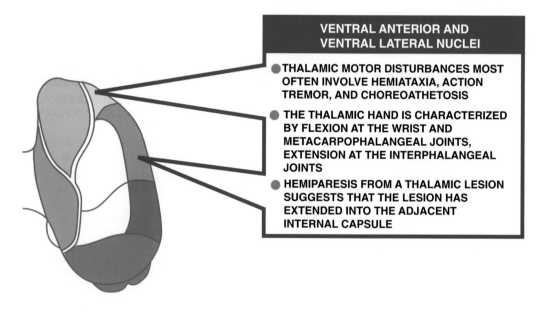

VENTRAL ANTERIOR AND VENTRAL LATERAL NUCLEI

- THALAMIC MOTOR DISTURBANCES MOST OFTEN INVOLVE HEMIATAXIA, ACTION TREMOR, AND CHOREOATHETOSIS
- THE THALAMIC HAND IS CHARACTERIZED BY FLEXION AT THE WRIST AND METACARPOPHALANGEAL JOINTS, EXTENSION AT THE INTERPHALANGEAL JOINTS
- HEMIPARESIS FROM A THALAMIC LESION SUGGESTS THAT THE LESION HAS EXTENDED INTO THE ADJACENT INTERNAL CAPSULE

Disturbances of Alertness

See **Fig. 9.12**.

Disturbances of alertness result from lesions in the intralaminar nuclei, which interrupt the ascending reticular activating system.

Thalamic lesions extending into the rostral midbrain also result in disturbances of arousal. They are clinically distinguished from pure thalamic lesions as follows: midbrain involvement is accompanied by the presence of oculomotor nerve paresis (large pupils and ophthalmoparesis), whereas pure thalamic lesions exhibit small pupils ("diencephalic pupils") and a full range of extraocular movement.

Affective Disturbances

See **Fig. 9.13**.

Disturbances of affect result from lesions in the anterior and dorsomedial nuclei that interrupt their connections with limbic system structures and the frontal cortex.

Such disturbances include apathy, disinterest, and lack of initiative or drive. Less often, agitation and confusion develop instead.

Fig. 9.12 **Disturbances of alertness.**

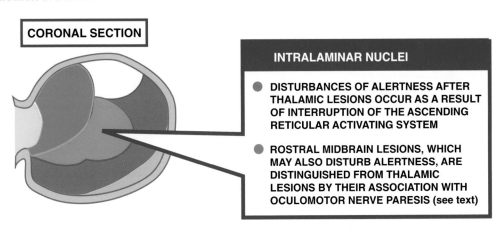

Fig. 9.13 **Affective disturbances.**

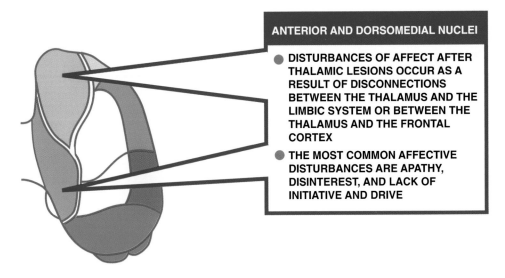

Memory Disturbances

See **Fig. 9.14**.

Disturbances of memory result from lesions in the dorsomedial nucleus.

Bilateral lesions are most often responsible, but memory loss may also follow a unilateral lesion.

Fig. 9.14 **Memory disturbances.**

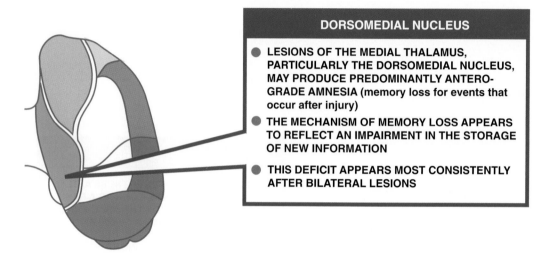

DORSOMEDIAL NUCLEUS

● LESIONS OF THE MEDIAL THALAMUS, PARTICULARLY THE DORSOMEDIAL NUCLEUS, MAY PRODUCE PREDOMINANTLY ANTERO-GRADE AMNESIA (memory loss for events that occur after injury)

● THE MECHANISM OF MEMORY LOSS APPEARS TO REFLECT AN IMPAIRMENT IN THE STORAGE OF NEW INFORMATION

● THIS DEFICIT APPEARS MOST CONSISTENTLY AFTER BILATERAL LESIONS

Visual Disturbances

See **Fig. 9.15**.

Disturbances of vision result from lesions in the lateral geniculate body. These consist of a hemianopsia in the opposite visual field.

Fig. 9.15 **Visual disturbances.**

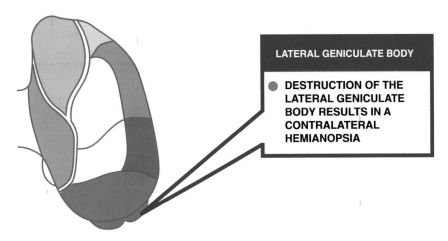

LATERAL GENICULATE BODY

● **DESTRUCTION OF THE LATERAL GENICULATE BODY RESULTS IN A CONTRALATERAL HEMIANOPSIA**

10 Hypothalamus

Hypothalamus

The hypothalamus is a small but crucial part of the diencephalon that lies below the thalamus and surrounds the lower part of the third ventricle.

From ventral to dorsal, the undersurface of the hypothalamus is marked by the optic chiasm, the tuber cinereum, the infundibulum, and the mammillary bodies.

The rostral border comprises the anterior commissure and the lamina terminalis; the caudal border merges with the tegmentum of the midbrain.

Laterally, the hypothalamus is flanked by the internal capsule; medially, it is flanked by the third ventricle.

The hypothalamus exerts its influence through three major systems: (1) the limbic, (2) the autonomic, and (3) the endocrine. It is composed of numerous nuclei of ill-defined boundaries that make connections with many parts of the central nervous system (CNS), including (1) limbic structures, (2) autonomic nuclei of the brainstem and spinal cord, and (3) the pituitary gland.

Although specific functions have not yet been assigned to individual hypothalamic nuclei, several afferent and efferent pathways of the hypothalamus have been described, and many functions have been identified.

This chapter describes the hypothalamic nuclei; the afferent and efferent connections of the hypothalamus; the limbic, autonomic, and endocrine hypothalamic functions; and the clinical manifestations of selected hypothalamic disorders.

Hypothalamic Nuclei

See **Fig. 10.1**.

The hypothalamus may be divided into a medial hypothalamic region that contains the majority of nuclei and a lateral hypothalamic region that contains the major fiber tracts (e.g., the medial forebrain bundle) and a group of diffuse nuclei.

The medial hypothalamic area is further subdivided into three regions: (1) the supraoptic region, which lies farthest anterior and includes the *supraoptic*, suprachiasmatic, and *paraventricular nuclei*; (2) the tuberal region, which lies just posterior to the supraoptic region and includes the *ventromedial, dorsomedial,* and *infundibular nuclei*; and (3) the mammillary region, which lies farthest posterior and includes the *mammillary body* to the *posterior nucleus.*

Fig. 10.1 **Hypothalamic nuclei.**

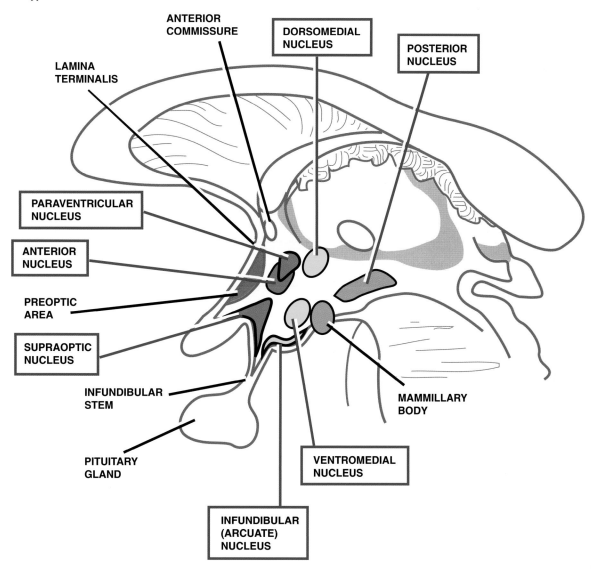

ANTERIOR
COMMISSURE

DORSOMEDIAL
NUCLEUS

POSTERIOR
NUCLEUS

LAMINA
TERMINALIS

PARAVENTRICULAR
NUCLEUS

ANTERIOR
NUCLEUS

PREOPTIC
AREA

SUPRAOPTIC
NUCLEUS

INFUNDIBULAR
STEM

MAMMILLARY
BODY

PITUITARY
GLAND

VENTROMEDIAL
NUCLEUS

INFUNDIBULAR
(ARCUATE)
NUCLEUS

Afferent Connections

See **Fig. 10.2**.

The hypothalamus is located in the center of the limbic system and receives numerous projections from limbic system structures. In addition, the hypothalamus receives ascending afferents from the brainstem reticular formation and descending afferents from the thalamus and cerebral cortex.

The major afferent connections of the hypothalamus include the following:

- *Olfactory and septal areas* These areas are concerned with smell and basic emotional drives. They send axons to the hypothalamus via the medial forebrain bundle.
- *Hippocampus* This limbic system structure is probably involved in a variety of behaviors, including learning and memory. The hippocampus sends axons to the *mammillary bodies* of the hypothalamus in a large fiber bundle called the *fornix*.
- *Amygdaloid nucleus* Like the hippocampus, the amygdaloid nucleus is associated with complex behaviors. It sends axons to the hypothalamus via the stria terminalis.
- *Midbrain tegmentum (reticular formation)* This includes a diffuse network of neurons concerned with a variety of autonomic functions. It sends axons to the hypothalamus through the *medial forebrain bundle*. Two additional brainstem nuclei, closely related to the reticular formation, also send axons to the hypothalamus. They are the raphe nucleus, which projects serotonin-containing fibers, and the nucleus ceruleus, which projects norepinephrine-containing fibers. Both fiber types project to the hypothalamus in the dorsal longitudinal fasciculus.
- *Dorsomedial and midline thalamic nuclei* These are concerned with emotional states and autonomic functions. They project axons to the hypothalamus via the thalamohypothalamic tract.

Fig. 10.2 **Afferent hypothalamic connections.**

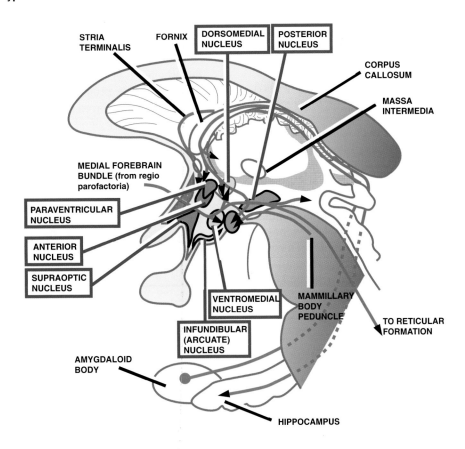

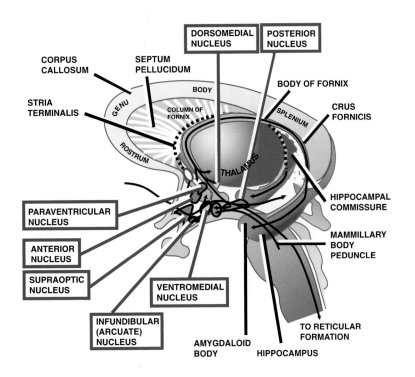

Efferent Connections

See **Figs. 10.3** and **10.4**.

The hypothalamus is a major output pathway of the limbic system. The efferent connections of the hypothalamus are largely reciprocal to the afferent projections. There are ascending connections to the cortex and thalamus as well as descending connections to the autonomic nuclei of the brainstem and spinal cord. Separately, two hypothalamic pathways project to the pituitary gland.

The major efferent connections of the hypothalamus include the following:

- *Olfactory and septal areas*   These areas are concerned with smell and basic emotional drives. They receive hypothalamic axons via the medial forebrain bundle.
- *Anterior thalamic nucleus*   This nucleus is the thalamic part of the limbic system. It is concerned with emotional states and memory. It receives hypothalamic axons via the *mammillothalamic tract* and projects in turn to the cingulate gyrus.

- *Preganglionic autonomic neurons of the brainstem and spinal cord*   These are concerned with various autonomic functions. They include the dorsal nucleus of the vagus (brainstem) and the intermediolateral cell column (spinal cord). Both receive input from the hypothalamus via the dorsal longitudinal fasciculus; the hypothalmic projections to the intermediolateral cell column are relayed in reticulospinal pathways.
- *Posterior pituitary gland*   The posterior pituitary gland receives direct axonal projections from large neurosecretory cells in the *paraventricular* and *supraoptic nuclei* of the hypothalamus. They are carried in the *supraoptic hypophyseal tract*. Neurons of the paraventricular and supraoptic nuclei synthesize and secrete the hormones oxytocin and antidiuretic hormone (ADH), which are involved in reproductive functions and water balance, respectively. They are discussed in greater detail later in the chapter.

Fig. 10.3 **Efferent hypothalamic connections.**

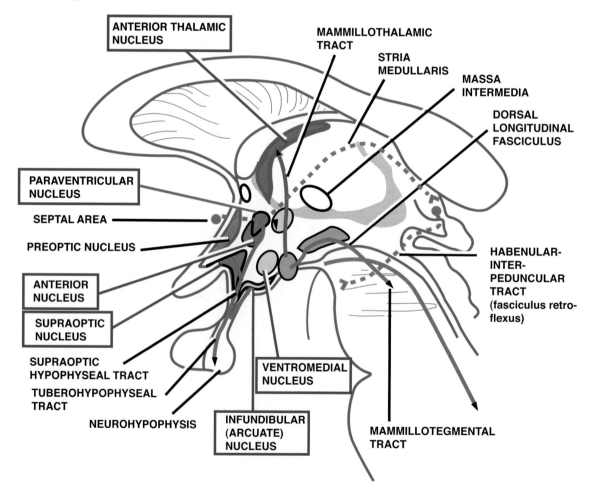

- *Anterior pituitary gland*   Neurosecretory cells in the *infundibular nucleus* of the hypothalamus produce releasing and inhibiting factors that influence the secretion of pituitary hormones. There are no direct axonal connections between the hypothalamus and the anterior pituitary gland. These factors are carried by axoplasmic transport in the *tuberoinfundibular tract* and are secreted into a capillary bed in the median eminence. From the median eminence, they are transported in *hypophyseal portal veins* to a second capillary bed in the anterior pituitary gland, where they modulate the secretion of trophic hormones, such as thyroid-stimulating hormone (TSH), adrenocorticotropic hormone (ACTH), follicle-stimulating hormone (FSH), luteinizing hormone (LH), growth hormone (GH), melanocyte-stimulating hormone (MSH), and prolactin.

Fig. 10.4 **Hypophyseal portal system.**

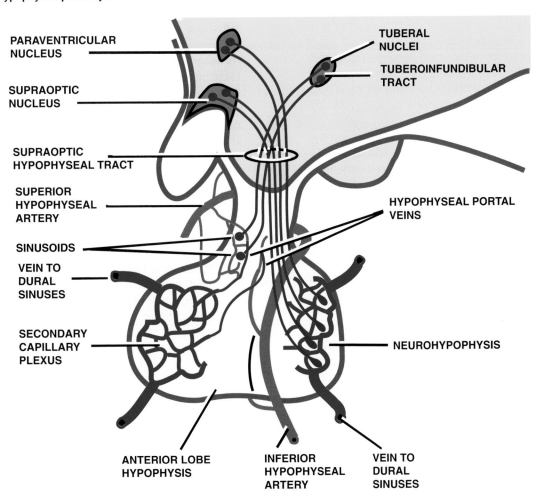

Functions of the Hypothalamus

The functions of the hypothalamus are centered on three "systems": (1) autonomic, (2) endocrine, and (3) limbic system (i.e., emotion and behavior). It should be emphasized that the hypothalamus integrates autonomic and emotional/behavioral functions (for example, the sympathetic discharge of the "fight or flight" response to fear).

Autonomic Functions

- *Cardiovascular regulation*   The hypothalamus exerts both sympathetic and parasympathetic influence on the cardiovascular system. Stimulation of the posterior hypothalamus produces primarily sympathetic effects, including increased arterial pressure and heart rate. By contrast, stimulation of the anterior hypothalamus produces primarily parasympathetic effects, including decreased arterial pressure and heart rate. These effects are mediated via cardiovascular control centers in the reticular formation of the brainstem.
- *Regulation of body temperature*   The anterior hypothalamus contains heat-sensitive neurons that sense the temperature of the blood passing through this area. As blood temperature rises, these neurons increase their rate of firing and stimulate vasodilatation and sweating (parasympathetic response). By contrast, cold-sensitive neurons located in the posterior hypothalamus increase their rate of firing when exposed to cold. The autonomic response to stimulated cold-sensitive neurons includes vasoconstriction, piloerection, and shivering (sympathetic response).
- *Regulation of water balance*   The lateral hypothalamus contains a "thirst center" that is made up of an ill-defined collection of neurons. As the electrolytes in the neurons of this area become too concentrated (due to increased serum osmolarity), the subject develops an intense sensation of thirst. The sensation of thirst persists until the electrolyte concentration is restored by drinking.
- *Regulation of food intake*   Several areas of the hypothalamus are concerned with the regulation of food intake. For example, the lateral hypothalamus appears to contain a "hunger center." Stimulation of the lateral hypothalamus causes excessive eating in an animal, whereas destructive lesions in the same result in loss of the desire for food. By contrast, the ventromedial nucleus appears to contain a "satiety center." Stimulation of the ventromedial nucleus causes loss of appetite in an animal, whereas a destructive lesion in this area is followed by excessive eating.

Endocrine Functions

There are two groups of endocrine functions performed by the hypothalamus:

- *Regulation of water balance*   Endocrine regulation of water balance is concerned with the control of renal excretion. This begins in the neurons of the supraoptic nuclei, which are sensitive to the concentration of body fluids (i.e., serum osmolarity). When the body fluids become too concentrated (increased serum osmolarity), these neurons synthesize ADH, which is carried by axoplasmic transport into the posterior pituitary gland. Because axon terminals lie adjacent to capillaries in the posterior pituitary gland, ADH enters into the bloodstream. It then acts on the collecting ducts of the kidney to cause reabsorption of water. This conserved "free water" acts to decrease the serum osmolarity with resultant increased urine concentration.
- *Regulation of reproductive functions*   Neurons of the paraventricular nuclei synthesize the hormone oxytocin, which is carried by axoplasmic transport into the posterior pituitary gland. From there it is secreted into the bloodstream, where it causes increased contractility of the uterus and contraction of the myoepithelial cells that surround the alveoli of the breasts. Large quantities of oxytocin are secreted at the end of pregnancy, causing contractions of the uterus during delivery. Separately, the hypothalamus releases oxytocin in response to the baby's attempt to breast feed. This leads to contraction of the myoepithelial cells, which in turn causes ejection of breast milk.

Emotional Behavior

Through its integration and control of the limbic and autonomic systems (both sympathetic and parasympathetic), the hypothalamus is concerned with the physiological expression of emotional states. Experiments show that stimulation of the lateral hypothalamus elicits rage and fear, whereas lesions in this area result in passive behavior. By contrast, stimulation of the ventromedial hypothalamus provokes placidity and tameness, whereas lesions in this area are followed by aggressiveness and rage.

Clinical Manifestations of Hypothalamic Lesions

Although the details of hypothalamic function are not precisely known, several symptoms and symptom complexes related to hypothalamic disorders have been described. These are primarily due to endocrine abnormalities and less often to autonomic dysfunction.

Disturbances of Water Balance

Hypothalamic dysfunction may result in one of two syndromes of altered water balance: (1) diabetes insipidus (DI), which is marked by a deficiency of ADH and is clinically characterized by the excretion of large volumes of dilute urine; and (2) the syndrome of inappropriate secretion of antidiuretic hormone (SIADH), which is marked by increased ADH secretion and is clinically characterized by water retention and dilutional hyponatremia.

Disturbances of Temperature Regulation

As noted, the anterior hypothalamus contains heat-sensitive neurons. Lesions in this area undercut the compensatory autonomic response to increased body temperature and thereby result in hyperthermia. By contrast, lesions in the "cold-sensitive" posterior hypothalamus may result in hypothermia.

Obesity

As noted, the ventromedial hypothalamus contains a so-called satiety center, which when stimulated inhibits the appetite for food. Destructive lesions in this area may result in excessive eating and lead to obesity.

Hypogonadotropic Hypogonadism

This condition may be caused by either hypothalamic or pituitary disorders. In women, it is manifested by amenorrhea; in men, it is manifested by gonadal dysfunction.

Disturbances of Emotional Behavior

Hypothalamic lesions, particularly in the ventromedial region, may cause episodic outbursts of rage and fear that are associated with a prominent autonomic component. Between outbursts, the behavior is normal and the patient may be remorseful.

11 Basal Ganglia

The *basal ganglia* are a collection of five subcortical nuclei located deep in the cerebral hemispheres. They play an important role in the control of posture and voluntary movement.

Like the cerebellum, the basal ganglia are components of the motor system that serve to influence the major descending tracts (i.e., the corticospinal and corticobulbar tracts). Unlike the cerebellum, however, the basal ganglia have no direct connections with the spinal cord. Instead, they act as regulators of cortical function via their influence on thalamocortical projections.

Thus, the major output of the basal ganglia is directed to the thalamus, which in turn projects to the frontal cortex; the major input is received from large cortical areas, forming a loop that may be summarized as follows: cortex–basal ganglia–thalamus–cortex.

The main components of the basal ganglia involved in this loop are (1) the caudate nucleus, (2) the putamen, and (3) the globus pallidus. Two related subcortical nuclei traditionally included among the basal ganglia are (4) the subthalamic nucleus and (5) the substantia nigra.

This chapter reviews the basic anatomy of the five main components of the basal ganglia, describes their main connections, and briefly reviews their neurochemistry and physiology. In closing, the chapter briefly reviews the clinical manifestations of basal ganglia lesions, which have played an important role in our current understanding of basal ganglia function.

Components of the Basal Ganglia

See **Figs. 11.1** and **11.2**.

As noted, the basal ganglia comprise five subcortical nuclei: (1) the *caudate nucleus*, (2) the *putamen*, (3) the *globus pallidus*, (4) the *subthalamic nucleus*, and (5) the substantia nigra. The caudate nucleus and the putamen have many functional and developmental similarities and are usually considered together as a single structure, the striatum.

Striatum

The striatum is composed of the caudate nucleus and the putamen. Both nuclei receive projections from the telencephalon, and together they constitute the input component of the basal ganglia.

The caudate nucleus is **C**-shaped and is closely related to the lateral ventricle. It lies lateral to the thalamus and medial to the fibers of the internal capsule. It is composed of three parts, which are related to the three main areas of the lateral ventricle, as follows:

- The head of the caudate nucleus forms the lateral wall of the anterior horn of the lateral ventricle, the body forms part of the floor of the body of the *lateral ventricle*, and the tail continues forward into the temporal lobe in the roof of the inferior horn of the lateral ventricle.
- The putamen is the largest and most lateral nucleus of the basal ganglia. It is partly separated from the caudate nucleus by the fibers of the internal capsule.

Globus Pallidus

In contrast to the striatum, the globus pallidus derives from the diencephalon. It is divided into external and internal parts. The latter constitutes the output component of the basal ganglia.

The globus pallidus is the smallest nucleus of the basal ganglia. Laterally, it is bordered by the putamen. Medially, it is bordered by the internal capsule. Together, the putamen and globus pallidus form a lens-shaped structure, which is sometimes called the lentiform nucleus—a purely structural designation not employed here.

Subthalamic Nucleus

The subthalamic nucleus forms a side loop with the globus pallidus. It is a lens-shaped nucleus located on the medial side of the internal capsule at the border between the diencephalon and the mesencephalon. Caudally, it is continuous with the substantia nigra.

Substantia Nigra

The substantia nigra is located in the mesencephalon. It is divided into two regions: a dorsal pars compacta and a ventral pars reticulata. These two regions have distinct histological and functional characteristics.

The pars compacta is composed of neurons that contain the pigment melanin, giving the substantia nigra its dark color which is reflected in its name. These neurons project rostrally and form a side loop with the striatum.

The pars reticulata is directly continuous with the globus pallidus with which it shares both histological and functional characteristics.

Fig. 11.1 **Basal ganglia.**

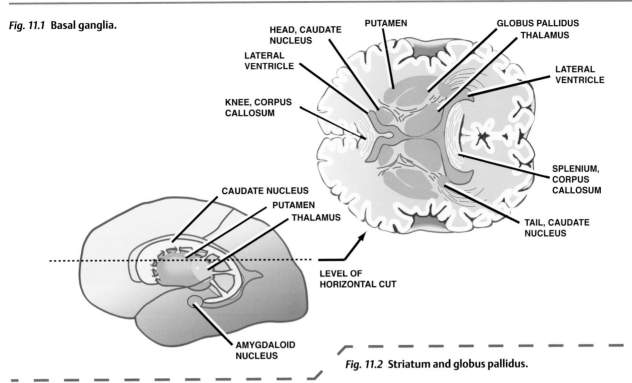

Fig. 11.2 **Striatum and globus pallidus.**

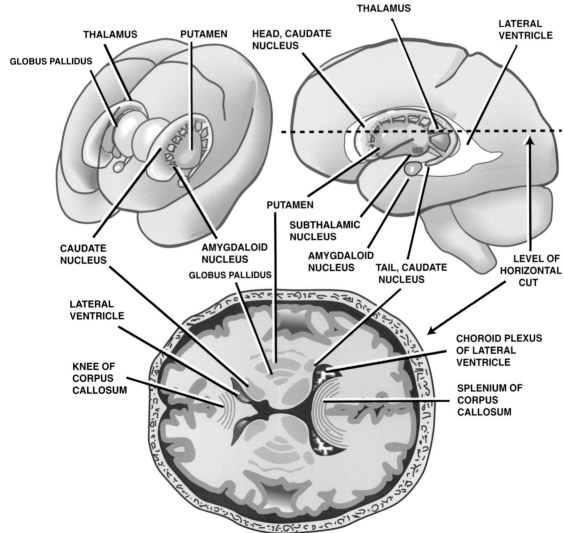

Connections of the Basal Ganglia

All input into the basal ganglia terminates in the striatum; all output projects from the globus pallidus and the pars reticulata of the substantia nigra.

Striatum

Afferents

See **Fig. 11.3**.

There are three major sources of input to the striatum:

- *Cerebral cortex* This is the dominant source of input to the basal ganglia. Large areas of the cortex are involved, including the motor, sensory, and association cortices. Corticostriate projections are organized topographically (i.e., specific parts of the cortex project onto specific regions of the striatum).
- *Intralaminar nuclei of the thalamus* The centromedian nucleus provides the most important thalamic input. Because the thalamus receives input from the cortex, thalamostriate projections represent another means by which the cortex influences the striatum.
- *Pars compacta of the substantia nigra* The substantia nigra is involved in a major side loop with the striatum (see later discussion).

Fig. 11.3 **Afferent connections of the striatum.**

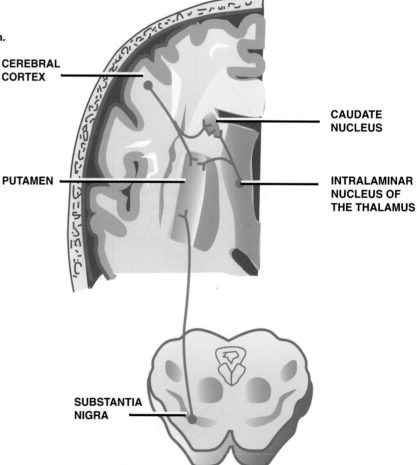

Efferents

See **Fig. 11.4**.

There are two major destinations of striatal efferents:

- *Globus pallidus* This is the dominant striatal projection. The fibers in this pathway are topographically organized. They contribute to the major cortex–basal ganglia–thalamus–cortex loop.
- *Substantia nigra (both parts)* Both the pars compacta and the pars reticularis receive striatonigral fibers. As mentioned, the pars compacta is involved in a side loop with the striatum. The pars reticulata is the functional equivalent of the globus pallidus.

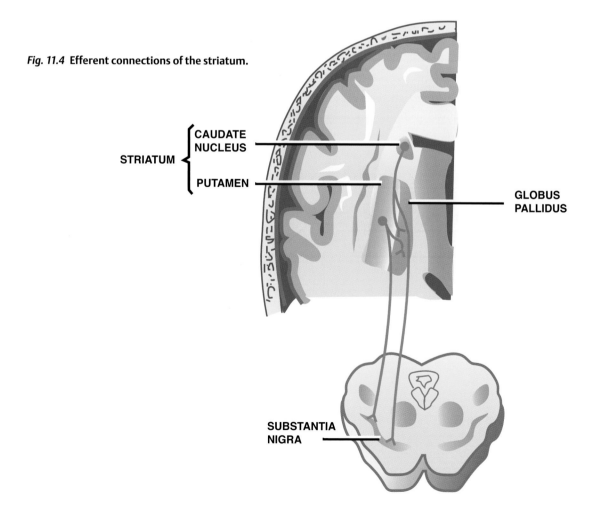

Fig. 11.4 **Efferent connections of the striatum.**

Globus Pallidus

Afferents

See **Fig. 11.5**.

There are two major sources of input to the globus pallidus:

- *Striatum* (putamen and striate nucleus) Fibers from the striatum are projected topographically onto the *globus pallidus*. The pars reticulata of the substantia nigra, which is functionally similar to the globus pallidus, also receives topographically organized afferents from the striatum (not shown in this figure).
- *Subthalamic nucleus* The subthalamic nucleus projects topographically organized fibers on the globus pallidus as part of a major side loop.

Fig. 11.5 Afferent connections of the globus pallidus.

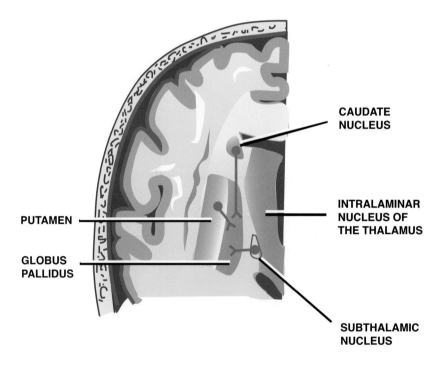

Efferents

See **Fig. 11.6**.

There are three major destinations for pallidal efferents:

- *Ventral lateral and ventral anterior thalamic nuclei* This is the major outflow pathway of the basal ganglia. Fibers projected from the globus pallidus to the thalamus are carried in two fiber bundles, the *ansa lenticularis* and the *lenticular fasciculus*. These fiber bundles later fuse to reach the thalamus as the *thalamic fasciculus*. Fibers of the ventral anterior (VA) and ventral lateral (VL) thalamic nuclei project, in turn, to the prefrontal and premotor cortex to complete the cortex–basal ganglia–thalamus–cortex loop.
- *Subthalamic nucleus* The globus pallidus projects fibers to the subthalamic nucleus as part of the globus pallidus–subthalamic nucleus–globus pallidus side loop, as already mentioned.
- *Brainstem reticular formation* The nuclei in this region receive fibers from the globus pallidus and in turn project to other nuclei that give rise to descending motor tracts (e.g., the rubrospinal, reticulospinal, and vestibulospinal tracts).

Fig. 11.6 **Efferent connections of the globus pallidus.**

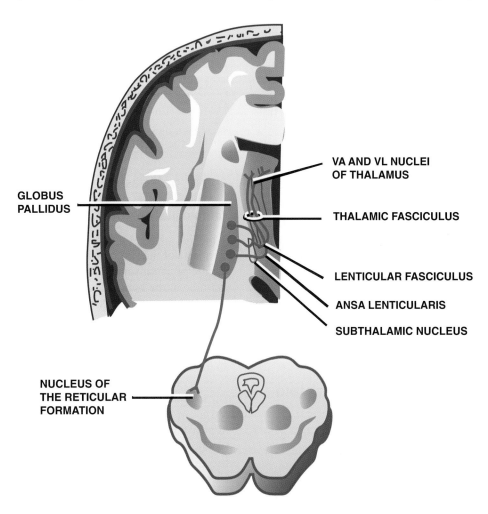

Physiology and Neurochemistry of the Basal Ganglia

See **Fig. 11.7**.

The primary function of the basal ganglia is in the control of posture and voluntary movement. The basic means by which the basal ganglia carry out this function is through the influence they exert on the cerebral cortex. As mentioned, this influence is primarily made via the cortex–basal ganglia–thalamus–cortex loop, which is modulated by two additional side loops: the striatum-substantia nigra–striatum loop and the globus pallidus-subthalamic nucleus–globus pallidus loop. Interruptions of these loops, or alterations in their neurotransmitter systems, are responsible for the clinical manifestations, which will be considered in the following section.

The Cortex–Basal Ganglia–Thalamus–Cortex Loop

As mentioned, this is the major loop by which the basal ganglia exert their influence on the cortical neurons that contribute to the corticospinal and corticobulbar tracts.

At one point of this loop, the corticostriate neurons release the excitatory neurotransmitter glutamate. Within the basal ganglia, neurons in the striatum and the globus pallidus contain the inhibitory neurotransmitter gamma-aminobutyric acid (*GABA*), creating a two-step sequence of double inhibition. Closing the loop, the thalamocortical neurons, like the corticostriate neurons, release the excitatory neurotransmitter *glutamate*.

Because the basal ganglia contain a double inhibitory pathway, the excitatory drive from the cortex disinhibits thalamocortical fibers, which finally project to and excite the cortex. The upshot of the loop: excitation of the cortex.

This at least appears to be the case shortly before and during a movement, as shown by electrical recordings in animals. These recordings further show that when no movements are being made, the neurons of the striatum are quiescent and those of the globus pallidus are active, which allows the globus pallidus to inhibit the thalamocortical fibers.

Modulating this circuit are two additional side loops, as described next.

The Striatum–Substantia Nigra–Striatum Loop

The precise modulatory effect of this loop is unknown. What is known is that the *striatum* projects inhibitory, GABA-containing neurons onto the *pars compacta* of the *substantia nigra*. In turn, the pars compacta projects *dopamine*-containing neurons on the striatum, where they exert varying effects on different subpopulations of striatal neurons.

The Globus Pallidus–Subthalamic Nucleus–Globus Pallidus Loop

The globus pallidus projects inhibitory, GABA-containing neurons onto the *subthalamic nucleus*. In turn, the subthalamic nucleus projects excitatory, glutamate-containing neurons on the *globus pallidus*. The consequence of this circuit is to increase the inhibitory effect of the globus pallidus on the thalamus.

Clinical Manifestations of Basal Ganglia Disease

The clinical manifestations of basal ganglia disease result from (1) **the presence of an abnormal increase or decrease in movement** and (2) **the presence of an abnormal increase or decrease in tone**.

Because decreased movement/increased tone and increased movement/decreased tone are common combinations in basal ganglia disease, the following two syndromes have been identified: (1) the hypokinesia-hypertonia syndrome, of which parkinsonism is an example, and (2) the hyperkinesia-hypotonia syndrome, of which chorea, athetosis, dystonia, and ballismus are examples.

Although the details of the pathogenesis of these two syndromes are not well known, it is thought that the hypokinesia-hypertonia syndrome is due to disease of the substantia nigra, whereas the hyperkinesia-hypotonia syndrome is related to lesions of the striatum.

This section briefly describes the clinical features of basal ganglia disease and discusses current thoughts regarding their pathological anatomy.

The Hypokinesia-Hypertonia Syndrome

Pathological Anatomy

It has long been known that degeneration of the pars compacta of the substantia nigra is the chief pathological feature of parkinsonism, which is the most characteristic example of the hypokinesia-hypertonia syndrome. More recent studies offer further insights into the pathological anatomy of parkinsonism.

The subthalamic nucleus increases the excitatory drive of the globus pallidus. The globus pallidus, in turn, exerts an inhibitory effect on thalamocortical neurons.

In parkinsonism, these pathways become more active. The loss of (inhibitory) dopaminergic nigrostriatal fibers causes an increase in the GABAergic striatal output. This, in turn, inhibits the GABAergic pallidal output to the subthalamic nucleus, which causes an increase in activity of the globus pallidus. This causes an increase in the inhibition of thalamocortical neurons, and thus a decrease in voluntary movement (hypokinesia) and an increase in tone (hypertonia).

Fig. 11.7 Neurochemistry of the basal ganglia.

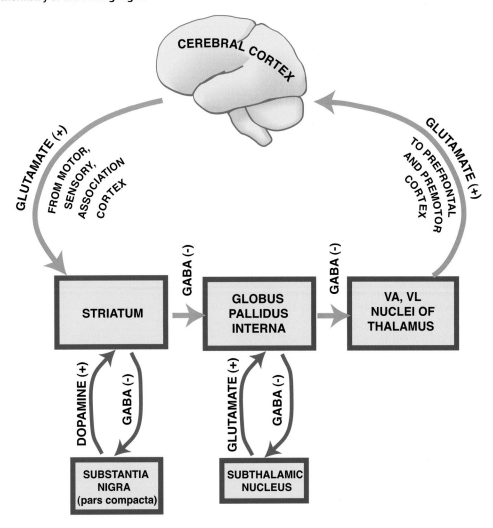

Parkinsonism

See **Fig. 11.8**.

Clinically, parkinsonism is characterized by the triad of **hypokinesia**, **rigidity**, and resting **tremor**.

Hypokinesia is the most disabling symptom. It is marked by a slowness of movement that interferes with all acts of daily living: walking becomes a shuffle, and arm swings are greatly reduced; small adjustive movements are no longer made, making it awkward to arise from a chair; meals are consumed slowly, facial expressions become fixed ("masked facies"); speech is monotonous and markedly reduced in volume; and the head does not turn to accommodate new directions of gaze.

Rigidity consists of a resistance to passive movement. It is present from the start of a movement and continues throughout the movement. This is in contrast to spasticity, in which resistance is often greatest at the beginning of a passive movement (clasp-knife phenomenon). Further, the resistance in parkinsonism has a characteristic ratchet-like quality, which is probably related to an underlying tremor (cogwheel phenomenon).

The tremor of parkinsonism is most conspicuous at rest and characteristically improves during voluntary movement (hence the term *resting tremor*). It typically consists of a 4 to 6 Hz tremor involving the hand or foot in a rhythmic oscillation between agonist and antagonist muscles.

CARDINAL FEATURES

- CHIEF PATHOLOGICAL FEATURE: DEGENERATION OF PARS COMPACTA OF SUBSTANTIA NIGRA

- NEUROCHEMICAL ABNORMALITY: SELECTIVE DEPLETION OF DOPAMINE

- CLINICAL TRIAD: TREMOR, RIGIDITY, AND BRADYKINESIA

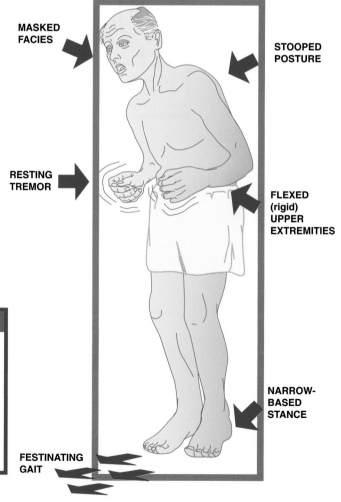

Fig. 11.8 Parkinsonism disease.

MASKED FACIES

STOOPED POSTURE

RESTING TREMOR

FLEXED (rigid) UPPER EXTREMITIES

NARROW-BASED STANCE

FESTINATING GAIT

The Hyperkinesia-Hypotonia Syndrome

Pathological Anatomy

The hyperkinesia-hypotonia syndrome is represented by various movement disorders described here. It is thought to be related to lesion(s) of the striatum or the subthalamic nucleus.

Lesions of the subthalamic nucleus produce a loss of excitatory projections to the globus pallidus. This results in a decrease in the activity of GABAergic globus pallidus neurons that project on the thalamus and causes disinhibition of thalamocortical neurons.

Lesions of the striatum cause a loss of GABAergic output to the globus pallidus. This disinhibits GABAergic fibers from the globus pallidus that project on the subthalamic nucleus. Diminished activity in the subthalamic nucleus disinhibits thalamocortical neurons, as already described.

Chorea

See **Fig. 11.9**.

Chorea consists of **involuntary, arrhythmic movements of a forcible, rapid, jerky type**. The distal parts of the extremities are typically involved early, but spread to more proximal parts often follows. Tongue movements and facial grimacing occur in more florid cases. Voluntary movements may be distorted by the superimposed involuntary ones, and the patient may incorporate the latter into the former, as if to make them less noticeable. Although power is generally unaffected, there may be difficulty maintaining muscular contraction, giving the appearance of diminished power.

Fig. 11.9 **Huntington's chorea.**

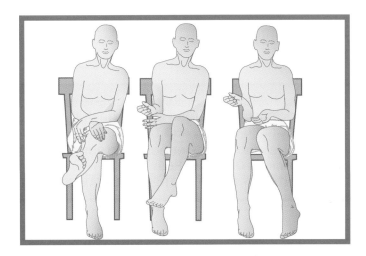

CARDINAL FEATURES

- CHARACTERIZED BY INVOLUNTARY ARRHYTHMIC MOVEMENTS OF A FORCIBLE, RAPID, JERKY TYPE
- TYPICALLY INVOLVES DISTAL PARTS OF EXTREMITIES EARLY, PROXIMAL PARTS LATER
- TONGUE MOVEMENTS AND FACIAL GRIMACING ARE MANIFEST IN ADVANCED CASES
- OFTEN INCORPORATED INTO NORMAL VOLUNTARY MOVEMENTS TO MAKE LESS NOTICEABLE
- HUNTINGTON'S CHOREA, A GENETICALLY DETERMINED PROGRESSIVE DEGENERATIVE CONDITION ASSOCIATED WITH EVENTUAL COGNITIVE DECLINE, IS CLASSIC EXAMPLE

Athetosis

See **Fig. 11.10.**

Athetosis is characterized by **slow, sinuous, involuntary movements** that tend to flow into one another. They often involve the extremities, the face, and the tongue. Compared with chorea, athetotic movements are slower and more continuous.

Dystonia

Dystonia is characterized by slow, sustained, involuntary movements or postures. As compared with athetosis, dystonic movements differ only in their more persistently sustained postures and their tendency to involve the larger muscles of the trunk and limb girdles.

Fig. 11.10 Athetosis.

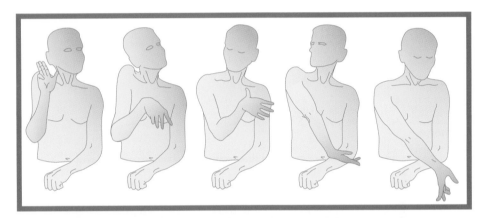

CARDINAL FEATURES
- MAY AFFECT ALL FOUR LIMBS OR MAY BE UNILATERAL; MAY AFFECT NECK, FACE, AND TONGUE
- MOVEMENTS ARE SLOW, SINUOUS, AND PURPOSELESS; MAY FLOW INTO ONE ANOTHER
- MOVEMENTS MAY END IN EXTREME, SUSTAINED POSTURES

Ballism

See **Fig. 11.11**.

Ballism is a form of chorea. It is distinguished by movements that are flinging and violent in nature. It predominantly affects the proximal extremities and is usually unilateral (hemiballism).

Fig. 11.11 **Hemiballism.**

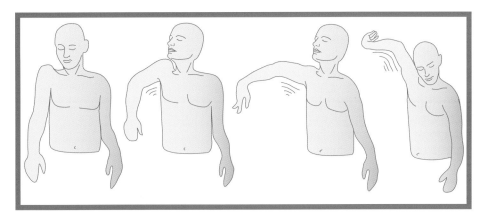

CARDINAL FEATURES

● **LESION IN CONTRALATERAL SUBTHALAMIC NUCLEUS**
● **PRIMARILY AFFECTS PROXIMAL LIMB MUSCLES**
● **MOVEMENTS ARE VIOLENT AND FLINGING IN NATURE**
(high velocity, high amplitude)

12 Limbic System

Many structures have been included in various accounts of the limbic system, but for our purpose the limbic system means (1) the limbic lobe, (2) the hippocampal formation, (3) the amygdaloid nucleus, (4) the hypothalamus, and (5) the anterior nucleus of the thalamus.

Functional studies suggest the limbic system participates in emotion and emotional behaviors (e.g., anger, fear, and sexuality), which appear to be important in the preservation of the individual and of the species. In addition, these studies suggest the limbic system is important in coordinating the emotion and autonomic responses such as changes in blood pressure, respiration, pupillary dilation, and bowel and bladder control. More recently appreciated is the important role of the limbic system, in particular the hippocampus, regarding learning and memory.

It should be emphasized that, despite the persistent use of the term *limbic system*, which includes, as noted, several structures that appear to share some common functions, the idea that it represents an independent functional system can no longer be maintained. Indeed, the individual structures of the limbic system are now known to be involved in a wide variety of functions and connections.

With this in mind, the major components of the limbic system are addressed separately. Further, because the thalamus and the hypothalamus are discussed at length elsewhere (Chapters 9 and 10), this chapter concentrates on the limbic lobe, the hippocampal formation, and the amygdaloid nucleus.

In 1878, the French anthropologist Pierre Paul Broca introduced the term *limbic lobe* to describe a ring of gray matter that surrounded the rostral brainstem. The term, which comprised the subcallosal, the cingulate, and the parahippocampal gyri, was applied to characterize these structures as phylogenetically primitive.

In 1937, the American anatomist James Papez transformed the limbic lobe from an evolutionary concept into a physiological one. In an attempt to explain the relationship between consciousness and the emotions, he described a circuit of neuronal connections between the limbic lobe and the hypothalamus. The circuit of Papez is described later in this chapter. One of the historical consequences of Papez's efforts was to enlarge the concept of a "limbic lobe" into a "limbic system," which encompasses the limbic lobe as well as associated subcortical structures.

Structures of the Limbic System

Limbic Lobe

See **Fig. 12.1**.

As noted, the limbic lobe consists of (1) the *subcallosal*, (2) the *cingulate*, and (3) the *parahippocampal gyri*. Collectively, these gyri form a ring around the rostral portion of the brainstem.

The limbic system is formed by the limbic lobe and associated subcortical structures, the amygdala, habenula, mammillary bodies, septal nuclei, portions of the thalamus, hypothalamus, and midbrain. The hippocampus is part of the limbic lobe and is situated on the inferomedial aspect of the hemisphere in the temporal lobe.

Fig. 12.1 **Limbic lobe.**

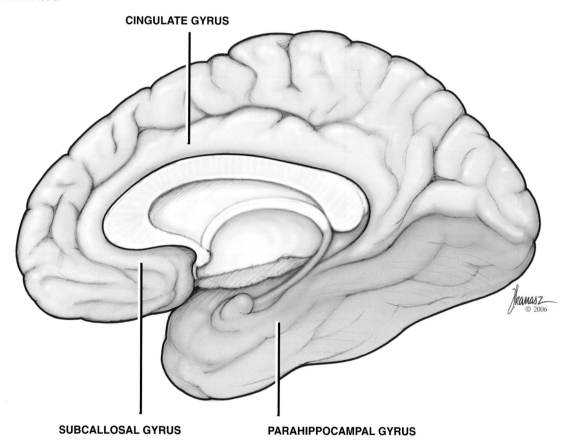

CINGULATE GYRUS

SUBCALLOSAL GYRUS   PARAHIPPOCAMPAL GYRUS

Hippocampal Formation

See **Figs. 12.2** and **12.3**.

The hippocampal formation consists of (1) the *hippocampus*, (2) the *dentate gyrus*, and (3) the *parahippocampal gyrus*. The hippocampus has the appearance of a sea horse. It bulges out into the temporal horn of the lateral ventricle and is arched around the mesencephalon. It is divided into three anatomic segments: head, body, and tail.

Fig. 12.2 **The hippocampus.**

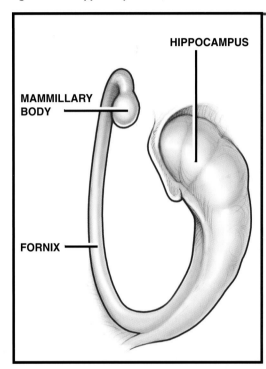

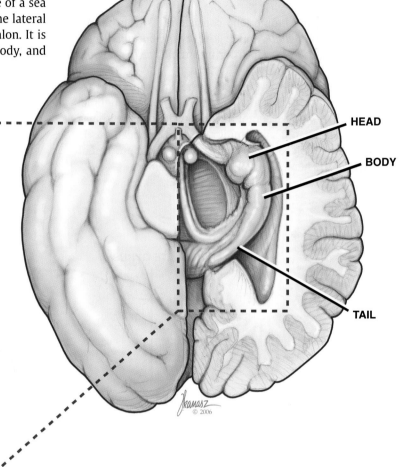

Fig. 12.3 **Hippocampal micro-anatomy.**
The hippocampus is a bilaminar archicortical (archicortex) structure consisting of Ammon's horn (hippocampus proper) and the dentate gyrus with one lamina rolled up in the other.

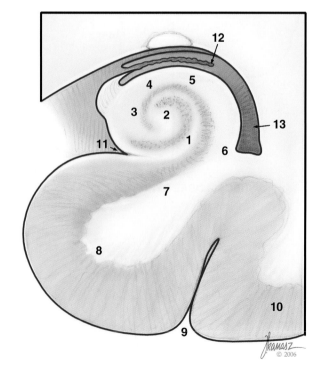

Key

1. Dentate gyrus
2. Hilum
3. CA3
4. CA2
5. CA1
6. Prosubiculum
7. Presubiculum
8. Parahippocampal gyrus
9. Collateral sulcus
10. Fusiform gyrus
11. Hippocampal sulcus
12. Choroid plexus
13. Temporal horn

Hippocampus

The hippocampus is composed of an intraventricular expansion of the temporal lobe cortex. It forms the floor of the inferior horn of the lateral ventricle and is **C**-shaped in the coronal section. Anteriorly, it enlarges to form the pes hippocampus. Posteriorly, it terminates beneath the splenium of the corpus callosum.

Fig. 12.4 **Hippocampal histology.**

Histology of the Hippocampus

Histologically, the hippocampus is an example of the three-layered archicortex, which is phylogenetically older than the six-layered neocortex (**Fig. 12.4**). The three layers of the hippocampus are described as follows:

- The molecular layer contains nerve fibers and small neurons and is continuous with the outermost layer of the neocortex.
- The pyramidal layer contains pyramidal-shaped neurons that send dendrites into the molecular layer, and axons, destined for the fornix, into the alveus. This layer is continuous with layer 5 (internal pyramidal) of the neocortex.
- The polymorphic layer is similar to the innermost layer (layer 6) of the neocortex.

Key

1. Alveus fibers
2. Stratum oriens of CA1 → CA4
3. Stratum pyramidal
4. Stratum lucidum
5. Stratum radiatum
6. Stratum moleculare
7. Vestigal hippocampal sulcus
8. Stratum moleculare of dentate sulcus
9. Dentate gyrus granule cells
10. Polymorphic layer of dentate gyrus
11. Fibers of the fimbria that form the fornix

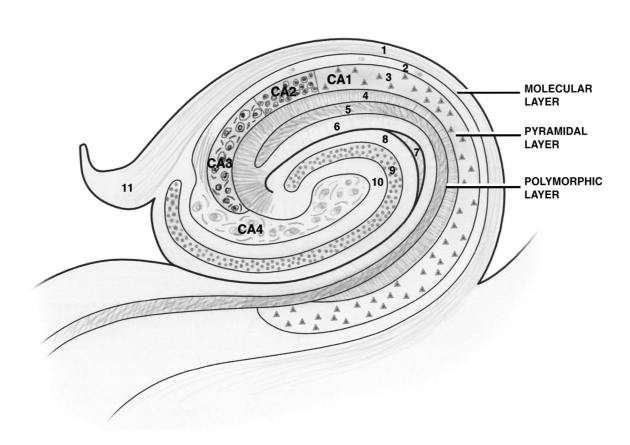

Afferent and Efferent Connections

See **Figs. 12.5, 12.6, 12.7,** and **12.8.**

Afferent fibers are received from the *entorhinal area* (lateral olfactory cortex), the septal area, the anterior thalamic nucleus, and the mammillary bodies. Noradrenergic fibers are projected from the locus ceruleus, and serotonergic fibers are projected from the raphe nuclei. Finally, the fornix carries commissural fibers that originate in the hippocampus on the opposite side.

Fig. 12.5 **Parahippocampal-intrahippocampal connection.**

Key

A—Perforant pathway that connects the entorhinal cortex (parahippocampal gyrus) to the dentate gyrus
B—Mossy fibers that connect the dentate gyrus to CA3
C—Schaeffer collaterals that connect CA3 to CA1
D—Fibers that emerge from the alveus that form the fimbria and later emerge (posteriorly) as an anteriorly ascending pathway that forms the fornix
E—Fornix

The predominant efferent fibers of the hippocampus are projected in the fornix as follows:

- The ventricular surface of the hippocampus is covered by a thin layer of white matter called the *alveus*, which contains fibers that originate in the large pyramidal cells of the hippocampus. These fibers converge on the medial border of the hippocampus and then continue posteriorly as the *fimbria*.

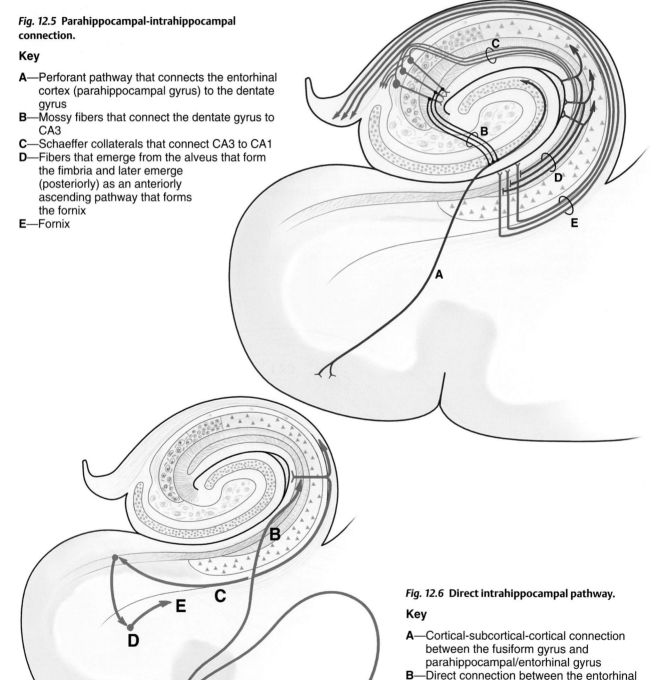

Fig. 12.6 **Direct intrahippocampal pathway.**

Key

A—Cortical-subcortical-cortical connection between the fusiform gyrus and parahippocampal/entorhinal gyrus
B—Direct connection between the entorhinal area (layer III) and CA1 subfield pyramidal cells
C, D, E—Direct connection between the pyramidal cells of CA1 and the deep layers of the neocortex

- The fimbria continues as the *crus of the fornix*, beginning at the posterior end of the hippocampus beneath the splenium of the corpus callosum. The two crura from each hemisphere converge to form the *body of the fornix*, which then continues anteriorly along the undersurface of the corpus callosum. At its anterior extent, the body of the fornix diverges into two *columns*, which terminate in the mammillary bodies of the hypothalamus and the septal region of the frontal lobe.

- Along the way the fornix also sends fibers to the anterior thalamic nucleus, the midbrain reticular formation, and the hippocampus on the opposite side (via the *commissure of the fornix*).

Fig. 12.7 **Cortical connections of the direct intrahippocampal pathway.**

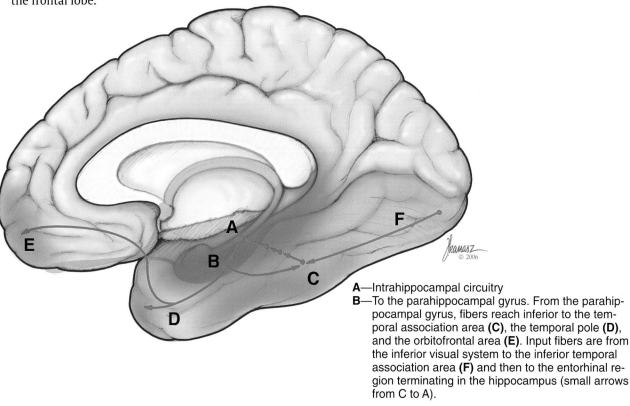

A—Intrahippocampal circuitry
B—To the parahippocampal gyrus. From the parahippocampal gyrus, fibers reach inferior to the temporal association area **(C)**, the temporal pole **(D)**, and the orbitofrontal area **(E)**. Input fibers are from the inferior visual system to the inferior temporal association area **(F)** and then to the entorhinal region terminating in the hippocampus (small arrows from C to A).

Fig. 12.8 **Cortical connections of the polysynaptic intrahippocampal pathway.**

Output pathways
(1) Output fibers from the hippocampus that reach the fornix **(2)**, then the mammillary bodies **(3)**, the anterior nucleus of the thalamus **(4)**, and later the cingulum **(6)**.

Input pathways
The input to the hippocampus for this pathway is from the visual cortex to the parietal association area **(A)**, then to the parahippocampal/entorhinal cortex **(B)**, then to the hippocampus **(D)** through the perforant path **(C)**.

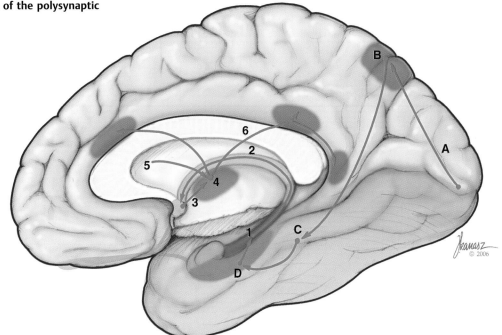

Dentate Gyrus

The dentate gyrus is a narrow band of cortex with a notched appearance. It is located between the fimbria of the hippocampus and the parahippocampal gyrus. Anteriorly, it is continuous with the uncus of the parahippocampal gyrus; posteriorly, it is continuous with the indusium griseum, a thin layer of gray matter that covers the corpus callosum.

Histologically, the dentate gyrus, like the hippocampus, is composed of three layers. However, in contrast to the hippocampus, the pyramidal cell layer is replaced by a granule cell layer, which sends axons to terminate upon dendrites of the pyramidal cells in the hippocampus. All dentate gyrus efferents are confined to the hippocampal formation.

Parahippocampal Gyrus

See **Fig. 12.3**, p. 340.

The parahippocampal gyrus is located between the hippocampal fissure and the collateral sulcus. It is continuous with the hippocampal formation along the medial-inferior border of the temporal lobe. Most of the cortex of the parahippocampal gyrus is six-layered. However, in the region of the gyrus known as the subiculum there is a transition between the neocortex and the three-layered archicortex of the hippocampus.

Amygdaloid Nucleus

The amygdaloid nucleus, a large gray mass covered by rudimentary cortex, lies in the anterior pole of the temporal lobe. It is located in front of and above the tip of the inferior horn of the lateral ventricle and just below the uncus of the parahippocampal gyrus.

The amygdaloid nucleus is divided into two nuclear groups: (1) the corticomedial group, which lies just below the pyriform area of the temporal lobe and receives fibers from the olfactory bulb and the olfactory cortex; and (2) the basolateral group, which has reciprocal connections with the visual, auditory, and somatosensory cortices, as well as the thalamus and the brainstem reticular formation.

In addition to the fibers it sends back upon its sources of input, the amygdaloid nucleus projects a major efferent tract, the stria terminalis, upon the hypothalamic nuclei. The fibers of the stria terminalis accompany the **C**-shaped caudate nucleus as the caudate nucleus loops around the thalamus.

Interconnections in the Limbic System

Many interconnections between various parts of the limbic system have been described. The best known of these is the circuit of Papez.

The Circuit of Papez

As an anatomist, Papez was interested in the anatomic substrate by which cognitive functions influence emotions and their autonomic effects, a relationship that earlier experimental studies had suggested. Papez postulated that limbic structures occupied an intermediate position between cognitive cortical effects and the emotional and autonomic effects of the hypothalamus. The pathway he described, known as the circuit of Papez, interconnects the association areas of the cerebral cortex with the hypothalamus as follows.

The association areas of the prefrontal, parietal, temporal, and occipital cortices send fibers to the cingulate gyrus. The cingulate gyrus then projects to the parahippocampal gyrus, which in turn projects to the hippocampus. Fibers from the cingulate and parahippocampal gyri are carried in the **C**-shaped cingulum bundle. Information in the hippocampus is then relayed in the mammillary bodies of the hypothalamus via the **C**-shaped fornix. It is projected from the mammillary bodies, via the mammillothalamic tract, to the anterior nucleus of the thalamus. Finally, information in the thalamus is projected back on the cingulate gyrus, bringing the circuit to an effective close.

Functions of the Limbic System

Our knowledge of the functions of the limbic system is incomplete. It is primarily based on animal experiments involving ablation and stimulation of limbic structures, and clinicopathologic correlates in patients with memory loss, emotional disturbance, and temporal lobe epilepsy.

Hippocampus: Recent Memory

The hippocampus has been implicated in the execution of recent memory.

Recent memory is the ability to learn and retrieve material after an interval of minutes, hours, or days. (Immediate memory refers to an interval of seconds; remote memory refers to an interval of weeks or more.)

In addition to the hippocampus, two other structures are involved in the execution of recent memory: (1) the mammillary bodies of the hypothalamus and (2) the dorsomedial nucleus of the thalamus. The mammillary bodies receive fibers, via the fornix, from the hippocampus, and the dorsomedial nucleus contains fibers from the mammillothalamic tract on their way to the anterior thalamic nucleus from the mammillary bodies.

These three limbic structures, the hippocampi, the mammillary bodies, and the dorsomedial nuclei, appear to store and retrieve memories from the cerebral cortex.

Their putative role in recent memory is in part suggested by two amnestic syndromes. These syndromes are marked by recent memory loss with preservation of immediate and remote memory. They are (1) the Korsakoff syndrome, which consists of bilateral destruction of the mammillary bodies and the dorsomedial nuclei, and (2) the surgical destruction of hippocampi performed on patients with medically intractable epilepsy (an example of the latter is described in the Clinical Manifestations section).

Amygdaloid Nucleus: Emotions and Autonomic Effects

The amygdaloid nucleus is thought to be concerned with the emotions and their autonomic consequences.

This is in contrast to the more "cognitive" role of the hippocampus, which is primarily associated with memory and learning.

As noted, the amygdaloid nucleus receives sensory input from areas of the cortex representing all sensory modalities. The precise pattern of neuronal connections that are involved in the processing of this information is not understood. However, the amygdala does not appear to play an important role in fashioning an emotional or behavioral response that is appropriate to the sensory input.

An important part of this response involves autonomic effects such as changes in blood pressure, respiration, and bowel and bladder control. These effects are mediated by the hypothalamus, which receives fibers from the amygdaloid nucleus via the stria terminalis.

Emotional and behavioral responses may include expressions of fear, anxiety, placidity, or sexual activity. Some of these will be considered in more detail in the following section.

Clinical Manifestations of Lesions in the Limbic System

One of the striking characteristics of limbic structures is their low threshold for epileptic seizures. At a cellular level, so-called temporal lobe seizures represent excessive, synchronized neuronal discharges in limbic and neocortical structures. Clinically, these are expressed by an alteration in consciousness, accompanied by a combination of sensory, motor, psychic, and autonomic manifestations.

This symptomatology, as illustrated in the following case study, provides important insights into the signs and symptoms of dysfunction in several limbic structures. We will first consider the clinical syndrome of a temporal lobe seizure and then discuss some individual signs and symptoms.

Case Example: Temporal Lobe Epilepsy

While talking to her neighbor on the porch outside her house, Lauren suddenly noticed a rising epigastric sensation, accompanied by a fleeting, inexplicable sense of fear.

A minute later, the neighbor observed that Lauren was staring blankly into space and not responding appropriately to the conversation. What is more, Lauren fumbled with her dress in a purposeless and uncoordinated manner. She appeared pale and sweaty, and her breathing pattern seemed to be irregular. Three minutes after she assumed her spacey look, Lauren regained her responsiveness and stopped her stereotypic fumbling. She was amnestic for the episode, although she vaguely recalled anxiety and a rising abdominal distress. She remained mildly confused for several hours after the event.

As noted earlier, so-called temporal lobe seizures are often expressed clinically by sensory, motor, psychic, and autonomic manifestations. All of these manifestations contributed to Lauren's seizure: the rising epigastric sensation (sensory); the fumbling movements (motor); the feelings of anxiety and fear (psychic); and the pallor, sweating, and respiratory abnormalities (autonomic).

Of these, the psychic and autonomic symptoms appear to arise, particularly (though by no means exclusively) as a result of abnormal discharge in the amygdaloid nucleus.

Disturbances of Emotion and Emotional Behavior

Fear is the most common emotion produced by temporal lobe seizures. The clinical observation of the connection between fear and temporal lobe seizures is supported by animal experiments where stimulation of the amygdaloid nucleus sometimes elicits fearful behavior. Such behavior is usually accompanied by autonomic hyperactivity (see below).

Less commonly, sexual emotions and behavior, which may be associated with autonomic changes such as erections or vulvovaginal secretions, are manifest during temporal lobe seizures. Like the emotion of fear, sexual emotions have been reproduced by stimulation of the amygdaloid nucleus.

Disturbances of Autonomic Function

As discussed earlier, disturbances of autonomic function consist of changes in (1) blood pressure, (2) heart rate, (3) respiration, (4) gastrointestinal motility and secretion, (5) bowel and bladder control, (6) pupillary dilatation, and (7) piloerection.

These autonomic changes may occur in isolation. More commonly they occur in an appropriate emotional context. For example, an increase in blood pressure, heart rate, and respiratory rate may accompany a feeling of fear, or vulvovaginal secretions may accompany sexual feelings.

In addition to these physical changes, autonomic sensations may also occur. A rising epigastric sensation, as mentioned in the case study, is most common, but other autonomic sensory phenomena such as nausea, palpitations, and a feeling of warmth or cold occur too.

Stimulation of the amygdaloid nucleus may produce these autonomic effects, presumably by its projection (via the stria terminalis) on the hypothalamus.

Disturbances of Memory

Deficits of memory related to temporal lobe lesions may result from bilateral destruction of the hippocampi.

Evidence for this comes from the small group of patients who have undergone bilateral anterior temporal lobectomies as a treatment for psychiatric disease or for medically intractable temporal lobe epilepsy (surgical treatment for these patients is usually by unilateral temporal lobectomies).

The most famous patient studied after a bilateral operation, case H.M., illustrates the memory deficit caused by bilateral destruction of the hippocampi.

Immediately after surgery, H.M. exhibited both a retrograde and an anterograde amnesia—a loss of memory for events both prior to and following the operation.

In time, the retrograde amnesia cleared, and he was left with a severe, persistent, anterograde amnesia. Immediate recall and remote memory were both preserved, but he showed an almost total lack of recent memory. As a result, he failed to remember almost anything following the time of the operation and seemed quite unable to learn any new information.

He would reread the same papers and repeat the same tasks without any knowledge that he had done so before. He could not learn the location of his house or the location of the objects within it, nor could he learn the names or recognize the faces of individuals who frequently visited him.

13 Cerebral Cortex

Major Sulci and Fissures

See **Fig. 13.1**.

The *frontal, temporal, parietal,* and *occipital lobes* are delimited by the *lateral, parieto-occipital, central (rolandic),* and *calcarine sulci.* The lateral sulcus, or sylvian fissure as it is also known, is the most constant fissure in the brain. It begins as a deep furrow on the inferior surface of the hemisphere and extends laterally between the frontoparietal and temporal lobes.

The central sulcus vertically separates the frontoparietal cortices and, therefore, the motor (ventral) from the sensory (dorsal) cortex. It slopes downward from the cerebral convexity and forward 70 degrees to the horizontal plane and runs ~2 cm deep. The central sulcus is mainly a continuous sulcus. It rarely dips into the sylvian fissure.

The walls of the calcarine sulcus, which lies on the medial surface of the occipital lobe, are formed by the visual cortex. It begins at the dorsal end of the *corpus callosum* and follows an arched course from the parieto-occipital sulcus to the *occipital pole.*

The parieto-occipital sulcus extends vertically from the calcarine sulcus to the rostral border of the hemisphere to separate the parietal and occipital lobes. It begins ~4 cm from the occipital pole.

The interhemispheric fissure divides the cerebrum into two hemispheres (right and left). The caudal border of the interhemispheric fissure is formed by the corpus callosum, a white matter tract that contains fibers that cross from one hemisphere to the other. The falx cerebri is a dural fold that extends into the interhemispheric fissure and serves to anatomically separate the right from the left cerebral hemispheres.

The transverse cerebral fissure marks the separation between the cerebral hemispheres above and the cerebellum, midbrain, and diencephalon below. The dorsal portion of the transverse cerebral fissure intervenes between the occipital lobe above and the cerebellum below. It contains the tentorium cerebelli, a dural fold. The ventral aspect of the transverse cerebral fissure separates the corpus callosum above from the diencephalon below. It contains the tela choroidea, a vascular plexus derived from pia mater.

Fig. 13.1 Major sulci and fissures.

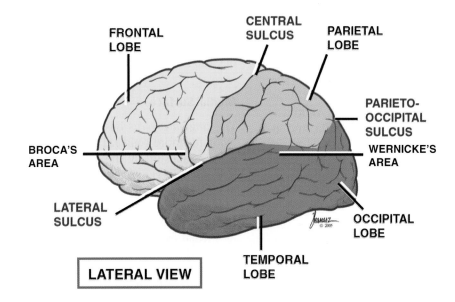

LATERAL VIEW

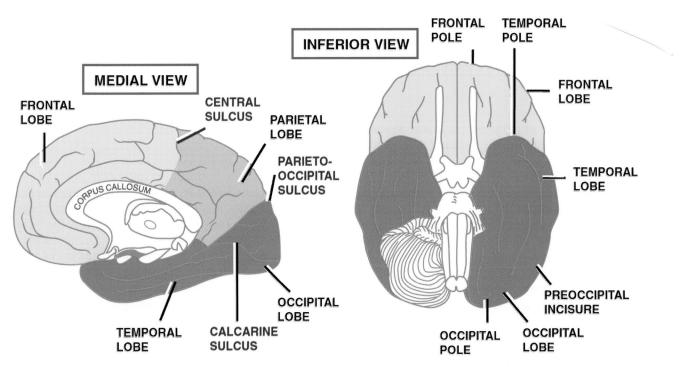

MEDIAL VIEW

INFERIOR VIEW

Gyri and Sulci

See **Fig. 13.2.**

Frontal Lobe

The precentral sulcus is discontinued and runs parallel to the central sulcus, just ventral to the precentral gyrus, which comprises the primary motor cortex. Ventral to the precentral sulcus are the superior, middle, and inferior frontal gyri, which are separated by the superior and inferior frontal sulci. In the dominant hemisphere, the posterior part of the inferior frontal gyrus contains Broca's area, which controls expressive speech function.

Parietal Lobe

The postcentral gyrus runs parallel and dorsal to the central sulcus. It comprises the primary sensory cortex. The intraparietal sulcus, which extends from the postcentral sulcus dorsally, separates the dorsal parietal cortex into the superior and inferior parietal lobules. The inferior parietal lobule contains the supramarginal and angular gyri, which make up part of the receptive language area (*Wernicke's area*) in the dominant hemisphere.

Temporal Lobe

The lateral surface of the temporal lobe comprises the *superior*, *middle*, and *inferior temporal gyri*, which are separated by the *superior* and *inferior temporal sulci*. The *transverse temporal gyri* (*Heschl's convolutions*) lie adjacent to that portion of the superior temporal gyrus that forms the floor of the lateral sulcus. Heschl's gyri are buried in the temporal operculum (within the insular cortex). They are not visualized on inspection of the lateral cerebral hemisphere. The cerebral hemispheres contain the primary auditory cortex on each side. The dorsal aspect of the superior temporal gyrus contains part of the receptive language region (Wernicke's area) in the dominant hemisphere.

Occipital Lobe

Aside from the calcarine sulcus already described, the occipital cortex contains minor and extremely variable sulci that may rarely result in the definition of superior, middle, and inferior occipital gyri.

Medial Surface

The *cingulate gyrus* lies rostral to the *corpus callosum* along its entire course. The gyrus is separated from the corpus callosum by the sulcus of the corpus callosum (*callosal sulcus*) and the indusium griseum, a thin layer of cortical gray matter that lies on the superior surface of the corpus callosum. The *paracentral lobule* surrounds the indentation made by the central sulcus. It is formed by medial extensions of the precentral and postcentral gyri of the lateral hemisphere. The paracentral lobule contains parts of the primary motor and primary sensory cortices. In addition, the supplementary motor area lies in the anterior aspect of the paracentral lobule. The *precuneus* is located just dorsal to the paracentral lobule. It is formed by medial extensions of the superior parietal lobule of the lateral hemisphere. The *cuneus* is located in the occipital lobe just dorsal to the precuneus. The precuneus is separated from the cuneus by the *parieto-occipital sulcus*.

Inferior Surface

A convolution on the inferior undersurface of the hemisphere extends from the occipital pole almost to the temporal pole. Ventrally, it contains the *parahippocampal gyrus*; dorsally, it contains the medial *occipitotemporal gyrus*. Deep to the parahippocampal gyrus is the hippocampus. The ventromedial extent of the parahippocampal gyrus contains the uncus. Herniation of the uncus as the result of increased intracranial pressure results in early oculomotor nerve palsy that may progress into a coma and cardiorespiratory compromise. Laterally, these gyri are bounded by the *collateral sulcus*. Just lateral to the collateral sulcus is the lateral occipitotemporal gyrus and the inferior part of the *inferior temporal gyrus*. The *lingual gyrus* extends forward into the temporal lobe, where it is continuous with the parahippocampal gyrus.

The inferior frontal lobe is marked by the *olfactory sulcus*, which contains the olfactory bulb and tract. The olfactory sulcus is bordered medially by the *gyrus rectus* and laterally by the *orbital gyri*.

Fig. 13.2 Gyri and sulci.

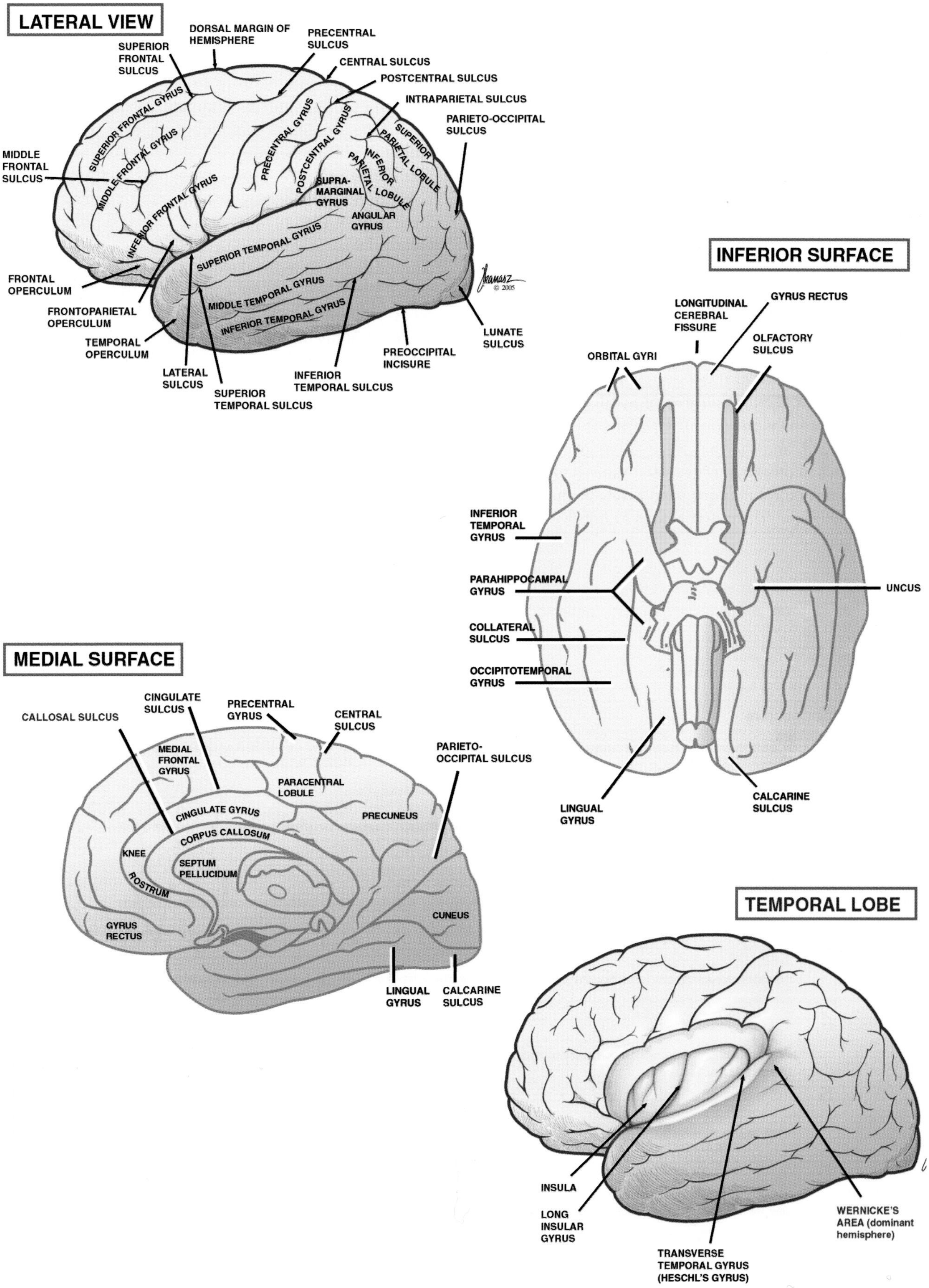

LATERAL VIEW

DORSAL MARGIN OF HEMISPHERE
PRECENTRAL SULCUS
SUPERIOR FRONTAL SULCUS
CENTRAL SULCUS
POSTCENTRAL SULCUS
INTRAPARIETAL SULCUS
PARIETO-OCCIPITAL SULCUS
SUPERIOR FRONTAL GYRUS
MIDDLE FRONTAL SULCUS
MIDDLE FRONTAL GYRUS
SUPERIOR FRONTAL GYRUS
PRECENTRAL GYRUS
POSTCENTRAL GYRUS
SUPERIOR PARIETAL LOBULE
INFERIOR PARIETAL LOBULE
INFERIOR FRONTAL GYRUS
SUPRA-MARGINAL GYRUS
ANGULAR GYRUS
FRONTAL OPERCULUM
FRONTOPARIETAL OPERCULUM
TEMPORAL OPERCULUM
SUPERIOR TEMPORAL GYRUS
MIDDLE TEMPORAL GYRUS
INFERIOR TEMPORAL GYRUS
LUNATE SULCUS
PREOCCIPITAL INCISURE
LATERAL SULCUS
SUPERIOR TEMPORAL SULCUS
INFERIOR TEMPORAL SULCUS

INFERIOR SURFACE

LONGITUDINAL CEREBRAL FISSURE
GYRUS RECTUS
OLFACTORY SULCUS
ORBITAL GYRI
INFERIOR TEMPORAL GYRUS
PARAHIPPOCAMPAL GYRUS
UNCUS
COLLATERAL SULCUS
OCCIPITOTEMPORAL GYRUS
LINGUAL GYRUS
CALCARINE SULCUS

MEDIAL SURFACE

CALLOSAL SULCUS
CINGULATE SULCUS
PRECENTRAL GYRUS
CENTRAL SULCUS
PARIETO-OCCIPITAL SULCUS
MEDIAL FRONTAL GYRUS
PARACENTRAL LOBULE
PRECUNEUS
CINGULATE GYRUS
CORPUS CALLOSUM
KNEE
SEPTUM PELLUCIDUM
ROSTRUM
GYRUS RECTUS
CUNEUS
LINGUAL GYRUS
CALCARINE SULCUS

TEMPORAL LOBE

INSULA
LONG INSULAR GYRUS
TRANSVERSE TEMPORAL GYRUS (HESCHL'S GYRUS)
WERNICKE'S AREA (dominant hemisphere)

Histology of the Cortex

Cortical Neurons

See **Fig. 13.3**.

A variety of cells make up the cerebral cortex. These include both neurons and glia. Glial cells, which include oligodendrocytes, astrocytes, and microglial cells, serve to support the neurons. Examples of these roles include providing metabolic support, scavenging neurotransmitters, and providing myelination. Neurons are the targets or cells of origin of all of the information traveling into and out of the cerebral cortex, respectively. The *pyramidal cell neurons*, which are the most numerous cells of the cerebral cortex, constitute about two thirds of the cortical neurons. The pyramidal cells communicate with other neurons in one of three ways: (1) projection neurons send axons out of the cerebral hemisphere to such areas of the brain as the corpus striatum, the brainstem, the spinal cord, and the thalamus; (2) association neurons connect to other neurons in the same hemisphere; and (3) commissural neurons send axons to the contralateral hemisphere. The most obvious example is the corpus callosum.

Stellate cells are interneurons present in the cerebral cortex. They are smaller in size (compared with pyramidal cells), polygonal in shape, and possess multiple branching dendrites with a relatively short axon. They are the only excitatory interneurons in the cerebral cortex that use the neurotransmitter glutamate. All other cortical interneurons are gamma-aminobutyric acid (GABA)–containing inhibitory neurons.

Fusiform cells are also interneurons and are concentrated mainly in the deepest layers of the cortex (i.e., farthest from the cortical surface). They send dendrites toward the surface of the cortex to branch and influence neurons in the superficial cortical layers.

The *horizontal cells* are confined to the most superficial layer of the cortex. They are small fusiform cells that are horizontally oriented. These axons run parallel to the surface of the cortex, making contact with the ascending dendrites of pyramidal cells.

The *cells of Martinotti* are present at many levels of the cortex. They send axons that end in the most superficial layers of the cortex.

Fig. 13.3 **Cortical neurons.**

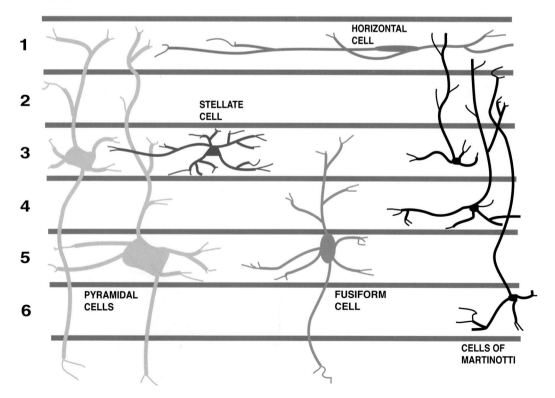

Cortical Layers

See **Fig. 13.4**.

The thickness of the cerebral cortex varies from 1.5 to 4.5 mm. The full complement of cortical neurons is present by the 18th week of gestation, and by the ninth month the cortex comprises six distinguishable layers:

1. *Molecular layer*   This is the most superficial layer of the cortex. Its sparse population of cells gives it its name. It contains dendrites of the pyramidal and fusiform cells (see below) and axons of the stellate cells and the cells of Martinotti. Occasional horizontal cells of Cajal are also present. Many synaptic connections are formed in the molecular layer.

2. *External granular layer*   This layer contains many small pyramidal cells and interneurons.

3. *External pyramidal layer*   This layer contains pyramidal cells. The dendrites of these neurons pass superficially to enter the molecular layer, whereas the axons pass deep to enter the white matter as projection, association, or commissural fibers.

4. *Internal granular layer*   This layer consists mostly of stellate cells and a small number of other interneurons.

5. *Internal pyramidal layer*   This layer contains many large pyramidal cells. Axons from pyramidal cells project to the deep structures/nuclei of the brain and nervous system. These projections constitute the bulk of the white matter. The giant pyramidal cells (of Betz) are located in this layer, in the primary motor area of the cortex.

6. *Multiform layer*   This layer is composed mainly of fusiform cells and a smaller number of pyramidal cells and interneurons.

Granular and Agranular Cortex

The cerebral cortex is composed of two cell types: granular and agranular. Granular cortex is so-called because it contains a large percentage of granule cells, which receive afferent impulses. This type of cortex is located mainly in primary sensory regions, such as visual, auditory, and somatosensory cortices. Granular cortex contains strongly developed layers II and IV (refers to cortical layers).

Agranular cortex is so-called because it contains a high percentage of pyramidal cells (as compared with granule cells). It is located mainly in areas that give rise to efferent impulses, such as the motor cortex, and the frontal eye field, which gives rise to prominent corticobulbar and corticospinal projections. Agranular cortex is characterized by strongly developed pyramidal layers III and V and less well developed granular layers.

Fig. 13.4 **Cortical layers.**

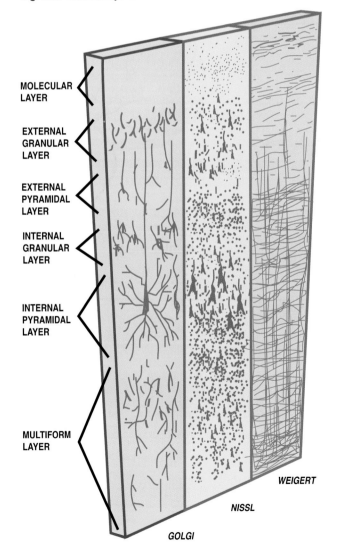

MOLECULAR
LAYER

EXTERNAL
GRANULAR
LAYER

EXTERNAL
PYRAMIDAL
LAYER

INTERNAL
GRANULAR
LAYER

INTERNAL
PYRAMIDAL
LAYER

MULTIFORM
LAYER

WEIGERT

NISSL

GOLGI

Brodmann's Map

See **Fig. 13.5**.

In 1909, the German histologist Korbinian Brodmann distinguished over 50 different regions of the cerebral cortex. He based these divisions on variations in cytoarchitectural features, such as relative thickness, density, size, shape, and arrangement of cortical neurons. Brodmann believed that these variations in cytoarchitecture should correspond to distinct physiological functions. In fact, only a limited number of the Brodmann's areas have been related to specific functions. Among the most important are the following: somatosensory cortex (areas 3, 1, and 2); primary motor and premotor cortex (areas 4 and 6, respectively); the frontal eye field (area 8); primary visual cortex (area 17); visual association cortex (areas 18 and 19); auditory cortex (areas 41 and 42); auditory association cortex (area 22, part of Wernicke's language comprehension area); Broca's speech area (area 44); sensory association cortex (areas 5 and 7); and prefrontal cortex (areas 9, 10, 11, and 12).

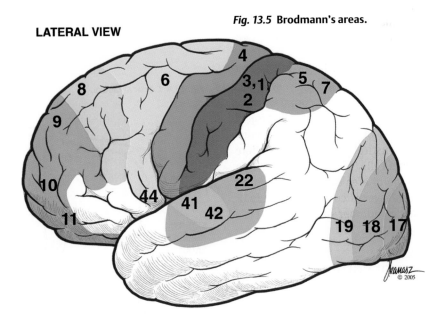

Fig. 13.5 **Brodmann's areas.**

LATERAL VIEW

MEDIAL VIEW

Subcortical White Matter

Projection Fibers

A variety of projection fibers originate in the cerebral cortex. Examples of these corticofugal projections include the corticostriatal and corticothalamic pathways; cortical projections to the amygdaloid body and the hippocampus; and corticospinal, corticoreticular, and corticopontine pathways. Many of the corticofugal projections, including the latter three named pathways, pass through the corona radiata and then the internal capsule. Other parts of the cortical projection system include the optic radiation, connecting the lateral geniculate body with the visual cortex, and the acoustic radiation, connecting the medial geniculate body with the auditory cortex.

Association Fibers

See **Fig. 13.6**.

The association fibers constitute most of the cerebral white matter. They provide connections between both adjacent and remote areas of the cortex. Among the most important association fibers are the following.

The *arcuate fibers*, also known as U-fibers, occupy the immediate subcortical white matter. They interconnect adjacent cortical fields. The *superior longitudinal fasciculus* connects the frontal lobes with portions of the parieto-occipital and temporal convolutions. It lies just dorsal to the level of the insula. The frontotemporal portion of this projection system is called the *arcuate fasciculus* and is believed to connect the temporal (Wernicke) and frontal (Broca) areas of speech. The temporo-occipital or *inferior longitudinal fasciculus* connects the temporal and occipital lobes; and the *uncinate fasciculus* connects the frontal lobe with the temporal pole. The *cingulum* is one of the association bundles of the limbic system. It connects the subcallosal area with the parahippocampal gyrus.

Fig. 13.6 Association fibers.

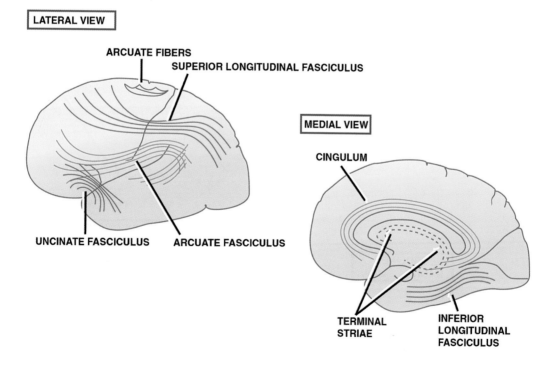

Commissural Fibers

See **Fig. 13.7**.

The commissural fibers cross the midline between the two cerebral hemispheres, providing interconnections between them. Important groups of commissural fibers include the following:

- The *corpus callosum*, which is the largest commissure, comprises connections between the two hemispheres. Although most regions of the cortex are interrelated through commissural fibers, areas that do not receive commissural fibers from the contralateral hemisphere include the primary visual cortex (area 17) and the hand and foot areas in the somatosensory cortex.
- The *anterior commissure* traverses the midline just anterior to the fornix column in the lamina terminalis. It comprises fibers that connect the middle and inferior temporal gyri of the two sides. Other fibers interconnect the olfactory cortex of the temporal lobes (the lateral olfactory area), including the uncus. A small ventral portion of the anterior commissure runs between the olfactory bulbs on each side.

- The *hippocampal commissure* traverses the midline inferior to the splenium of the corpus callosum. It contains fibers that connect the posterior columns of the fornix.
- The *posterior commissure* is located in the border between the diencephalon and mesencephalon, just anterior to the superior colliculus. It contains a complex mixture of fibers related to adjacent structures.
- The *habenular commissure* is located just superior to the pineal gland. It contains the fibers of the stria medullaris, which interconnects the habenular complex on each side.

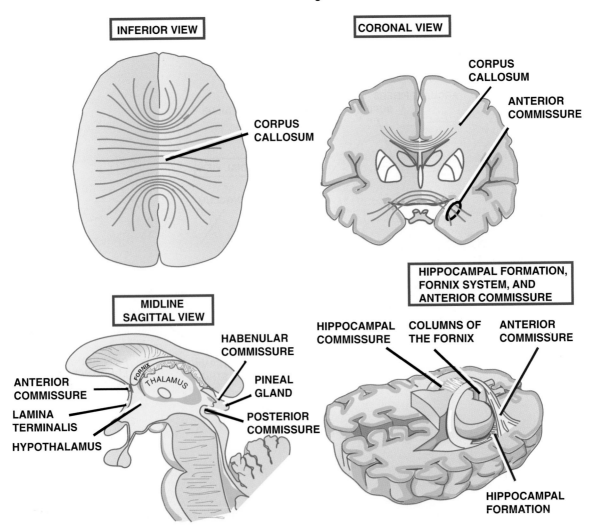

Fig. 13.7 **Commissural fibers.**

Cortical Localization

In 1861, before the Société d'Anthropologie in Paris, Pierre Paul Broca demonstrated on a human brain that the cerebral cortex has localized functions. Subsequent investigations by Broca and others provided further support for localization in other functional areas. By the turn of the twentieth century, sufficient evidence had accrued to convince the majority of the neurological community of the concept of cerebral localization.

The widespread acceptance of this doctrine motivated neuroanatomists to establish cortical maps that related cortical brain structures and functions. In the 1930s, for example, Wilder Penfield and colleagues at the Montreal Neurological Institute, under the influence of training in Germany with Dr. Foerster, created maps of human motor-sensory functions through the systematic electrical stimulation of the exposed brains of conscious epileptic patients undergoing epilepsy surgery. The human homunculus is an example of the results of Penfield's studies. With these historical considerations in mind, the major functions of the cerebral cortex are reviewed in relation to their anatomic substrate.

Frontal Cortex

The frontal lobe contains several cortical areas that are involved in motor functions. These include the primary motor cortex (Brodmann's area 4), the premotor cortex (area 6), the prefrontal area (areas 9, 10, 11, 12, 45, 46, 47), and the supplementary motor area.

Primary Motor Cortex

See **Fig. 13.8**.

The primary motor cortex (Brodmann's area 4) is located in the precentral gyrus and extends over the superomedial border of the hemisphere into the anterior portion of the paracentral lobule. The cytoarchitecture of the cortex in this area is of the agranular type, containing a preponderance of the giant pyramidal cells of Betz.

The function of the primary motor cortex is related to the execution of movement on the contralateral side of the body. The body is represented on the cortex in an inverted orientation, such that the sequence from below upward (i.e., beginning at the sylvian fissure inferiorly and ending at the superior interhemispheric fissure in the following order) is pharynx, larynx, tongue, face, head, neck, hand, arm, shoulder, trunk, and thigh. Continuing on the adjacent region of the medial aspect of the hemisphere are the leg and foot. Some areas of the body, such as the fingers and hands, show disproportionate representatives in the homunculus.

Afferent fibers that assist in the function of the primary motor cortex are derived from a complex network that includes the premotor area (see below), the somatosensory cortex, the posterior division of the ventrolateral (VL) nucleus of the thalamus, the cerebellum, and the basal ganglia.

Fig. 13.8 **Primary motor cortex.**

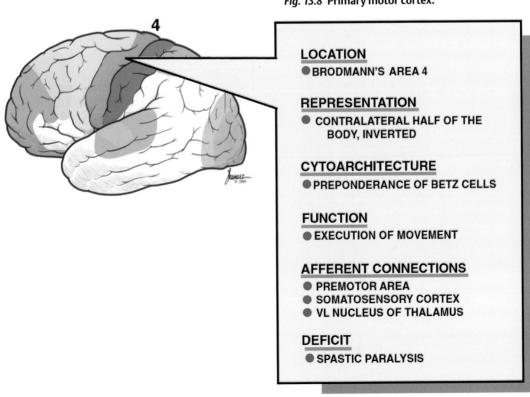

LOCATION
- BRODMANN'S AREA 4

REPRESENTATION
- CONTRALATERAL HALF OF THE BODY, INVERTED

CYTOARCHITECTURE
- PREPONDERANCE OF BETZ CELLS

FUNCTION
- EXECUTION OF MOVEMENT

AFFERENT CONNECTIONS
- PREMOTOR AREA
- SOMATOSENSORY CORTEX
- VL NUCLEUS OF THALAMUS

DEFICIT
- SPASTIC PARALYSIS

Supplementary Motor Area

See **Fig. 13.9**.

The supplementary motor area (SMA) is located in that part of area 6 that occupies the medial surface of the hemisphere, just anterior to the precentral gyrus in the paracentral lobule. The body is represented bilaterally in the SMA. The primary purpose of the SMA is to plan and program movements to be executed by the primary motor cortex. Lesions in area 6 often present with a so-called SMA syndrome. Patients are often acutely mute with contralateral paresis; both resolve over weeks to months. Interestingly, patients with an acute SMA syndrome are not able to initiate a voluntary movement, but when the movement is passively initiated (with the help of the examiner), both the movement and strength are within normal limits.

Fig. 13.9 **Supplementary motor area.**

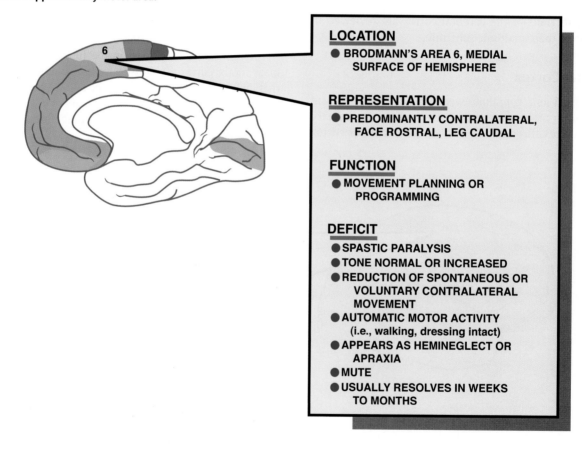

LOCATION
- BRODMANN'S AREA 6, MEDIAL SURFACE OF HEMISPHERE

REPRESENTATION
- PREDOMINANTLY CONTRALATERAL, FACE ROSTRAL, LEG CAUDAL

FUNCTION
- MOVEMENT PLANNING OR PROGRAMMING

DEFICIT
- SPASTIC PARALYSIS
- TONE NORMAL OR INCREASED
- REDUCTION OF SPONTANEOUS OR VOLUNTARY CONTRALATERAL MOVEMENT
- AUTOMATIC MOTOR ACTIVITY (i.e., walking, dressing intact)
- APPEARS AS HEMINEGLECT OR APRAXIA
- MUTE
- USUALLY RESOLVES IN WEEKS TO MONTHS

Premotor Cortex

See **Fig. 13.10.**

The premotor cortex corresponds roughly to Brodmann's area 6 and is also represented on the lateral hemisphere. It contains no giant pyramidal cells of Betz. Although electrical stimulation of this region of the cortex produces movement on the contralateral side of the body, a greater stimulus is required in this region to produce a comparable movement.

Afferent fibers to the premotor cortex are derived from the somatosensory cortex, the anterior division of the ventrolateral nucleus of the thalamus, and the basal ganglia. Like the supplementary motor area, the premotor area is concerned with the planning and programming of movements. It helps to store programs of motor activity that have been developed as a result of past experiences. Thus, whereas the primary motor cortex is responsible for the execution of movements, the supplementary and premotor areas help direct the primary motor area in its execution. *Apraxia* refers to impairment in the performance of a movement in the absence of paralysis. For example, a person is able to describe the process of unlocking the front door of the house with a key but is unable to physically perform the task. Such is the deficit associated with a lesion that is isolated to the premotor area.

Fig. 13.10 Premotor cortex.

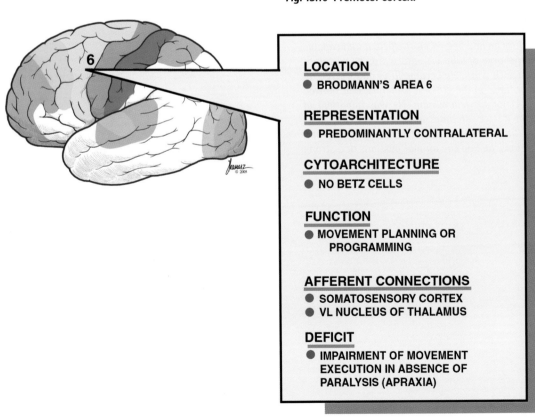

LOCATION
- BRODMANN'S AREA 6

REPRESENTATION
- PREDOMINANTLY CONTRALATERAL

CYTOARCHITECTURE
- NO BETZ CELLS

FUNCTION
- MOVEMENT PLANNING OR PROGRAMMING

AFFERENT CONNECTIONS
- SOMATOSENSORY CORTEX
- VL NUCLEUS OF THALAMUS

DEFICIT
- IMPAIRMENT OF MOVEMENT EXECUTION IN ABSENCE OF PARALYSIS (APRAXIA)

Prefrontal Cortex (Frontal Association Cortex)

See **Fig. 13.11.**

The prefrontal cortex comprises a large cortical area in the frontal lobe that covers the frontal pole. It roughly corresponds to Brodmann's areas 9, 10, 11, and 12. Because the prefrontal region is an association cortex, its electrical stimulation does not produce a motor response. The prefrontal cortex receives afferent fibers from the cortex of the parietal, temporal, and occipital lobes, which provide a source of sensory data derived from past experiences. What is more, the prefrontal cortex also receives afferents from the amygdaloid body of the temporal lobe and the mediodorsal thalamic nucleus. These fibers provide a source of affective reactions that may indirectly influence the execution of movements. In addition, the prefrontal cortex may play a role in the determination of an individual's personality. It may also play important roles in the makeup of such higher mental faculties as judgment and foresight and in the determination of the intellectual and emotional aspects of behavior.

An illustration of these functions is perhaps best demonstrated by the case of the nineteenth-century New England railroad worker Phineas Gage. The unfortunate Gage was struck by a rod that penetrated his forehead and destroyed a significant portion of his left frontal lobe. Remarkably, Gage survived. The personality changes that subsequently emerged, however, serve to underline some of the functions of the prefrontal cortex. As recorded in a contemporary medical journal:

> *Gage lived for twelve years afterwards; but whereas before the injury he had been a most efficient and capable foreman in charge of laborers, afterwards he was unfit to be given such work. He became fitful and irreverent, indulged at times in the grossest profanity, and showed little respect for his fellow man. He was impatient of restraint or advice, at times obstinate, yet capricious and vacillating. A child in his intellectual capacity and manifestations, he had the animal passions of a strong man.*

Fig. 13.11 Prefrontal cortex.

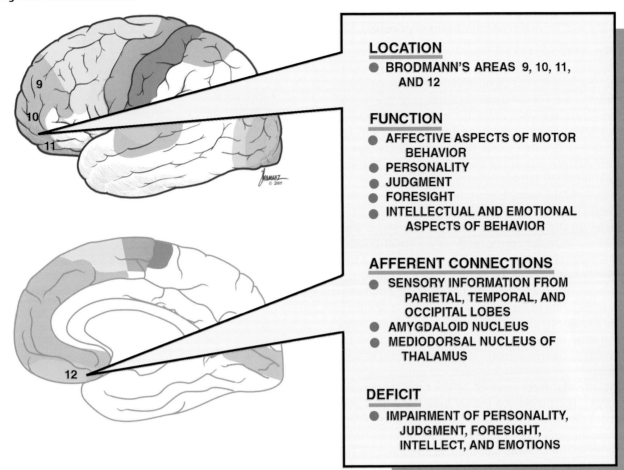

LOCATION
- BRODMANN'S AREAS 9, 10, 11, AND 12

FUNCTION
- AFFECTIVE ASPECTS OF MOTOR BEHAVIOR
- PERSONALITY
- JUDGMENT
- FORESIGHT
- INTELLECTUAL AND EMOTIONAL ASPECTS OF BEHAVIOR

AFFERENT CONNECTIONS
- SENSORY INFORMATION FROM PARIETAL, TEMPORAL, AND OCCIPITAL LOBES
- AMYGDALOID NUCLEUS
- MEDIODORSAL NUCLEUS OF THALAMUS

DEFICIT
- IMPAIRMENT OF PERSONALITY, JUDGMENT, FORESIGHT, INTELLECT, AND EMOTIONS

Parietal, Occipital, and Temporal Cortex

Primary and Secondary Somatosensory Cortex

See **Figs. 13.12** and **13.13.**

The primary somatosensory cortex occupies the postcentral gyrus on the lateral surface of the hemisphere and the dorsal aspect of the paracentral lobule on the medial surface. It encompasses areas 3, 1, and 2 of Brodmann's cytoarchitectural map. Electrical stimulation of this region produces sensations on the corresponding part of the contralateral side of the body. The configuration and orientation of the sensory homunculus roughly approximate those of the motor homunculus in the primary motor area of the precentral gyrus.

Histologically, the primary somatosensory area consists of the granular cortex, with only a small number of pyramidal cells. Although this area represents a histologically and functionally distinct region of the cortex, stimulation of this area may elicit a motor response; likewise, stimulation of the primary motor area may elicit a sensory response. Thus, these two regions of the cortex demonstrate overlap in function, providing support for the concept of a sensorimotor strip surrounding the central sulcus.

The afferent fibers received by the primary somatosensory cortex are derived mainly from the *ventral posterior (VP) nucleus of the thalamus.* This nucleus in turn receives afferents that include all the terminating fibers of the medial lemniscus and most of the fibers of the spinothalamic and trigeminothalamic tracts. Cortical projections of the ventral posterior nucleus traverse the internal capsule to terminate in the primary somatosensory cortex.

Although the primary somatosensory cortex is necessary for the appreciation of discriminative sensation related to touch, position, and movement of the parts of the body, a crude form of awareness of pain and temperature sensations persists despite destruction of the primary somatosensory cortex. Awareness of pain and temperature is apparent at the level of the thalamus.

A secondary somatosensory area occupies the rostral lip of the dorsal limb of the lateral fissure. The homunculus is oriented so that the face is most ventral and the leg is dorsal. Although the contralateral side is dominant, the body is bilaterally represented. Afferent fibers are received from the intralaminar nuclei and from the posterior group of nuclei of the thalamus. Efferent fibers are projected onto the ipsilateral primary somatosensory area and the ipsilateral primary motor and supplementary motor areas. The function of the secondary somatosensory area is not well described, but it appears to be involved in the elaboration of the less discriminative aspects of sensation.

Fig. 13.12 **Primary somatosensory cortex.**

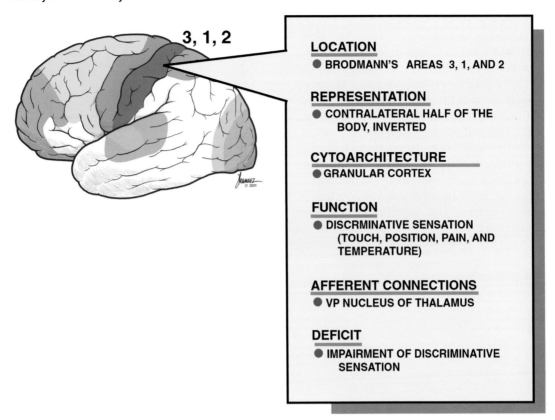

3, 1, 2

LOCATION
- BRODMANN'S AREAS 3, 1, AND 2

REPRESENTATION
- CONTRALATERAL HALF OF THE BODY, INVERTED

CYTOARCHITECTURE
- GRANULAR CORTEX

FUNCTION
- DISCRMINATIVE SENSATION (TOUCH, POSITION, PAIN, AND TEMPERATURE)

AFFERENT CONNECTIONS
- VP NUCLEUS OF THALAMUS

DEFICIT
- IMPAIRMENT OF DISCRIMINATIVE SENSATION

Fig. 13.13 **Secondary somatosensory areas.**

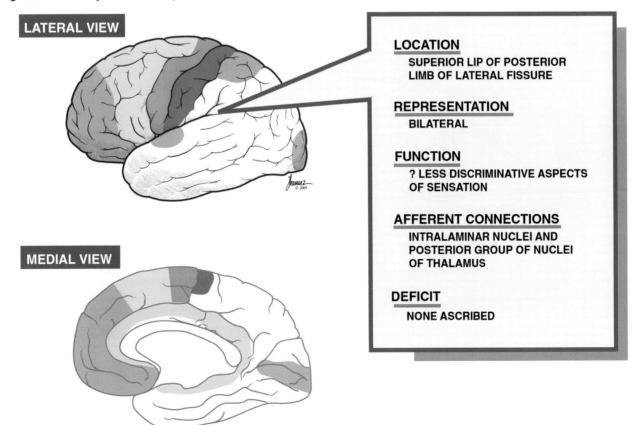

LATERAL VIEW

MEDIAL VIEW

LOCATION
SUPERIOR LIP OF POSTERIOR LIMB OF LATERAL FISSURE

REPRESENTATION
BILATERAL

FUNCTION
? LESS DISCRIMINATIVE ASPECTS OF SENSATION

AFFERENT CONNECTIONS
INTRALAMINAR NUCLEI AND POSTERIOR GROUP OF NUCLEI OF THALAMUS

DEFICIT
NONE ASCRIBED

The Somatosensory Association Area

See **Fig. 13.14.**

The somatosensory association area comprises Brodmann's areas 5 and 7, which occupy most of the parietal lobe posterior to the postcentral gyrus. The function of this region of the cortex is not well described. However, it has been suggested that this area receives afferent impulses from the primary somatosensory area, which are analyzed and integrated to relate new sensory experiences to previously learned ones. This provides for higher level sensory interpretations, such as the identification of an object by touch alone. Destruction of this area of the cortex does not result in numbness but does diminish one's ability to understand the significance of sensory information (agnosia).

Fig. 13.14 **Somatosensory association area.**

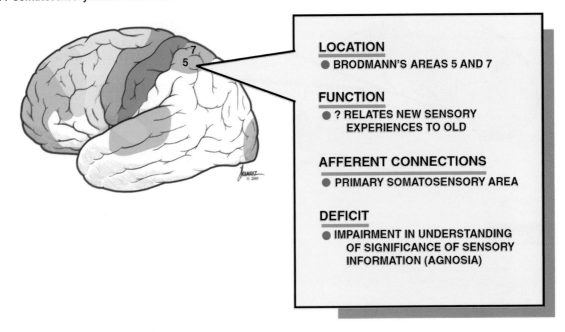

LOCATION
- BRODMANN'S AREAS 5 AND 7

FUNCTION
- ? RELATES NEW SENSORY EXPERIENCES TO OLD

AFFERENT CONNECTIONS
- PRIMARY SOMATOSENSORY AREA

DEFICIT
- IMPAIRMENT IN UNDERSTANDING OF SIGNIFICANCE OF SENSORY INFORMATION (AGNOSIA)

Primary Visual Cortex

See **Fig. 13.15.**

The primary visual cortex occupies the cortex surrounding the calcarine sulcus on the medial surface of the occipital lobe. It consists of Brodmann's area 17 and is sometimes referred to as the striate area. It receives most of its afferent fibers from the lateral geniculate body via the geniculocalcarine tract.

The visual cortex in each hemisphere receives input from the temporal half of the ipsilateral retina and the nasal half of the contralateral retina. Thus, the left visual field is portrayed in the right visual cortex, and the right visual field is portrayed in the left visual cortex.

Furthermore, the lower quadrant of the retinal field (upper visual field) is represented in the lower wall of the calcarine sulcus, and the upper quadrant of the retinal field (lower visual field) is represented in the upper wall of the calcarine sulcus. Central and peripheral fields of vision are also encoded in a topographical fashion.

The macula lutea of the retina, which is responsible for central vision of maximal discrimination, is represented in the dorsal aspect of area 17. The representation of the macula is of clinical significance because (for reasons that are unclear) lesions that involve either the geniculocalcarine tract or the visual cortex tend to be associated with central vision (macular) sparing.

Fig. 13.15 **Primary visual cortex.**

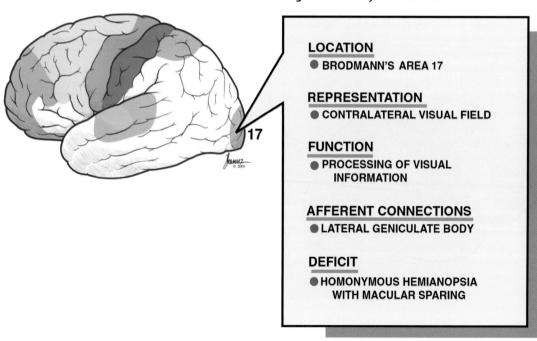

LOCATION
● BRODMANN'S AREA 17

REPRESENTATION
● CONTRALATERAL VISUAL FIELD

FUNCTION
● PROCESSING OF VISUAL INFORMATION

AFFERENT CONNECTIONS
● LATERAL GENICULATE BODY

DEFICIT
● HOMONYMOUS HEMIANOPSIA WITH MACULAR SPARING

Visual Association Cortex

See **Fig. 13.16.**

The visual association cortex is located in Brodmann's areas 18 and 19. These areas receive afferent fibers from area 17 and make reciprocal connections with other cortical areas and the pulvinar of the thalamus. Like the somatosensory association cortex, the visual association cortex functions in part by relating new visual representations to old ones and by recognizing the significance of what is seen.

Primary Auditory Cortex

See **Fig. 13.17.**

The primary auditory cortex occupies Heschl's transverse convolutions in Brodmann's areas 41 and 42 of the temporal lobe. Histologically, this cortex is of the granular type. It receives afferent fibers from the medial geniculate body in tonotopic order. This means that impulses related to low frequencies are located in the anterolateral portion of the cortex, whereas impulses related to high frequencies are located in the posteromedial portion of the auditory cortex. Afferents to the medial geniculate body are derived from the organs of Corti via bilateral projections in the lateral lemniscus. Thus, lesions involving the auditory cortex result in a decrease in the perception of sound direction only.

Fig. 13.16 **Visual association cortex.**

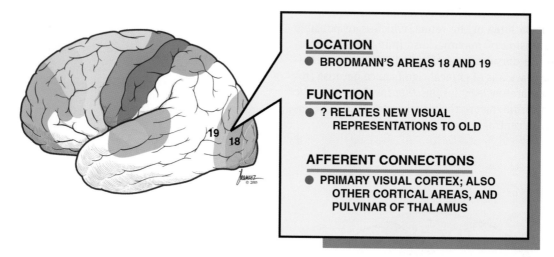

LOCATION
- BRODMANN'S AREAS 18 AND 19

FUNCTION
- ? RELATES NEW VISUAL REPRESENTATIONS TO OLD

AFFERENT CONNECTIONS
- PRIMARY VISUAL CORTEX; ALSO OTHER CORTICAL AREAS, AND PULVINAR OF THALAMUS

Fig. 13.17 **Primary auditory cortex.**

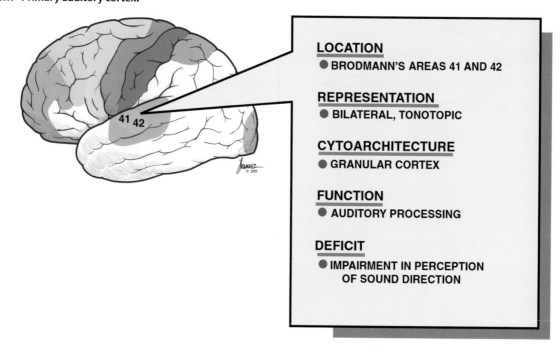

LOCATION
- BRODMANN'S AREAS 41 AND 42

REPRESENTATION
- BILATERAL, TONOTOPIC

CYTOARCHITECTURE
- GRANULAR CORTEX

FUNCTION
- AUDITORY PROCESSING

DEFICIT
- IMPAIRMENT IN PERCEPTION OF SOUND DIRECTION

Auditory Association Cortex

See **Fig. 13.18.**

The auditory association cortex occupies the dorsal aspect of Brodmann's area 22 on the lateral surface of the superior temporal gyrus. Included in this region is Wernicke's area, the major receptive sensory area for language.

Language Areas

The anatomic substrate of our capacity for language occupies two principal areas of the cortex of the dominant hemisphere (usually left). Wernicke's area, or the receptive language area, occupies the dorsal region of the superior temporal gyrus, extending onto the upper surface of the temporal lobe. Stimulation studies showed that Wernicke's area is much more widespread. It may involve parts of the supramarginal and angular gyri (inferior parietal lobule), the superior temporal gyrus, and at times the posterior end of the middle temporal gyrus. Included in this area is Brodmann's area 22. Wernicke's area is responsible for the reception and comprehension of both written and spoken language. It therefore receives fibers from the auditory cortex in the superior temporal gyrus and the primary visual cortex in the occipital lobe. The supramarginal (Brodmann's area 40) and angular (Brodmann's area 38) gyri of the inferior parietal lobule participate in the process of receptive speech.

Fibers that originate in Wernicke's area are projected in the arcuate fasciculus to the expressive language area, or Broca's area. Broca's area corresponds to Brodmann's areas 44 and 45 and is located in the inferior frontal gyrus. Broca's area is formed of two minor gyri, called pars opercularis and pars triangularis, that lie in the posterior end of the inferior frontal gyrus. In the Wernicke–Geschwind model for language, Wernicke's receptive language area contains memory images of a word as seen or heard. These images are conveyed, via the arcuate fasciculus, to Broca's expressive language area, which translates them into the grammatical structure of a phrase. This information about the pattern of a phrase is then conveyed to the facial area of the motor cortex, which is responsible for word articulation. The Wernicke–Geschwind model for the faculty of language is predictive of the clinical deficit caused by lesions in the language area (see later discussion).

Fig. 13.18 **Auditory association cortex.**

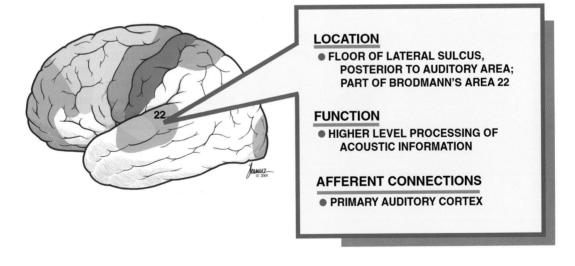

LOCATION
- FLOOR OF LATERAL SULCUS, POSTERIOR TO AUDITORY AREA; PART OF BRODMANN'S AREA 22

FUNCTION
- HIGHER LEVEL PROCESSING OF ACOUSTIC INFORMATION

AFFERENT CONNECTIONS
- PRIMARY AUDITORY CORTEX

Cortical Syndromes

Right Hemisphere Syndromes

Constructional Apraxia

See **Fig. 13.19.**

Constructional apraxia refers to an inability to draw or construct two- or three-dimensional objects as a result of a disorder in learned movements. It is implied that this disorder cannot be explained by a disturbance in strength, coordination, sensation, lack of comprehension, or attention. Although constructional apraxia may occur as a result of a dominant hemisphere lesion, a higher incidence and greater severity of constructional deficits are associated with parietal lesions in the right nondominant hemisphere.

Fig. 13.19 **Constructional apraxia.**

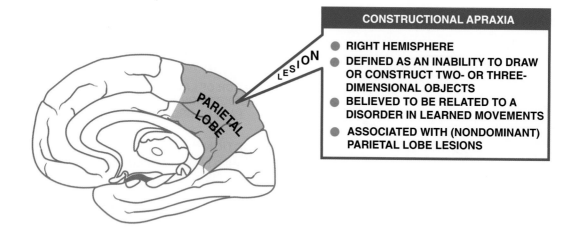

CONSTRUCTIONAL APRAXIA

● RIGHT HEMISPHERE
● DEFINED AS AN INABILITY TO DRAW OR CONSTRUCT TWO- OR THREE-DIMENSIONAL OBJECTS
● BELIEVED TO BE RELATED TO A DISORDER IN LEARNED MOVEMENTS
● ASSOCIATED WITH (NONDOMINANT) PARIETAL LOBE LESIONS

LESION

PARIETAL LOBE

Dressing Apraxia

See **Fig. 13.20.**

Patients with dressing apraxia are unable to properly clothe themselves. Most often this involves leaving the left side partly undressed. It occurs most frequently as a result of parietal lesions in the right nondominant hemisphere. It should be considered as part of the neglect syndrome (see later discussion), rather than as a disorder of learned movement.

Neglect and Denial

See **Fig. 13.21.**

When asked to perform a task in space, the patient with neglect tends to neglect the half of space contralateral to the lesion. Thus, the patient may draw a clock with the numbers densely crowded on one side (i.e., the side ipsilateral to the parietal lesion). The patient may shave only half of his face. Or patients may not use one side of their body, even though paralysis is not present. The neglect syndrome may be accompanied by the denial disorder. The most severe expression of denial consists of a complete denial of illness in the presence of an obvious disability. This syndrome is known as anosognosia. Thus, hemiplegic patients may deny that their limbs are paralyzed and may even deny that the hemiplegic limbs are their own. The neglect syndrome is most commonly associated with nondominant hemisphere lesions. A more specific locus of the lesion has not been established.

Fig. 13.20 **Dressing apraxia.**

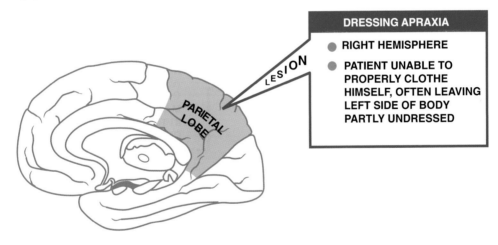

Fig. 13.21 **Neglect and denial.**

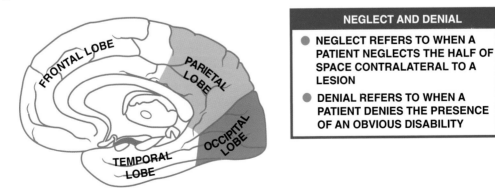

Color Blindness

See **Fig. 13.22.**

Patients with color blindness, or achromatopsia, cannot sort colors according to hue. This deficit is usually the result of a bilateral or a nondominant inferior occipitotemporal lesion. Infarction in the territory of the inferior occipital branch of the posterior cerebral artery may be responsible. This lesion spares the primary visual cortex, which is supplied by the calcarine branch of the posterior cerebral artery. The presence of color blindness should be distinguished from color agnosia, which is typically associated with a dominant hemisphere lesion. Color agnosia refers to an inability to name or point to colors, without loss of the ability to sort colors according to hue.

Fig. 13.22 **Color blindness.**

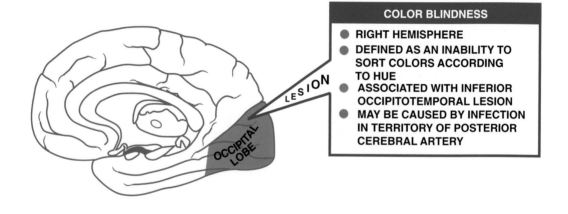

COLOR BLINDNESS

- RIGHT HEMISPHERE
- DEFINED AS AN INABILITY TO SORT COLORS ACCORDING TO HUE
- ASSOCIATED WITH INFERIOR OCCIPITOTEMPORAL LESION
- MAY BE CAUSED BY INFECTION IN TERRITORY OF POSTERIOR CEREBRAL ARTERY

Dominant Hemisphere Syndromes

Ideomotor Apraxia

Ideomotor apraxia is the most common type of apraxia. It refers to an inability to perform previously learned motor acts that cannot be explained by elementary disturbances in sensation, strength, or comprehension. The simplest test for the presence of an ideomotor apraxia is to ask the patient to perform a simple motor command, such as "brush your teeth," or "comb your hair." Patients with apraxias who are asked to do these things typically demonstrate fundamental errors, such as gripping the toothbrush inaccurately, failing to open their mouth, or missing the mouth entirely. Patients who are asked to comb their hair may respond by simply smoothing it.

The anatomic substrate of these learned motor acts has been described in the model of Geschwind. According to this model, a command is first processed in Wernicke's area, the area for receptive language. It is then conveyed, via the arcuate fasciculus, to the premotor cortex in the frontal lobe. The left hemisphere is considered dominant for learned motor acts. If the motor command requires activity involving the right extremities, then the left premotor cortex activates the appropriate motor neurons in the left primary motor cortex, which executes the command. If the motor command requires activity involving the left extremities, then the left premotor cortex activates the right premotor cortex via fibers in the anterior corpus callosum. This information is then relayed to the appropriate neurons in the right primary motor cortex, which executes the commanded movements in the left extremities. As illustrated, this model is predictive of the various combined deficits in language and movement that may result from lesions in the involved areas.

Visual Agnosia

See **Fig. 13.23.**

Visual agnosia refers to the inability to recognize objects visually, in the absence of an elementary disturbance in visual acuity or general intellectual function. Two types of visual agnosia are identified. In the first type, a defect in visual perception results in poor visual pattern recognition despite normal performance in visual acuity and visual field testing. Affected patients are unable to name objects pointed to or point to objects named. Bilateral involvement of the visual association cortex (Brodmann's areas 18 and 19) is typically responsible.

The second type of visual agnosia involves a defect in association. Although visual perception is intact in these patients, there is a disconnection between the visual cortex and the language area or visual memory stores. Thus, these patients are unable to name objects presented visually, but they are able to draw them or point to them. The locus of the lesion responsible for this disorder is either (1) bilateral, involving the inferior temporal and occipital lobes, or (2) dominant hemisphere, involving the occipital lobe and the posterior corpus callosum. The latter lesion disconnects visual input from language and visual memory areas and is the same lesion that causes alexia without agraphia. Most patients affected by associative visual agnosia are alexic.

Fig. 13.23 **Visual agnosia.**

VISUAL AGNOSIA

- BILATERAL VISUAL ASSOCIATION CORTEX OR DOMINANT OCCIPITAL CORTEX AND POSTERIOR CORPUS CALLOSUM
- OFTEN ASSOCIATED WITH ALEXIA WITHOUT AGRAPHIA

LESION

LESION

OCCIPITAL LOBE

TEMPORAL LOBE

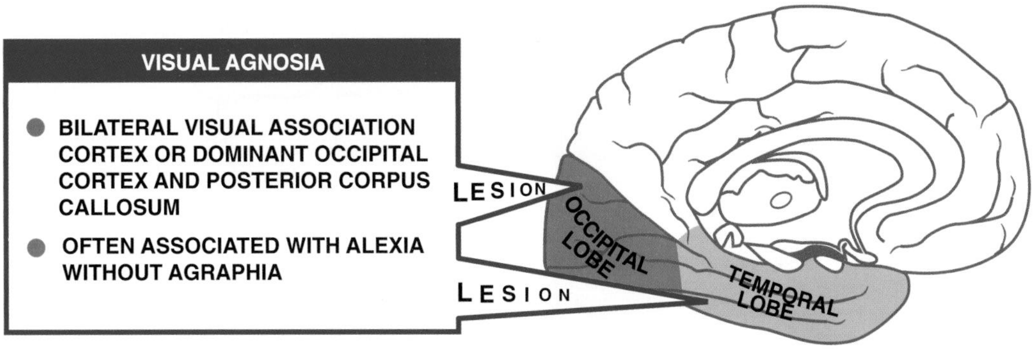

Alexia without Agraphia

See **Fig. 13.24.**

Alexia without agraphia refers to a syndrome in which the affected individual is unable to read but is still able to write. The causative lesion involves the dominant occipital cortex and the posterior corpus callosum. Most commonly this lesion is the result of an infarction in the territory of the left posterior cerebral artery.

The anatomic substrate of alexia without agraphia is as follows. Because the left visual cortex is damaged, it is unable to receive visual information. The right visual cortex can receive visual information, but it cannot transmit this information to the left (dominant) hemisphere due to disruption of crossing corpus callosum pathways. Alexia occurs in these patients because the dominant inferior parietal lobule (angular gyrus), which is responsible for processing the auditory and visual information necessary for reading and writing, is cut off from all visual input. The patient with alexia without agraphia retains the ability to write because the inferior parietal lobule is itself preserved.

Fig. 13.24 **Alexia without agraphia.**

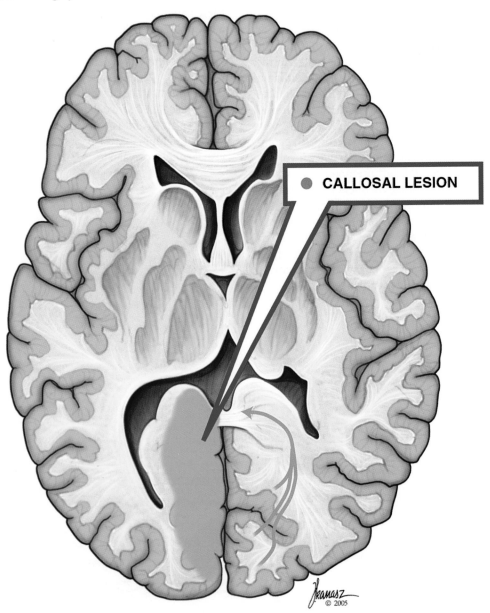

CALLOSAL LESION

Gerstmann's Syndrome

See **Fig. 13.25.**

Gerstmann's syndrome comprises the following four clinical deficits: (1) dyscalculia, (2) finger agnosia, (3) left–right disorientation, and (4) dysgraphia. The classic lesion associated with Gerstmann's syndrome is the left (dominant) angular gyrus. Since the syndrome was originally described by Gerstmann, however, other studies have shown that the angular gyrus need not be disturbed. It appears that the syndrome may be caused by either dominant or bilateral parietal lesions.

Color Agnosia

See **Fig. 13.26.**

As already described, color agnosia consists of an inability to name or point to colors in the presence of an intact ability to sort colors according to hue. It is most commonly caused by a dominant hemisphere lesion in the inferomedial aspect of the occipital and temporal lobes. Frequently it is associated with a right homonymous hemianopsia. The latter deficit is due to additional involvement of the lateral geniculate body, optic radiations, or calcarine cortex.

Fig. 13.25 **Gerstmann's syndrome.**

GERSTMANN'S SYNDROME

- LEFT HEMISPHERE
- ASSOCIATED WITH ANGULAR GYRUS (PART OF INFERIOR PARIETAL LOBULE)
- DEFINED BY FOUR SYMPTOMS:
  1. DYSCALCULIA
  2. FINGER AGNOSIA
  3. LEFT-RIGHT DISORIENTATION
  4. DYSGRAPHIA

LESION

SUPERIOR PARIETAL LOBULE
INFERIOR PARIETAL LOBULE

ANGULAR GYRUS

SUPRAMARGINAL GYRUS

Fig. 13.26 **Color agnosia.**

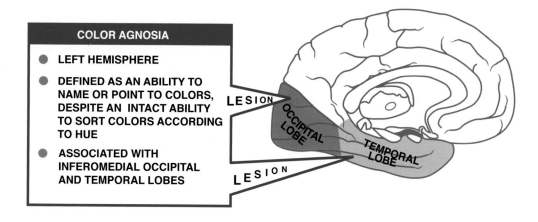

COLOR AGNOSIA

- LEFT HEMISPHERE
- DEFINED AS AN ABILITY TO NAME OR POINT TO COLORS, DESPITE AN INTACT ABILITY TO SORT COLORS ACCORDING TO HUE
- ASSOCIATED WITH INFEROMEDIAL OCCIPITAL AND TEMPORAL LOBES

LESION

OCCIPITAL LOBE

TEMPORAL LOBE

LESION

Aphasias

Aphasia is a disturbance in language function that is characterized by an impairment in word choice or grammar or a defect in comprehension. Several types of aphasia are identified on the basis of their clinical findings.

Global Aphasia

Global aphasia is characterized by a disturbance in all aspects of language, including comprehension, repetition, and expression. It is caused by a lesion that encompasses both Wernicke's and Broca's areas. Most commonly it is caused by an infarction in the left hemisphere secondary to occlusion of the internal carotid artery or the middle cerebral artery. It is almost always accompanied by a right hemiparesis.

Broca's Aphasia

Broca's aphasia is a nonfluent aphasia that is characterized by agrammatic or telegraphic speech. Both spontaneous speech and repetition are impaired, although comprehension is preserved. The halting, effortful speech of a Broca's patient comprises a disproportionate number of nouns and verbs (high content words), with too few grammatical fillers. It is caused by a lesion in Broca's motor speech area in the inferior frontal gyrus. It is frequently associated with a right hemiparesis.

Wernicke's Aphasia

Wernicke's aphasia is a fluent aphasia that is characterized by an effortless spontaneous speech that contains many paraphasic errors. The verbal output in this aphasia may be excessive, but it is often devoid of substance. Although severely impaired comprehension is the hallmark of this aphasia, repetition, naming, reading, and writing are also markedly impaired. Because the comprehension deficit may not be recognized, and the speech pattern may be pressured (rapid and voluminous), the patient may be mistakenly deemed psychotic. The lesion that is responsible for Wernicke's aphasia is located in the posterior superior temporal gyrus (Wernicke's area). Hemiparesis is typically not present.

Conduction Aphasia

Conduction aphasia is characterized by a fluent (though perhaps halting) pattern of speech that is marked by significant word-finding difficulties and paraphasias. Comprehension is intact, naming is mildly impaired, and repetition is markedly defective. The lesion responsible for conduction aphasia may involve the supramarginal gyrus and the arcuate fasciculus. The effect of this lesion is to disconnect Wernicke's area of language comprehension from the motor speech area of Broca.

Transcortical Sensory Aphasia

The transcortical sensory aphasia is characterized by intact repetition but impaired comprehension. As in Wernicke's aphasia, speech and naming are fluent but paraphasic. The responsible lesion in this aphasia is a crescent that lies within the border zone between the anterior and middle cerebral arteries. Both Wernicke's area and Broca's area are preserved.

Transcortical Motor Aphasia

The transcortical motor aphasia is characterized by intact repetition but impaired spontaneous speech. As in Broca's aphasia, comprehension is intact. The lesion associated with the transcortical motor aphasia is similar to that described for the transcortical sensory aphasia.

Bihemispheric Syndromes

Ideational Apraxia

Ideational apraxia represents a defect in motor planning of a higher order than that associated with ideomotor apraxia. Patients with this deficit are able to perform individual motor acts but are unable to coordinate the complex sequences of acts that constitute many of our everyday motor tasks. For example, patients with ideational apraxia may be able to light a match or put a cigarette in their mouth but be unable to open a pack of cigarettes, remove a single cigarette, light it with a match, place the cigarette in their mouth, and begin to smoke. The anatomic substrate of this disorder is bilateral brain disease or any process of diffuse cortical involvement.

Anton's Syndrome

Anton's syndrome consists of the denial of blindness in a patient who is cortically blind. Frequently, patients will confabulate what they "see." The responsible lesion involves the occipital lobes bilaterally. It extends beyond the primary visual cortices to involve the visual association areas.

III
System-based Anatomy and Differential Diagnosis

14 Somatosensory System

Testing the somatosensory system constitutes one of the most difficult but most important aspects of the neurologic examination. A logical approach to this examination requires an understanding of the basic modalities of sensation, the major fiber tracts that they follow, and the primary fiber types in which they are carried.

This chapter describes two major components of the somatosensory systems: (1) the spinothalamic system, which is responsible for pain, temperature, light touch, and pressure sensation; and (2) the dorsal column–medial lemniscus system, which is responsible for position sense, vibratory sense, and discriminative touch. Sensory pathways for the face and cortical processing of sensory information are also described.

Spinothalamic System

The spinothalamic system may be divided into two sensory pathways: the lateral spinothalamic tract, which mediates pain and temperature sensation, and the anterior spinothalamic tract, which mediates light touch and pressure sensation.

Lateral Spinothalamic Tract

See **Fig. 14.1**.

Receptors

Sensory receptors that mediate pain and temperature sensation are known as nocireceptors and thermoreceptors, respectively. Nociceptors (pain receptors) and thermoreceptors (temperature receptors) are free nerve endings of axons in the A-delta and C fiber classes. A-delta fibers are slightly myelinated compared with C fibers, which are unmyelinated. The abrupt, sharp, and well-localized sensation of so-called fast pain, carried by A-delta fibers, is commonly followed by the noxious and burning sensation of slow pain, carried by C fibers.

Spinal Pathways

Pain and temperature sensation are carried in spinal pathways. The cell bodies of pain- and temperature-related fibers (A-delta and C fibers) are located in the *dorsal root ganglia*. These first-order neurons send central processes through the lateral portions of the dorsal roots to enter the *dorsolateral tract* (of Lissauer) of the spinal cord.

In the dorsolateral tract these neurons ascend or descend one to three spinal segments from their level of entry and then synapse in the *substantia gelatinosa* (lamina II of the dorsal gray horn), the *posteromarginal nucleus* (lamina I), and/or the *nucleus proprius* (laminae III and IV).

After synapsing in the dorsal horn, *second-order neurons* send axons to the contralateral *lateral spinothalamic tract*, often crossing through the *anterior white commissure*. Because the tract is formed by crossed fibers that are added medially as the spinal cord is ascended, the central fibers of cells (whose peripheral fibers supply the legs) are located lateral to those that supply the arms. Therefore, the spinothalamic tract is somatotypically arranged, with the upper extremities represented medially and the lower extremities and sacrum laterally.

During its passage through the brainstem, the lateral spinothalamic tract is known as the spinal lemniscus. The spinal lemniscus is located lateral to the *medial lemniscus* and contains fibers of the spinotectal tract destined for the superior colliculus. The spinal lemniscus also gives off collateral branches to the reticular formation at several levels of the brainstem.

Fibers of the second-order neurons of the lateral spinothalamic tract terminate in the *ventral posterolateral (VPL) nucleus* of the thalamus. The perception of pain and temperature is initiated in the VPL nucleus and later modified in the cerebral cortex. Somatotopic order is maintained in the thalamus.

Thalamocortical Projections

The cell bodies of third-order neurons are located in the VPL nucleus of the thalamus. These cell bodies project axons through the dorsal limb of the internal capsule and the corona radiata to reach the primary somatosensory cortex I in the postcentral gyrus (Brodmann's areas 3, 2, and 1) and somatosensory area II in the anterior aspect of the parietal speculum. Sensory information is distributed from these areas to other regions of the cortex, including motor areas and the parietal association areas.

Fig. 14.1 **Lateral spinothalamic tract.**

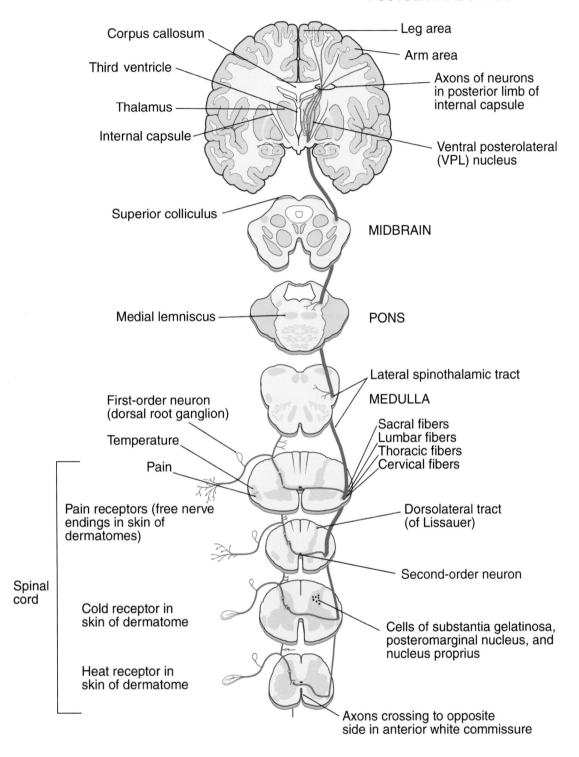

POSTCENTRAL GYRUS

Leg area

Arm area

Corpus callosum

Third ventricle

Axons of neurons
in posterior limb of
internal capsule

Thalamus

Internal capsule

Ventral posterolateral
(VPL) nucleus

Superior colliculus

MIDBRAIN

Medial lemniscus

PONS

Lateral spinothalamic tract

MEDULLA

First-order neuron
(dorsal root ganglion)

Sacral fibers
Lumbar fibers
Thoracic fibers
Cervical fibers

Temperature

Pain

Pain receptors (free nerve
endings in skin of
dermatomes)

Dorsolateral tract
(of Lissauer)

Spinal
cord

Second-order neuron

Cold receptor in
skin of dermatome

Cells of substantia gelatinosa,
posteromarginal nucleus, and
nucleus proprius

Heat receptor in
skin of dermatome

Axons crossing to opposite
side in anterior white commissure

Anterior Spinothalamic Tract

See **Fig. 14.2**.

Receptors

Light touch and pressure sensation are mediated by specialized receptors in the skin. Among these are free nerve endings, such as Merkel's cells, and encapsulated endings, such as Meissner's corpuscles.

Spinal Pathways

The *anterior spinothalamic tract* runs ventromedially in relation to the lateral spinothalamic tract. First-order neurons located in the dorsal root ganglia send central processes though the dorsal roots that enter the dorsolateral tract of the spinal cord, ascend or descend one to three segments, and synapse on dorsal horn cells. These dorsal horn cells, constituting the second-order neurons, project axons that traverse the anterior white commissure to contribute to the contralateral anterior spinothalamic tract, which maintains the same somatotopic order as the lateral spinothalamic tract. After ascending the spinal cord and traversing the brainstem (as part of the spinal lemniscus), these fibers terminate on third-order neurons in the *VPL nucleus of the thalamus.*

Thalamocortical Projections

Third-order neurons in the VPL thalamic nucleus project axons through the dorsal limb of the *internal capsule* and the corona radiata to reach the *postcentral gyrus* of the cerebral cortex.

Fig. 14.2 **Anterior spinothalamic tract.**

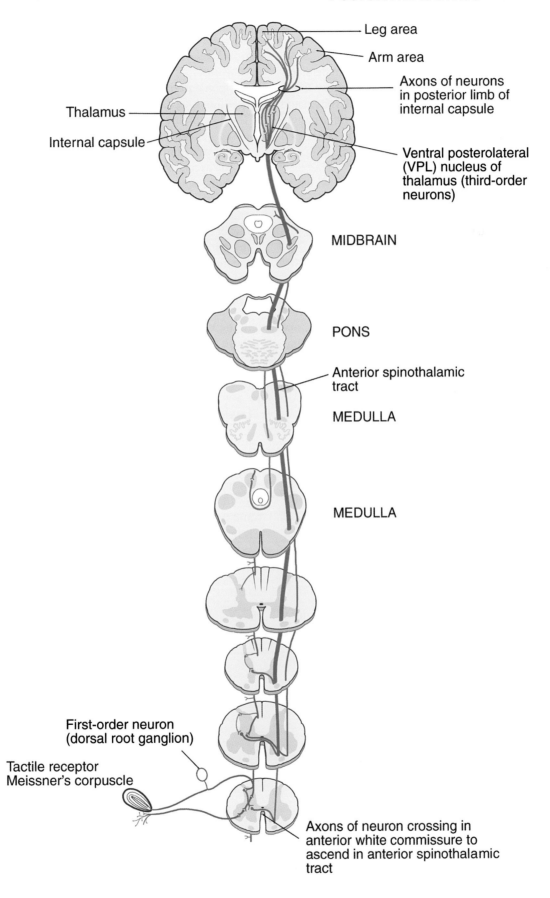

POSTCENTRAL GYRUS

Leg area

Arm area

Axons of neurons
in posterior limb of
internal capsule

Thalamus

Internal capsule

Ventral posterolateral
(VPL) nucleus of
thalamus (third-order
neurons)

MIDBRAIN

PONS

Anterior spinothalamic
tract

MEDULLA

MEDULLA

First-order neuron
(dorsal root ganglion)

Tactile receptor
Meissner's corpuscle

Axons of neuron crossing in
anterior white commissure to
ascend in anterior spinothalamic
tract

Dorsal Column–Medial Lemniscal System

See **Fig. 14.3**.

The dorsal column–medial lemniscal system mediates impulses concerned with position sense, vibratory sense, and discriminative touch. Although both this system and the spinothalamic system transmit touch information, the dorsal columns alone carry information concerned with detailed localization, spatial forms, and temporal patterns of tactile stimuli.

In contrast to the spinothalamic system in which fibers cross the midline of the spinal cord almost upon entering it, dorsal column fibers ascend on the ipsilateral side of the cord and decussate in the caudal medulla.

Receptors

Although the various histologic types of mechanoreceptors are not specific for sensory modality, it is at least known that the *pacinian corpuscle* mediates vibratory sense; that the *Meissner's corpuscle* mediates discriminative touch; and that a variety of proprioceptors of muscle, tendon, and joint mediate position sense.

In contrast to the thin, unmyelinated (slowly conducting) A-delta and C fibers that carry pain and temperature sensation, vibratory, position, and discriminative touch sensations are carried in large, myelinated (fast-conducting) fibers in the A-alpha and A-beta range.

Spinal Pathways

The cell bodies of these fibers, located in the dorsal root ganglia, constitute the first-order neurons of the dorsal column–medial lemniscus system. Central processes of these neurons pass through the medial portion of the dorsal root, then directly enter and ascend in the dorsal columns of the ipsilateral side of the spinal cord.

As fibers enter the spinal cord, they are added in a medial to lateral fashion, creating a somatotopy in which long sacral fibers occupy the most medial aspect, and shorter cervical fibers occupy the most lateral aspect of the dorsal funiculus.

At the T6 level and above, this funiculus is divided into two adjacent fasciculi by a septum. The dorsal column fibers entering at the T6 level and below thus form the *fasciculus gracilis*; dorsal column fibers entering above this level form the more laterally situated *fasciculus cuneatus*.

Upon entering these fasciculi, fibers at all levels bifurcate into long ascending and short descending branches. The descending branches travel down a variable number of segments to synapse on interneurons and ventral horn cells involved in intersegmental reflexes.

The ascending branches travel upward into the caudal medulla, where fibers of the fasciculus gracilis and fasciculus cuneatus synapse with cells of the *nucleus gracilis* and *nucleus cuneatus*, respectively. These dorsal column nuclei contain second-order neurons whose axons cross the midline as *internal arcuate fibers*, which join to form the *medial lemniscus* on the contralateral side of the spinal cord.

The medial lemniscus ascends the contralateral half of the brainstem and terminates on third-order neurons in the VPL nucleus of the thalamus. Central processes of these neurons traverse the posterior limb of the internal capsule and corona radiata to reach the postcentral gyrus of the cerebral cortex.

Lesions

Knowledge of the anatomy of the spinothalamic and dorsal column systems aids the clinician in localizing central nervous system (CNS) lesions. A lesion of the left hemicord results in a loss of pain and temperature sensation on the contralateral side (right) and a loss of vibration and position sense on the ipsilateral side (left). Weakness is ipsilateral. If the sensory deficits are both on the same side, the lesion must be above the spinal cord and located in the brainstem or cortex.

Fig. 14.3 Dorsal column–medial lemniscal system.

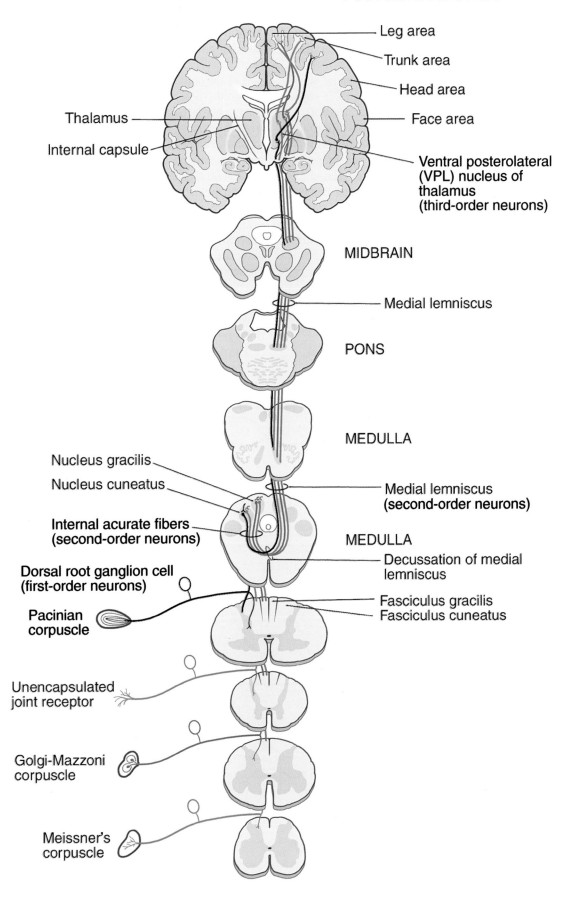

POSTCENTRAL GYRUS

Leg area

Trunk area

Head area

Face area

Thalamus

Internal capsule

Ventral posterolateral (VPL) nucleus of thalamus (third-order neurons)

MIDBRAIN

Medial lemniscus

PONS

MEDULLA

Nucleus gracilis

Nucleus cuneatus

Medial lemniscus (second-order neurons)

Internal acurate fibers (second-order neurons)

MEDULLA

Decussation of medial lemniscus

Dorsal root ganglion cell (first-order neurons)

Pacinian corpuscle

Fasciculus gracilis

Fasciculus cuneatus

Unencapsulated joint receptor

Golgi-Mazzoni corpuscle

Meissner's corpuscle

Sensory Pathways for the Face

Sensory input from most of the head and much of the external ear is carried in the second and third cervical nerves in the spinothalamic and dorsal column–medial lemniscal pathways, as already described. General sensory innervation of the face, on the other hand, is supplied entirely by the trigeminal nerve (cranial nerve V).

The three divisions of the trigeminal nerve (ophthalmic, maxillary, and mandibular) each contain fibers concerned with pain and temperature, touch, and proprioception. Afferent fibers that conduct impulses related to pain and temperature and touch have their cell bodies in the trigeminal (gasserian) ganglion—the cranial nerve counterpart of the spinal ganglion. Uniquely, the cell bodies of axons carrying proprioceptive information are located in the brainstem (mesencephalic nucleus).

Pain and Temperature

See **Fig. 14.4**.

Pain and temperature sensation is mediated by axons that have cell bodies in the trigeminal ganglion. The central processes of these cell bodies traverse the lateral part of the *pons* to enter the pontine tegmentum. Within the pons, these axons descend in the *spinal trigeminal tract* to reach the associated nucleus (*nucleus of the spinal trigeminal tract*), where they terminate in a somatotopic fashion. Fibers of the mandibular division occupy the most dorsal aspect; fibers of the ophthalmic division, the most ventral aspect; and fibers of the maxillary division, an intermediate position in the nucleus.

Trigeminothalamic axons arising from the second-order neurons in the spinal trigeminal nucleus project ventromedially, cross the midline, and come into close association with the contralateral medial lemniscus. These second-order fibers ascend with the medial lemniscus in the *ventral trigeminothalamic tract* to terminate in the ventral posteromedial (VPM) nucleus of the thalamus. Recall that the medial lemniscal and spinothalamic tracts terminate in the VPL thalamic nucleus.

Third-order neurons in the VPM thalamic nucleus project axons through the internal capsule to the somatosensory cortex.

Fig. 14.4 Sensory pathways for the face.

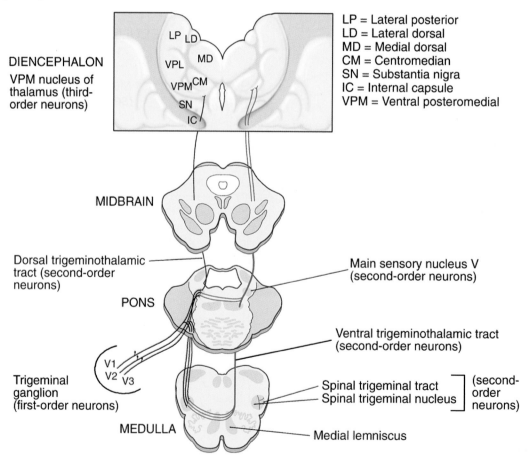

LP = Lateral posterior
LD = Lateral dorsal
MD = Medial dorsal
CM = Centromedian
SN = Substantia nigra
IC = Internal capsule
VPM = Ventral posteromedial

Touch

Afferent fibers that mediate touch and pressure sense, the latter a sustained form of touch, have cell bodies in the trigeminal ganglion. The central processes of these first-order neurons enter the pontine tegmentum and ascend to the upper pons, where they synapse with second-order neurons in the *main sensory nucleus* and the rostral part of the nucleus of the spinal trigeminal tract. The topographic organization of cell bodies in the main sensory nucleus is identical to that in the nucleus of the spinal trigeminal tract.

Unlike the caudal portion of the nucleus of the spinal trigeminal tract, in which all of the axons are crossed, secondary trigeminal fibers from the main sensory nucleus and the rostral part of the spinal trigeminal tract are both crossed and uncrossed. They form the *dorsal trigeminothalamic tract.*

Both crossed and uncrossed fibers synapse with cell bodies in the contralateral and ipsilateral VPM thalamic nucleus, respectively. These third-order cell bodies project axons through the internal capsule to the postcentral gyrus of the cerebral cortex.

Proprioception

Proprioceptive information from the face is carried by afferent fibers that innervate the teeth, periodontium, hard palate, joint capsules, and muscles of mastication. Unlike the bipolar trigeminal neurons concerned with pain, temperature, and touch, these unipolar neurons have their cell bodies in a ganglion that has been "displaced" into the brainstem. This is the mesencephalic nucleus, which is contained in the periaqueductal gray of the midbrain. (It is termed mesencephalic nucleus, rather than ganglion, because it lies within the CNS.)

The central pathways of axons projected from the mesencephalic nucleus are not known. Collateral fibers derived from proprioceptive afferents synapse with cells of the trigeminal motor nucleus, forming thus the anatomic basis of the jaw jerk reflex.

Cortical Sensation and Sensory Representation

Three regions of the cerebral cortex are especially important for general somatic sensation.

Primary Somesthetic Area

The primary somesthetic area occupies the postcentral gyrus on the lateral cerebral surface and the paracentral lobule on the medial surface (Brodmann's areas 3, 1, and 2). Projections from the VPL and VPM thalamic nuclei constitute the major source of afferent fibers.

The somatotopic organization of this area is similar to that found in the motor cortex. The size of cortical representation of particular body parts is proportionate to the density of sensory afferents that innervate it. The cortical regions that represent the face, hand, and mouth, therefore, occupy a disproportionately large area of the cortex.

Topographically, the contralateral half of the body is represented as inverted (upside down). From ventral to dorsal on the postcentral gyrus are the pharyngeal region, face, hand, arm, trunk, and thigh; extending onto the paracentral lobule are the leg and the foot.

Although crude awareness of pain and temperature sensation may occur in the absence of the cerebral cortex, detailed localization and the perception of more discriminative qualities (e.g., position sense and fine touch) requires an intact primary somesthetic area. Ablation of the postcentral gyrus thus results in a loss of these "cortical sensations."

Secondary Somesthetic Area

The secondary somesthetic area lies in the superior lip of the lateral cerebral fissure. Its function is less clear than the primary somesthetic area, but it appears to be involved in the further elaboration of sensory data received from the first area and may play a role in somatotopic pars representation. Efferent fibers are projected to the ipsilateral primary somesthetic area and the ipsilateral motor and supplementary motor areas.

Although the contralateral side predominates, body parts are bilaterally represented in the secondary somesthetic area. Regions representing the face are most ventral in position, followed by the hand, arm, trunk, and legs, in that order.

Somesthetic Association Area

The somesthetic association area occupies the superior parietal lobule of the lateral cerebral surface extending onto the adjacent medial surface. Receiving afferents from the first somesthetic area, the association area serves to integrate various types of sensory input and to relate new sensory experiences to learned ones. Thus, handled objects may be identified, without visual aid, on the basis of their texture, size, and shape and by comparison with previously experienced sensations.

Destructive lesions of the association area (or the primary somesthetic area, from which it receives its input) result in clinical deficits of "cortical sensation." Astereognosis is the inability to identify a common object when held in the hand while the eyes are closed. Agraphesthesia is the inability to recognize letters or numbers drawn on the hand.

15 Visual System

The visual system transforms visual representations of the external world into patterns of neural activity. As a peripheral receptor organ, the eye contains nonneural elements that transmit light stimuli. These stimuli impinge on the neural elements of the eye, which respond by giving rise to impulses that are carried and processed in central pathways.

The testing of vision constitutes one of the most sensitive and important parts of the neurologic examination. It is sensitive because the visual pathways traverse the brain's entire horizontal axis and are thus vulnerable to a wide range of anatomic lesions. It is important because such lesions tend to produce discrete visual deficits that facilitate their localization.

The Retina

See **Fig. 15.1**.

The *optic nerve* and retina represent outgrowths of the forebrain that are specially adapted for light sensitivity, for modifying light information, and for transmitting the modified information to the thalamus and occipital cortex.

The area of the retina where the optic nerve fibers exit the eye is called the *optic disc*. Because it contains only nerve fibers, the optic disc is a blind spot. Radiating from the center of the disc are the retinal vessels.

Roughly two temporal disc diameters away from the optic disc lies the *macula lutea*, which occupies the center of the retina and is specialized for visual acuity. The greatest visual acuity occurs at a depression in the center of the macula, the fovea centralis, the central part of which contains only cone receptors (one of the two photoreceptor types).

The basic cell layers of the retina, from outside in, are the *pigment epithelium*, *rods* and *cones*, *bipolar cells*, and *ganglion cells*. Interneurons (i.e., *horizontal cells* and *amacrine cells*) and neuroglial cells are also present.

There are many more rods than cones. They are more concentrated in the periphery of the retina, and because they exhibit more convergence on bipolar cells (several rods synapsing with a single bipolar cell), they are also more sensitive to low levels of light (e.g., night vision). Cones, which are concentrated more centrally than rods, exhibit less convergence. They sometimes make one-to-one synaptic contacts with bipolar cells, and they therefore provide greater discrimination (i.e., acuity) compared with rods. Cones alone are responsible for color vision.

Bipolar neurons connect rods and cones to the ganglion cells. Ganglion cell axons pass dorsally in the optic nerve and terminate in the lateral geniculate body of the thalamus. They transmit information laterally within individual layers of the retina.

Fig. 15.1 **Retina.**

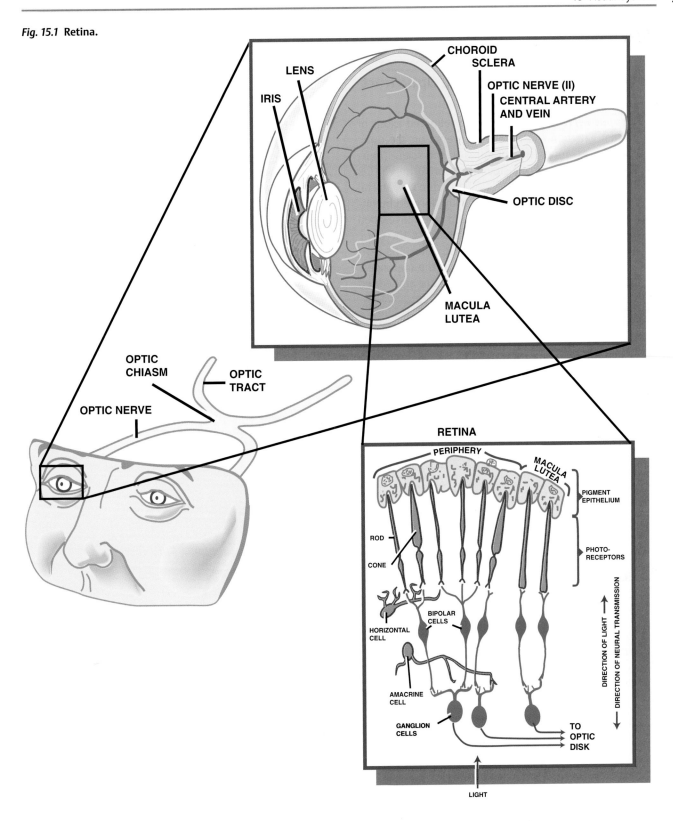

Visual Pathways

Optic Nerve, Optic Chiasm, and Optic Tract

See **Fig. 15.2**.

The *optic nerve* is formed by the myelinated axons of the retinal ganglion cells, which converge on the optic disc and pass through the foramina in the sclera (lamina cribrosa). Although considered a cranial nerve (CN II), the optic nerve is more like a tract within the central nervous system, its myelin sheaths being formed by oligodendrocytes rather than by Schwann cells. Enveloped by the meninges, which fuse with the sclera, the optic nerve leaves the orbit through the optic canal. The central retinal artery and vein are carried in the meningeal sheaths surrounding the optic nerve and are embedded in the ventral portion of the nerve.[1]

The *optic chiasm* constitutes a partial crossing of optic nerve fibers. Fibers of the nasal half of each optic nerve decussate to join the uncrossed temporal fibers on the opposite side. The optic tracts, which constitute a continuation of the optic nerves just dorsal to their partial decussation in the optic chiasm, are thus formed by temporal fibers of the ipsilateral optic nerve and nasal fibers of the contralateral optic nerve. In this manner, images in the left field of vision are represented in the right cerebral hemisphere, and vice versa.

The *optic tract* courses dorsolaterally around the cerebral peduncles, where most of its fibers terminate in the *lateral geniculate body* (LGB) of the thalamus. Other fibers that are specialized for control of eye movements and the pupillary light reflex terminate in the *superior colliculus* and the *pretectal region*, respectively.

---

[1]Increased intracranial pressure is transmitted to the central vein by its surrounding cerebrospinal fluid. Given a sufficient increase in intracranial pressure, obstruction of the venous return from the retina may develop, thus engorging the optic disc. The funduscopic picture of a disc that is swollen secondary to increased intracranial pressure is referred to as papilledema.

Fig. 15.2 **Optic nerve, optic chiasm, and optic tract.**

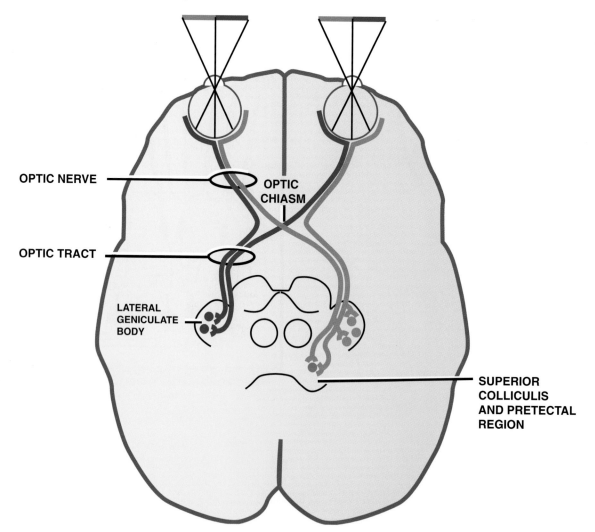

OPTIC NERVE

OPTIC CHIASM

OPTIC TRACT

LATERAL GENICULATE BODY

SUPERIOR COLLICULIS AND PRETECTAL REGION

Optic Radiation and Visual Cortex

See **Fig. 15.3**.

The LGB cells that receive impulses from the retinal ganglion cells in turn project axons in the *optic radiation* (geniculocalcarine tract), which passes dorsally through the retro- and sublenticular parts of the internal capsule and then around the lateral ventricle to terminate in the *visual cortex* (Brodmann's area 17) of the occipital lobe. Those fibers of the optic radiation that form the so-called *Meyer's loop* pass through the temporal lobe en route to the visual cortex, where they terminate below the *calcarine sulcus*.

The primary visual cortex occupies the medial aspect of the occipital lobe in the region of the calcarine sulcus.

As a result of the decussation of nasal fibers at the optic chiasm, each visual cortex receives information only from the opposite visual field. Furthermore, impulses initiated in the inferior retinal quadrants (upper field of vision) are projected on the lower bank of the calcarine sulcus; those initiated in the superior retinal quadrants (lower field of vision) are projected on the upper bank. In sum, cortical representation of the visual field is inverted and reversed from right to left.

The primary visual cortex sends impulses to the surrounding association visual cortex (Brodmann's areas 18 and 19), which is responsible for higher visual functions such as recognition of objects and perception of depth and color.

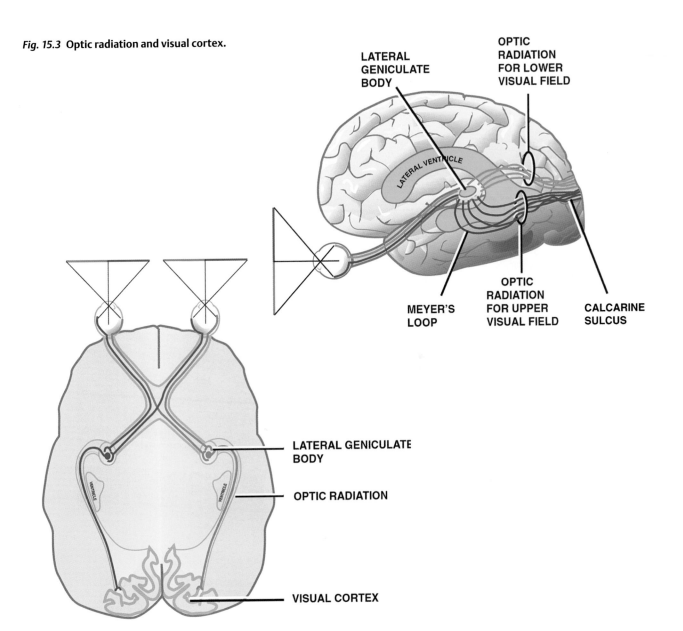

Fig. 15.3 **Optic radiation and visual cortex.**

Topographic Organization of the Visual Pathways

There is a point-to-point projection from the retina to the LGB, and from the LGB to the visual cortex. Because of the highly organized topography of the visual projections, localized lesions tend to produce distinctive visual symptoms.

Vascular Supply to the Visual Pathway

See **Fig. 15.4**.

The retina and orbital portion of the *optic nerve* are supplied by the *ophthalmic artery*, which is the most proximal branch of the *internal carotid artery*. The intracranial portion of the optic nerve is fed by the internal carotid, *anterior cerebral*, and *anterior communicating arteries*. The *optic chiasm* is perfused by the internal carotid, anterior cerebral, and anterior communicating arteries, and, to a lesser extent, the *posterior communicating, posterior cerebral*, and *basilar arteries*. The *optic tract* receives its major supply from the *anterior choroidal artery*. The *lateral geniculate body* is fed by the anterior choroidal artery laterally and the *posterior choroidal artery* medially. The major supply of the *optic radiations* is from branches of the *middle cerebral artery* rostrally and the *posterior cerebral artery* caudally. The majority of the *visual cortex* is fed by the posterior cerebral artery.

Fig. 15.4 **Vascular supply to the visual pathway.**

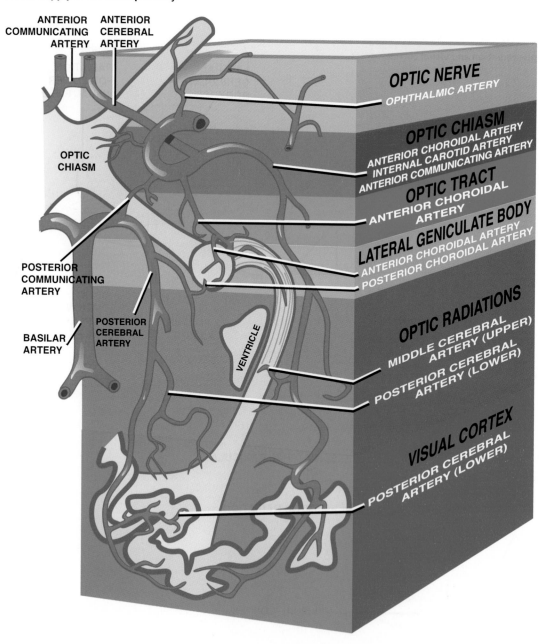

Visual Reflexes

Certain fibers of the optic tract do not terminate in the LGB, but rather enter the superior brachium to reach the pretectal area and the superior colliculus. They form the afferent limb of the visual reflex arcs.

Pupillary Light Reflex

See **Fig. 15.5**.

The pupillary light reflex describes the response of the pupil (constriction) to a stimulus of bright light shone into the eye. On receiving the light stimulus, the retina sends impulses to the *pretectal area* of the midbrain, which relays the impulses to the *Edinger-Westphal nucleus*

of the oculomotor complex. *Parasympathetic preganglionic fibers* from the Edinger-Westphal nucleus (traveling in the oculomotor nerve) in turn stimulate postganglionic neurons in the *ciliary ganglion*, which projects fibers (*short ciliary nerve*) to the sphincter pupillae muscle in the iris.

Normally, both pupils constrict when light is shone in only one eye because neurons in the pretectal area project to both the ipsilateral and the contralateral Edinger-Westphal nuclei, the latter via the posterior commissure. The response of the eye into which the light was shone is termed the direct light reflex; the response of the contralateral eye is termed the consensual light reflex.

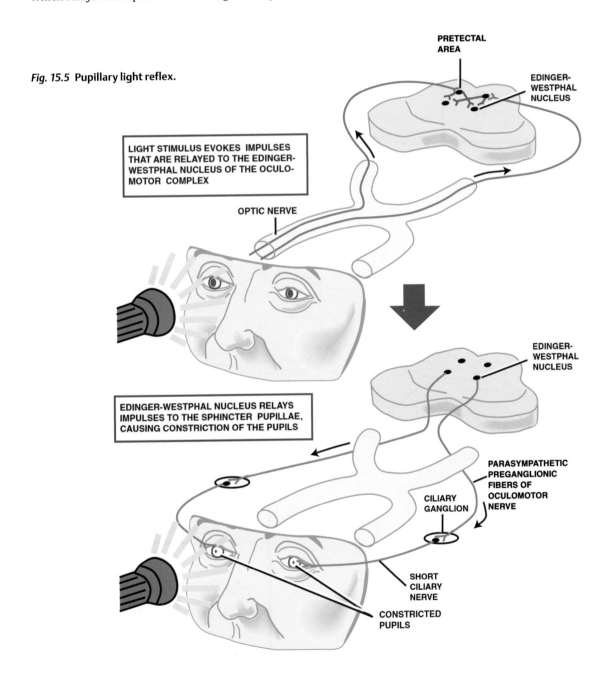

Fig. 15.5 **Pupillary light reflex.**

PRETECTAL AREA

EDINGER-WESTPHAL NUCLEUS

LIGHT STIMULUS EVOKES IMPULSES THAT ARE RELAYED TO THE EDINGER-WESTPHAL NUCLEUS OF THE OCULO-MOTOR COMPLEX

OPTIC NERVE

EDINGER-WESTPHAL NUCLEUS

EDINGER-WESTPHAL NUCLEUS RELAYS IMPULSES TO THE SPHINCTER PUPILLAE, CAUSING CONSTRICTION OF THE PUPILS

PARASYMPATHETIC PREGANGLIONIC FIBERS OF OCULOMOTOR NERVE

CILIARY GANGLION

SHORT CILIARY NERVE

CONSTRICTED PUPILS

Accommodation Reflex

See **Fig. 15.6**.

This reflex consists of pupillary constriction, ocular convergence, and thickening of the lens as an adaptation of the eyes for near vision. An example of this reflex is looking at an object at the tip of your nose.

The visual pathways of this reflex include impulses that originate in the *visual association cortex*, traverse the *superior brachium*, and terminate in the *pretectal area* and the superior colliculus. The superior colliculus in turn stimulates the cranial nerve nuclei involved in extraocular eye movement and the *Edinger-Westphal nucleus*. The result of the reflex is constriction of the pupils, convergence (adduction) of the eyes, and contraction of the *ciliary muscle*, which results in a "rounding up" or thickening of the lens to accommodate near vision.

Fig. 15.6 **Accommodation reflex.**

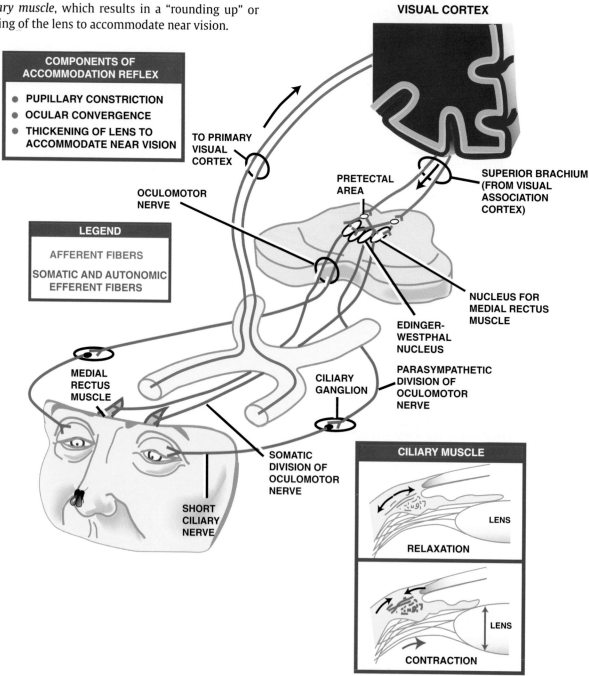

Approach to the Patient with a Visual Field Defect

Because the shape and distribution of a visual field deficit closely reflect the site of a lesion in the visual pathway, visual field testing is an important aspect of even a basic neurologic examination. Such testing is most commonly performed by a bedside confrontation test, although a formal visual field test using the Goldmann perimeter may provide a more accurate assessment of a visual field defect. The common sites of lesions and associated visual field defects are described here.

Optic Nerve Lesions

See **Fig. 15.7**.

Complete optic nerve lesions result in *monocular blindness*. Partial lesions of the optic nerve result in scotomas—the loss of function in the central or peripheral parts of the visual field. Typically, loss of central vision (*central scotoma*) occurs first when an extrinsic mass causes compression of an optic nerve. This is because the papillomacular bundle conveying central vision is very vulnerable to extrinsic compression. Thus, the visual loss associated with a compressive mass spreads from the central to the peripheral part of the visual field, rather than the other way around, as would be expected on purely anatomic grounds.

Fig. 15.7 **Optic nerve lesions.**

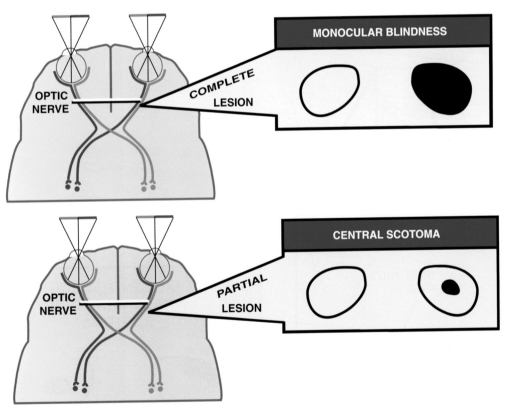

Junctional Lesions

See **Fig. 15.8**.

Lesions at the junction between the optic nerve and chiasm may cause damage to both the optic nerve and the fibers of *Wilbrand's knee* (i.e., the retinal fibers of the inferonasal quadrant of the optic nerve that project into the base of the opposite optic nerve). The visual field deficit associated with a junctional lesion comprises loss of function in the ipsilateral eye (optic nerve lesion) and a defect in the contralateral superotemporal quadrant (Wilbrand's knee lesion).

Fig. 15.8 Junctional lesions.

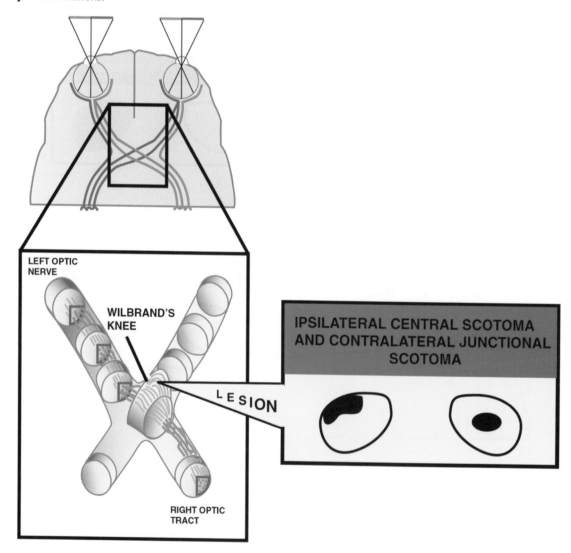

Chiasmal Lesions

See **Fig. 15.9**.

Lesions of the *optic chiasm* involve the nasal fibers of both optic nerves as they decussate to the opposite side. The associated visual field deficit is a *bitemporal hemianopsia*, which is classic for a lesion in the optic chiasm. Most commonly, the optic chiasm lies above the diaphragm sellae and the pituitary gland, tumors of which are the most common compressive masses of the optic chiasm. Anatomic variations do exist, however, and thus a *prefixed chiasm* refers to one that overlies the *tuberculum sellae*, and a *postfixed chiasm* refers to one that overlies the *dorsum sellae*.

Fig. 15.9 **Chiasmal lesions.**

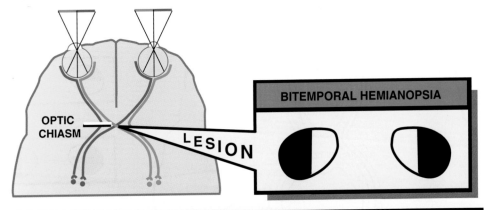

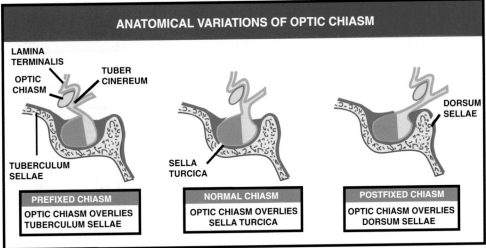

Retrochiasmal Lesions

In general, retrochiasmal lesions produce homonymous hemianopsias. Those lesions affecting the anterior retrochiasmal pathway (i.e., optic tract and lateral geniculate body) tend to produce incongruous hemianopsias, whereas those lesions affecting the posterior pathway (i.e., optic radiation and visual cortex) tend to produce more congruous hemianopsias. A congruous defect suggests that the shape of the defect is the same in both eyes, whereas an incongruous defect implies that the defect is different in the two half fields.

Lesions Affecting the Anterior Retrochiasmal Pathway

See **Fig. 15.10**.

Optic Tract Lesions

Lesions of the optic tracts produce very incongruous *homonymous hemianopsias*.

Lateral Geniculate Body Lesions

Lesions of the lateral geniculate body are rare. Like optic tract lesions, they produce incongruous homonymous hemianopsias.

Fig. 15.10 **Optic tract and lateral geniculate body lesions.**

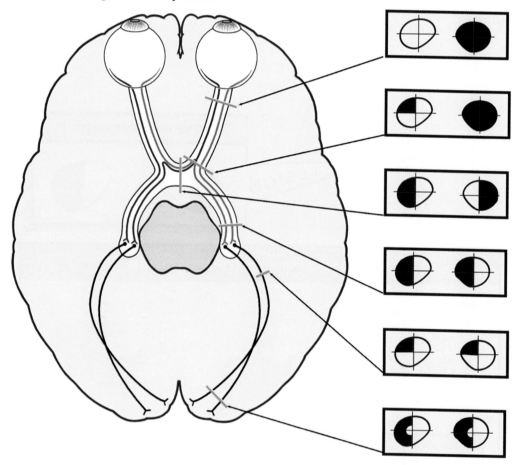

Optic Radiation Lesions

See **Fig. 15.11**.

Lesions of the optic radiations produce congruous homonymous quadranopsias. Those lesions affecting the temporal lobe (Meyer's loop) produce superior quadrantic defects, whereas partial lesions affecting the parietal lobe produce inferior quadrantic defects. Most lesions involving the optic radiations affect fibers that represent both the superior and inferior visual fields, and therefore result in homonymous hemianopsias.

Fig. 15.11 **Optic radiation lesions.**

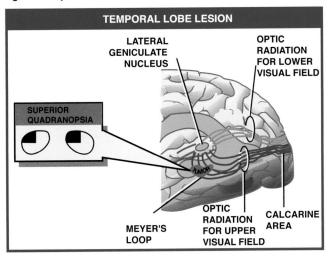

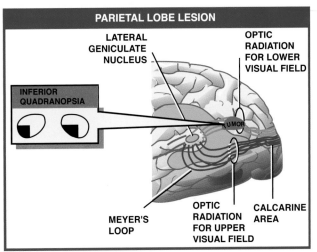

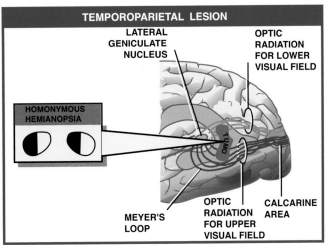

Visual Cortex

See **Fig. 15.12**.

Large lesions affecting the visual cortex on one side will produce a very congruous homonymous hemianopsia. Smaller lesions, particularly those that spare the occipital pole, tend to cause defects that spare central (or macular) vision. The explanation of this phenomenon is not entirely clear, although it is believed that there is extensive representation of macular vision at the occipital pole. Lesions that selectively involve the lower bank of the calcarine cortex are associated with an upper quadrantic defect, whereas lesions that selectively involve the upper bank of the calcarine cortex are associated with a lower quadrantic defect. In each case there is commonly macular sparing.

Loss of Color Perception

Loss of color perception may accompany partial defects in the visual field or may decline, more generally, in parallel with visual acuity loss. The presence of complete color blindness in the face of normal visual acuity, however, suggests a bilateral lesion in the inferomedial temporo-occipital region.

Fig. 15.12 **Visual cortex lesions.**

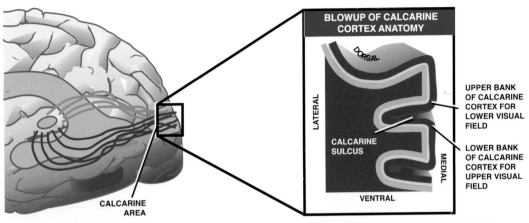

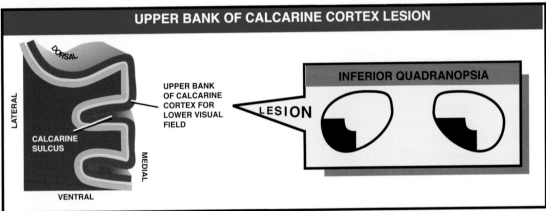

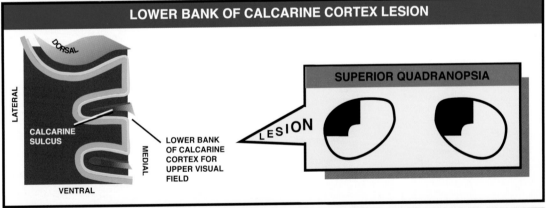

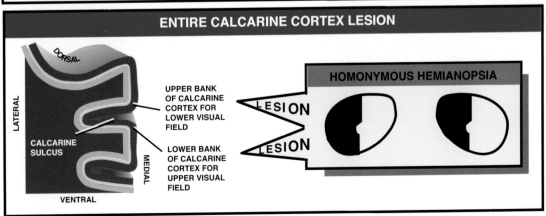

16 Auditory System

The auditory system consists of the external ear, middle ear, cochlea of the inner ear, cochlear nerve, and central auditory pathways.

Functional Anatomy of the Auditory System

The External and Middle Ear

See **Fig. 16.1**.

The external ear comprises the *auricle* and the *external auditory meatus*. It is separated from the middle ear by the *tympanic membrane*. The *middle ear* comprises three main chambers: the tympanic cavity, the *mastoid antrum*, and the *eustachian tube*. The tympanic cavity contains three ossicles that transmit vibrations from the tympanic membrane to the auditory labyrinth. The *malleus* abuts the tympanic membrane, the *stapes* abuts the oval window, and the *incus* is set between the two. The mastoid antrum communicates with pneumatized spaces of the mastoid. The eustachian tube connects the tympanic cavity with the pharynx.

Fig. 16.1 **External, middle, and inner ear.**

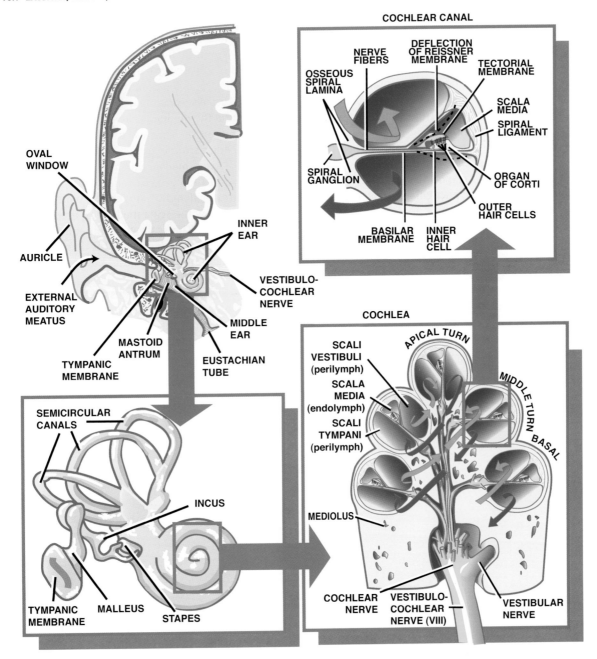

The Inner Ear

See **Figs. 16.1** and **16.2**.

The inner ear comprises two parts: a bony labyrinth formed by cavernous openings in the petrous portion of the temporal bone and a membranous labyrinth formed by a simple epithelial membrane. The membranous labyrinth, which is filled with a fluid called endolymph, lines the contours of the bony labyrinth from which it is separated by a fluid called perilymph.

The membranous labyrinth consists of the *cochlea*, the *utricle* and *saccule*, and the *semicircular canals*. The cochlea, or auditory labyrinth, is responsible for hearing. The utricle and saccule and the semicircular canals make up the vestibular labyrinth.

Cochlea

See **Figs. 16.1** and **16.2**.

The cochlea is the auditory part of the membranous and bony labyrinth. It is shaped like the shell of a snail. It consists of (1) a bony core called the *mediolus*, which contains the cochlear part of the vestibulocochlear nerve, and (2) a *cochlear canal*, which winds two and one-half times around the mediolus like the threads of a screw.

The cavity of the cochlear canal is divided into three compartments: scala vestibuli, scala tympani, and scala media. The *scala media*, which is situated in the middle portion of the cochlear canal, contains endolymph. The *scala vestibuli* and *scala tympani*, which are situated above and below the scala media, respectively, are filled with perilymph. The scala vestibuli and scala tympani communicate with each other at the apex of the cochlea called the *helicotrema*; the scala media ends in a blind sac.

Reissner's membrane separates the scala vestibuli from the scala media; the *basilar membrane* separates the scala tympani from the scala media. These membranes are attached to the bony wall of the cochlear canal by the *spiral ligament*.

Fig. 16.2 Middle and inner ear.

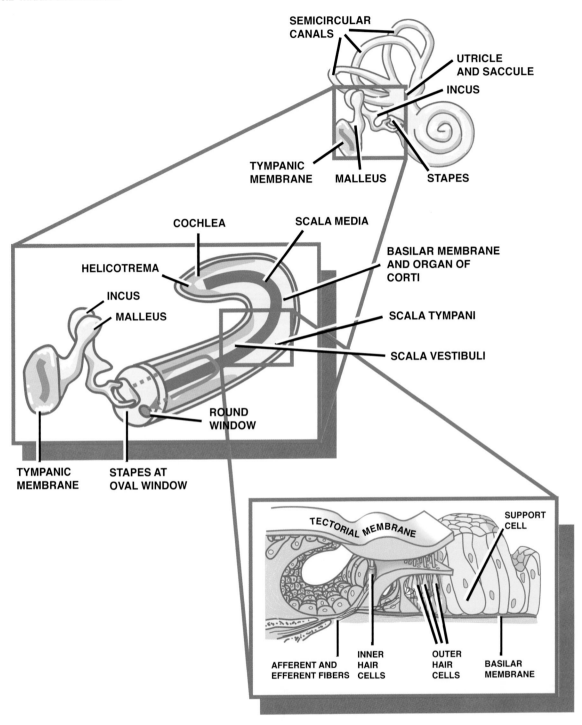

Organ of Corti

See **Fig. 16.3**.

The organ of Corti is composed of sensory *hair cells*. It is situated on the scala media side of the *basilar membrane*. The hair cells of the organ of Corti contain *stereocilia* that project into an overlying gelatinous structure called the *tectorial membrane*. The sequence of steps involved in the transduction of fluid wave energy into electric action potentials is described as follows.

Inward movement of the oval window by the stapes sets up a complicated fluid wave. The fluid wave travels along the scala vestibuli and scala tympani and across the scala media to cause upward displacement of the basilar membrane. As the basilar membrane is forced upward against a fixed tectorial membrane, shearing forces are exerted on the intervening stereocilia, causing excitation of the sensory hair cells.

The point of maximum displacement along the basilar membrane is determined by the sound frequency transmitted: low-frequency sounds result in maximum displacement near the apex; high-frequency sounds result in maximum displacement near the base. Excitability of cochlear nerve fibers is also frequency dependent. Each fiber is most sensitive at a specific frequency. This spatial distribution of sound frequency within the cochlea is clinically manifest by cochlear lesions that result in threshold losses for certain parts of the auditory spectrum.

Fig. 16.3 **Organ of Corti.**

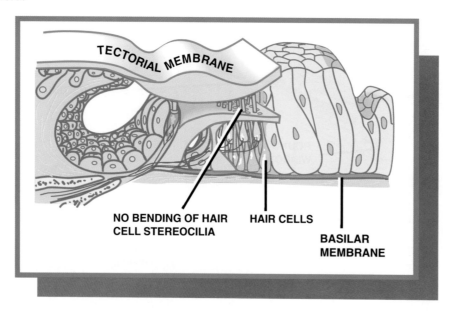

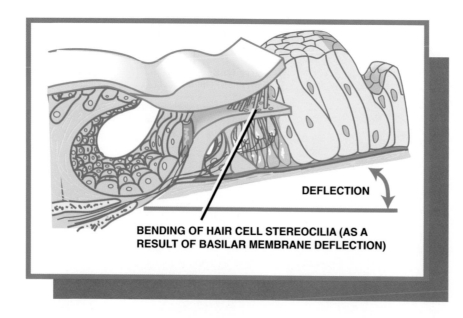

Conductive Hearing

See **Fig. 16.4**.

The mechanical events involved in the transduction of sound waves into chemoelectrical potentials occur as follows:

1. The auricle of the external ear collects sound waves that enter the external acoustic meatus and cause the tympanic membrane to vibrate.
2. This vibration is transmitted through the middle ear by the malleus, incus, and stapes.
3. Oscillation of the stapes at the oval window of the inner ear causes fluid waves to develop within the cochlea.
4. The fluid waves are carried in the cochlea by perilymph.
5. High-frequency (short) waves are carried at the base of the cochlea.
6. Low-frequency (long) waves are carried to the apex of the cochlea.
7. The energy of the fluid waves are transmitted across the scala media from the scala vestibuli to the scala tympani. In the process, the fluid waves stimulate the sensory epithelium in the organ of Corti, which transduces the mechanical energy of fluid waves into chemoelectrical potentials.
8. After crossing the scala media to reach the scala tympani, the fluid waves descend to reach the oval window.
9. The fluid wave causes the round window membrane to move in and out.

Two features of the middle ear enhance the efficiency of the energy transfer from air to fluid: (1) because the area of the oval window is substantially smaller than the area of the tympanic membrane, the vibratory force

Fig. 16.4 **Conductive hearing.**

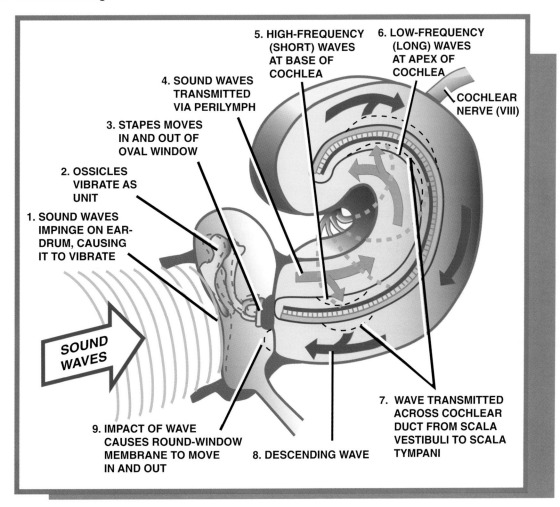

created by sound waves at the tympanic membrane is greatly magnified at the fluid interface of the oval window; (2) because fluid has a higher acoustic impedance than air, the direct transfer of sound waves to the fluid-filled cochlea would result in a substantial loss of energy. The transfer of sound energy to the fluid-filled cochlea via the tympanic membrane and ossicles ameliorates this potential loss of energy.

Central Auditory Pathways

See **Fig. 16.5**.

Brainstem

Central fibers of the cochlear nerve enter the brainstem at the level of the pontomedullary junction. As they enter the brainstem, these fibers bifurcate and are distributed to both dorsal and ventral cochlear nuclei that are located in the medulla adjacent to the inferior cerebellar peduncles. The cochlear nuclei maintain the tonotopic organization present in the cochlea and the primary auditory fibers, as described earlier.

The basic anatomy of the central auditory pathway in the brainstem is described as follows:

- Neurons in the *dorsal cochlear nucleus* project axons across the midline in the dorsal acoustic stria. These axons then ascend in the contralateral *lateral lemniscus* to terminate in the *inferior colliculus*.
- Neurons in the *ventral cochlear nucleus* project axons to the ipsilateral and contralateral *superior olivary nucleus*, the latter via the *trapezoid body*. These axons then ascend in the contralateral lateral lemniscus to terminate in the inferior colliculus.
- Neurons in the inferior colliculus project axons to the *medial geniculate body* via the brachium of the inferior colliculus.

The superior olivary nucleus and the nucleus of the lateral lemniscus are pontine nuclei that serve as relay and integration centers. They are situated between the cochlear nuclei in the medulla and the inferior colliculi in the midbrain.

The superior olivary nucleus is concerned with sound localization. This is accomplished by comparing differences in timing and intensity of sounds received in each ear. The superior olivary nucleus receives input from the ipsilateral and contralateral ventral cochlear nuclei (the latter via the trapezoid body) and projects to the nucleus of the lateral lemniscus and the inferior colliculus. The nucleus of the lateral lemniscus receives fibers from the lateral lemniscus and contributes fibers to the same.

The inferior colliculi are two rounded elevations located in the tectum of the midbrain. They project primarily to the ipsilateral medial geniculate bodies via the brachium of the inferior colliculus.

Thalamus

The medial geniculate bodies are located in the posterior thalamus. All secondary cochlear fibers synapse first in one of the pontine nuclei or the inferior colliculus before reaching the medial geniculate body. No fiber in the auditory pathway bypasses the medial geniculate body. Unlike the rest of the auditory pathway in the brainstem and cortex, the medial geniculate bodies do not possess commissural connections.

Auditory Cortex

The auditory cortex is located in the superior temporal gyrus, along the lateral (sylvian) fissure. It receives fibers from the medial geniculate body. These fibers ascend in the auditory radiation through the posterior limb of the internal capsule. Connections between the primary auditory cortex and adjacent association areas provide higher levels of integration. Thus, electrical stimulation in the area of the primary auditory cortex produces the sensation of simple sounds such as buzzing or ringing, whereas stimulation in the auditory association areas results in complex sounds such as that of a dog barking or a familiar voice.

Like the rest of the auditory system, the auditory cortex is organized tonotopically: neurons concerned with low-frequency sounds are located anteriorly; neurons concerned with high-frequency sounds are located posteriorly. Moreover, like the somatosensory and visual cortices, the auditory cortex is organized into functional columns. These include summation columns, which are primarily concerned with binaural input, and suppression columns, which are primarily concerned with monaural (contralateral) input.

Furthermore, the auditory cortex is functionally organized by layers: layer IV receives afferents and layer V sends efferents to the inferior colliculus. Functional layers, like functional columns, are also characteristic of the somatosensory and visual cortices.

Input in each ear is received bilaterally in the auditory system, beginning above the level of the cochlear nuclei. Commissural fibers connect multiple levels of the brainstem, including the superior olivary nuclei (pons), the nuclei of the lateral lemniscus (pons), the nuclei of the inferior colliculi (midbrain), and the auditory cortices (via the corpus callosum). As a result, lesions affecting the central auditory fibers do not produce clinically evident loss of hearing.

Like the visual cortex, where form, color, and stereopsis are processed in anatomically discrete areas of the brain, the auditory cortex deconstructs complex sounds into their elements of timing, intensity, and frequency. These are processed in parallel by functionally designated areas of the auditory cortex.

Fig. 16.5 Central auditory pathways.

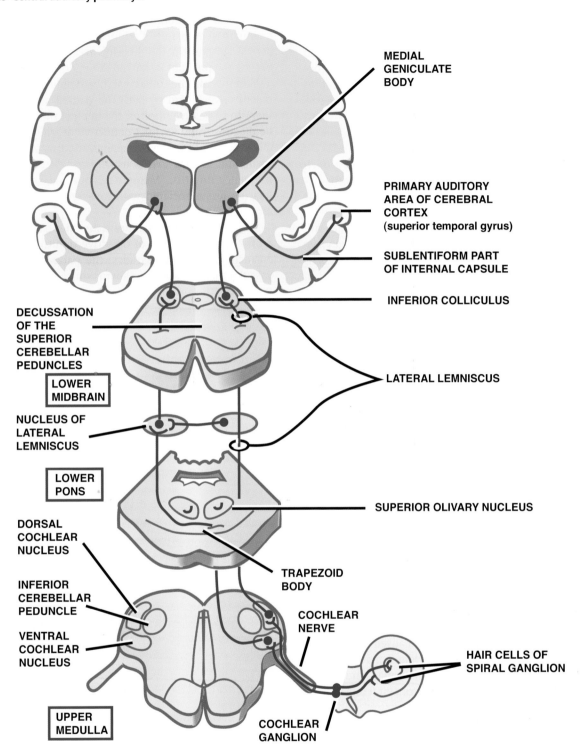

MEDIAL
GENICULATE
BODY

PRIMARY AUDITORY
AREA OF CEREBRAL
CORTEX
(superior temporal gyrus)

SUBLENTIFORM PART
OF INTERNAL CAPSULE

INFERIOR COLLICULUS

DECUSSATION
OF THE
SUPERIOR
CEREBELLAR
PEDUNCLES

LATERAL LEMNISCUS

LOWER
MIDBRAIN

NUCLEUS OF
LATERAL
LEMNISCUS

LOWER
PONS

SUPERIOR OLIVARY NUCLEUS

DORSAL
COCHLEAR
NUCLEUS

TRAPEZOID
BODY

INFERIOR
CEREBELLAR
PEDUNCLE

COCHLEAR
NERVE

VENTRAL
COCHLEAR
NUCLEUS

HAIR CELLS OF
SPIRAL GANGLION

UPPER
MEDULLA

COCHLEAR
GANGLION

Approach to the Patient with Hearing Loss

The mechanisms of hearing loss are divided into two main categories: conductive and sensorineural. Conductive and sensorineural hearing loss is commonly accompanied by tinnitus, a buzzing or ringing sound in the ear.

Conductive Hearing Loss

In conductive hearing loss, the mechanism by which sound is transformed and conducted to the cochlea is impaired. This results from lesions involving the external or middle ear.

Normally, the tympanic membrane and ossicles are responsible for transforming and amplifying sound wave energy and transmitting it to a fluid medium in the cochlea of the inner ear. This pathway provides for an efficient transfer of energy from sound to fluid.

In the absence of this normal pathway, transmission of sound energy from the environment to the fluid-filled cochlea is provided by bones of the skull. This occurs at the expense of considerable energy loss, which is clinically expressed as a decrease in hearing. Patients with conductive hearing loss maintain good ability to hear loud noises, and they hear better in the setting of noisy backgrounds.

Common causes of conductive hearing loss include impacted cerumen in the external ear, inflammation of the middle ear (otitis media), and bony overgrowth and immobility of the stapes (otosclerosis).

Sensorineural Hearing Loss

Sensorineural hearing loss refers to hearing loss that is caused by a deficit in the auditory pathway that occurs central to the oval window. Such a deficit may occur in the cochlea, the cochlear nerve or nuclei, or the central auditory pathway. The presentation of sensorineural hearing loss helps establish its etiology. Thus, bilateral and progressive deafness may be caused by ototoxic drugs, unilateral and progressive deafness may be caused by Meniere's disease or acoustic neuromas, and unilateral and acute deafness may result from viral infection or ischemic infarction

Clinically, sensorineural hearing loss is suggested by a selective difficulty hearing high-pitched sounds and vowels. Formal audiometric testing of individuals with sensorineural hearing loss demonstrates a loss of speech discrimination that is out of proportion to associated pure-tone deafness. Indeed, patients with sensorineural deafness complain of difficulty hearing speech that is mixed with background noise. Conversely, pure tones may be distorted into a complex mixture of noisy, rough, or buzzing tones.

Tinnitus

Tinnitus aurium literally means "ringing in the ears." It is a common complaint in adults and is frequently associated with sensorineural hearing loss. Most commonly, it occurs as a result of lesions in the middle or inner ear.

Tinnitus may be subjective (heard only by the patient) or objective (heard by both the patient and the examiner). In subjective tinnitus, the pitch of the tinnitus may be diagnostically useful. Conductive hearing loss is usually associated with low-frequency tinnitus, whereas sensorineural hearing loss is usually associated with high-frequency tinnitus. (Meniere's syndrome, sensorineural hearing loss associated with low-frequency tinnitus, is an exception.)

Objective tinnitus signifies a disorder outside the auditory system. Sources of objective tinnitus include the eustachian tube, the ossicles, the palate, and cerebral vascular malformations or aneurysms.

Bedside Tests

The Weber Test

See **Fig. 16.6**.

The Weber test involves placing a vibrating tuning fork on the midline of the forehead and asking the patient to indicate on which side, if any, the sound is loudest (to lateralize, if possible, the sound). Normally, the sound is heard with equal force on both the right and the left sides (i.e., no sound lateralization). However, patients with conductive hearing loss will lateralize the sound to the side of the affected ear, whereas patients with sensorineural hearing loss will lateralize the sound to the normal ear.

The Rinne Test

See **Fig. 16.7**.

The Rinne test involves a two-step process in which air conduction is compared with bone conduction. The test is performed as follows: Place the stem of a vibrating tuning fork on the mastoid bone of the subject and count the number of seconds the vibration is heard. When the subject no longer hears the tuning fork (bone conduction), place the tines of the fork near the ear (air conduction). Then count the number of seconds the sound is heard by air conduction. Normally, air conduction is better than bone conduction, and thus the sound continues to be heard at the ear after it is no longer detectable at the mastoid bone, essentially twice as long, or a 2:1 ratio.

Fig. 16.6 **Weber test.**

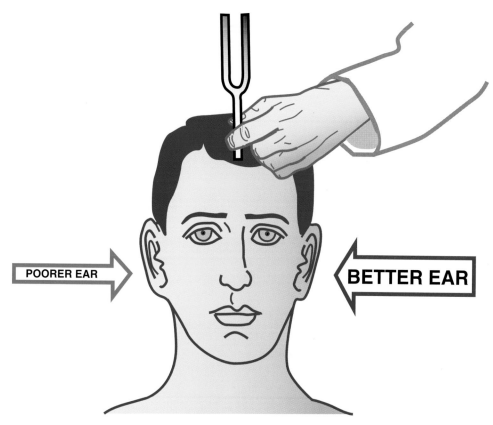

- **CONDUCTION DEAFNESS: PATIENT LATERALIZES SOUND TO THE AFFECTED EAR**
- **SENSORINEURAL DEAFNESS: PATIENT LATERALIZES SOUND TO THE NORMAL EAR**
- **NORMALLY, SOUND IS HEARD EQUALLY ON BOTH THE LEFT AND RIGHT SIDE**

In the presence of sensorineural hearing loss, there is an equal decrement in both air and bone conduction, and thus air conduction remains greater than bone conduction, although in a less than 2:1 ratio. In the presence of conductive hearing loss, however, bone conduction is better than air conduction, and thus the tuning fork cannot be heard at the ear after it is no longer heard at the mastoid bone.

Because the cochlea and cochlear nerve are tonotopically organized, lesions affecting these structures produce frequency-specific hearing loss. For example, lesions at the base of the cochlea result in threshold losses for high-frequency tones, whereas lesions at the apex of the cochlea result in threshold losses for low-frequency tones. Moreover, the timing for different frequencies of the auditory spectrum may be altered.

Central Hearing Loss

Central hearing loss results from lesions in the central auditory pathway, including the brainstem, thalamus, auditory cortex, and their connections.

Because the central auditory structures above the level of the cochlear nucleus receive bilateral innervation, unilateral lesions do not cause clinically significant hearing loss.

Although bilaterally innervated, the auditory cortex on one side is primarily responsible for localizing sounds from the opposite side. Thus, lesions in the auditory cortex may impair ability to localize sounds and may make it difficult for a listener to ignore background noise or competing messages.

Fig. 16.7 **Rinne test.**

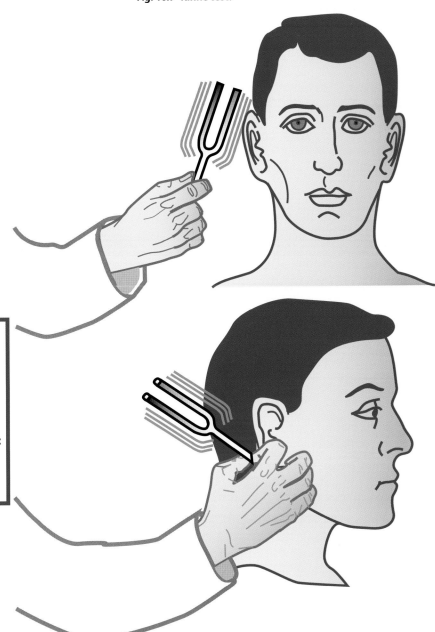

- ● NORMAL: AIR CONDUCTION LONGER THAN BONE CONDUCTION, 2:1 RATIO

- ● CONDUCTION DEAFNESS: CONDUCTION BETTER THAN AIR IN AFFECTED EAR

- ● SENSORINEURAL DEAFNESS: EQUAL DECREMENT IN AIR AND BONE CONDUCTION, ALTHOUGH RATIO < 2:1

17 Vestibular System

Dizziness is one of the most common complaints for which patients seek the attention of a neurologist. Often the underlying disorder causing patients to experience dizziness is disequilibrium, which represents malfunction in one of three separate but communicating systems: the visual system, the proprioceptive system, or the vestibular system.

As will be seen, the diagnosis of disequilibrium as a disturbance of the vestibular system is based on a constellation of signs and symptoms elicited from the patient at bedside.

Much is understood about the anatomy and physiology of the vestibular system, the basic functions of which include the coordination of motor control, posture, equilibrium, and eye movements.

This chapter begins with a description of the functional anatomy of the peripheral vestibular system. Next, central connections with the spinal cord, cerebellum, and oculomotor system are discussed, followed by a practical approach to the dizzy patient.

Functional Anatomy

The Peripheral Vestibular System

See **Fig. 17.1**.

The peripheral vestibular system detects movement and position of the head in space.

The inner ear, or labyrinth, is composed of two parts: a bony labyrinth formed by cavernous openings in the petrous portion of the temporal bone, and a membranous labyrinth formed by a simple epithelial membrane. The membranous labyrinth, which is filled with a fluid called *endolymph*, lines the contours of the bony labyrinth from which it is separated by a fluid called *perilymph*.

Peripheral receptors of the vestibular and auditory systems are contained within the membranous labyrinth. Two sets of structures comprise the vestibular portion of the labyrinth: (1) the *utricle* and *saccule* and (2) the *semicircular canals*.

Fig. 17.1 **Peripheral vestibular system.**

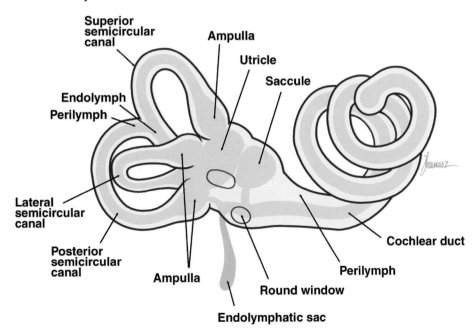

The Utricle and Saccule

See **Figs. 17.2, 17.3, 17.4,** and **17.5**.

The utricle and saccule detect linear acceleration and the position of the head in space.

These structures are dilatations of the membranous labyrinth, separated (by perilymph) from the bony labyrinth. They are filled with endolymph and lined by simple cuboidal epithelium except at receptor-rich regions called maculae.

Utricular and saccular maculae are histologically identical. They contain the following four elements: (1) *supporting cells*, which consist of simple columnar epithelial cells that are continuous with the simple cuboidal epithelial cells that line the utricle and saccule; (2) *hair cells*, which are specialized receptor cells intercalated between the supporting cells; (3) an otolithic membrane, which is a gelatinous mass embedded with crystals of calcium carbonate (*otoliths*) that covers the hair cells; and (4) dendrites of cells in the vestibular ganglion, which carry afferent impulses from the hair cells to the vestibular nuclei of the brainstem.

The "hairs" of a macular hair cell are microvilli. Each hair cell contains ~40 to 80 microvilli together with a single *kinocilium* that arises from a centriole. One kinocilium is located in the periphery of each hair cell, thus polarizing the hair cell in the direction of the kinocilium.

The kinocilia of the maculae of the utricle and saccule are arranged in such a way as to polarize the maculae in relation to an imaginary curved line called the *striola*. Utricular maculae are polarized toward the striola, saccular maculae are polarized away from the striola. The functional significance of this arrangement is as follows.

The weight of the otolithic membrane exerts a gravitational pull on hair cells. The orientation of the hair cells relative to this gravitational force determines the direction of their displacement. For example, when the head is held in the horizontal plane, the vertical gravity vector is perpendicular to the hair cell, and no displacement occurs. When the head is tilted, say, to the left, hair cells follow, and the gravitational force of the otoliths, now at an angle to the cells, deflects them further in this direction.

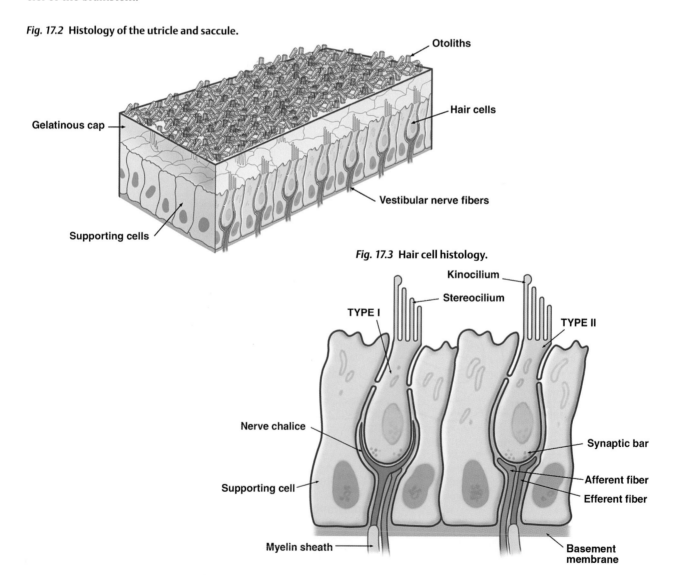

Fig. 17.2 **Histology of the utricle and saccule.**

Otoliths

Hair cells

Gelatinous cap

Vestibular nerve fibers

Supporting cells

Fig. 17.3 **Hair cell histology.**

Kinocilium

Stereocilium

TYPE I

TYPE II

Nerve chalice

Synaptic bar

Supporting cell

Afferent fiber

Efferent fiber

Myelin sheath

Basement membrane

Displacement of hair cells along the axis of polarization depolarizes the cells and initiates excitatory impulses that are carried in afferent fibers to the vestibular nuclei.

Displacement of hair cells in the direction opposite to the axis of polarization hyperpolarizes the cells and initiates inhibitory impulses.

Thus, in response to a tilt of the head, certain hair cells depolarize, whereas others hyperpolarize—depending on their axis of polarization (i.e., the relation of their kinocilium to the striola). Because of their multiple axes of polarization (a product of the curved striola), the utricle and saccule detect changes of head position in any direction in the vertical (saccule) and horizontal (utricle) planes. The overall pattern of macular activity—of excitation and inhibition in both the utricle and the saccule—is finally relayed to the vestibular nuclei, where it signals the position of the head in space. Although they predominantly function as sensors of static position, the utricle and saccule detect linear acceleration as well.

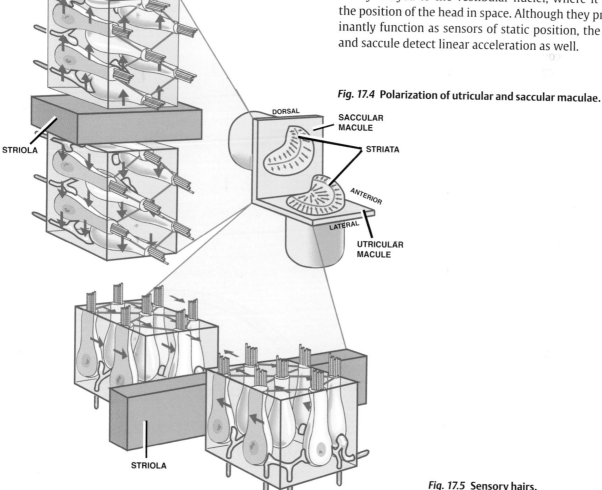

Fig. 17.4 **Polarization of utricular and saccular maculae.**

Fig. 17.5 **Sensory hairs.**

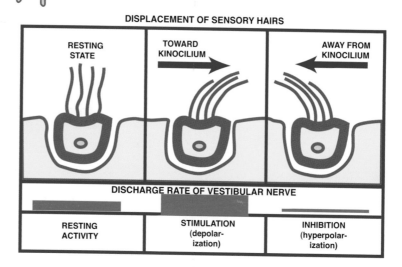

The Semicircular Ducts

See **Figs. 17.1, 17.6, 17.7,** and **17.8**.

The three endolymph-containing semicircular ducts detect angular acceleration of the head in space are formed by the membranous labyrinth, in direct continuation with the utricle. Because the ducts lie in planes oriented at right angles to one another, they provide information about the angular acceleration of the head in any direction, though they lack the ability of the utricle and saccule to detect its static position.

One end of each duct enlarges at its point of attachment to the utricle. These enlargements, or *ampullae*, are the functional counterparts of the maculae of the utricle and saccule. They contain a thickened sensory epithelium called the ampullary crest, which is composed of columnar epithelial supporting cells with interspersed kinocilia-containing hair cells. These hair cells are embedded in a gelatinous mass termed the *cupula*. They fill the space between the crest and the roof the ampulla. (The cupula is the equivalent of the otolithic membrane but lacks its high-specific-gravity calcium carbonate crystals.)

Angular acceleration of the head causes displacement of endolymphatic fluid and movement of the cupula, which stimulates the hair cells.

The kinocilia of the *horizontal ducts* are polarized in the direction of the utricle. Bending hair cells of these ducts in the direction of the utricle thus results in excitatory output. Conversely, the kinocilia of the vertical ducts are polarized in the direction opposite the utricle. Bending hair cells in these ducts in the direction of the utricle thus results in inhibitory output.

In a given plane, the axis of polarization of the ampullae of a pair of ducts, one in the right ear and one in the left, are mirror images of one another. Deflection of their cupulae by the clockwise or counterclockwise flow of endolymphatic fluid excites the duct whose hair cells are deflected toward the axis of polarization, while inhibiting the duct whose hair cells are deflected opposite their axis of polarization. The combined effect of excitatory and inhibitory input from paired semicircular ducts on opposite sides of the head apprises the brain of the head's rotary movements.

Fig. 17.6 **Histology of ampullae.**

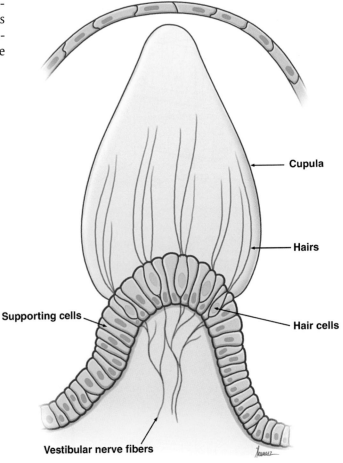

Cupula

Hairs

Supporting cells

Hair cells

Vestibular nerve fibers

Fig. 17.7 Vestibular system and brainstem connections.

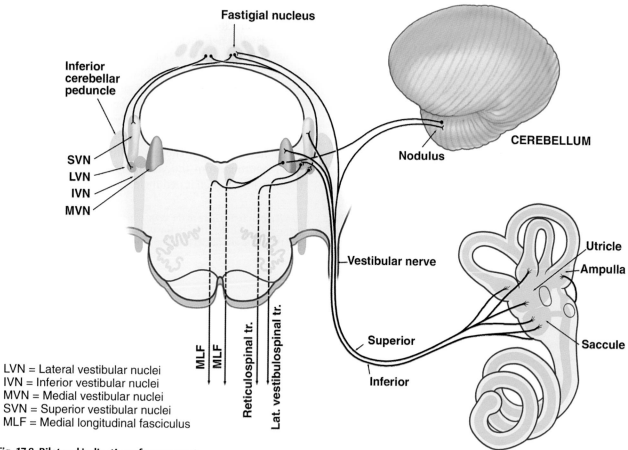

LVN = Lateral vestibular nuclei
IVN = Inferior vestibular nuclei
MVN = Medial vestibular nuclei
SVN = Superior vestibular nuclei
MLF = Medial longitudinal fasciculus

Fig. 17.8 Bilateral indication of movement.

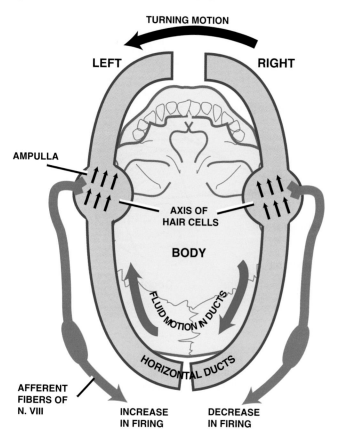

Vestibular System Connections

Vestibular–Central Nervous System

See **Fig. 17.9**.

Central projections of the vestibular system terminate in three major areas: (1) the spinal cord, (2) the cerebellum, and (3) the oculomotor nuclei[1] of the brainstem (III, IV, VI).

These areas are reached by second-order neurons whose cell bodies make up the superior, inferior, medial, and lateral vestibular nuclei (*SVN, IVN, MVN, LVN*). Input from the vestibular labyrinth is transmitted by first-order (bipolar) neurons whose cell bodies are located in the *vestibular ganglion* (Scarpa's ganglion), which lies at the base of the internal auditory canal.

Vestibular nerve fibers enter the brainstem between the medulla and pons. Part of these fibers terminate on vestibular nuclei, and part continue on through the inferior cerebellar peduncle to terminate in the cerebellum.

Second-order neurons of the vestibular nuclei project descending fibers to the spinal cord via the *vestibulospinal tract* (lateral vestibular or Deiters' nucleus exclusively) as well as ascending fibers to the oculomotor nuclei, some directly, some via the medial longitudinal fasciculus (*MLF*). In addition to receiving fibers from the vestibular labyrinth, the cerebellum receives second-order neurons from the vestibular nuclei, also through the inferior cerebellar peduncle.

---

[1]*Oculomotor* refers here to the cranial nerve nuclei that innervate the extraocular muscles, that is, the oculomotor (III), the trochlear (IV), and the abducens nuclei (VI), and not the oculomotor nucleus alone.

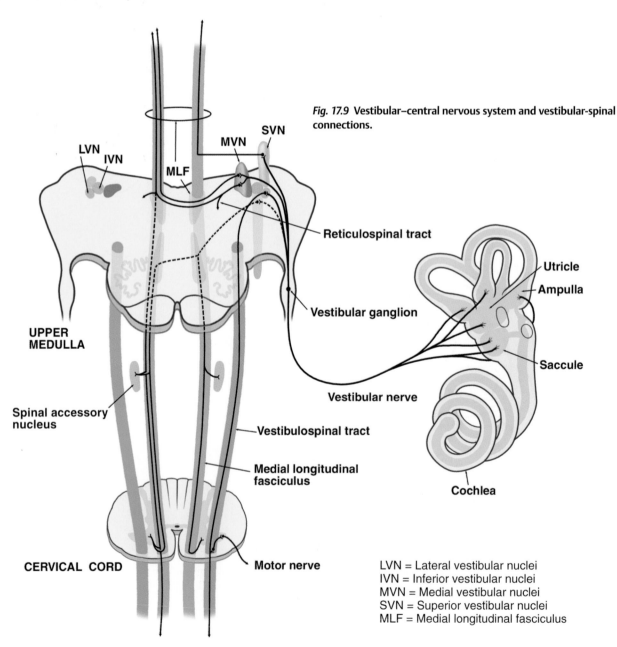

Fig. 17.9 Vestibular–central nervous system and vestibular-spinal connections.

LVN = Lateral vestibular nuclei
IVN = Inferior vestibular nuclei
MVN = Medial vestibular nuclei
SVN = Superior vestibular nuclei
MLF = Medial longitudinal fasciculus

Vestibular-Spinal Connections

See **Fig. 17.9**.

Two spinal pathways originate in the vestibular nuclear complex: the medial vestibulospinal tract and the lateral vestibulospinal tract. These pathways are responsible for upright posture.

The medial vestibulospinal tract arises in the medial vestibular nucleus. It projects crossed and uncrossed fibers in the descending *MLF* as far as the cervical spinal segments.

The larger lateral vestibulospinal tract arises in the lateral vestibular nucleus (Deiters' nucleus). It projects primarily uncrossed fibers to all levels of the spinal cord.

Both vestibulospinal tracts terminate on interneurons in laminae VII and VIII, which exert a facilitatory influence on α and γ motor neurons, particularly those that innervate extensor muscles. The tonic excitation of extensor (antigravity) motor neurons provides the physiological basis for the maintenance of extensor muscle tone that is required for an upright body posture.

Because unopposed tonic facilitatory influence on spinal motor neurons would result in muscular rigidity, the facilitatory influence of the vestibulospinal tract is modified by the inhibitory influence of the reticulospinal tract.

Separation of the reticulospinal tract from its excitatory cortical input, as occurs in transection of the rostral brainstem, alters the balance of inhibitory and facilitatory influences on the extensor motor neurons in favor of facilitation. Decerebrate rigidity—an exaggerated tone of upper and lower limb extensors seen in patients with massive cerebral lesions that effectively disconnect the brainstem from the cerebrum—results from this unopposed facilitatory action of the lateral vestibulospinal tract on spinal motor neurons.

Vestibular-Cerebellar Connections

The connections between the cerebellum and the vestibular system are conducted via the inferior cerebellar peduncle. They are reciprocal in the sense that the cerebellum receives input from the vestibular system, and vice versa. These connections are responsible for body posture, equilibrium, and the control of eye movements.

Cerebellar afferents from the vestibular system include both first-order neurons that originate in the vestibular labyrinths as well as second-order neurons that originate in the ipsilateral vestibular nuclei.

The vestibulocerebellum, which is the part of the cerebellum that reciprocates with the vestibular system, includes the flocculonodular lobe and the vermis. Through its innervation of the vestibular nuclei the vestibulocerebellum helps to control body posture, equilibrium, and eye movements.

Fig. 17.10 **Vestibulo-ocular anatomy.**

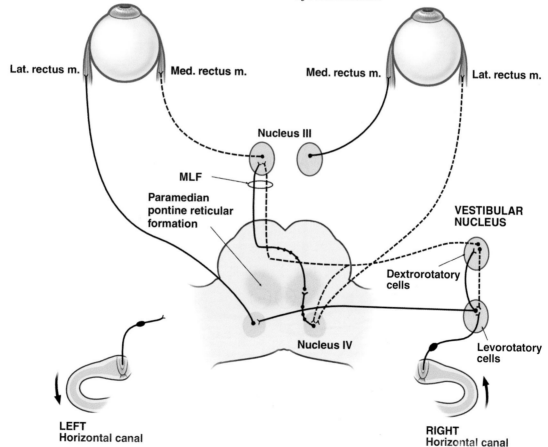

Vestibulo-ocular Reflexes

See **Figs. 17.10** (page 417) and **17.11**.

Movements of the head excite and inhibit the semicircular ducts. These semicircular ducts in turn initiate impulses that are relayed in the *vestibular nuclei* to terminate in the oculomotor nuclei (III, IV, VI). This provides a mechanism for compensatory eye movements during movement of the head, as follows.

Imagine a woman reading a novel when she is suddenly interrupted by the call of her roommate from another room. While maintaining visual fixation on the passage she is reading, she rotates her head leftward in the horizontal plane to better hear her roommate's call. Unbeknownst to her, our reader's leftward head rotation in the horizontal plane results in the flow of endolymphatic fluid in the direction opposite the head rotation, causing stimulation of the left horizontal duct (fluid flowing toward the utricle) and inhibition of the right (fluid flowing away from the utricle). A stimulated left horizontal duct increases the impulse frequency of its afferent output, which is transmitted to vestibular nuclei via first-order vestibular neurons.

Second-order neurons in the vestibular nuclei in turn project to the contralateral abducens nucleus, which innervates the right *lateral rectus*. This produces abduction of the right eye.

The ipsilateral oculomotor nucleus, which innervates the left *medial rectus*, receives input from the contralateral abducens nucleus via the crossed *MLF* as well as input from the vestibular nuclei directly. This produces adduction of the left eye.

Because the labyrinths work in pairs, an increase in afferent output of the left *horizontal semicircular duct* is accompanied by diminished afferent output in the same receptor on the opposite side of the head. The combined effect of these two pathways is simultaneous contraction of the left medial rectus (adduction of the left eye) and the right lateral rectus (abduction of the right eye) associated with relaxation of the left lateral rectus and the right medial rectus. As she rotates her head to the left, the eyes of our reader conjugately turn to the right, enabling her to maintain visual fixation on her novel.

Fig. 17.11 **Vestibulo-ocular reflex.**

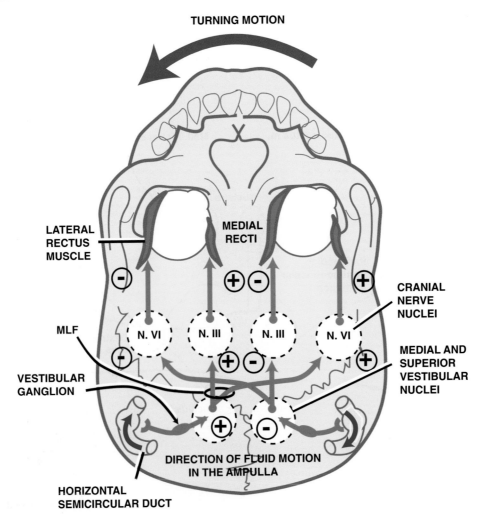

Nystagmus

See **Fig. 17.12**.

In our example, the angle of head rotation was small enough that compensatory eye movements enabled our reader to keep her eyes on her novel even as she turned her head away from it. But what if the angle of a head movement is too wide for the motion of the eyes in the orbits to compensate?

Such is the case when a subject is rotated 360 degrees around a vertical axis. In this case, slow vestibular-induced compensatory eye movements are interrupted by quick movements in the opposite direction.

Rhythmic alternation of such slow and quick movements is termed nystagmus. By convention, the direction of nystagmus is named for the fast phase, although the slow phase represents the true labyrinth-stimulated movement.

Physiological stimulation of a labyrinth produces nystagmus in the plane of that labyrinth with a conjugate slow movement away from the stimulated labyrinth followed by a quick component in the opposite direction.

Spontaneous (pathological) nystagmus likewise results when the balance of tonic activity in the labyrinth is altered. Damage to the left vestibular labyrinth or nerve, for example, results in unopposed right-sided tonic ac-

tivity with nystagmus that is indistinguishable from that produced by right-sided stimulation.

Compared with peripheral vestibular nystagmus, central-induced nystagmus due to interruption of central vestibulo-ocular pathways is distinctive in the following two respects: (1) the direction of central-induced nystagmus is less predictable and may vary with the subject's direction of gaze; and (2) visual fixation, which inhibits peripheral vestibular nystagmus, does not inhibit nystagmus due to central lesions.

The best way to anticipate the direction of pathological nystagmus due to labyrinthine disease is to remember that it represents unopposed tonic activity of its counterpart on the opposite side. Because the horizontal semicircular ducts are most important clinically, it is also useful to remember that, when stimulated, they contract the ipsilateral medial rectus and the contralateral lateral rectus, and that they thus produce, when stimulated, a slow conjugate movement away from the stimulated duct followed by a quick movement in the opposite direction. It is emphasized, however, that rote memorization of various patterns of pathological nystagmus, here as elsewhere in neuroscience, is a recipe for frustration and failure.

Fig. 17.12 **Physiologic and spontaneous nystagmus.**

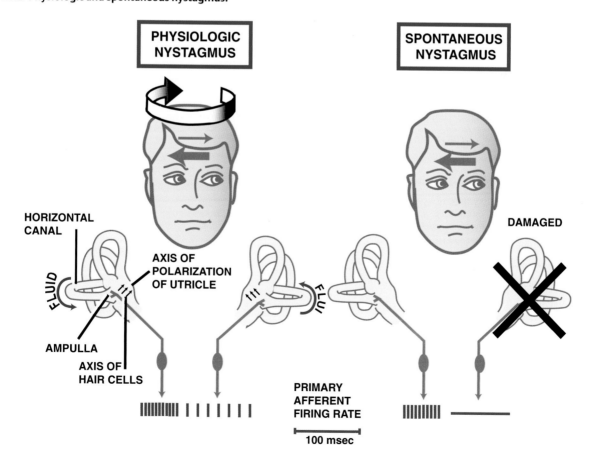

Approach to the Dizzy Patient

The common denominator of symptoms caused by vestibular system dysfunction is vertigo: the illusion of movement of self or environment.

In practice, true vertigo is a far less common complaint as compared with dizziness, a term that encompasses a wide array of meanings. The initial task in the diagnostic approach to dizziness thus consists of querying patients about what they means by "dizziness." Descriptions that suggest a nonvestibular pathophysiology such as orthostatic hypotension, visual impairment, or proprioceptive loss will redirect the diagnostic evaluation accordingly.

The approach to the dizzy patient of evident vestibular origin begins with the anatomic localization of the responsible lesion. Such lesions are conveniently categorized as systemic, peripheral, or central in origin on the basis of the history and physical examination.

Systemic disorders, including cardiovascular, endocrine, and metabolic diseases that secondarily affect the vestibular system, are identified by their systemic signs and symptoms (**Table 17.1**).

Peripheral and central vestibular lesions are further subdivided as follows.

Table 17.1 Signs and Symptoms of Peripheral and Central Vestibular Lesions

Peripheral Vestibular
• Pathology affects the vestibular labyrinth and/or ganglia
• May present with hearing loss, tinnitus, ear pressure, and/or pain with labyrinth lesions
• May present with facial weakness with hearing loss and tinnitus with ganglia lesions
• Often see past-pointing to the affected side
• Nystagmus is often rotary and inhibited by visual fixation
• Associated autonomic symptoms—sweating, pallor, nausea, and vomiting
Central Vestibular
Cerebellopontine angle lesions
• Hearing loss and tinnitus
• Loss of corneal reflex (ipsilateral) and facial numbness
• Facial weakness
• Ispilateral ataxia and intention tremor
Brainstem and cerebellar lesions
• Vertigo mild
• Other cranial nerves affected—diplopia, dysarthria, perioral numbness
• Long-tract signs—hemiparesis, hemisensory loss, hyperreflexia
• Hearing loss and tinnitus absent

Peripheral Vestibular Lesions

Peripheral vestibular lesions occur in two major areas: the vestibular labyrinth and the vestibular ganglia and nerve within the internal auditory canal.

Lesions in the Vestibular Labyrinth

In addition to episodic vertigo, damage to the labyrinth most commonly presents with hearing loss, tinnitus, ear pressure, and pain.

On examination the patient points to the affected side. There is spontaneous nystagmus, with the quick component directed away from the affected side. The nystagmus, which is usually rotary due to involvement of ducts in both the vertical and the horizontal planes, is inhibited by fixation.

Vertigo, nystagmus, and associated autonomic symptoms such as sweating, pallor, nausea, and vomiting are typically pronounced.

Common causes of lesions in the vestibular labyrinth include viral and bacterial infections and drug toxicity. (The aminoglycosides are notoriously ototoxic.)

Lesions in the Vestibular Ganglia and Nerve within the Internal Auditory Canal

The close proximity of the vestibulocochlear (VIII) and facial (VII) nerves, which come together within the internal auditory canal, accounts for the constellation of symptoms that accompany lesions in this site.

Ipsilateral facial weakness (VII) is characteristic. Hearing loss and tinnitus are often present, but vertigo is less prominent, and ear pressure and pain are usually absent.

Central Vestibular Lesions

Central vestibular lesions occur in two major areas: the cerebellopontine angle (CPA) and the brainstem and cerebellum.

Lesions in the Cerebellopontine Angle

The CPA is bounded by the cerebellum, the pons, and the petrous portion of the temporal bone. The facial (VII) and vestibulocochlear (VIII) nerves traverse this angle in their stretch between exiting the pontomedullary junction and entering the internal auditory canal.

Tumors, most commonly the vestibular schwannoma, are the major source of lesions in this area.

They cause (1) progressive hearing loss and tinnitus due to compression of the cochlear nerve (VIII), (2) loss of the ipsilateral corneal reflex and facial numbness due to compression of afferent fibers of the trigeminal nerve (V), and (3) facial weakness due to compression of the facial nerve (VII).

Ipsilateral limb ataxia and intention tremor signal compression of the cerebellum, and long-tract signs such as contralateral hemiparesis and hemisensory loss signal compression of the brainstem.

Compared with peripheral lesions, vertigo, nystagmus, and autonomic symptoms are mild.

Lesions in the Brainstem and Cerebellum

Isolated vestibular symptoms are rarely the result of lesions in the brainstem or cerebellum.

Rather, vertigo, which tends to be mild, is associated with other cranial nerve signs such as diplopia (III, IV, VI), dysarthria (IX and X), and perioral numbness (V), as well as long-tract signs such as hemiparesis (corticospinal tract) and hemisensory loss (spinothalamic tract).

Typically, hearing loss and tinnitus are absent in brainstem lesions, and autonomic symptoms are mild.

Vertebrobasilar insufficiency, a diminished flow of blood in the vertebrobasilar arterial system, is a common cause of the brainstem vestibular syndrome.

Interruption of vestibular pathways due to cerebellar lesions, such as infarction in the territory of the posteroinferior cerebellar artery, commonly results in limb ataxia and vertigo.

18 Oculomotor System

This chapter discusses the ocular motor system. It is organized into six sections: (1) a description of the four types of eye movements, including saccades, smooth pursuit, vestibular-optokinetic, and vergence movements; (2) a discussion of the anatomy and disorders of the supranuclear control system; (3) a discussion of the anatomy and localization of lesions involving the oculomotor nerves; (4) a description of the clinical features and anatomic localization of nystagmus; (5) a description of the anatomy and disorders of pupillary function; and (6) a discussion of the anatomy and disorders of the eyelid.

Four Types of Eye Movements

Saccades

See **Fig. 18.1.**

The major function of saccadic eye movements is to rapidly place the object of interest on the fovea. Saccadic eye movements may be volitional (voluntary refixations) or involuntary (quick phases of vestibular and optokinetic nystagmus). The stimulus required to elicit a saccade consists of an object of interest in the peripheral eye field. From stimulus to onset of eye movement, the latency of saccadic eye movements is ~200 msec; a typical velocity is ~400 degrees/s (but may be as high as 600 to 700 degrees/s.)

One hypothesis suggests that saccadic movements are ballistic; that is, they are not modifiable once begun. In support of this hypothesis, it is argued that visual information is sampled by the saccadic system. Once an object of interest is identified in the visual periphery, a decision is made to generate a saccade that will bring the object into focus on the fovea. Depending on the retinal error (i.e., the distance between the retinal location of an image and the fovea), the size, direction, and duration of a saccade are automatically calculated, and an irrevocable decision is made to generate the saccade. Once the saccade is completed, the visual world is again sampled, and the process is then repeated.

The anatomic substrate for volitional saccades originates in the *frontal eye fields* (*Brodmann's area 8*), which can initiate saccades in the contralateral direction, via descending pathways to the *superior colliculi*. The superior colliculus receives an orderly retinal projection such that the visual field can be mapped onto its surface. Stimulation of the superior colliculus drives the eyes toward a point in the visual field that corresponds to the retinal projection to that site. When the image of the target reaches the fovea, a negative feedback system involving the superior colliculus causes the eye movement to end.

Examination of saccadic eye movements is best performed at the bedside by instructing the patient to fixate alternatively on two targets, such as the tip of a pen and the examiner's nose. Saccadic eye movements should be examined in each field of gaze in both the horizontal and vertical planes. The examination should determine whether the saccades are normal, whether they are promptly initiated, and whether they are accurate.

Fig. 18.1 **Saccades.**

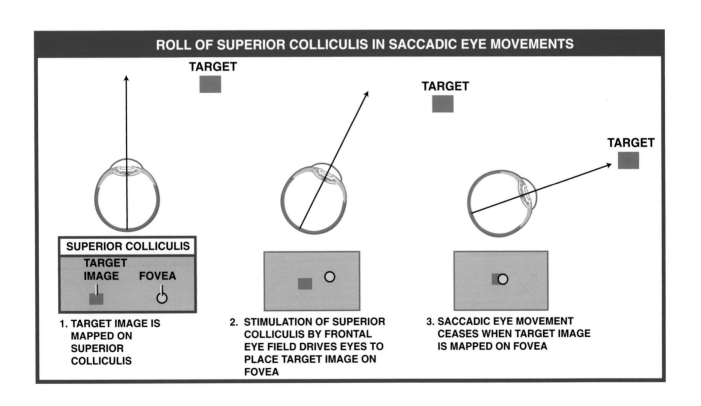

SACCADIC EYE MOVEMENTS

FUNCTION :	**TO RAPIDLY PLACE THE OBJECT OF INTEREST ON THE FOVEA,**
STIMULUS :	**AN OBJECT IN THE PERIPHERAL EYE FIELD**
LATENCY :	**200 msec**
VELOCITY :	**AVERAGES 400 degrees/sec**

FRONTAL EYE FIELDS
(Brodmann's area 8)

CEREBRAL

SUPERIOR COLLICULI

MIDBRAIN

OCULO-MOTOR NUCLEI

PONS

ROLL OF SUPERIOR COLLICULIS IN SACCADIC EYE MOVEMENTS

TARGET

TARGET

TARGET

SUPERIOR COLLICULIS

TARGET IMAGE   **FOVEA**

1. **TARGET IMAGE IS MAPPED ON SUPERIOR COLLICULIS**

2. **STIMULATION OF SUPERIOR COLLICULIS BY FRONTAL EYE FIELD DRIVES EYES TO PLACE TARGET IMAGE ON FOVEA**

3. **SACCADIC EYE MOVEMENT CEASES WHEN TARGET IMAGE IS MAPPED ON FOVEA**

Smooth Pursuits

See **Fig. 18.2.**

The major function of the smooth pursuit system is to maintain the object of regard near the fovea, matching the eye with the target. The stimulus for smooth pursuit is the image of an object moving across the retina, usually within or near the fovea. The image of the object may not cover the fovea (it may be smaller) and may indeed project outside the margin of the fovea, in the parafoveal region. This is preferential under conditions of poor ambient light because rods are more efficient photoreceptors than are cones. In certain circumstances, the stimulus is not a visual image at all. Nonvisual stimuli, such as proprioceptive information related to the movement of one's own limbs, may be sufficient to generate smooth tracking movements.

The latency from stimulus to onset of smooth pursuit movements is 125 msec. The velocity of smooth pursuit movements matches the velocity of the target, which is typically less than 10% of saccadic eye movements (around 30 degrees/s). The feedback substrate is usually continuous and slow; objects that move fast may require a combination of pursuit and saccadic movements. Saccadic movements in these instances allow the eye to keep up with the object.

The neural substrate for smooth pursuit involves the following sequence: Retinal information on the speed and direction of a moving target is projected on the striate visual cortex of the occipital lobes. This information is relayed to the ipsilateral middle temporal visual area, the frontal eye fields, and the pontine nuclei in a retinotopic fashion. After modification of the visual impulses in the cerebellum and vestibular nuclei, they are finally projected to the ocular motor nuclei. *Note that smooth pursuit movements are identified with the ipsilateral occipital lobes, in contrast to saccadic movements, which are identified with the contralateral frontal lobes.*

To examine smooth pursuits, ask the patient to hold the head still while tracking a small target, such as the tip of a pencil, held at least a meter in front of the patient. Move the target at a slow, uniform speed, and observe whether the eye movements match the velocity and direction of the target. If the pursuit gain is low, then catch-up saccades are noted; if the pursuit gain is too high, then backup saccades are noted. When evaluating a patient, it should be kept in mind that execution of smooth pursuits requires that a patient is able to normally attend and that pursuit movements naturally deteriorate with age. Smooth pursuit movements are also particularly sensitive to drugs, which may affect the results of testing. Such drugs include phenytoin, barbiturates, diazepam, chloral hydrate, methadone, alcohol, and marijuana.

Fig. 18.2 **Smooth pursuits.**

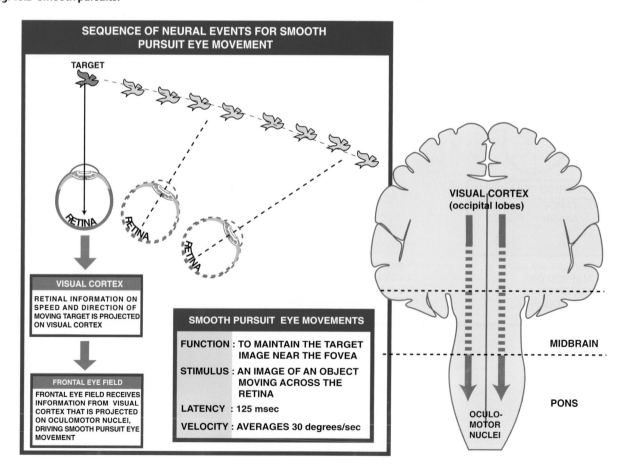

Vestibular-Optokinetic Eye Movements

See **Fig. 18.3.**

The function of vestibular-optokinetic eye movements is to maintain eye position with respect to changes in head and body position. To hold images on the retina, compensatory eye movements must be made to counteract the effects of head movement. To compensate for loss of sensory input, and to counteract the entire range of different head movements, a redundant system of sensory signals contribute to the programming of compensatory eye movements. These sensory signals include inputs from the labyrinthine semicircular canals, the otoliths, vision, and somatosensors that include muscle spindles and joint receptors.

Thus, the vestibulo-ocular reflex (VOR), which depends on the semicircular canals, generates compensatory eye movements during high-frequency rotational head movements. The latency of these movements is extremely short, on the order of 10 msec, and the frequency is as high as 300 degrees/sec. Visual inputs form the stimulus for the optokinetic and smooth pursuit systems, which supplement the VOR during sustained (low-frequency) head movements. The otolithic organs, by virtue of their sensitivity to linear acceleration, generate compensatory eye movements during translational movements of the head. The combined inputs from the semicircular canals, the otolithic organs, the visual system, and the somatosensors are relayed together in the vestibular nuclei, where a best estimate of the head's movement is determined.

As part of the clinical examination of vestibular-optokinetic movements, bedside caloric testing is a relatively simple method of determining the side of a peripheral vestibular lesion. If examination verifies the integrity of the tympanic membranes, the patient is positioned supine, with the head flexed 30 degrees. Flexion of the head places the lateral semicircular canals in a vertical position. Irrigate the external auditory canals on each side with a small amount of ice water (a normal response can be elicited with as little as 0.2 mL). Normally, the ear that is irrigated exhibits nystagmus with its quick phase in the opposite direction. Failure to elicit this response indicates loss of unilateral vestibular function.

Fig. 18.3 **Vestibular-optokinetic eye movements.**

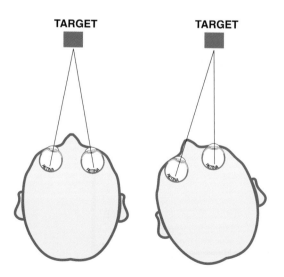

VESTIBULAR-OPTOKINETIC EYE MOVEMENTS

FUNCTION : TO MAINTAIN EYE POSITION WITH RESPECT TO CHANGES IN HEAD AND BODY POSITION

STIMULUS : CHANGE IN HEAD AND BODY POSTURE

LATENCY : 10 msec

VELOCITY : AS HIGH AS 300 degrees/sec

RETINAL IMAGE IS MAINTAINED BY COMPENSATORY EYE MOVEMENTS THAT COUNTERACT THE EFFECTS OF HEAD MOVEMENT. WHEN HEAD MOVEMENT OCCURS, COMPENSATORY EYE MOVEMENTS ARE STIMULATED BY SENSORY SIGNALS FROM THE VESTIBULAR SYSTEM, THE VISUAL SYSTEM, AND THE SOMATOSENSORY SYSTEM.

Vergence Eye Movements

See **Fig. 18.4**.

Vergence movements align the visual axes to maintain bifoveal fixation so that an object seen by both eyes is perceived as a single object. This requires that the object of interest to fall on corresponding retinal points. In the event that two images of an object fall on noncorresponding retinal areas in each eye, one of two possibilities may occur. Either the object is perceived to exist in two separate locations simultaneously, causing diplopia, or the perception is created that two objects are located in the same position in space, causing visual confusion. Normally, when retinal disparity develops, it is so short-lived that it produces neither diplopia nor visual confusion. The latency of vergence movements is ~160 msec, and the velocity is around 20 degrees/s.

The two primary stimuli of vergence movements are retinal disparity and retinal blur. *Retinal disparity* refers to a disparity between the location of images on the two retinas, and *retinal blur* refers to defocused images. Whereas retinal disparity is associated with fusional vergence (in which the two retinal images are perceived as one), retinal blur leads to accommodation-linked vergence. This latter type of vergence is associated with pupillary constriction and lens accommodation in response to the retinal blur associated with near vision. Other vergence stimuli include the sense of nearness (proximal vergence), which is related to cues such as perspective and size, and an underlying level of vergence tone (tonic vergence).

As mentioned, when the eyes focus on a near object, the response that occurs is the so-called near reflex or accommodation reflex. This reflex consists of (1) convergence of the eyes, (2) accommodation of the lens, and (3) pupillary constriction. As always, the purpose of the vergence component of this reflex is to maintain the image of the object on the fovea of each eye. Accommodation of the lens involves contraction of the ciliary muscle, which reduces the tension on the suspensory ligaments of the lens. This causes the lens to become more spherical to accommodate near vision. Constriction of the pupil helps to produce a sharper image, which also contributes to near accommodation.

Fig. 18.4 **Vergence eye movements.**

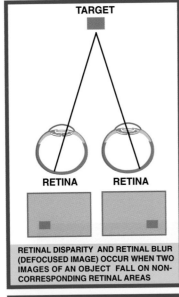

RETINAL DISPARITY AND RETINAL BLUR (DEFOCUSED IMAGE) OCCUR WHEN TWO IMAGES OF AN OBJECT FALL ON NON-CORRESPONDING RETINAL AREAS

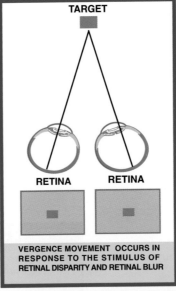

VERGENCE MOVEMENT OCCURS IN RESPONSE TO THE STIMULUS OF RETINAL DISPARITY AND RETINAL BLUR

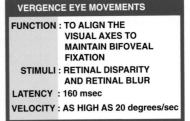

VERGENCE EYE MOVEMENTS	
FUNCTION :	TO ALIGN THE VISUAL AXES TO MAINTAIN BIFOVEAL FIXATION
STIMULI :	RETINAL DISPARITY AND RETINAL BLUR
LATENCY :	160 msec
VELOCITY :	AS HIGH AS 20 degrees/sec

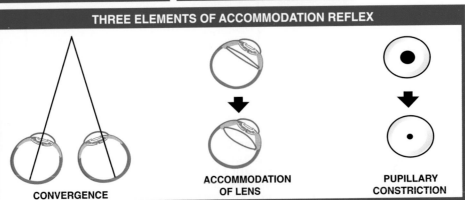

THREE ELEMENTS OF ACCOMMODATION REFLEX

CONVERGENCE   ACCOMMODATION OF LENS   PUPILLARY CONSTRICTION

Supranuclear Control of Eye Movements

In the broadest sense, there are two types of eye movements, horizontal and vertical, that provide useful clinicoanatomic correlates. The following section describes the anatomy of these two types of movements and their associated clinical disorders.

Horizontal Eye Movements

Anatomy

See **Fig. 18.5**.

Horizontal eye movements originate in either the frontal lobe contralaterally (for saccades) or the ipsilateral occipital lobe (for smooth pursuits). The impulses carrying information about these movements travel through the internal capsule to the *paramedian pontine reticular formation* (PPRF) in the *pons*. The left gaze center controls saccades to the left and smooth pursuit to the left. The converse is true for the right gaze center. The tract begins in the frontal lobe gaze center and projects first to the PPRF and then to the ipsilateral sixth nerve nucleus. The projection then reaches the contralateral third nerve nucleus via the *medial longitudinal fasciculus* (MLF).

Fig. 18.5 **Anatomy of horizontal eye movements.**

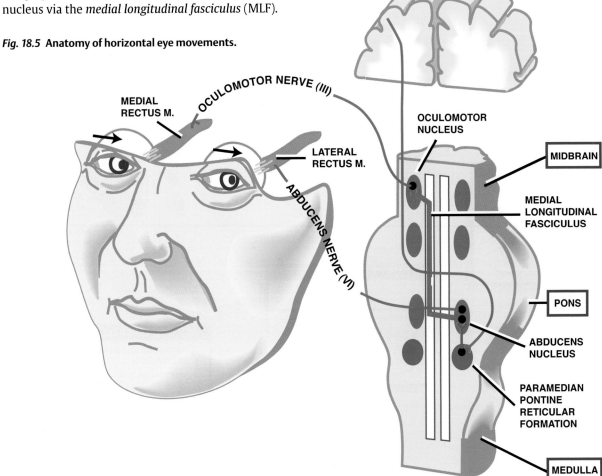

Disorders

There are three major types of horizontal eye movement disorders: internuclear ophthalmoplegia (INO), a gaze palsy, and one and a half syndrome.

Internuclear Ophthalmoplegia

See **Fig. 18.6.**

An INO represents a lesion of the MLF producing failure of adduction on the side of the lesion and nystagmus of the abducting eye. In a posteriorly located INO, the vergence system is intact; in a centrally located INO, the vergence system is impaired.

Fig. 18.6 Internuclear ophthalmoplegia.

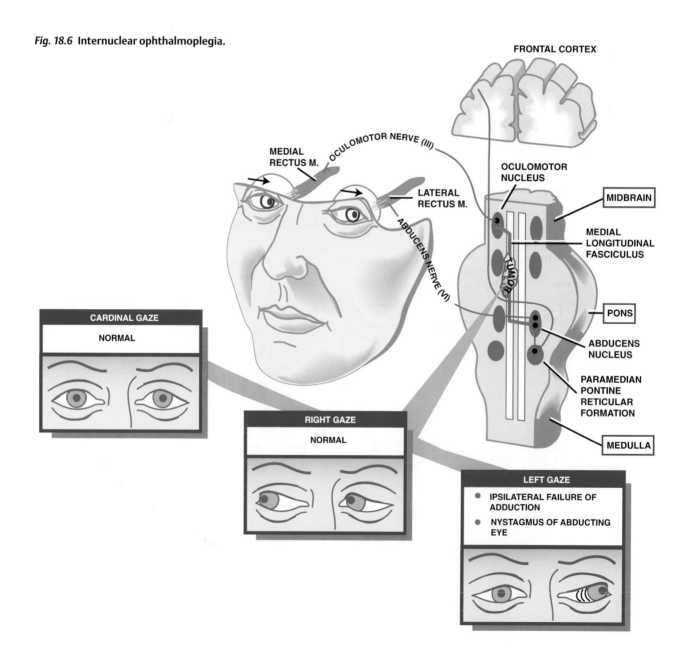

Gaze Palsy

See **Fig. 18.7.**

Gaze palsy is characterized by impairment of the conjugate horizontal gaze to one side or the other.

Fig. 18.7 **Gaze palsy.**

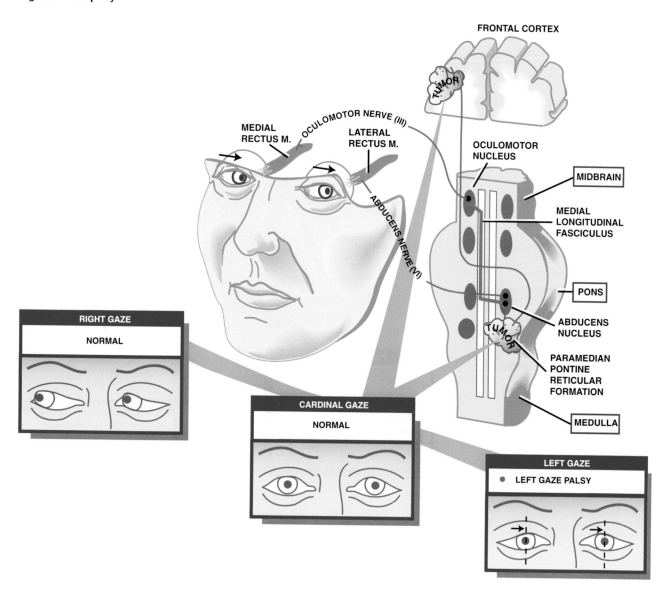

One and a Half Syndrome

See **Fig. 18.8.**

One and a half syndrome consists of (1) impairment of conjugate horizontal gaze to the side ipsilateral to the lesion, and (2) an INO on gaze to the side contralateral to the lesion. This is due to simultaneous involvement of the PPRF (paramedian pontine reticular formation) and ipsi-

lateral MLF by a lesion located in the pons. Thus, as illustrated by **Fig. 18.8**, a lesion involving the right PPRF and right MLF will result in the impairment of right lateral conjugate gaze (due to interruption of the right PPRF) and an INO on left lateral gaze (due to interruption of the right MLF).

Fig. 18.8 **One and a half syndrome.**

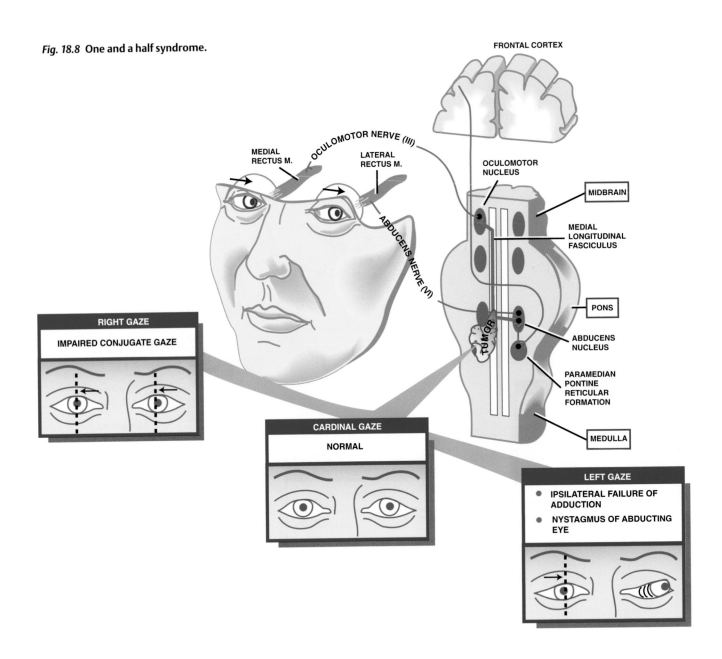

Vertical Eye Movements

Anatomy

Vertical eye movements originate bilaterally and pass to the pretectal area (vertical gaze center) and thence to the third nerve and sixth nerve nuclei.

Disorders

See **Fig. 18.9**.

There are two major types of vertical gaze palsy, Parinaud's syndrome and the Steele-Richardson-Olszewski syndrome.

Parinaud's Syndrome

Also known as the sylvian aqueduct syndrome, Parinaud's syndrome constitutes a problem with the upward gaze and is associated with hydrocephalus secondary to dilation of the sylvian aqueduct. The complete syndrome is characterized by the following problems: (1) vertical gaze paresis, (2) pupillary abnormalities, (3) retraction nystagmus, (4) lid retraction (Collier's sign) when the patient looks up, (5) loss of convergence, and (6) loss of accommodation.

Steele-Richardson-Olszewski's Syndrome

Steele-Richardson-Olszewski's syndrome (primary supranuclear palsy) constitutes a problem with downward gaze and is associated with nuchal rigidity and progressive dementia.

Fig. 18.9 **Disorders of vertical gaze.**

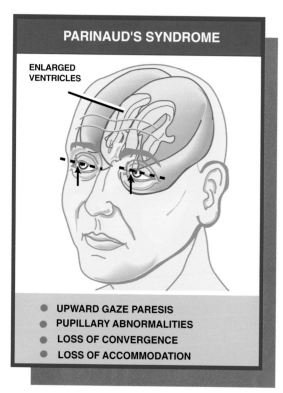

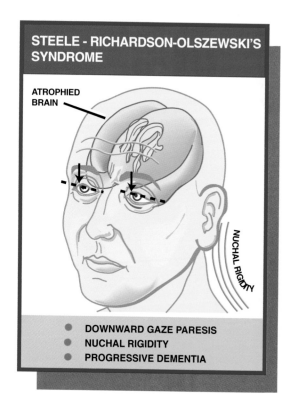

Ocular Motor Nerves and Localization of Lesions

The ocular motor nerves comprise the third, fourth, and sixth cranial nerves.

Third Nerve

Anatomy

See **Fig. 18.10**.

The third nerve nuclear complex is located near the midline at the level of the *superior colliculus* in the midbrain. It lies ventral to the *cerebral aqueduct* and dorsal to the medial longitudinal fasciculus. The Edinger-Westphal nuclei are most rostral. They contain parasympathetic neurons that mediate constriction of the pupil. The subnuclei that subserve the levator palpebrae muscle are most caudal. They provide bilateral innervation. All the other subnuclei provide ipsilateral innervation except the superior rectus subnucleus, which innervates the contralateral side.

The fascicles of the third nerve exit the midbrain in close association with the *red nucleus* and the *cerebral peduncle*.

In the subarachnoid space, the third nerve runs between the *superior cerebellar artery* and the *posterior cerebral artery*. It also runs in close association with the posterior communicating artery and the medial temporal lobe before piercing the dura just lateral to the *posterior clinoid* process to enter the lateral wall of the *cavernous sinus*.

Within the cavernous sinus, the third nerve separates into a *superior* and an *inferior division*. After traversing the cavernous sinus, both divisions pass through the superior orbital fissure to enter the orbit. The superior division innervates the *superior rectus* and *levator palpebrae superioris muscles*. The inferior division innervates the *inferior rectus*, the *inferior oblique*, and the *medial rectus muscles*. The inferior division also contains parasympathetic fibers that mediate pupillary constriction and accommodation.

Fig. 18.10 Anatomy of third nerve.

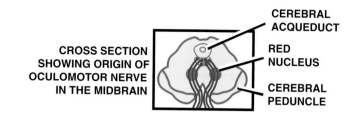

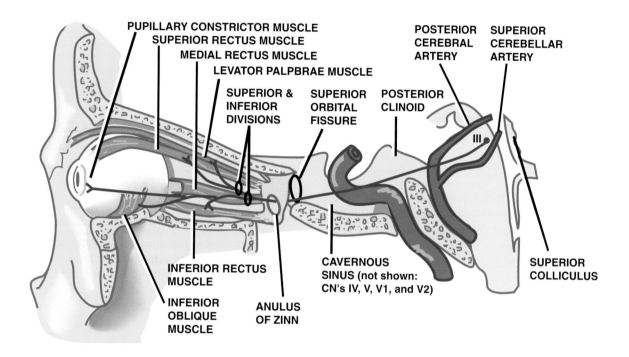

Topographic Localization of Third Nerve Lesions

See **Fig. 18.11**.

There are three major regions where a third nerve lesion may be produced: (1) nuclear, or within the third nerve nucleus; (2) fascicular, or involving the fibers of the third nerve within the brainstem; and (3) subarachnoid, or involving the third nerve as it passes through the subarachnoid space.

Nuclear Third Nerve Lesions

Nuclear third nerve lesions are rare. Nevertheless, three major patterns of deficits are associated with nuclear third nerve lesions: (1) complete third nerve palsy (including ptosis) on the ipsilateral side, plus ptosis and superior rectus palsy on the opposite side; (2) bilateral ptosis with normal extraocular movements; and (3) bilateral third nerve palsy with lid sparing.

Fascicular Third Nerve Lesions

Two brainstem lesions that involve the fascicular third nerve are (1) Benedikt's syndrome, which comprises an ipsilateral third nerve palsy and a contralateral tremor, usually due to involvement of the red nucleus; and (2) Weber's syndrome, which comprises an ipsilateral third nerve palsy and a contralateral hemiparesis due to involvement of the ipsilateral cerebral peduncle.

Subarachnoid Third Nerve Lesions

Involvement of the third nerve in the subarachnoid space results in symmetric involvement of all divisions of the third nerve, with one exception. The exception is an ischemic lesion. These lesions disproportionately affect the internal portion of the nerve but spare the more peripherally located parasympathetic fibers. The result is a pupil-sparing third nerve palsy.

Cavernous Sinus Third Nerve Lesions

In the cavernous sinus, a third nerve palsy from a compressive lesion is frequently accompanied by other ocular motor nerve lesions and an impairment in the ophthalmic division of the trigeminal nerve. Usually the third nerve palsy is of the pupil-sparing type because compressive lesions in the cavernous sinus preferentially involve only the superior division of the oculomotor nerve, which contains no pupillomotor fibers. Finally, the fronto-orbital pain that is often associated with a cavernous sinus lesion may be the result of the fact that sensory fibers from the ophthalmic division of the trigeminal nerve join the oculomotor nerve within the lateral wall of the cavernous sinus.

Superior Orbital Fissure Third Nerve Lesions

Lesions of the third nerve in this location tend to be indistinguishable from lesions in the cavernous sinus, except that the former lesions are more likely to be associated with proptosis.

Orbital Third Nerve Lesions

Lesions that involve the third nerve in the orbit are frequently associated with other ocular motor signs as well as optic atrophy and proptosis. Isolated involvement of either the superior or inferior division of the oculomotor nerve is most commonly associated with lesions in the orbit.

Fig. 18.11 **Localization of third nerve lesions.**

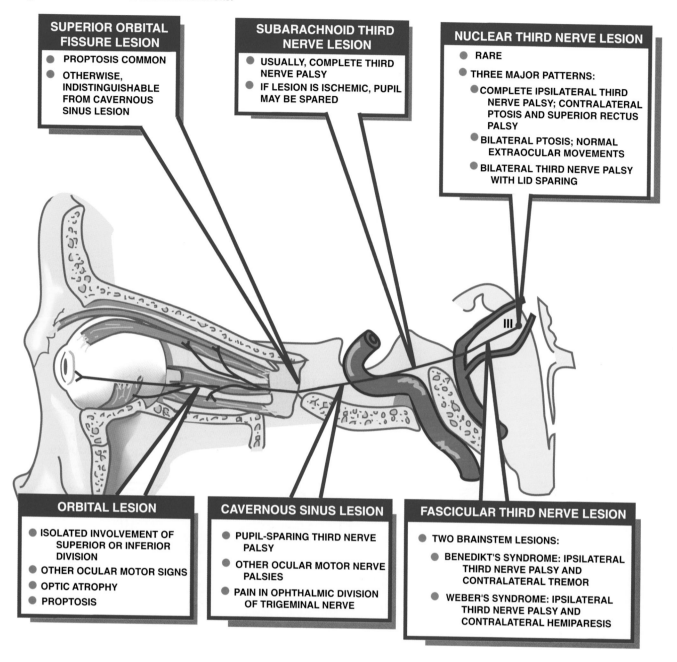

SUPERIOR ORBITAL FISSURE LESION
- PROPTOSIS COMMON
- OTHERWISE, INDISTINGUISHABLE FROM CAVERNOUS SINUS LESION

SUBARACHNOID THIRD NERVE LESION
- USUALLY, COMPLETE THIRD NERVE PALSY
- IF LESION IS ISCHEMIC, PUPIL MAY BE SPARED

NUCLEAR THIRD NERVE LESION
- RARE
- THREE MAJOR PATTERNS:
  - COMPLETE IPSILATERAL THIRD NERVE PALSY; CONTRALATERAL PTOSIS AND SUPERIOR RECTUS PALSY
  - BILATERAL PTOSIS; NORMAL EXTRAOCULAR MOVEMENTS
  - BILATERAL THIRD NERVE PALSY WITH LID SPARING

III

ORBITAL LESION
- ISOLATED INVOLVEMENT OF SUPERIOR OR INFERIOR DIVISION
- OTHER OCULAR MOTOR SIGNS
- OPTIC ATROPHY
- PROPTOSIS

CAVERNOUS SINUS LESION
- PUPIL-SPARING THIRD NERVE PALSY
- OTHER OCULAR MOTOR NERVE PALSIES
- PAIN IN OPHTHALMIC DIVISION OF TRIGEMINAL NERVE

FASCICULAR THIRD NERVE LESION
- TWO BRAINSTEM LESIONS:
  - BENEDIKT'S SYNDROME: IPSILATERAL THIRD NERVE PALSY AND CONTRALATERAL TREMOR
  - WEBER'S SYNDROME: IPSILATERAL THIRD NERVE PALSY AND CONTRALATERAL HEMIPARESIS

Fourth Nerve

Anatomy

See **Fig. 18.12**.

The fourth nerve originates in the caudal midbrain. Two unique anatomic features of the fourth nerve are (1) that its fibers exit dorsally and (2) that they decussate, via the superior medullary velum, to the opposite side. The fibers course ventrally along the edge of the tentorium, to enter the *cavernous sinus*. Within the cavernous sinus, the fourth nerve courses ventral to the third nerve and dorsal to the ophthalmic division of the fifth nerve. After exiting the cavernous sinus, the nerve passes through the *superior orbital fissure* to enter the orbit, where it innervates the *superior oblique muscle*. The superior oblique muscle depresses and intorts the eye.

Fig. 18.12 **Anatomy of fourth nerve.**

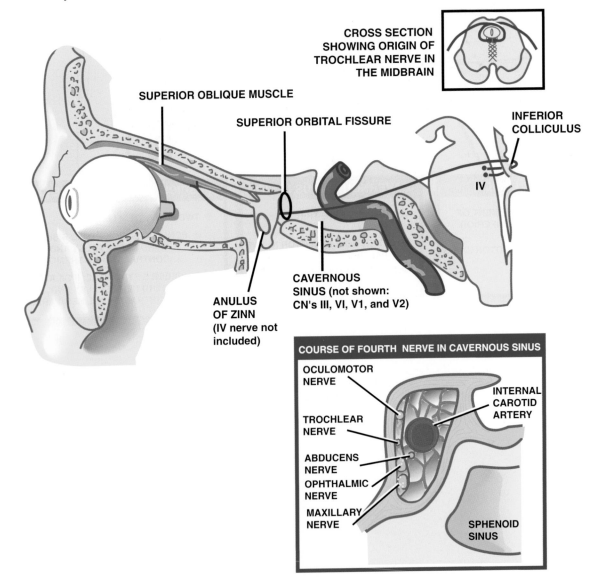

Topographic Localization of Fourth Nerve Lesions

See **Fig. 18.13**.

Isolated nuclear or fascicular lesions of the fourth nerve are rare. The most common fourth nerve lesion is a contusion of the nerve in its subarachnoid course against the edge of the tentorium. Bilateral lesions are not rare.

In a unilateral palsy (**Fig. 18.14**), the patient complains of vertical diplopia that is made worse when the gaze is directed down and to the opposite side (such as is required to walk down stairs). These patients tilt their heads to the side opposite the paretic muscle to decrease the degree of diplopia. Isolated lesions of the fourth nerve in the cavernous sinus or the superior orbital fissure are uncommon. Vertical diplopia due to a lesion in the orbit is more often caused by direct damage to the superior oblique muscle or trochlea.

Fig. 18.13 Localization of fourth nerve lesions.

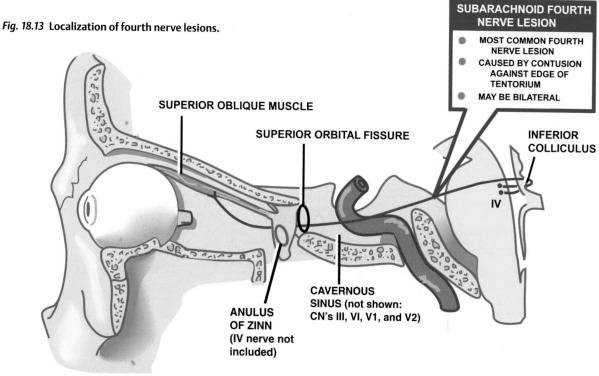

Fig. 18.14 Unilateral fourth nerve palsy.

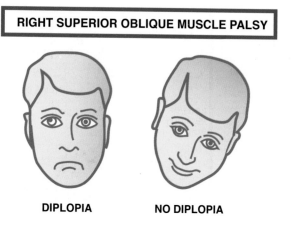

Sixth Nerve

Anatomy

See **Fig. 18.15**.

The sixth nerve originates in the pons. It exits ventrally in the pons in the horizontal sulcus between the pons and medulla. In its subarachnoid course, the sixth nerve ascends along the base of the pons in the prepontine cistern and enters Dorello's canal beneath *Grüber's (petroclinoid) ligament*. It travels in the subarachnoid space along the clivus before it enters the *cavernous sinus*. In the cavernous sinus, the sixth nerve lies between the carotid artery medially and the ophthalmic branch of the *trigeminal nerve* laterally. Thus, unlike the other cranial nerves, which are located in the dural wall, the sixth nerve is more free floating in the cavernous sinus. After passing through the *superior orbital fissure* to enter the orbit, the sixth nerve innervates the *lateral rectus muscle*.

Fig. 18.15 Anatomy of sixth nerve.

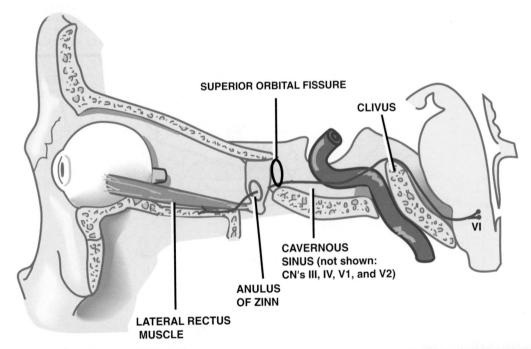

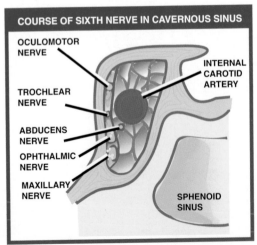

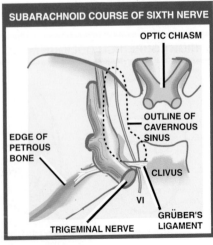

Topographic Localization of Sixth Nerve Lesions

See **Fig. 18.16**.

The sixth nerve palsy is the most common isolated ocular motor nerve palsy. Lesions involving the sixth nerve nucleus cause both an ipsilateral lateral rectus palsy and an ipsilateral gaze palsy. The latter occurs because of involvement of the abducens interneurons. These interneurons send their axons to the contralateral third nerve nucleus via the contralateral medial longitudinal fasciculus.

Lesions of the sixth nerve fascicles are frequently associated with an ipsilateral seventh nerve palsy and a contralateral hemiparesis (Millard-Gubler syndrome).

The most common cause of a sixth nerve lesion in its subarachnoid course is increased intracranial pressure. This results in a sixth nerve palsy that may be associated with ipsilateral facial pain due to stretching of the root of the trigeminal nerve.

Fig. 18.16 Localization of sixth nerve lesions.

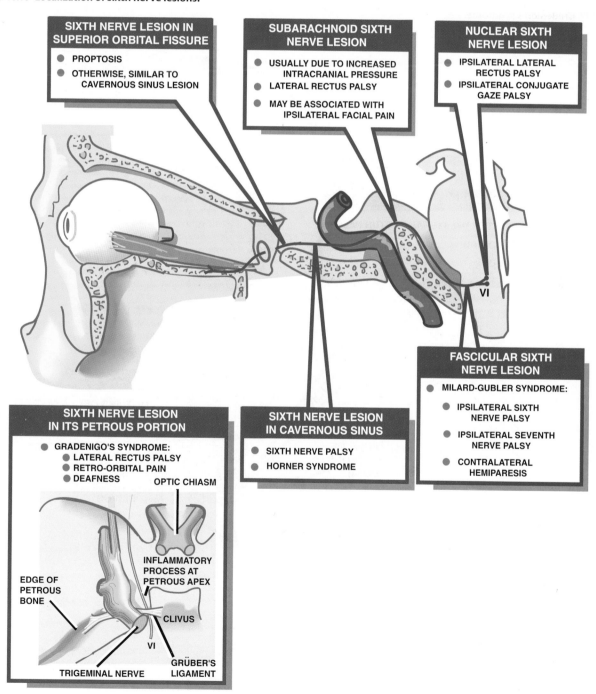

SIXTH NERVE LESION IN SUPERIOR ORBITAL FISSURE
- PROPTOSIS
- OTHERWISE, SIMILAR TO CAVERNOUS SINUS LESION

SUBARACHNOID SIXTH NERVE LESION
- USUALLY DUE TO INCREASED INTRACRANIAL PRESSURE
- LATERAL RECTUS PALSY
- MAY BE ASSOCIATED WITH IPSILATERAL FACIAL PAIN

NUCLEAR SIXTH NERVE LESION
- IPSILATERAL LATERAL RECTUS PALSY
- IPSILATERAL CONJUGATE GAZE PALSY

FASCICULAR SIXTH NERVE LESION
- MILARD-GUBLER SYNDROME:
  - IPSILATERAL SIXTH NERVE PALSY
  - IPSILATERAL SEVENTH NERVE PALSY
  - CONTRALATERAL HEMIPARESIS

SIXTH NERVE LESION IN ITS PETROUS PORTION
- GRADENIGO'S SYNDROME:
  - LATERAL RECTUS PALSY
  - RETRO-ORBITAL PAIN
  - DEAFNESS

OPTIC CHIASM
INFLAMMATORY PROCESS AT PETROUS APEX
EDGE OF PETROUS BONE
CLIVUS
VI
TRIGEMINAL NERVE
GRÜBER'S LIGAMENT

SIXTH NERVE LESION IN CAVERNOUS SINUS
- SIXTH NERVE PALSY
- HORNER SYNDROME

A lesion of the sixth nerve in its petrous portion (i.e., in Dorello's canal) may result in Gradenigo's syndrome (**Fig. 18.17**). Gradenigo's syndrome is a clinical triad caused by an inflammatory process at the petrous apex (petrous apicitis). The triad comprises a lateral rectus palsy (due to involvement of the sixth nerve), retro-orbital pain (due to involvement of the fifth nerve), and deafness (due to involvement of the eighth nerve).

Fig. 18.17 **Gradenigo's syndrome.**

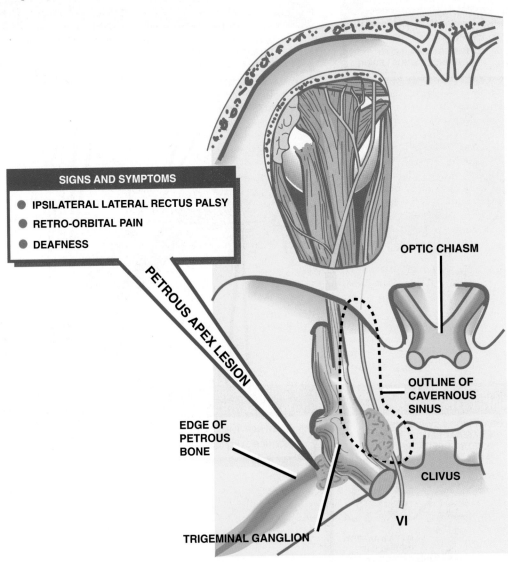

SIGNS AND SYMPTOMS

- IPSILATERAL LATERAL RECTUS PALSY
- RETRO-ORBITAL PAIN
- DEAFNESS

PETROUS APEX LESION

OPTIC CHIASM

OUTLINE OF CAVERNOUS SINUS

EDGE OF PETROUS BONE

CLIVUS

VI

TRIGEMINAL GANGLION

Involvement of the sixth nerve within the *cavernous sinus* typically results in Horner syndrome, in addition to a sixth nerve palsy (Parkinson's syndrome). This is because the sympathetic fibers to the eye join the sixth nerve for a short distance within the cavernous sinus. A similar syndrome may be caused by a lesion at the *superior orbital fissure* (**Fig. 18.18**), although this is frequently associated with proptosis.

Fig. 18.18 **Superior orbital fissure syndrome.**

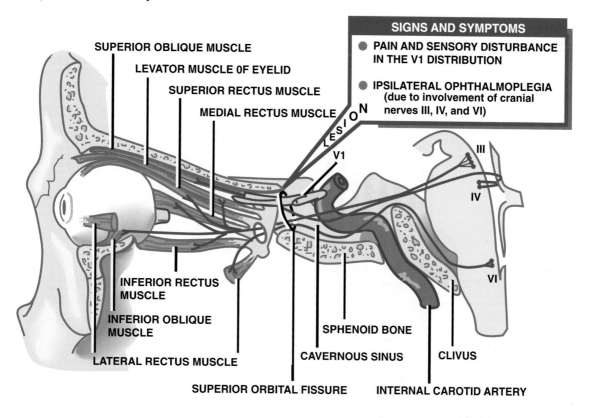

SIGNS AND SYMPTOMS

- PAIN AND SENSORY DISTURBANCE IN THE V1 DISTRIBUTION
- IPSILATERAL OPHTHALMOPLEGIA (due to involvement of cranial nerves III, IV, and VI)

SUPERIOR OBLIQUE MUSCLE

LEVATOR MUSCLE OF EYELID

SUPERIOR RECTUS MUSCLE

MEDIAL RECTUS MUSCLE

LESION

V1

III

IV

VI

INFERIOR RECTUS MUSCLE

INFERIOR OBLIQUE MUSCLE

LATERAL RECTUS MUSCLE

SPHENOID BONE

CAVERNOUS SINUS

SUPERIOR ORBITAL FISSURE

CLIVUS

INTERNAL CAROTID ARTERY

Nystagmus

Nystagmus is a biphasic ocular oscillation that comprises a fast component and a slow component. By convention, the direction of the nystagmus is defined as the direction of the fast component. The neurophysiological basis of nystagmus is described in Chapter 17. In this section, the identifying features and the localizing value of the common and classic forms of nystagmus are briefly described.

Optokinetic Nystagmus

See **Fig. 18.19**.

Optokinetic nystagmus is elicited by moving a repetitive visual stimulus through the visual field. The slow phase of this nystagmus comprises a pursuit movement that follows the moving target. The fast phase comprises a saccade in the opposite direction. A lesion that involves the pursuit or saccadic pathways will disrupt this induced form of physiological nystagmus.

Fig. 18.19 **Optokinetic nystagmus.**

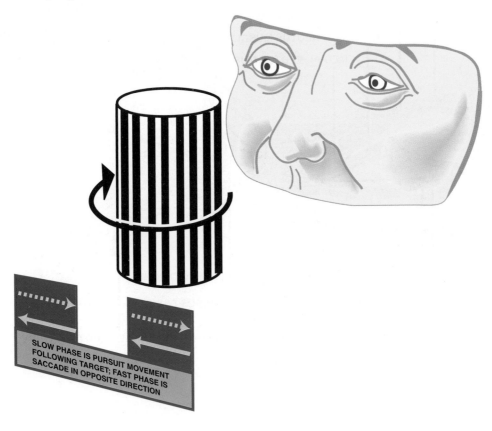

SLOW PHASE IS PURSUIT MOVEMENT FOLLOWING TARGET; FAST PHASE IS SACCADE IN OPPOSITE DIRECTION

Vestibular Nystagmus

See **Fig. 18.20**.

Normally, the vestibular apparatus sends impulses to the paramedian pontine reticular formation (PPRF). In turn, the PPRF sends impulses that reach the ipsilateral lateral rectus muscle and the contralateral medial rectus muscle via the medial longitudinal fasciculus. Any disturbance in the balance of vestibular input between the two sides will result in vestibular nystagmus with a slow component to the side opposite the lesion. This nystagmus is typically associated with a rotatory component. It may be induced by caloric stimulation or rotation of the head.

Fig. 18.20 **Vestibular nystagmus.**

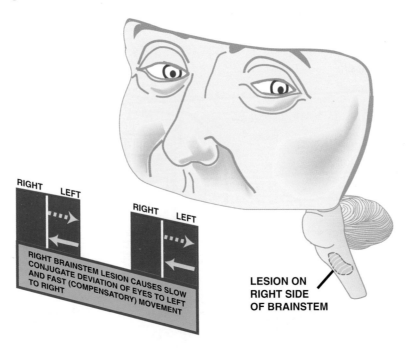

Drug-Induced Nystagmus

See **Fig. 18.21**.

Drug-induced nystagmus is the most common type of nystagmus seen in clinical practice. It is characterized by a horizontal gaze–evoked nystagmus. The drugs that most commonly cause drug-induced nystagmus are alcohol, phenytoin (Dilantin), and barbiturates. Phenytoin toxicity may be quantitated by the degree of associated nystagmus. Barbiturate intoxication will cause degeneration of smooth pursuit movements, followed later by degeneration of saccadic eye movements. Finally, severe barbiturate intoxication eliminates even caloric responses. Thus, the patient with absent caloric responses but an intact pupillary light reflex may be in a metabolic (barbiturate) coma.

Fig. 18.21 **Drug-induced nystagmus.**

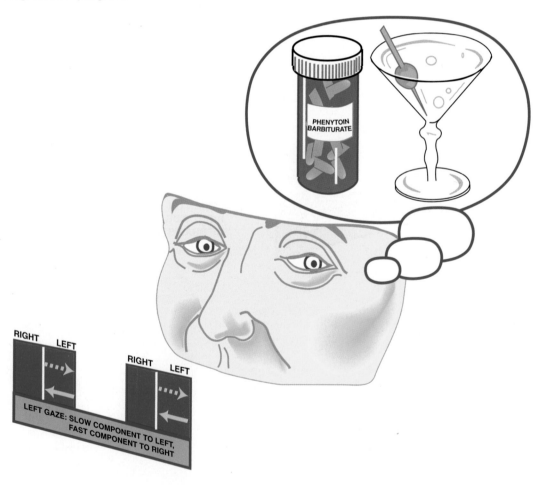

Physiologic End-Point Nystagmus

See **Fig. 18.22**.

Physiologic end-point nystagmus is observed on extreme lateral or upward gaze. It is distinguished from pathological nystagmus by its symmetry on the right and left side and by the absence of associated neurologic signs.

Fig. 18.22 **Physiologic end-point nystagmus.**

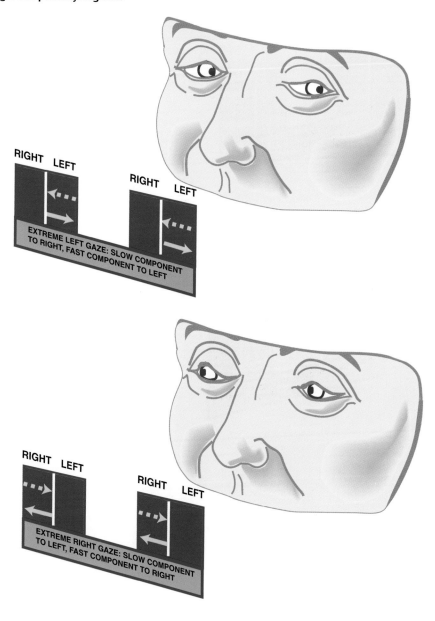

Gaze-Evoked Nystagmus

See **Fig. 18.23**.

Gaze-evoked nystagmus is similar to that induced by drugs. Typically, it is associated with *brainstem* or *cerebellar disease*. Bilateral horizontal gaze–evoked nystagmus is usually also associated with nystagmus on upgaze, but rarely is there downbeat nystagmus on downgaze.

Fig. 18.23 **Gaze-evoked nystagmus.**

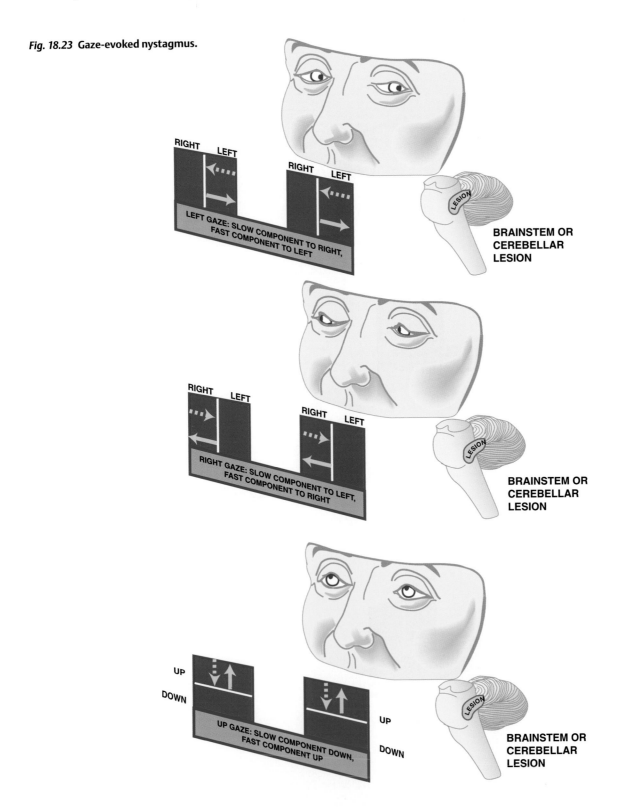

Gaze-Paretic Nystagmus

See **Fig. 18.24**.

Gaze-paretic nystagmus occurs in persons who seem unable to sustain an eccentric gaze. The eyes have a tendency to wander toward the primary position. Corrective saccadic movements to the eccentric position define this type of nystagmus. The most common cause of gaze-paretic nystagmus is drug intoxication.

Fig. 18.24 **Gaze-paretic nystagmus.**

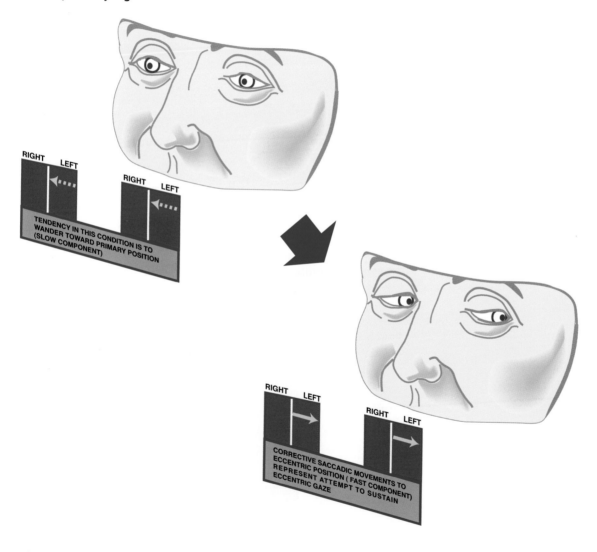

Rebound Nystagmus

See **Fig. 18.25**.

Rebound nystagmus is a horizontal jerk nystagmus that is associated with cerebellar disease. It characteristically appears to fatigue and change direction when lateral gaze is sustained or when the eyes are returned to primary position.

Fig. 18.25 **Rebound nystagmus.**

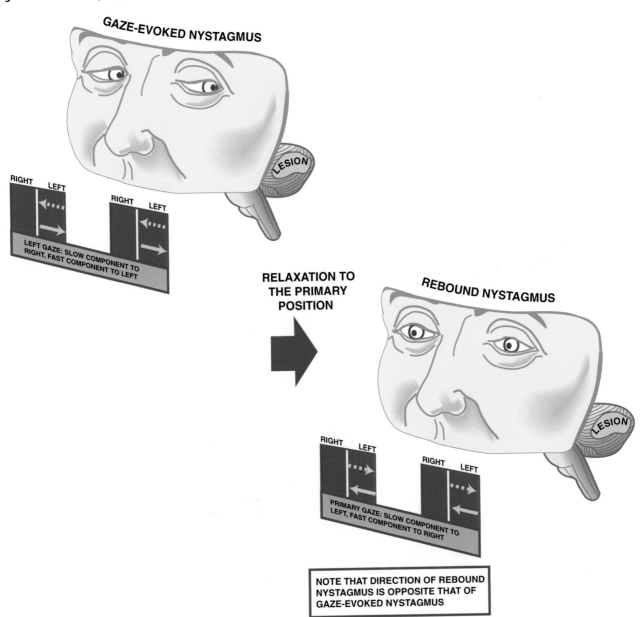

GAZE-EVOKED NYSTAGMUS

RIGHT LEFT RIGHT LEFT

LEFT GAZE: SLOW COMPONENT TO RIGHT, FAST COMPONENT TO LEFT

LESION

RELAXATION TO THE PRIMARY POSITION

REBOUND NYSTAGMUS

RIGHT LEFT RIGHT LEFT

PRIMARY GAZE: SLOW COMPONENT TO LEFT, FAST COMPONENT TO RIGHT

LESION

NOTE THAT DIRECTION OF REBOUND NYSTAGMUS IS OPPOSITE THAT OF GAZE-EVOKED NYSTAGMUS

Downbeat Nystagmus

See **Fig. 18.26**.

Downbeat nystagmus is associated with lesions at the *foramen magnum*. It is characterized by a slow component in the upward direction and a fast component in the downward direction. Unlike gaze-evoked downbeat nystagmus, which only occurs when the eyes are not in the primary position, true downbeat nystagmus is present in the primary position.

Fig. 18.26 **Downbeat nystagmus.**

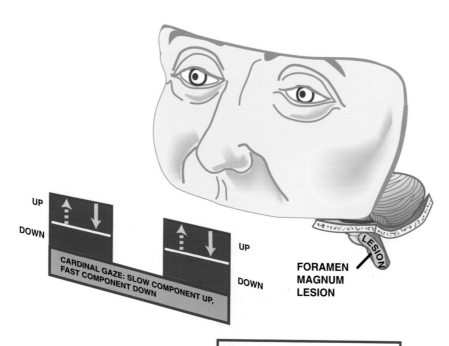

UP
DOWN

UP
DOWN

CARDINAL GAZE: SLOW COMPONENT UP, FAST COMPONENT DOWN

FORAMEN
MAGNUM
LESION

LESION

NOTE THAT DOWNBEAT NYSTAGMUS OCCURS WHEN EYES ARE IN PRIMARY POSITION. COMPARE GAZE-EVOKED NYSTAGMUS, WHICH OCCURS IN VERTICAL GAZE.

Upbeat Nystagmus

See **Fig. 18.27**.

Upbeat nystagmus is associated with medullary lesions. It is characterized by a slow component in the downward direction and a fast component in the upward direction. Unlike gaze-evoked upbeat nystagmus, which only occurs when the eyes are not in the primary position, true upbeat nystagmus is present in the primary position.

Fig. 18.27 **Upbeat nystagmus.**

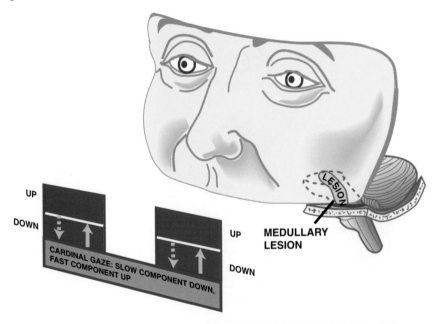

UP

DOWN

CARDINAL GAZE: SLOW COMPONENT DOWN, FAST COMPONENT UP

UP

DOWN

MEDULLARY LESION

NOTE THAT UPBEAT NYSTAGMUS OCCURS WHEN EYES ARE IN PRIMARY POSITION. COMPARE GAZE-EVOKED NYSTAGMUS, WHICH OCCURS IN VERTICAL GAZE.

Periodic Alternating Nystagmus

See **Fig. 18.28**.

Periodic alternating nystagmus is characterized by a horizontal jerk nystagmus that periodically (e.g., every 60 to 90 s) changes direction. It is most commonly associated with *foramen magnum lesions*.

Fig. 18.28 **Periodic alternating nystagmus.**

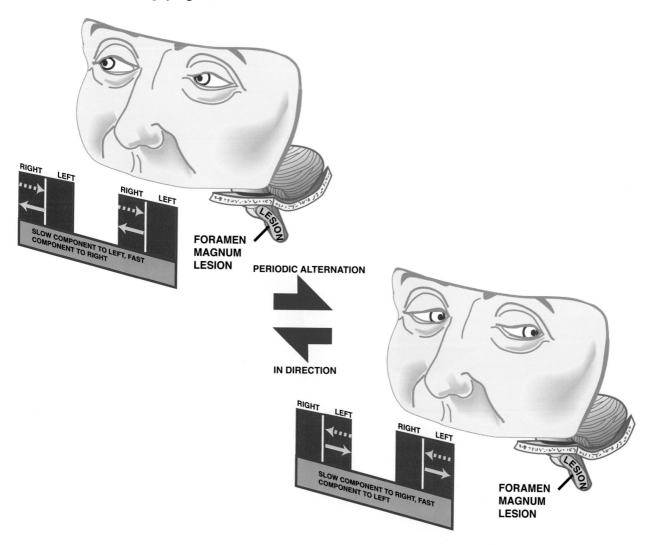

Seesaw Nystagmus

See **Fig. 18.29**.

Seesaw nystagmus is a dysconjugate nystagmus in which one eye rises and intorts while the other eye falls and extorts. It is most commonly associated with *diencephalic* and *midbrain lesions*.

Spasmus Nutans

See **Fig. 18.30**.

Spasmus nutans is a syndrome of infancy, which typically resolves spontaneously when the child is 3 or 4 years old. It comprises a clinical triad of head nodding, nystagmus, and head turning. The nystagmus is frequently monocular and variable.

Fig. 18.29 **Seesaw nystagmus.**

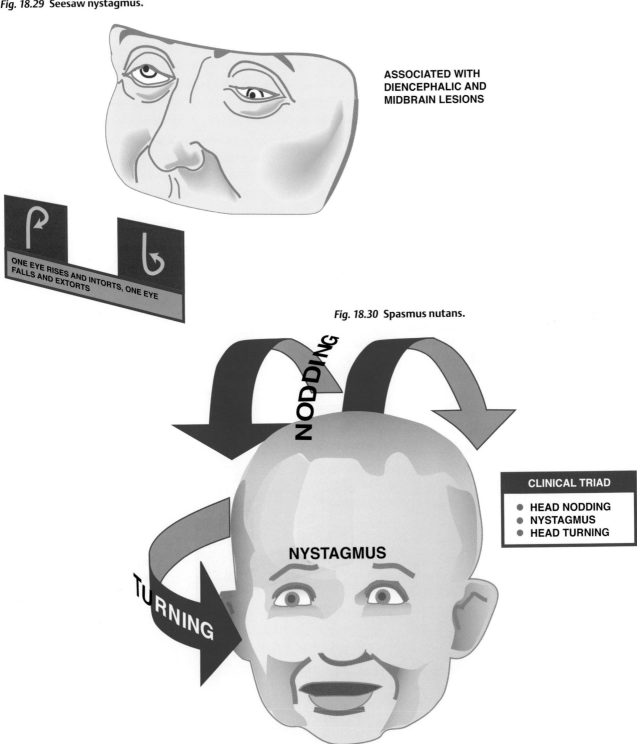

ASSOCIATED WITH DIENCEPHALIC AND MIDBRAIN LESIONS

ONE EYE RISES AND INTORTS, ONE EYE FALLS AND EXTORTS

Fig. 18.30 **Spasmus nutans.**

NODDING

TURNING

NYSTAGMUS

CLINICAL TRIAD
- HEAD NODDING
- NYSTAGMUS
- HEAD TURNING

Convergence Retraction Nystagmus

See **Fig. 18.31**.

Convergence retraction nystagmus is associated with dorsal midbrain lesions (Parinaud's syndrome). Attempts to gaze upward, in this condition, elicit jerky bilateral eye movements of retraction or convergence or both.

Ocular Bobbing

See **Fig. 18.32**.

Ocular bobbing is associated with massive *pontine lesions*. It is characterized by rapid downward movements of the eyes with a slow return to the primary position.

Fig. 18.31 **Convergence retraction nystagmus.**

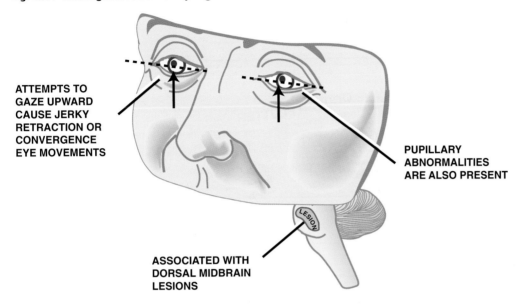

ATTEMPTS TO GAZE UPWARD CAUSE JERKY RETRACTION OR CONVERGENCE EYE MOVEMENTS

PUPILLARY ABNORMALITIES ARE ALSO PRESENT

ASSOCIATED WITH DORSAL MIDBRAIN LESIONS

Fig. 18.32 **Ocular bobbing.**

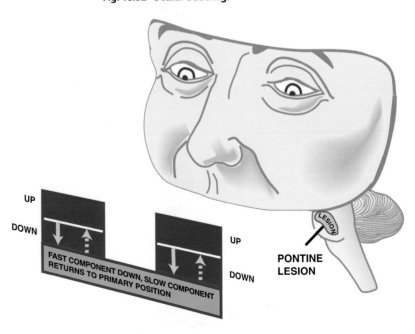

UP

DOWN

UP

DOWN

FAST COMPONENT DOWN, SLOW COMPONENT RETURNS TO PRIMARY POSITION

PONTINE LESION

Ocular Flutter and Opsoclonus

See **Fig. 18.33**.

Ocular flutter comprises a series of small saccades with normal intervening movements that occur upon attempts at fixation.

Opsoclonus is characterized by repetitive, chaotic, saccadic movements that occur in all directions (dancing eyes), preventing fixation. In an adult or older child, opsoclonus may be associated with a postinfectious encephalopathy. In younger children, opsoclonus may develop as a remote effect of neuroblastoma.

Fig. 18.33 Ocular flutter and opsoclonus.

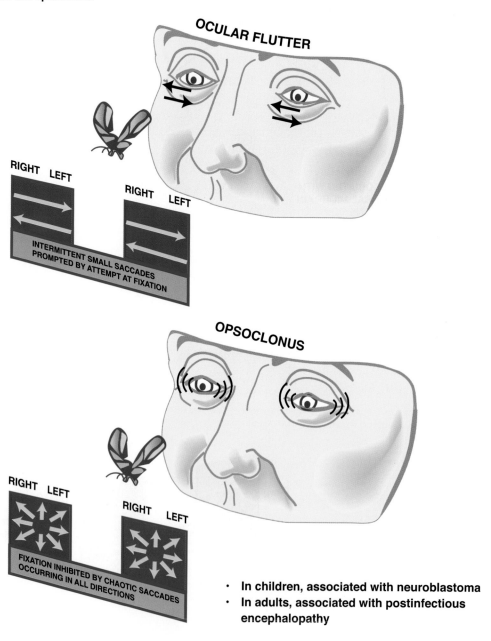

Ocular Dysmetria

See **Fig. 18.34**.

Ocular dysmetria is characterized by a series of undershooting and overshooting saccades that occur on attempts at refixation. Like limb dysmetria, it is associated with lesions of the cerebellar pathways.

Square Wave Jerks

See **Fig. 18.35**.

Square wave jerks comprise pairs of saccades that are directed away from and then back to fixation. Although they may occur in normal persons, they are associated with *cerebellar lesions*.

Fig. 18.34 Ocular dysmetria.

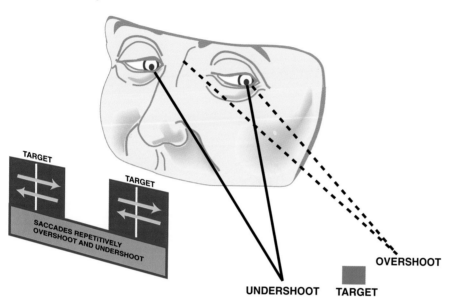

Fig. 18.35 Square wave jerks.

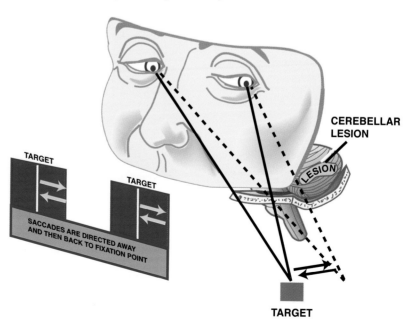

Ocular Myoclonus

See **Fig. 18.36**.

Ocular myoclonus is characterized by a continuous rhythmic oscillation of the eyes. It is invariably accompanied by myoclonic movements of the branchial musculature, such as the palate, the pharynx, or the face. Associated structural lesions typically involve the myoclonic triangle, which comprises the red nucleus, the ipsilateral inferior olive, and the contralateral dentate nucleus.

The Pupil

Innervation of the pupil comprises both sympathetic and parasympathetic input. These two sources of input are reciprocal in action: sympathetic activation causes pupillary dilatation; parasympathetic activation causes pupillary constriction.

Fig. 18.36 **Ocular myoclonus.**

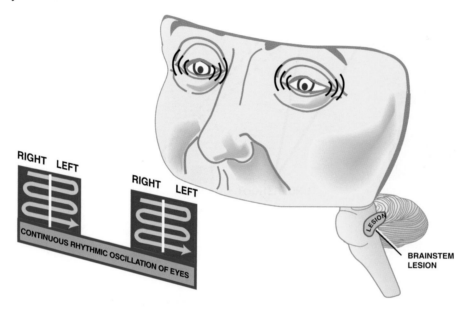

Sympathetic Innervation

See **Fig. 18.37**.

The sympathetic innervation of the pupil originates in the posterior hypothalamus. The *first-order neuron* that is projected by the hypothalamus proceeds through the lateral tegmentum of the brainstem to reach the *intermediolateral gray matter* of the *C8–T2* segments of the spinal cord. The intermediolateral gray matter projects a *second-order neuron*, which sends fibers through the sympathetic chain to reach the *superior cervical ganglion*. The superior cervical ganglion projects a *third-order neuron*, which joins the internal *carotid artery* to enter the *cavernous sinus*. The third-order neuron joins the ophthalmic branch of the trigeminal nerve to enter the orbit, reaching the pupillodilator muscles via the *long ciliary nerve*.

In addition to the sympathetic fibers that innervate the pupil, there are two other groups of sympathetic fibers that travel only part of the distance of the pupillodilator pathway. The first of these groups of fibers follows the *external carotid artery*, rather than the internal carotid artery, to innervate the sweat glands of the face (sudomotor and vasomotor fibers to the face). A second group of fibers continues along the internal carotid artery past the cavernous sinus to follow the ophthalmic artery to the orbit. These fibers supply the superior tarsal muscles, which are responsible for elevation of the upper eyelid.

Fig. 18.37 **Sympathetic innervation of pupil.**

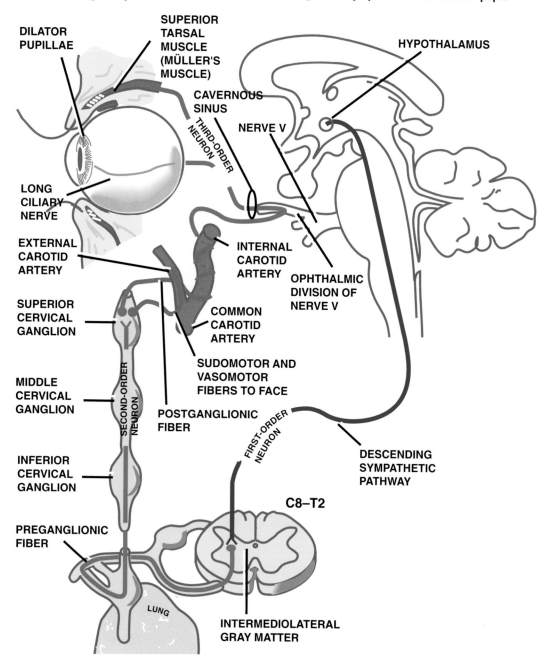

Parasympathetic Innervation

See **Fig. 18.38**.

Parasympathetic pupilloconstrictor fibers originate in the *Edinger-Westphal nucleus* of the oculomotor complex. These preganglionic fibers accompany the oculomotor nerve through the subarachnoid space, *cavernous sinus*, and *superior orbital fissure* and into the orbit. Within the orbit these fibers follow the inferior division of the oculomotor nerve until they terminate in the *ciliary ganglion*. The ciliary ganglion is located on the temporal side of the ophthalmic artery between the optic nerve and the lateral rectus muscle. Postganglionic neurons in the ciliary ganglion reach the pupilloconstrictor muscles via the short ciliary nerves.

Pupillary Abnormalities

A few of the pupillary abnormalities described here are frequently seen in clinical practice. Several other of the abnormalities are described more often than seen but are included in this discussion because they are classic clinical findings that tend to appear on board examinations.

Fig. 18.38 **Parasympathetic innervation of pupil.**

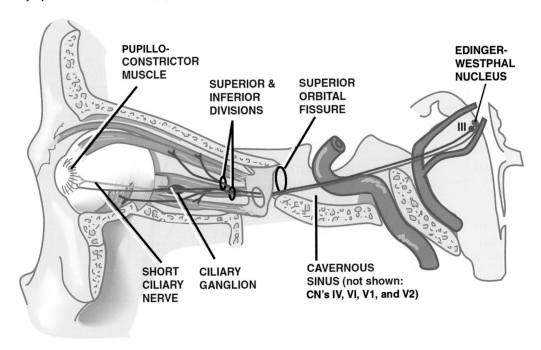

Marcus Gunn Pupil

See **Fig. 18.39**.

The Marcus Gunn pupil is associated with an afferent pupillary defect. An afferent pupillary defect is a dysfunction in the afferent fiber anatomy of the pupil, that is, the optic nerve. It may be seen in conditions such as optic atrophy. In fact, the Marcus Gunn pupil is one of the most sensitive indicators of optic nerve dysfunction. This pupillary abnormality may be detected on examination by the so-called swinging flashlight test, as follows. Normally, when a flashlight is shone on one eye and then moved quickly to the other, the degree of pupillary constriction that is elicited with each maneuver is equal (i.e., pupillary size remains constant after the flashlight is swung). By contrast, when a flashlight is shone on a good eye and then a bad one (i.e., one with an optic nerve lesion), a transient dilatation of the pupils will be seen as the flashlight is swung to the bad eye. This is because a decreased amount of light is conveyed to the system when a flashlight is shone on the affected eye, due to the affected optic nerve (afferent signal).

Fig. 18.39 **Marcus Gunn pupil.**

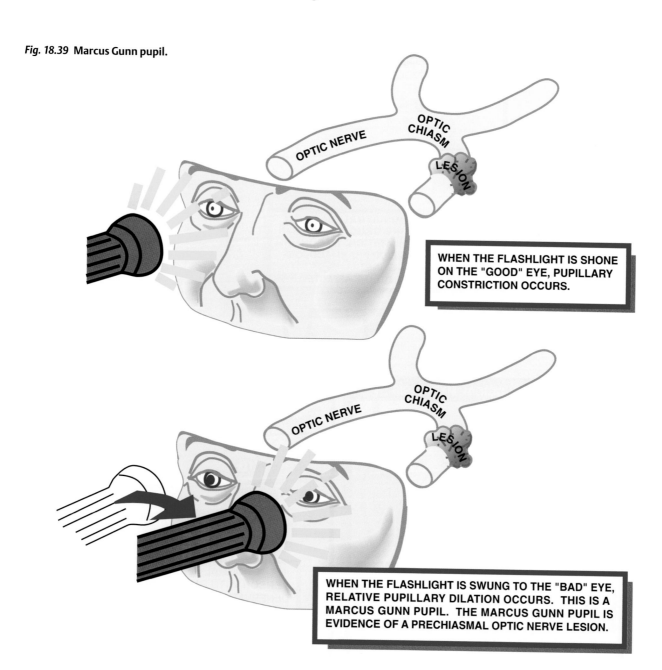

WHEN THE FLASHLIGHT IS SHONE ON THE "GOOD" EYE, PUPILLARY CONSTRICTION OCCURS.

WHEN THE FLASHLIGHT IS SWUNG TO THE "BAD" EYE, RELATIVE PUPILLARY DILATION OCCURS. THIS IS A MARCUS GUNN PUPIL. THE MARCUS GUNN PUPIL IS EVIDENCE OF A PRECHIASMAL OPTIC NERVE LESION.

Pharmacological Mydriasis

See **Fig. 18.40**.

Topical administration of an atropine-like drug will cause pupillary dilatation (mydriasis or cycloplegia) unresponsive to light. The diagnosis of pharmacological blockade requires a high index of suspicion. If suspected, this diagnosis may be confirmed by a pharmacological test, as follows. Instill 1% pilocarpine (acetylcholine) into the affected eye or eyes. In the normal person or in the person with interruption of parasympathetic innervation, the pupil will constrict because the drug acts directly at the neuromuscular junction. In the patient with pharmacological blockade at the neuromuscular junction, however, no pupillary constriction will be observed.

Fig. 18.40 Pharmacological mydriasis.

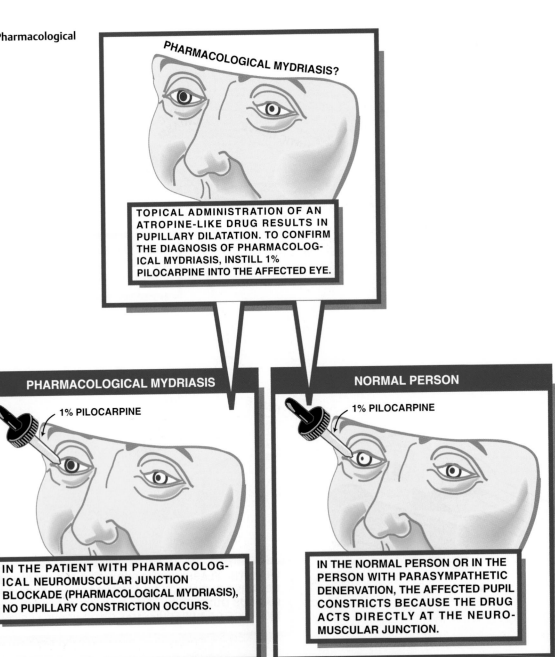

PHARMACOLOGICAL MYDRIASIS?

TOPICAL ADMINISTRATION OF AN ATROPINE-LIKE DRUG RESULTS IN PUPILLARY DILATATION. TO CONFIRM THE DIAGNOSIS OF PHARMACOLOGICAL MYDRIASIS, INSTILL 1% PILOCARPINE INTO THE AFFECTED EYE.

PHARMACOLOGICAL MYDRIASIS

1% PILOCARPINE

IN THE PATIENT WITH PHARMACOLOGICAL NEUROMUSCULAR JUNCTION BLOCKADE (PHARMACOLOGICAL MYDRIASIS), NO PUPILLARY CONSTRICTION OCCURS.

NORMAL PERSON

1% PILOCARPINE

IN THE NORMAL PERSON OR IN THE PERSON WITH PARASYMPATHETIC DENERVATION, THE AFFECTED PUPIL CONSTRICTS BECAUSE THE DRUG ACTS DIRECTLY AT THE NEUROMUSCULAR JUNCTION.

Traumatic Mydriasis

See **Fig. 18.41**.

Ocular trauma may result in a fixed and dilated pupil by one of two mechanisms of injury. A transient loss of parasympathetic tone may accompany ocular trauma in the same manner that loss of sympathetic tone occurs in patients with spinal shock. Alternatively, direct injury to the pupillary sphincter may result in pupillary dilatation. Whereas weak miotics may cause constriction in the former group of patients, patients in the latter group will not respond.

Fig. 18.41 **Traumatic mydriasis.**

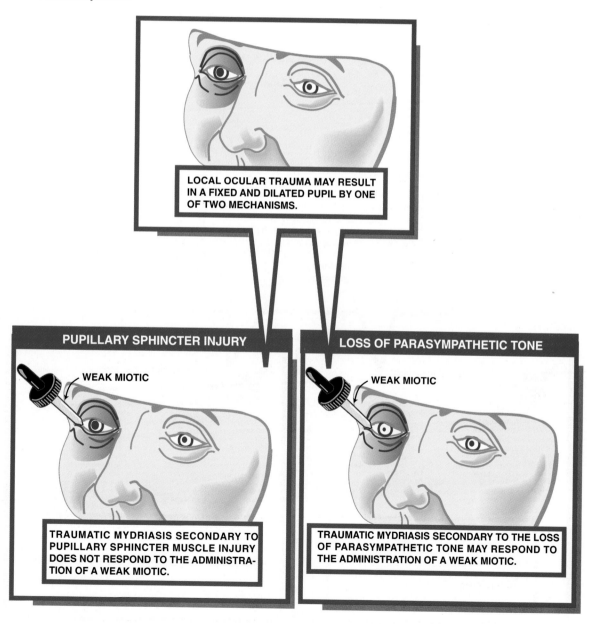

Adie's Tonic Pupil

See **Fig. 18.42**.

The Adie's tonic pupil is a fixed and dilated pupil that is usually unilateral. The underlying defect is a lesion of the ciliary ganglion. The diagnosis of an Adie's pupil may be established by the administration of a very weak parasympathetic (0.125% pilocarpine). Although this solution is ineffective as a pupillary constrictor in normal persons, patients with a tonic pupil exhibit parasympathetic supersensitivity, which leads to pupillary constriction after the instillation of the weak miotic agent.

Fig. 18.42 **Adie's tonic pupil.**

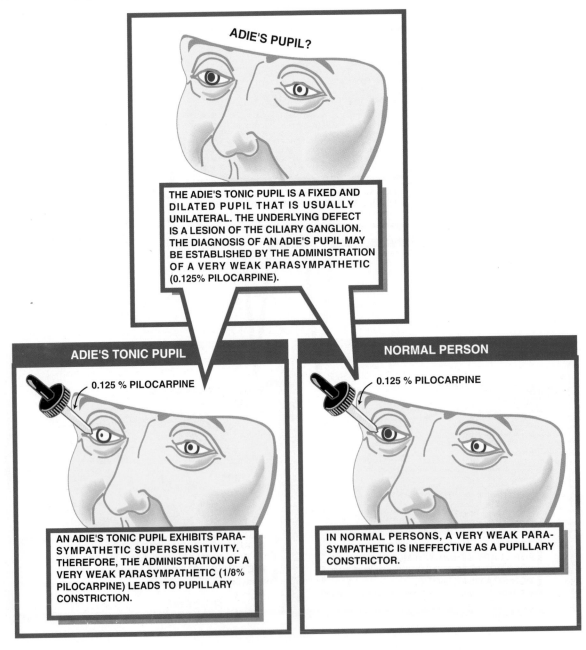

Hutchinson's Pupil ("Blown Pupil")

See **Fig. 18.43**.

In the presence of an expanding supratentorial mass, a central herniation syndrome may cause compression of the third cranial nerve, which gets caught between the herniating uncus and the tentorial edge. Because the parasympathetic fibers of the oculomotor nerve are located peripherally, pupillary dilatation may develop in the absence of other signs of a third nerve palsy. In clinical parlance, this is colloquially referred to as a blown pupil, a cardinal sign of a neurosurgical emergency.

Fig. 18.43 **Hutchinson's pupil.**

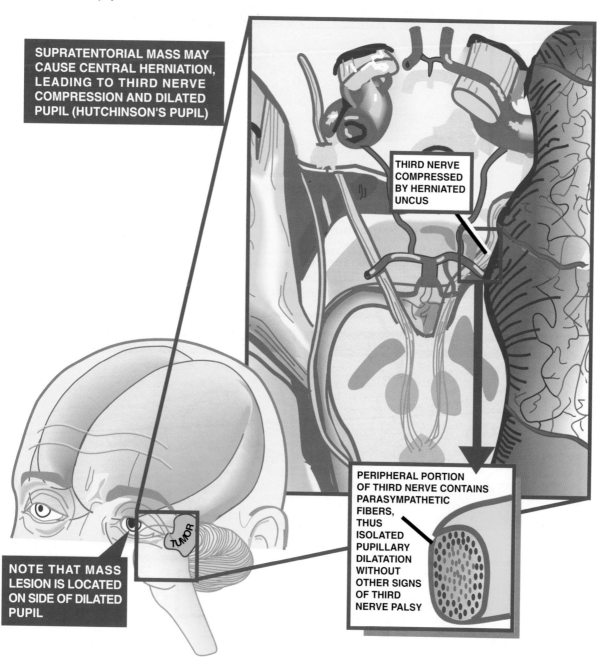

SUPRATENTORIAL MASS MAY CAUSE CENTRAL HERNIATION, LEADING TO THIRD NERVE COMPRESSION AND DILATED PUPIL (HUTCHINSON'S PUPIL)

THIRD NERVE COMPRESSED BY HERNIATED UNCUS

PERIPHERAL PORTION OF THIRD NERVE CONTAINS PARASYMPATHETIC FIBERS, THUS ISOLATED PUPILLARY DILATATION WITHOUT OTHER SIGNS OF THIRD NERVE PALSY

NOTE THAT MASS LESION IS LOCATED ON SIDE OF DILATED PUPIL

TUMOR

Argyll Robertson Pupil

See **Fig. 18.44**.

This condition is associated with neurosyphilis. It is characterized by reaction to near association in the absence of reaction to light. That is, the pupil fails to constrict to light but does react during convergence. This has been referred to as light-near dissociation. The Argyll Robertson pupil tends to be miotic and irregular. Most commonly, there is bilateral involvement.

Fig. 18.44 **Argyll Robertson pupil.**

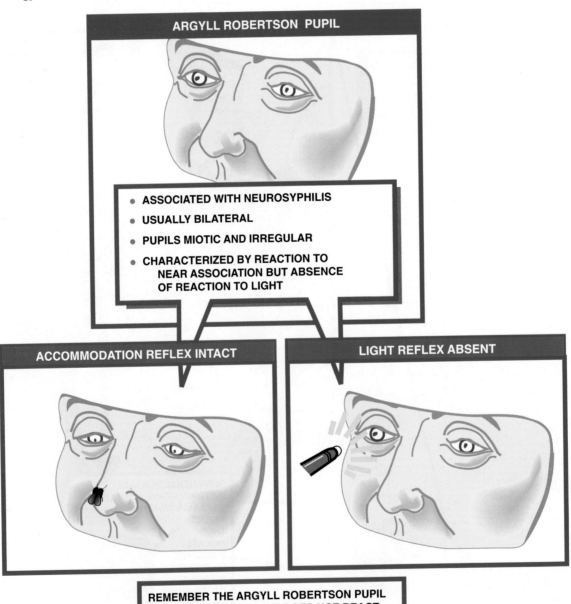

Midbrain Pupillary Abnormalities

See **Fig. 18.45**.

Lesions in the region of the sylvian aqueduct are associated with light-near dissociation (see p. 464). These abnormalities are typically seen as part of a Parinaud's syndrome.

Fig. 18.45 **Midbrain pupillary abnormalities.**

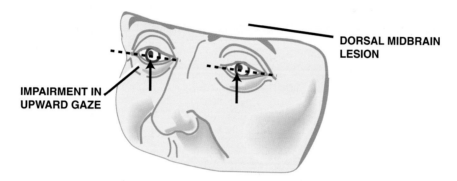

DORSAL MIDBRAIN LESION

IMPAIRMENT IN UPWARD GAZE

MIDBRAIN PUPILLARY ABNORMALITIES

- **ASSOCIATED WITH DORSAL MIDBRAIN LESION** (hydrocephalus, or pineal region tumor)

- **USUALLY PART OF PARINAUD'S SYNDROME**
  - impairment in upgaze
  - pupils react to near vision (accommodation) but not to light

Pinpoint Pupils

See **Fig. 18.46**.

The classic structural lesion associated with pinpoint pupils is a pontine lesion. Other causes of pinpoint pupils are eyedrops and narcotics.

Fig. 18.46 **Pinpoint pupils.**

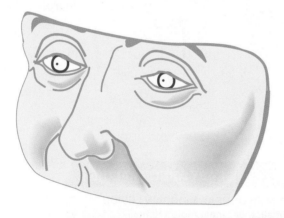

PINPOINT PUPILS

- PONTINE LESION IS MOST COMMON CAUSE
- OTHER CAUSES ARE EYEDROPS AND NARCOTICS

Horner Syndrome

See **Fig. 18.47**.

The underlying defect in Horner syndrome is a lesion in the sympathetic pathway. For lesions of the sympathetic pathway that occur below the bifurcation of the carotid artery, the classic findings of Horner syndrome are (1) ptosis, (2) miosis, and (3) anhydrosis. There may also be apparent enophthalmos, as a result of the narrow palpebral fissure (an appearance that the affected eye is located deeper, "sunken in," compared with the unaffected eye). For lesions that occur above the carotid bifurcation, Horner syndrome comprises only ptosis and miosis. Anhydrosis is absent in lesions at the level of the internal carotid artery or above (e.g., carotid dissection) because sudomotor and vasomotor fibers to the face follow the external carotid artery at the bifurcation.

Pharmacological testing may aid in the establishment of Horner syndrome. The test is performed as follows. Instillation of 10% cocaine solution into each eye blocks reuptake of norepinephrine at the neuroeffector junction. In normal persons, this causes pupillary dilatation. The pupils dilate in normal persons because of the accumulation of norepinephrine (a sympathomimetic) at the pupillodilator muscle. In the patient with Horner syndrome, however, the pupils do not dilate because there is no accumulation of norepinephrine. Blockade of the reuptake of norepinephrine does not cause accumulation of norepinephrine in the Horner patient because they do not release enough norepinephrine for it to accumulate.

Identification of the level of lesion in Horner syndrome (i.e., first neuron, second neuron, or third neuron) may usually be determined on clinical grounds. First-neuron lesions are typically accompanied by other signs of brainstem involvement, such as long tract signs or cranial nerve signs. Second-neuron lesions are usually associated with chest surgery, chest trauma, or pulmonary neoplasms involving the sympathetic plexus. Third-neuron lesions are most common. They are usually caused by pathology in the neck, such as neck trauma, carotid vascular disease, or cervical bony abnormalities. Typically, ipsilateral facial sweating is spared.

Finally, to distinguish Horner syndrome from simple anisocoria (normal pupillary asymmetry), check the pupillary light reflex. If both pupils react normally to light, then the patient may have simple anisocoria. Turn the lights off in the examining room to distinguish between these two possibilities. If the smaller pupil is the abnormal one, then the anisocoria will become more pronounced when the lights are turned off. A "dilatation lag" of the smaller pupils implies poor sympathetic tone and suggests the diagnosis of Horner syndrome.

Fig. 18.47 **Horner syndrome.**

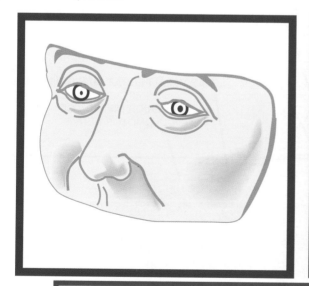 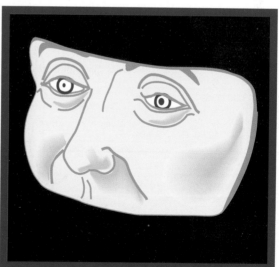

TO DISTINGUISH BETWEEN SIMPLE ANISOCORIA AND HORNER SYNDROME, TURN OFF THE LIGHTS IN THE EXAMINING ROOM. IF THE SMALLER PUPIL IS THE ABNORMAL ONE, HORNER SYNDROME, THEN THE ANISOCORIA, WILL BECOME MORE PRONOUNCED.

The Eyelids

Anatomy

See **Fig. 18.48**.

Eyelid opening is primarily a function of the *levator palpebrae superioris muscle*, which is innervated by the *superior division of the oculomotor nerve*. Two accessory muscles also contribute to eyelid opening. The *superior tarsal muscle*, or Müller's muscle, is embedded in the levator muscle and inserts on the tarsal plate. It is innervated by sympathetic fibers. The *frontalis muscle* helps to retract the eyelid in extreme upgaze. It is innervated by the facial nerve.

Both the levator and superior rectus are innervated by the superior division of the oculomotor nerve. To coordinate simultaneous eyelid opening and upward gaze, the tone of the levator and superior rectus must remain relatively equal and constant. During forced lid closure, however, there is an inverse relationship between these two muscles such that forced lid closure is accompanied by elevation of the eyes (Bell's phenomenon).

Normal eyelid closure is associated with loss of tone in the levator muscle. Forced eyelid closure is caused by contraction of the *orbicularis oculi muscle*, which is innervated by the facial nerve.

Fig. 18.48 **Eyelid anatomy.**

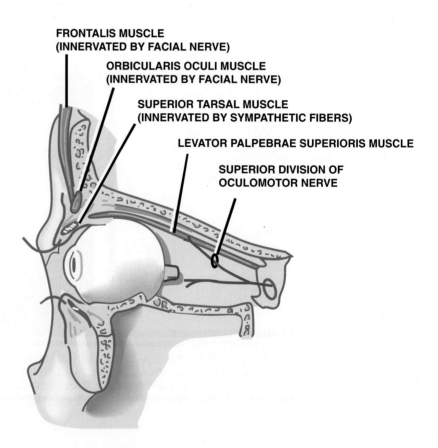

**FRONTALIS MUSCLE
(INNERVATED BY FACIAL NERVE)**

**ORBICULARIS OCULI MUSCLE
(INNERVATED BY FACIAL NERVE)**

**SUPERIOR TARSAL MUSCLE
(INNERVATED BY SYMPATHETIC FIBERS)**

LEVATOR PALPEBRAE SUPERIORIS MUSCLE

**SUPERIOR DIVISION OF
OCULOMOTOR NERVE**

Eyelid Abnormalities

See **Fig. 18.49**.

Ptosis is the paralytic drooping of the upper eyelid. Complete ptosis is usually caused by a third nerve palsy (loss of tone in the levator muscle), which is frequently also accompanied by pupillary dilatation and diplopia. Ptosis that is equal to or less than 2 mm may be caused by Horner syndrome (loss of tone in Müller's muscle), which is usually also accompanied by miosis and anhydrosis. There are many other causes of ptosis. Myasthenia gravis is typically associated with bilateral ptosis. Frequently it is also accompanied by weakness of eyelid closure and diplopia.

Eyelid retraction is present when there is sclera showing between the iris and the eyelid. Thyroid ophthalmopathy is a common cause of eyelid retraction. It is caused by a pathological shortening of the levator muscle. Bilateral eyelid retraction, or Collier's sign, is indicative of a dorsal midbrain lesion. It is frequently accompanied by light-near dissociation, and, unlike thyroid ophthalmopathy, there is no suggestion of lid retraction on downward gaze (Graefe's sign). Lower eyelid retraction may be the earliest clinical lid sign of a facial nerve lesion, which is the most common cause of lower eyelid retraction.

Fig. 18.49 **Ptosis.**

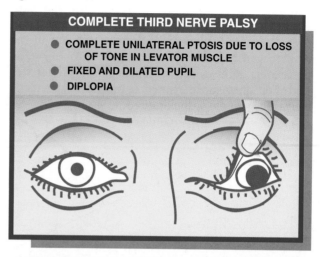

COMPLETE THIRD NERVE PALSY
- COMPLETE UNILATERAL PTOSIS DUE TO LOSS OF TONE IN LEVATOR MUSCLE
- FIXED AND DILATED PUPIL
- DIPLOPIA

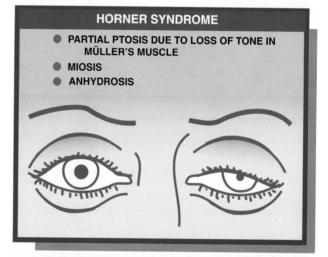

HORNER SYNDROME
- PARTIAL PTOSIS DUE TO LOSS OF TONE IN MÜLLER'S MUSCLE
- MIOSIS
- ANHYDROSIS

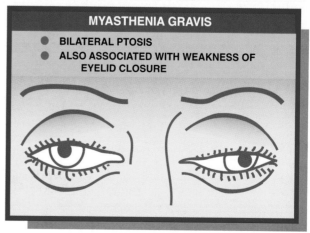

MYASTHENIA GRAVIS
- BILATERAL PTOSIS
- ALSO ASSOCIATED WITH WEAKNESS OF EYELID CLOSURE

19 Motor System

The motor system is complex and has many components. The system is composed of both supraspinal and spinal pathways. These may be further broken down into pathways that begin in the cortex and the brainstem. Moreover, there are cortical and subcortical regions of the brain that are concerned with higher order control of the descending pathways. This chapter presents a description of the anatomic integration of these components, as well as the neurologic implications.

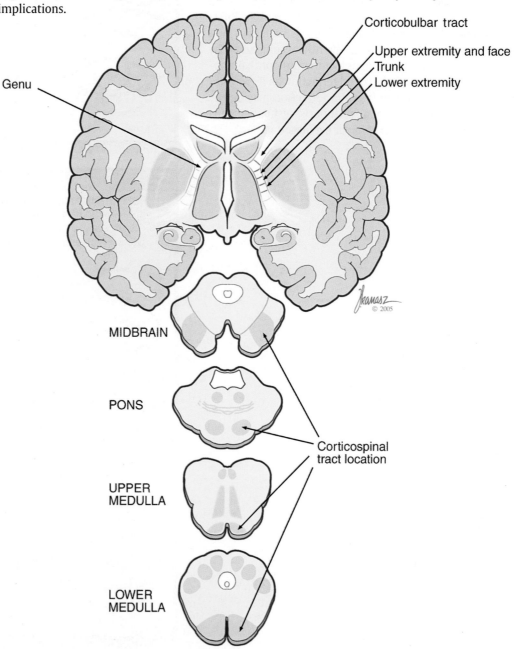

Fig. 19.1 Subcortical and corticospinal pathways.

Corticobulbar tract

Upper extremity and face
Trunk
Lower extremity

Genu

MIDBRAIN

PONS

Corticospinal tract location

UPPER MEDULLA

LOWER MEDULLA

Cortex

Corticospinal Tract

See **Figs. 19.1** and **19.2**.

The corticospinal (pyramidal) tract drives skilled and precise movement of the upper and lower extremities. Its mechanism of action is via the contraction of individual muscles.

The tract begins in the precentral gyrus (primary motor cortex, Brodmann's area 4). The primary motor cortex is arranged somatotopically. Stimulation of the primary motor cortex results in individual muscle contractions. These contractions, however, are only a small aspect of complex movements. Other regions of the cortex (i.e., premotor cortex) are involved in and help coordinate complex muscle activity (see later discussion).

The *corticospinal tract* is composed of ~1 million fibers. Approximately 30% arise from lamina V of the primary motor cortex, 30% from the premotor cortex, and 40% from the parietal lobe (sensory).

Fig. 19.2 **Corticospinal tract.**

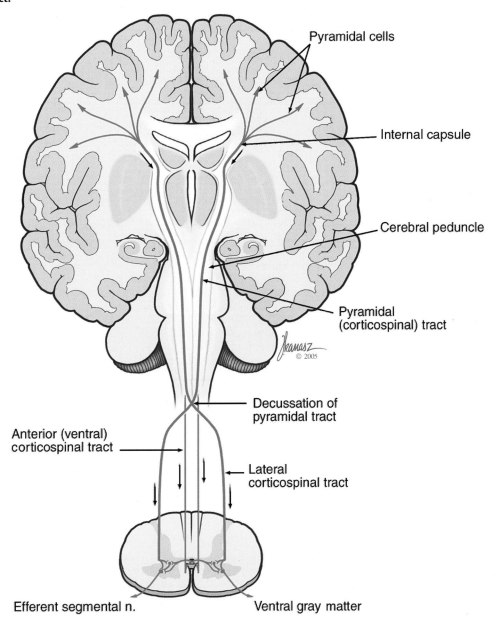

Pyramidal cells

Internal capsule

Cerebral peduncle

Pyramidal (corticospinal) tract

Decussation of pyramidal tract

Anterior (ventral) corticospinal tract

Lateral corticospinal tract

Efferent segmental n.

Ventral gray matter

Course of the Corticospinal Tract

See **Fig. 19.3**.

Axons leaving the cerebral cortex descend toward the brainstem by way of the *corona radiata*. They then converge and descend into and through the posterior limb of the *internal capsule*. The fibers in the posterior limb of the internal capsule are arranged topographically, with those of the upper extremity located in the rostral part and those of the lower extremity located more caudally.

Axons then pass through and form the *cerebral peduncles* of the midbrain along with other descending cortical fibers. The pyramidal fibers remain distinct and occupy the middle two thirds of the peduncles. Axons continue on as the descending *pyramidal tract* through the *pons* and form the pyramids on the ventral aspect of the *medulla*. In the lower medulla, ~90% of the fibers of the pyramids decussate. The decussated fibers then form the *lateral corticospinal tract* in the lateral funiculus of the spinal cord. These neurons are termed upper motor neurons. This terminology is important to note when evaluating a patient with motor weakness (see later discussion).

The upper motor neurons of the lateral corticospinal tract descend through the lateral funiculus of the spinal cord. At the appropriate levels, motor neurons (seated in the ventral gray matter) extended axons (lower motor neurons) to innervate the extremity vasculature. These motor neurons receive input from descending axons in the spinal cord. The synapse, from upper to lower motor neuron, is rarely direct (only in ~10% of cases). More often than not, there is a connection with interneurons in the intermediate spinal laminae prior to synapse with the lower motor neuron.

As previously mentioned, several corticospinal fibers do not cross at the lower medulla and descend uncrossed in the ventral funiculus as the anterior corticospinal tract.

The lower motor neuron (alpha motor neuron) is located in the nuclei of the medial (trunk) and lateral (extremity) portions of the *ventral gray matter*. The lower motor axons exit through the ventral roots and help form the spinal nerves at the appropriate levels. They then innervate the skeletal muscles of the trunk and extremities.

Fig. 19.3 **Corticospinal tract, axial view.**

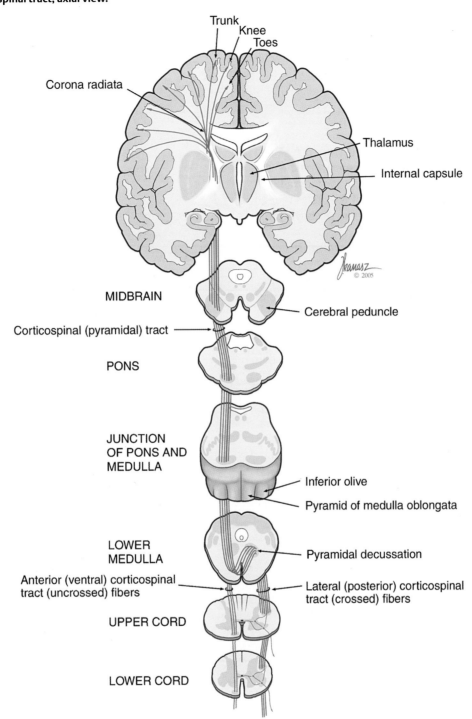

Corticobulbar Tract

Similar to the corticospinal tract anatomically and in function, the corticobulbar tract contributes to cranial nerve innervation, providing supply to the muscles of facial expression and mastication and the tongue.

Course of the Corticobulbar Tract

See **Fig. 19.4.**

Fibers leave the cortex (primary motor cortex) and converge and descend through the *corona radiata,* the anterior portion of the posterior limb of the *internal capsule,* and into the brainstem. The tract continues though the cerebral peduncle of the *midbrain,* occupying the middle two thirds.

In the brainstem, axons of the *corticobulbar tract* exit some distance above their respective cranial nerve nuclei and synapse on interneurons in the reticular formation. They may travel in the reticular formation, medial longitudinal fasciculus, and medial lemniscus to reach their cranial nerve nuclei.

The majority of the cranial nerve nuclei are innervated by both crossed and uncrossed fibers. Therefore, when one fiber is injured, innervation from the uninjured side (either crossed or uncrossed) still exists, and a deficit may not be observed. An important exception to this is the facial nucleus. The portion of the facial nucleus that innervates the lower facial muscles is supplied by crossed upper motor neuron fibers only, whereas those that subserve the upper facial muscles receive both crossed and uncrossed fibers. Thus, an injury to the corticobulbar tract will result in contralateral weakness of the lower facial muscles, leaving the upper facial muscles intact.

Fig. 19.4 **Corticobulbar tract.**

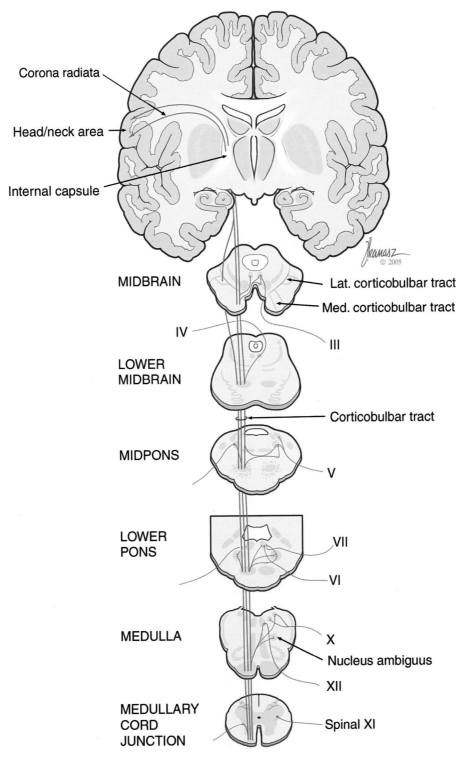

Brainstem

Several extrapyramidal motor tracts originate in the brainstem. The purpose of these tracts is to maintain muscle tone, posture, balance, and reflex movement. They are under supraspinal control, and their action is not at the conscious level. Injury may lead to disinhibition of these tracts and abnormal posture and tone.

Reticulospinal Tract

There are two components of the reticulospinal tract system. These are the pontine and medullary reticulospinal tracts. The pontine reticulospinal tract is thought to be an excitatory tract that innervates motor neurons supplying the axial and limb muscles. Its greatest effect is on the axial muscles in the neck. The medullary reticulospinal tract is an inhibitory tract. It may act to keep other facilitatory and inhibitory tracts in check and is under cortical control. Loss of cortical control, as with upper brainstem injury, is a component of the constellation of neural alterations that contribute to extensor (decerebrate) posturing.

Course of the Pontine Reticulospinal Tract

See **Fig. 19.5**.

The tract arises from cells in the pontine tegmentum. It descends ipsilaterally in the medial anterior funiculus traversing the length of the spinal cord, and in the process sending many branches to multiple spinal levels.

Fig. 19.5 **Pontine reticulospinal tract.**

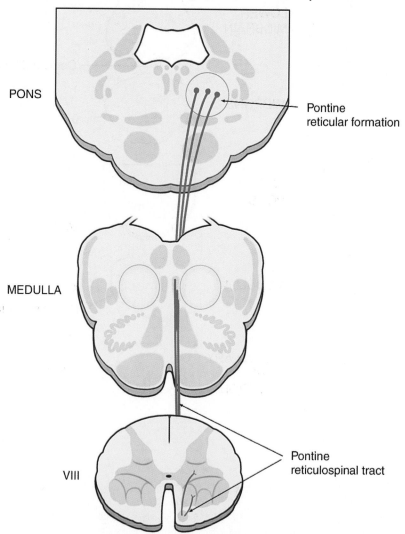

PONS

Pontine reticular formation

MEDULLA

VIII

Pontine reticulospinal tract

Course of the Medullary Reticulospinal Tract

See **Fig. 19.6**.

The tract arises from the medial two thirds of the medullary reticular formation. Most fibers originate from the nucleus reticularis gigantocellularis. The tract descends in the lateral funiculi and projects bilaterally to multiple spinal levels.

Fig. 19.6 **Medullary reticulospinal tract.**

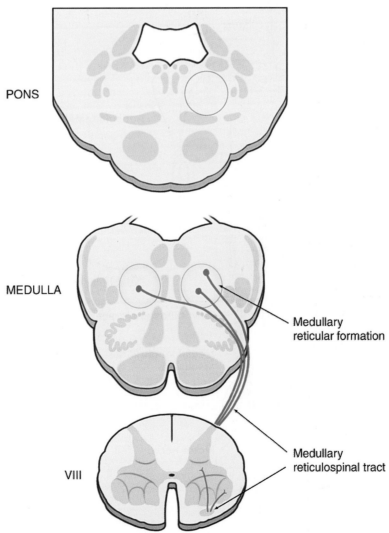

PONS

MEDULLA

Medullary
reticular formation

VIII

Medullary
reticulospinal tract

Vestibulospinal Tract

See **Fig. 19.7**.

The predominant contribution to this tract is from the *lateral vestibular nucleus* (Deiters' nucleus). The *vestibulospinal tract* is the main outflow of the vestibular nuclei. The tract descends ipsilaterally in the anterior funiculus. The tract terminates on interneurons at all spinal segments but has its strongest influence at cervical and lower lumbar regions. Stimulation of this tract results in excitation. The main function of this tract is to maintain extensor tone and, therefore, balance.

Fig. 19.7 **Vestibulospinal tract.**

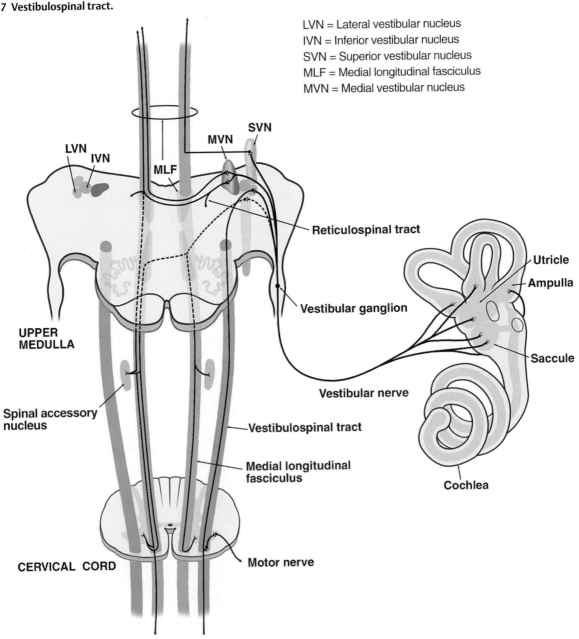

LVN = Lateral vestibular nucleus
IVN = Inferior vestibular nucleus
SVN = Superior vestibular nucleus
MLF = Medial longitudinal fasciculus
MVN = Medial vestibular nucleus

Rubrospinal Tract

See **Fig. 19.8**.

This tract originates from the magnocellular division of the *red nucleus* in the midbrain. The tract completely crosses in the ventral tegmentum and descends in the lateral funiculus in association with the lateral *corticospinal tract*. The tract descends to all spinal levels. The red nucleus receives input from the cortex and cerebellum, which then influences the rubrospinal tract. Stimulation of the tract results in excitation of motor neurons controlling contralateral flexion. The tract then acts to maintain tone in flexor muscle groups.

Fig. 19.8 **Rubrospinal tract.**

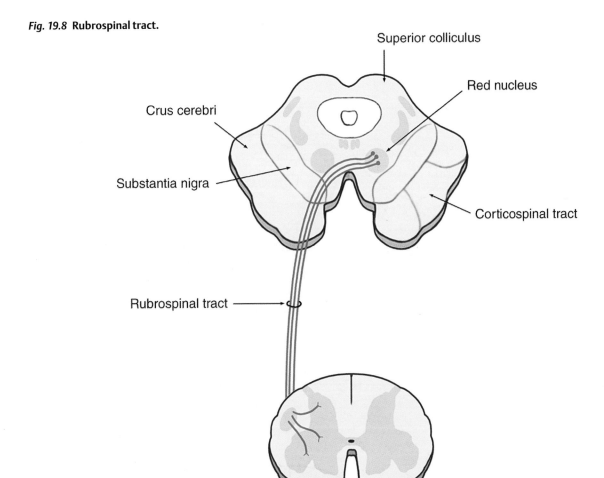

Superior colliculus

Red nucleus

Crus cerebri

Substantia nigra

Corticospinal tract

Rubrospinal tract

VIII

Tectospinal Tract

See **Fig. 19.9**.

This tract originates from cells deep in the *superior colliculus*. The tract crosses in the dorsal tegmentum and descends in the contralateral anterior funiculus. In the medulla, fibers become incorporated with the medial longitudinal funiculus. The tract continues only into cervical segments, mainly the upper four cervical segments. The tract mediates reflex and postural movements in response to visual and auditory stimuli.

Decerebrate Rigidity

The vestibulospinal and pontine reticulospinal tracts facilitate extensor tone, whereas the rubrospinal tract facilitates flexor tone. The medullary reticulospinal tract is inhibitory and acts in essence to maintain balance between extensor and flexor tone to permit smooth movement, posture, and balance. The medullary reticulospinal tract is under cortical control. An injury to the midbrain below the red nucleus injures the rubrospinal tract and the descending cortical control of the medullary reticulospinal tract. This leaves the vestibulospinal and pontine reticulospinal tracts unchecked and results in decerebrate posturing. Clinically, the patient demonstrates extension of the head and trunk. The upper and lower extremities are extended and internally rotated. Often the prognosis is poor.

Fig. 19.9 **Tectospinal tract.**

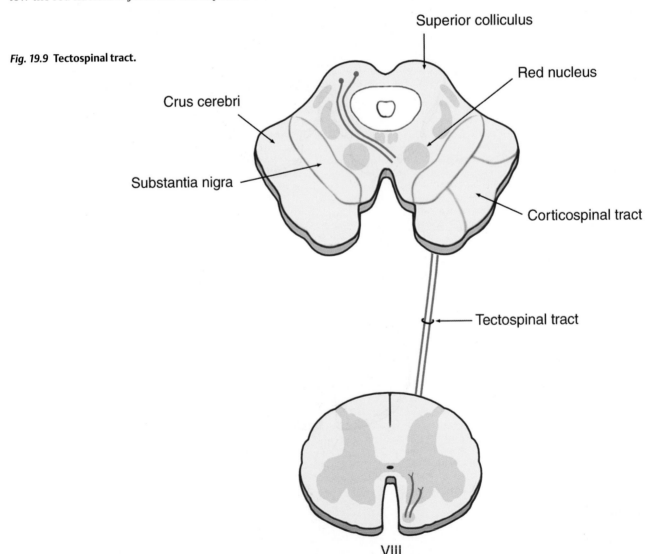

Superior colliculus

Red nucleus

Crus cerebri

Substantia nigra

Corticospinal tract

Tectospinal tract

VIII

Higher Orders of Control of the Descending Pathways

The motor system is under the influence of many extrapyramidal systems. These regions essentially initiate or reinforce postural movements of the trunk and limbs. The premotor and supplementary motor areas are located anterior to the primary motor cortex and contain reciprocal connections with each other and with other extrapyramidal and spinal tracts. These areas are involved with planning movement or keeping the primary motor neurons in a sense of readiness to visual, tactile, and auditory stimuli. In essence they demonstrate a neuronal discharge prior to the movement occurring. The cerebellum, with its connection to the cortex and extrapyramidal tracts, acts to regulate and control muscle tone, coordination of movement (especially skilled), and control of posture and gait. The basal ganglia is concerned with the initiation of movement, as well as coordinating movement and posture.

Damage to any of these areas of higher control will result in abnormal movement (e.g., tremor), posture (e.g., dystonia), or tone (e.g., hypotonia). Essentially, highly ordered, fine movements are impaired with such injuries.

Approach to the Patient with Weakness

Upper Motor Neuron Syndrome

The upper motor neuron (UMN) consists of the pyramidal and extrapyramidal motor systems. These include the cortex; the corticospinal tract (pyramidal system); and the rubrospinal, reticulospinal, vestibulospinal, and tectospinal tracts. In the spirit of practicality, however, the UMN is generally considered the corticospinal tract. It travels from the cortex through the subcortical white matter, the internal capsule, the brainstem, and the spinal cord. The UMN finally ends on the anterior horn cell. Injury to the UMN results in the upper motor neuron syndrome (UMNS).

UMN injury results in a typical clinical syndrome. The syndrome, in and of itself, is not specific for location. The general clinical features seen include weakness in the affected muscle groups (never individual muscles); spasticity with hyperactive reflexes, including Babinski's sign; normal nerve conduction studies; and lack of atrophy or fasciculations.

Although the UMNS is nonspecific, the patient's signs and symptoms may be helpful in localizing the pathological lesion to the cortex, internal capsule, brainstem, or spinal cord.

Lesions of the Cerebral Cortex

Lesions involving the cerebral cortex often lead to weakness of the contralateral arm, leg, and lower face. More often than not, weakness of only the contralateral leg, or only the arm and lower face, is observed, unless the lesion is large (e.g., a complete middle cerebral artery distribution stroke). If the lesion is large enough, there may also be alterations of sensation of the contralateral limbs. Rarely is complete loss of sensation observed. The key to localization in the cerebral cortex is the presence of "cortical findings." These include disorders of language (aphasia), loss of discriminative sensation (astereognosis), impairment of tactile localization (anosognosia), and homonymous visual field deficits.

Lesions of the Internal Capsule

Lesions of the internal capsule may also result in contralateral weakness of the arm, leg, and lower face. The weakness is usually equally distributed between the arm and leg. Sensory disturbances are often observed. "Cortical findings" such as aphasia are not observed.

Lesions of the Brainstem

Lesions of the brainstem are readily localized due to the involvement of the long descending and ascending tracts and associated cranial nerve findings. The level of the brainstem involved is discerned by the cranial nerve involved. For example, lesions of the brainstem are associated with contralateral weakness with ipsilateral third nerve palsy (Weber's syndrome). Lesions of the pons are associated with contralateral weakness of the arm and leg with ipsilateral weakness of the face or abducens nerve. (See **Figs. 6.17, 6.18, 6.19, 6.20, 6.21, 6.22, 6.23,** and **6.24** for a detailed review of brainstem syndromes.)

Lesions of the Spinal Cord

Lesions of the spinal cord involve only the upper or lower extremities; therefore, no alterations of cognition or other cortical or cranial nerve findings are observed. Findings of weakness or sensory changes are often located bilaterally. As opposed to supraspinal lesions, complete sensory loss may be observed with spinal cord lesions,

Lower Motor Neuron Syndrome

The lower motor neuron (LMN) consists of the anterior horn cell and its axon. LMN injury typically results in a clinical syndrome (LMNS). The LMNS consists of involvement of individual muscles, atrophy of the involved muscles, flaccidity, hypotonia, loss of reflexes, fasciculations, abnormal nerve conduction studies, and denervation potentials on electromyography.

The LMNS may result from damage to the anterior horn cell in the ventral gray matter of the spinal cord or to its associated root or peripheral nerve. Differentiation and localization may at times be difficult. The predominant differentiating factor is the presence or absence of sensory findings. If it is purely a motor syndrome, the lesion must be located in either the anterior horn cell or the anterior spinal root prior to exit of the spinal canal, or it must involve a purely motor peripheral nerve. If sensory findings are also observed, the lesion must involve a mixed motor and sensory peripheral nerve.

Approach to the Patient with Apraxia

Apraxia is a state in which a patient without an alteration of consciousness and without weakness, ataxia, extrapyramidal findings, or a sensory loss loses the ability to execute highly complex and previously learned skills and gestures. Visual, auditory, and somesthetic information is integrated in the parietal lobe and influences the planned action. The formation of engrams of skilled movement depends on the integrity of the dominant parietal lobe.

Apraxia has been further divided into ideational and ideomotor apraxia. Ideational apraxia is the failure to conceive and act, either when commanded or spontaneously, whereas ideomotor apraxia is the ability to conceive of the motor action to be executed but the inability to act.

Clinical Testing of Apraxia

The patient may be observed during dressing, washing, shaving, or eating. Certain tasks, such as waving goodbye and blowing a kiss, are encouraged. The patient is then asked to perform learned complex tasks, such as hammering a nail, unlocking and opening a door, combing the hair, opening a bottle, pouring the contents into a glass, and finally drinking from the glass. An inability to perform such tasks (complex) are examples of ideational apraxia, whereas the inability to perform the simpler tasks would be considered a manifestation of ideomotor apraxia.

20 Autonomic Nervous System

The autonomic nervous system comprises the central and peripheral components of the nervous system that regulate involuntary functions, such as those that are performed by smooth muscle, cardiac muscle, and glands.

Functionally, the two divisions of the autonomic nervous system (sympathetic and parasympathetic) are distinguished on the basis of their tendency to expand (sympathetic) and conserve (parasympathetic) energy. Thus, the activation of the sympathetic system stimulates an increase in heart rate and arterial blood pressure, dilatation of the pupils and bronchioles, and inhibition of the intestine and bladder wall, whereas the parasympathetic activation system exerts an opposing effect. In other words, the sympathetic system is the "fight or flight" system, whereas the parasympathetic system maintains vegetative functions (e.g., digestion, urination, etc.). It is the delicate balance between the sympathetic and parasympathetic outflow tracts that maintains the dynamic equilibrium of the internal environment.

In maintaining homeostasis, autonomic function is associated with several other responses. Thus, autonomic and endocrine activities are closely integrated in higher centers, as are psychological and emotional inputs. Together with the autonomic system, they contribute to the so-called limbic system. For example, smelling or remembering a disagreeable food may cause one to become nauseous, with pallor, sweating, and lightheadedness.

Anatomically, efferent pathways of the autonomic nervous system constitute a two-neuron limb that consists of fibers whose site of contact (i.e., synapse) lies outside the central nervous system (CNS) in the autonomic ganglia.

Preganglionic efferent neurons are typically small, myelinated group B fibers, whereas postganglionic efferents tend to comprise smaller, unmyelinated group C fibers. The preganglionic parasympathetic fibers are characteristically long, synapsing in or near their target organs. That is, their ganglia are often in the organ itself, for example, the myenteric plexus of the intestinal tract. The preganglionic sympathetic fibers have a very short course and terminate proximally, in a collection of ganglia that together form the sympathetic trunk (paravertebral ganglia). The paravertebral ganglia (or sympathetic chain) run along the lateral margin of the vertebral bodies. The postganglionic sympathetic fibers follow a long course that ends in their target organs. Occasionally preganglionic sympathetic fibers pass through the sympathetic chain and terminate in a more distal plexus, for example, the hypogastric plexus. These preganglionic fibers are known as splanchnic nerves.

Pharmacologically, acetylcholine is the neurotransmitter at all autonomic ganglia. The postganglionic parasympathetic fibers release acetylcholine as well. However, most postganglionic sympathetic fibers release norepinephrine. Select postganglionic sympathetic neurons, such as those that innervate sweat glands, release acetylcholine rather than norepinephrine.

The acetylcholine receptors on sympathetic postganglionic cell membranes are nicotinic, whereas the receptors on the parasympathetic postganglionic cells are muscarinic. The presence of dopaminergic interneurons in autonomic ganglia suggests that these ganglia are involved in the integration, rather than the simple relay, of information.

Efferent Pathways

Sympathetic Division

See **Fig. 20.1**.

The cell bodies of preganglionic sympathetic neurons are located in the intermediolateral cell column in the lateral horn of the spinal cord between levels T1 and L2–L3. The axons of these preganglionic neurons exit the spinal cord via the ventral roots, pass through the *white communicating rami* (remember these preganglionic fibers are myelinated), and synapse on postganglionic neurons in the paravertebral ganglia of the sympathetic trunk at their level of entry, or they may ascend or descend the sympathetic chain to finally synapse.

Alternatively, certain preganglionic fibers, which together form the *splanchnic nerve*, pass through the *paravertebral ganglion* without synapsing. Instead, they synapse in one of the prevertebral ganglia, which are distal to the spine, such as the *celiac ganglion* or the superior or inferior mesenteric ganglia. The neurotransmitter released by all preganglionic sympathetic neurons is acetylcholine.

Upon leaving the paravertebral or prevertebral ganglia, many postganglionic fibers accompany arteries as they pass peripherally to innervate various internal organs. Other postganglionic fibers leave the paravertebral ganglia to return to the spinal nerves via the *gray communicating rami,* so called because most of these postganglionic fibers are unmyelinated. These fibers innervate blood vessels, sweat glands, and erector pili muscles, structures that receive no parasympathetic innervation.

Because preganglionic neurons characteristically synapse on several postganglionic neurons, there is considerable divergence "built into the system." Functionally, this is evident in the widespread effect produced by sympathetic stimulation.

Further contributing to this widespread effect are a group of preganglionic fibers that accompany the splanchnic nerves and establish synaptic contacts with the secretory cells of the adrenal medulla. This neural crest structure represents a collection of specialized postganglionic sympathetic neurons that release epinephrine and, to a lesser extent, norepinephrine directly into the bloodstream.

Except for the cells of the adrenal medulla, which use epinephrine, and the fibers that innervate sweat glands, which use acetylcholine, the neurotransmitter released by all postganglionic sympathetic neurons is norepinephrine.

Fig. 20.1 Sympathetic outflow.

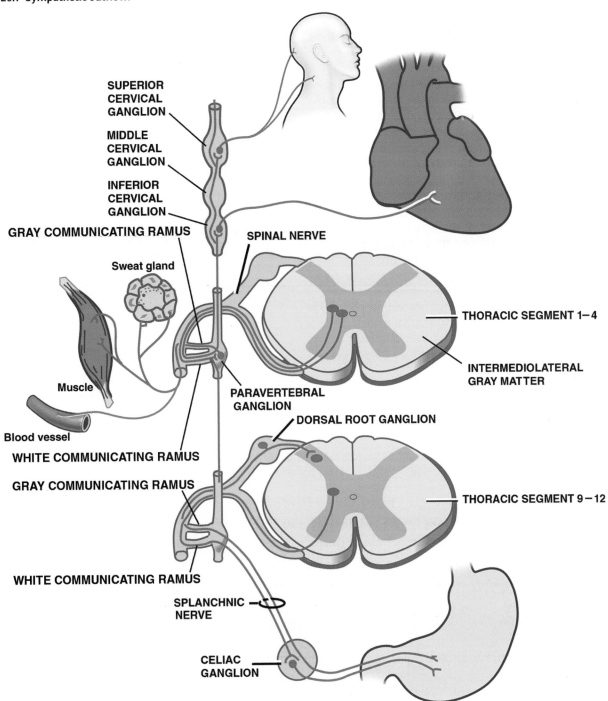

SUPERIOR
CERVICAL
GANGLION

MIDDLE
CERVICAL
GANGLION

INFERIOR
CERVICAL
GANGLION

GRAY COMMUNICATING RAMUS

SPINAL NERVE

Sweat gland

THORACIC SEGMENT 1–4

INTERMEDIOLATERAL
GRAY MATTER

Muscle

PARAVERTEBRAL
GANGLION

DORSAL ROOT GANGLION

Blood vessel

WHITE COMMUNICATING RAMUS

GRAY COMMUNICATING RAMUS

THORACIC SEGMENT 9–12

WHITE COMMUNICATING RAMUS

SPLANCHNIC
NERVE

CELIAC
GANGLION

Parasympathetic Division

See **Fig. 20.2**.

In contrast to the thoracolumbar distribution of the sympathetic division, the parasympathetic division is distributed both rostrally and caudally. The rostral component of the parasympathetic division contains preganglionic neurons that originate in the nuclei of cranial nerves III, VII, IX, and X. These preganglionic neurons project fibers that accompany their associated cranial nerves to terminate in ganglia comprising cell bodies of postganglionic neurons that innervate the eye, the salivary glands, and the viscera of the abdomen and thorax. Associated nuclei, nerves, ganglia, and effector organs are presented in **Table 20.1**.

The caudal component of the parasympathetic division comprises preganglionic fibers that originate in spinal segments S2 through S4, specifically in the intermediolateral cell columns. These fibers exit the spinal cord via the ventral roots to form long pelvic nerves that terminate in or near the pelvic viscera, where they synapse on short postganglionic fibers that innervate the proximal and distal *colon*, the *rectum*, the *bladder*, and the *genitalia*.

Compared with the sympathetic system, the parasympathetic system is capable of mounting a more discrete and localized response because there is less divergence in the contact between pre- and postganglionic neurons and between the postganglionic neurons and their target cells, and because acetylcholine is rapidly inactivated by acetylcholinesterase. Both the pre- and postganglionic neurons of the parasympathetic division use the neurotransmitter acetylcholine.

Table 20.1 Associated Nuclei, Nerves, Ganglia, and Effector Organs

Nerve (Nuclei)		Ganglia	Effector Organ(s)
CN III	Edinger-Westphal nucleus	Ciliary ganglia	Ciliary dilator pupillae
CN VII	Superior salivatory nucleus	Pterygopalatine ganglion Submandibular ganglion	Mucosa of mouth parotid gland Sublingual-submandibular glands
CN IX	Inferior salivatory nucleus	Otic ganglion	Mucosa of mouth Parotid gland
CN X	Dorsal motor nucleus of the vagus		Heart Larynx Trachea Bronchi Lung Liver Gallbladder Pancreas Spleen Kidney Esophagus Stomach Small intestines Ascending and transverse colon

Fig. 20.2 **Parasympathetic division.**

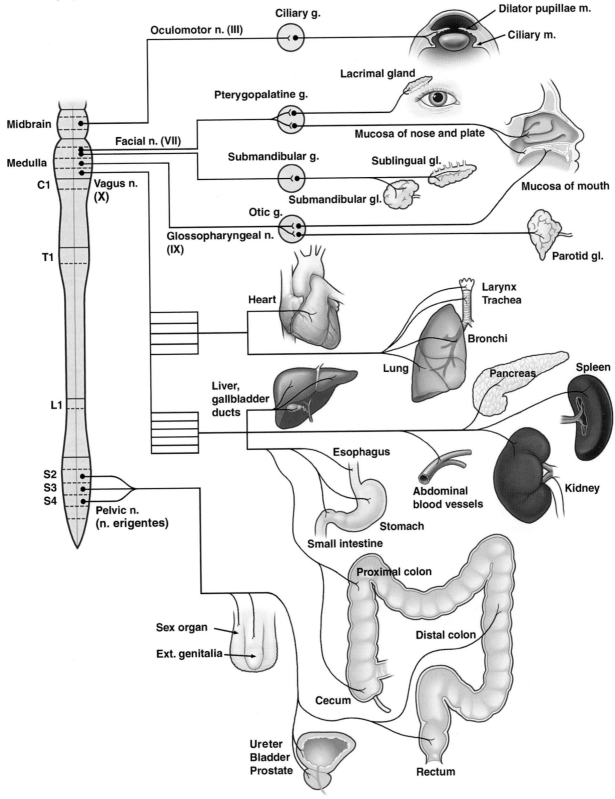

Afferent Pathways

Sympathetic and Parasympathetic Divisions

Both divisions of the autonomic nervous system contain afferent, as well as efferent, pathways. Afferent fibers in the sympathetic division pass through the sympathetic ganglia without synapsing. They enter the spinal nerves via the white communicating rami and synapse in the dorsal root ganglia of T1 through L2. By contrast, the cell bodies of the parasympathetic afferent fibers are located in the sensory ganglia of their associated cranial nerves and the dorsal root ganglia of segments S2 through S4.

The central branches of the autonomic afferent fibers travel alongside or are mixed with the somatic afferents (e.g., in the spinothalamic tract). Thus, the autonomic components of the general sensory system are fundamentally identical to their somatic counterparts, except that the former mediate stimuli such as stretch of the hollow organs and lack of oxygen, whereas the latter mediate stimuli such as heat and touch. Furthermore, some visceral afferents terminate in higher autonomic centers, such as the brainstem reticular formation and the hypothalamus, where they constitute the afferent limb of autonomic reflex mechanisms (e.g., those involved in the control of arterial blood pressure, heart rate, and respiration).

Thus, afferent pathways play an important role in various reflexes of the autonomic nervous system and are responsible as well for the conduction of visceral pain. Unlike the somatic sensory system, however, it is only in the presence of dysfunction or disease states that the impulses of the autonomic nervous system reach the level of consciousness.

Visceral pain exhibits several qualities that distinguish it from somatic pain. In particular, visceral pain is poorly localized and has a tendency to be felt on the body surface at a distance from its true source in the visceral organ (so-called referred pain). Also, visceral pain is aching in quality and characteristically stimulates autonomic responses (increased or decreased heart rate, sweating, etc.). Afferent fibers carrying visceral pain–related impulses run exclusively in the sympathetic system, whereas nearly all other visceral afferents run in the parasympathetic system.

Visceral pain is most commonly induced by distention of a hollow viscus, such as the intestine. Other causes of visceral pain include rapid stretching of a solid organ, peritoneal irritation, and the anoxia of ischemic cardiac muscle.

The anatomic substrate of referred pain comprises central axons of autonomic and somatic afferents that may terminate in identical spinal segments, although their peripheral branches supply structures that are widely separated. Thus, anginal pain, associated with ischemic heart disease, is often referred to the left side of the chest and to the inner aspect of the left arm, because the central branches of the sensory fibers that supply the heart originate in segments T1 through T4 or T5 of the spinal cord (segments that also receive sensory fibers from the chest wall and arm).

The Enteric Nervous System

The enteric nervous system is so called because it represents a form of visceral innervation that is histologically and pharmacologically distinct from both the sympathetic and the parasympathetic systems. Comprising a collection of neurons contained within the walls of the gastrointestinal tract, the enteric nervous system is capable of producing peristaltic activity in the absence of extrinsic stimulation.

The neurons of this system are organized into two nerve plexi: (1) the myenteric (Auerbach's) plexus, which lies between the longitudinal and circular muscle layers; and (2) the submucosal (Meissner's) plexus, which lies in the connective tissue between the circular muscle layer and the muscularis mucosae. A combination of bipolar and unipolar neurons, ensheathed by neuroglia-like cells, are represented, as are a constituency of interneurons. The intrinsic neurons that innervate the smooth muscle and glands within the walls of the gastrointestinal tract comprise excitatory neurons that release acetylcholine and inhibitory neurons that release a variety of peptides. Excitatory and inhibitory extrinsic inputs, which modulate the activity of the intrinsic neurons, are derived from cholinergic preganglionic parasympathetic neurons and noradrenergic postganglionic sympathetic neurons, respectively.

Central Control of Autonomic Function

Supraspinal control of autonomic spinal reflexes is mediated by the hypothalamus and cardiovascular and respiratory centers located in the reticular formation of the brainstem. Important spinal reflexes are discussed here.

Respiratory Center: Autonomic Control of Respiration

Respiration is coordinated by a respiratory center that consists of an aggregation of brainstem nuclei comprising the nucleus of the solitary tract, the nucleus ambiguus, and nuclei of the reticular formation. The cells of these nuclei are activated by vagal impulses, as well as by direct changes in their chemical environment, especially by the accumulation of carbon dioxide. Efferent impulses are carried in the reticulospinal pathway to lower motor neurons that innervate the diaphragm and the intercostal muscles.

Expiration is generally a passive action that results from recoil of the expanded chest after inspiration. The lung is protected from overinflation through a respiratory center control mechanism known as the Hering-Breuer reflex. As the lung is inflated to its volume, afferent impulses are sent to the expiratory center through a relay in the nucleus of the solitary tract. The expiratory center in turn inhibits the inspiratory center, and hence inspiration takes place. This is followed by a passive (elastic) expiratory movement. The rate of lung expansion also contributes to this process.

The rate and depth of respiratory movements are also mediated by reflexes involving chemoreceptors that are sensitive to decreases in arterial oxygen tension, such as occurs in the context of increased need (e.g., vigorous exercise) or decreased supply (e.g., lowered oxygen tension at high altitudes).

Cardiovascular Center: Autonomic Control of the Cardiovascular System

Under normal conditions the sympathetic cardiovascular center maintains a low-frequency tonic activity. However, an autonomic reflex arc permits the heart to respond appropriately to an increase or decrease in arterial blood pressure.

Thus, baroreceptors (those that respond to pressure) on the terminals of peripheral branches of the vagal and glossopharyngeal nerves supply the aortic arch and the carotid sinus at the bifurcation of the common carotid artery. The central processes of these nerves, whose cell bodies are located in cranial nerve ganglia, terminate in the nucleus of the solitary tract in the medulla (nucleus solitarius). Second-order fibers of the afferent limb originate in this nucleus to reach the cardiovascular center of the reticular formation, whence efferent fibers project to the nucleus ambiguus and the intermediolateral cell column of the spinal cord. By stimulating and inhibiting the sympathetic and parasympathetic supply to the heart, the autonomic cardiovascular center can compensate for changes in arterial blood pressure as detected by the baroreceptors and their vagal and glossopharyngeal afferents. As one assumes an upright position from lying down, blood is suddenly pooled in the numerous systems of the lower extremities. This pooling would result in a decrease in cerebral perfusion were it not for the autonomic reflex. In fact, an autonomic reflex usually compensates for a perceived decrease in blood pressure, thus avoiding the occurrence of orthostatic syncope. As it happens, the baroreceptors in the aortic arch and carotid sinus detect the sudden decrease in arterial wall tension (i.e., low blood pressure) and reflexively increase afferent impulses to the nucleus solitarius. The cardiovascular center, in turn, increases sympathetic outflow and decreases parasympathetic input, causing a constriction of the peripheral vasculature and increase in heart rate and stroke volume. The end result is maintenance of blood pressure and a balanced autonomic system.

Hypothalamus: Control and Mediation of Numerous Autonomic Functions

See **Fig. 20.3**.

By its direct and indirect influence on lower autonomic centers in the brainstem and spinal cord, and through its connections with the endocrine pituitary gland, the hypothalamus controls and integrates a large number of autonomic functions. In general, stimulation of the anterior hypothalamus results in a parasympathetic response, whereas stimulation of the posterior hypothalamus leads to a sympathetic response.

The hypothalamus receives input from multiple structures that it integrates in the visceral, limbic, and endocrine. This input is passed on directly or indirectly to lower autonomic centers in the brainstem and spinal cord to effect the desired physiological response(s).

Fig. 20.3 **Hypothalmus and endocrine control.**

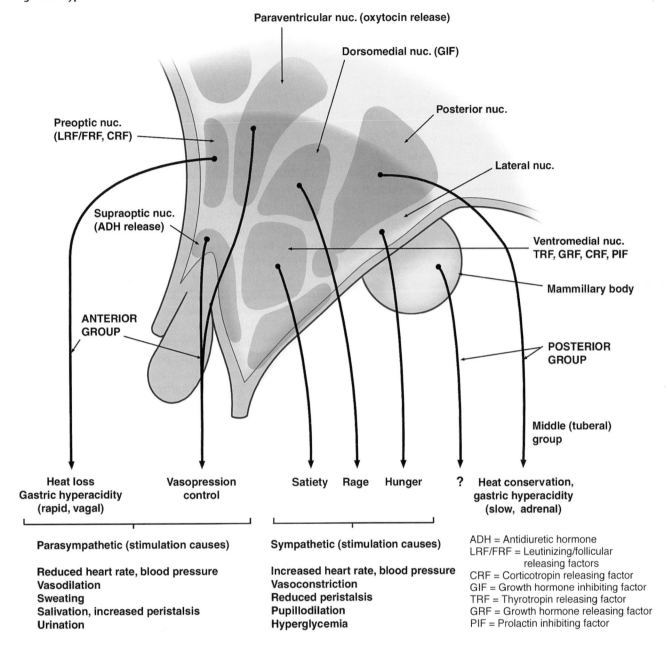

Paraventricular nuc. (oxytocin release)

Dorsomedial nuc. (GIF)

Posterior nuc.

Preoptic nuc.
(LRF/FRF, CRF)

Lateral nuc.

Supraoptic nuc.
(ADH release)

Ventromedial nuc.
TRF, GRF, CRF, PIF

Mammillary body

ANTERIOR
GROUP

POSTERIOR
GROUP

Middle (tuberal)
group

Heat loss
Gastric hyperacidity
(rapid, vagal)

Vasopression
control

Satiety   Rage   Hunger

?   Heat conservation,
gastric hyperacidity
(slow, adrenal)

Parasympathetic (stimulation causes)

Reduced heart rate, blood pressure
Vasodilation
Sweating
Salivation, increased peristalsis
Urination

Sympathetic (stimulation causes)

Increased heart rate, blood pressure
Vasoconstriction
Reduced peristalsis
Pupillodilation
Hyperglycemia

ADH = Antidiuretic hormone
LRF/FRF = Leutinizing/follicular
releasing factors
CRF = Corticotropin releasing factor
GIF = Growth hormone inhibiting factor
TRF = Thyrotropin releasing factor
GRF = Growth hormone releasing factor
PIF = Prolactin inhibiting factor

Autonomic Innervation: Some Examples

Eyes

See **Figs. 20.4** and **20.5**.

The preganglionic parasympathetic fibers that supply the eye originate in the *Edinger-Westphal nucleus* of the oculomotor complex and pass through the oculomotor nerve to reach the *ciliary ganglion*, where they synapse on postganglionic neurons. The postganglionic fibers travel within the short ciliary nerves to innervate the constrictor pupillae and the ciliary muscle. These parasympathetic fibers that supply the eye constitute the efferent limb of the pupillary light reflex. Activation of the parasympathetic system then results in constriction of the pupil (miosis) and contraction of the *ciliary muscle*, which results in a "rounding up" of the lens and hence accommodation for near vision.

The preganglionic sympathetic fibers that supply the eye originate in the intermediolateral cell column in segments T1 and T2. These fibers ascend in the sympathetic trunk and terminate on postganglionic neurons in the superior cervical ganglion. The postganglionic fibers first accompany the internal carotid and ophthalmic arteries, traverse the ciliary ganglion and the short and long ciliary nerves without synapsing, and innervate the *dilator pupillae* and the superior tarsal muscles. Activation of sympathetic fibers results in dilation of the pupil and maintenance of an elevated eyelid. Interruption of the sympathetic pathway to the eye results in the clinical constellation of ptosis, miosis, and apparent enophthalmos (i.e., the globe appears recessed in the face). If a more proximal sympathetic interruption occurs, anhidrosis (lack of sweating to the face) occurs, as well. This constellation is classically known as Horner syndrome. This syndrome may also occur as a consequence of interrupting sympathetic fibers descending on spinal levels from the hypothalamus.

Heart

Sympathetic supply to the heart begins with preganglionic fibers that arise in the intermediolateral cell column of segments T1 through T5. These fibers ascend in the sympathetic trunk to terminate on postganglionic neurons in the superior, middle, and inferior cervical ganglia and the upper thoracic ganglia. The postganglionic fibers leave these ganglia to form the cardiac nerves, which innervate the pacemaker cells and cardiac muscle. Activation of the sympathetic fibers increases both the heart rate and the force of cardiac muscle systolic contraction. In contrast, stimulation of the parasympathetic supply of the heart, which is carried in the vagus nerve, reduces the heart rate and may slightly decrease its force of contraction.

Lungs

Activation of the sympathetic fibers that originate in segments T2 through T5 of the sympathetic trunk that end on the bronchi and blood vessels of the lungs results in bronchodilation and vasoconstriction. In contrast, bronchoconstriction, vasodilation, and increased glandular secretion follow stimulation of the parasympathetic fibers that pass from the brainstem through the vagus to the lungs.

Gastrointestinal Tract

The parasympathetic supply to the gastrointestinal tract is derived from both the cranial and the spinal components of the autonomic nervous system. The cranial component contributes fibers that run in the vagus nerve to supply the length of the gastrointestinal system, excluding the descending and sigmoid colon and the rectum. The latter are supplied by spinal fibers that arise in the intermediolateral cell columns of S2 through S4 to form the pelvic splanchnic nerves.

The preganglionic parasympathetic fibers, both cranial and spinal, synapse on the postganglionic neurons that constitute the myenteric (Auerbach's) and submucosal (Meissner's) plexi in the gastrointestinal wall. Activation of the parasympathetic system stimulates peristaltic activity, relaxes the sphincters, and increases the secretion of gastric and intestinal walls.

In contrast, activation of the preganglionic sympathetic supply to the gastrointestinal system, which passes uninterruptedly through the sympathetic trunk to establish synaptic contact with postganglionic neurons in the prevertebral ganglia (the celiac ganglion and both the superior and inferior mesenteric ganglia), results in reduced peristalsis, sphincteric contraction, and decreased glandular secretion.

Adrenal Medulla

The adrenal medulla consists of secretory cells, derived from the neural crest, which represent specialized postganglionic sympathetic neurons that release epinephrine and, to a lesser extent, norepinephrine directly into the bloodstream, upon stimulation by cholinergic preganglionic sympathetic neurons. This neuroendocrine gland thus constitutes an important means for the initiation and maintenance of rapid and widespread sympathetic response to stressful situations.

Fig. 20.4 Preganglionic and postganglionic oculomotor complex.

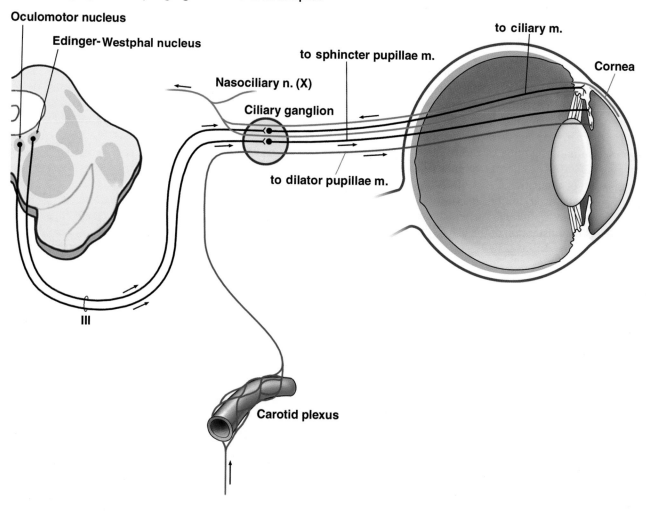

Fig. 20.5 Horner syndrome.

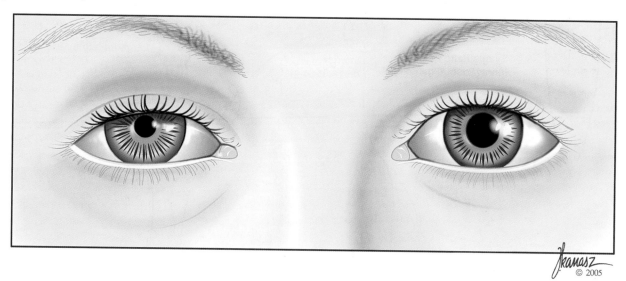

Urinary Bladder

See **Fig. 20.6**.

The urinary bladder receives both sympathetic and parasympathetic innervation, each division containing both afferents and efferents. Proprioceptive afferents in the parasympathetic fibers detect distention of the bladder and reflexively stimulate parasympathetic efferent fibers, which arise in spinal segments S2 through S4 and end in the *detrusor muscle* of the bladder wall to cause contraction and emptying of the bladder. In the adult, supraspinal influences permit voluntary bladder control. Stimulation of sympathetic efferent fibers that innervate the trigone (*sphincter*) inhibits micturition, whereas activated sympathetic afferents carry pain-related impulses that detect overdistention of the bladder.

Fig. 20.6 **(A) Autonomic innervation of the bowel and genitourinary system.**

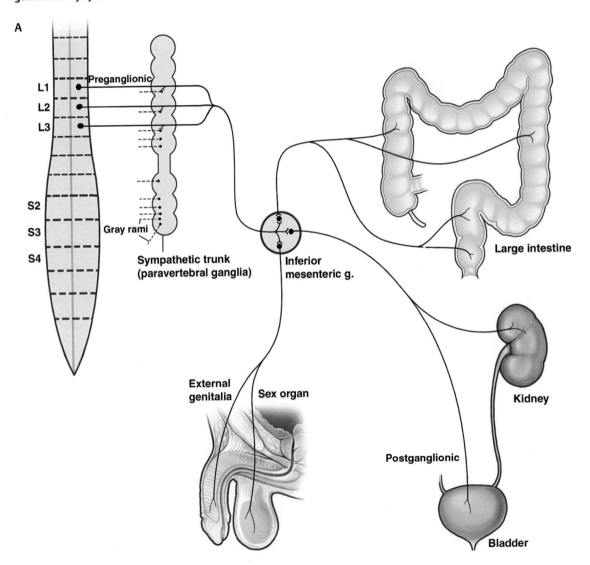

Fig. 20.6 (Continued) **(B)** Detailed innervation of the genitourinary system.

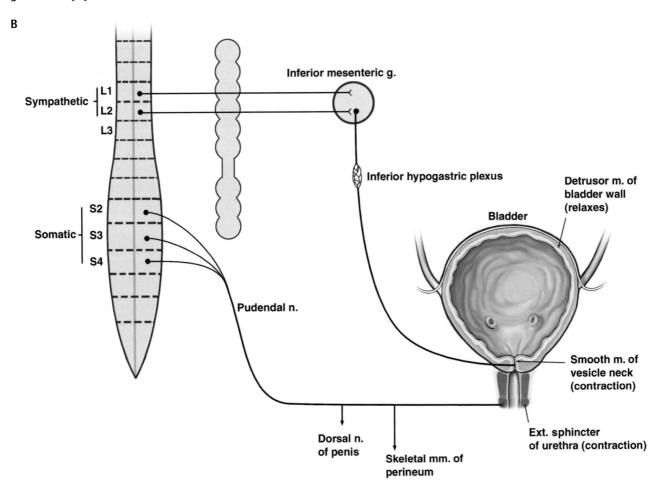

21 Consciousness

Consciousness means awareness of self and environment. The modern era of the study of consciousness began in the 1920s when it was discovered that awake and sleeping states were associated with distinctive electroencephalographic (EEG) patterns. These early EEG records showed that alertness was associated with low-voltage fast activity; sleep, with high-voltage slow activity (**Fig. 21.1**).

Later experiments demonstrated that the EEG pattern of sleep was replaced by a pattern of wakefulness after stimulation of the brainstem reticular formation. Further, this change resembled the EEG patterns during the transition between drowsy and awake states. Although these studies suggested that the reticular formation exerted broad and diffuse influence over the cerebral cortex, the anatomic and physiological mechanisms remained unclear. In particular, the connecting pathways between the reticular formation and the cerebral cortex were not well understood.

Two observations proved pivotal. First, it was noted that stimulation of the reticular formation activated the EEG, even after the placement of destructive lesions in the ascending sensory pathways (e.g., the medial lemniscus and the spinothalamic tract). Second, ascending sensory pathways conducted impulses normally, even when destructive lesions were placed in the reticular formation.

These observations implied that a second ascending system, anatomically and physiologically distinct from the "specific sensory pathways," carried impulses generated in the reticular formation. Two separate ascending pathways evidently existed: (1) a long ascending pathway concerned with specific sensory modalities and (2) an ascending reticular activating system (ARAS) concerned with arousal.

Further studies showed that both systems synapse in the diencephalon before reaching the cerebral cortex. However, the long ascending pathway synapses in "specific thalamic nuclei" (ventral posteromedial and ventral posterolateral nuclei), whereas the ARAS synapses in "nonspecific thalamic nuclei" (intralaminar, midline, and reticular nuclei). Furthermore, although both systems terminate in the cerebral cortex, the long ascending pathway terminates in the primary sensory cortex; the ARAS terminates diffusely throughout the cerebral cortex.

Clearly, then, the reticular formation, which was discussed in Chapter 6 in the context of the anatomy of the brainstem, is a morphological designation. It refers to a diffuse network of neurons with a wide variety of functions and connections. By contrast, the ARAS is a functional designation: it refers to a system of neurons concerned with arousal, some of which are found in the reticular formation.

Fig. 21.1 **Characteristic electroencephalographic (EEG) patterns associated with awake and sleeping states.**

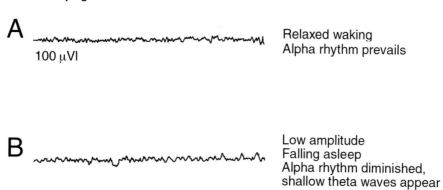

A

100 μVI

Relaxed waking
Alpha rhythm prevails

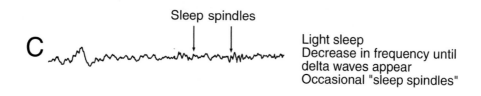

B

Low amplitude
Falling asleep
Alpha rhythm diminished,
shallow theta waves appear

Sleep spindles

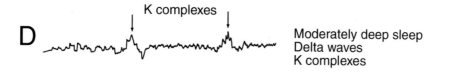

C

Light sleep
Decrease in frequency until
delta waves appear
Occasional "sleep spindles"

K complexes

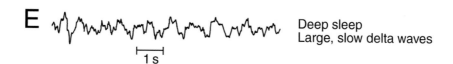

D

Moderately deep sleep
Delta waves
K complexes

E

Deep sleep
Large, slow delta waves

1 s

Ascending Reticular Activating System

See **Fig. 21.2**.

Several levels of the neuraxis contribute to the ARAS: (1) afferent sensory pathways, (2) the reticular formation, (3) the thalamus, and (4) the cerebral cortex.

Sensory Pathways

Widespread sources of sensory input are projected onto the reticular formation. These sensory stimuli possess varying capacities to arouse—some weak, such as a gentle whisper; some strong, such as a bucket of cold water thrown on a sleeping subject's head. Important sources of sensory input include (1) ascending tracts of the sensory system, (2) sensory cranial nerves, (3) the cerebellum, and (4) the cerebral cortex. Cortical input provides an important feedback mechanism that modifies other sources of sensory input.

Reticular Formation

The reticular formation is a diffuse aggregation of cells in the central brainstem that possesses an unusually wide range of neural connections. These connections involve the reticular formation in several functions, including motor control, control of the respiratory and cardiovascular system, sensory control, and consciousness. Reticular neurons that contribute to the ARAS are concerned with consciousness. They receive sensory inputs from multiple regions that project to the thalamus through long axons.

Thalamus

The thalamus contains three sets of functionally related nuclei: (1) the "specific thalamic nuclei," which receive sensory and motor input and project to specific areas of the cerebral cortex; (2) the "association thalamic nuclei," which receive input from other thalamic nuclei and project to association areas of the cerebral cortex; and (3) the "nonspecific thalamic nuclei," which receive input from the ARAS and project to large areas of the cerebral cortex.

The nonspecific thalamic nuclei, which contribute to the ARAS, are the intralaminar, midline, and reticular nuclei.

Cerebral Cortex

As noted, cortical electrical activity as recorded by the EEG correlates well with the behavioral expression of consciousness—the awareness of self and environment. The awake person demonstrates low-voltage, high-frequency EEG activity (α and β; > 8H3), whereas the sleeping patient demonstrates high-voltage, low-frequency EEG activity (δ 1 to 4H3). Activation of the cerebral cortex is dependent on thalamocortical innervation.

Specific sensory, motor, and cognitive functions have long been known to "localize" to specific areas of the brain. By contrast, no specific region of the brain is responsible for initiating or maintaining arousal. Rather, all areas of the cortex appear to contribute equally to consciousness. Thus, consciousness requires an intact cerebral cortex, and cerebral lesions, if sufficiently large, may impair consciousness. The degree of impairment is proportional to the size of the cerebral lesion and bears little relation to what area of the cortex has been lesioned.

Fig. 21.2 Ascending reticular activating system.

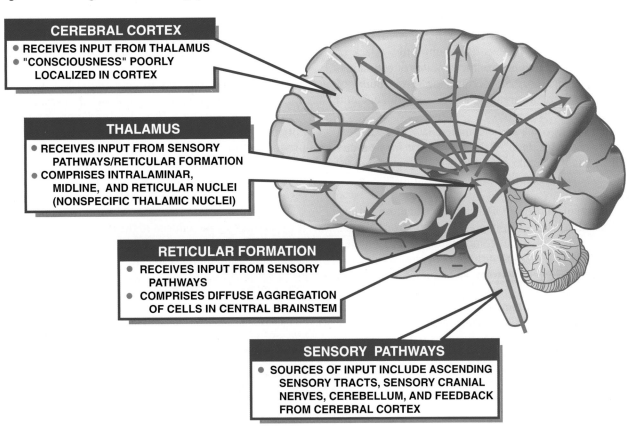

CEREBRAL CORTEX
- RECEIVES INPUT FROM THALAMUS
- "CONSCIOUSNESS" POORLY LOCALIZED IN CORTEX

THALAMUS
- RECEIVES INPUT FROM SENSORY PATHWAYS/RETICULAR FORMATION
- COMPRISES INTRALAMINAR, MIDLINE, AND RETICULAR NUCLEI (NONSPECIFIC THALAMIC NUCLEI)

RETICULAR FORMATION
- RECEIVES INPUT FROM SENSORY PATHWAYS
- COMPRISES DIFFUSE AGGREGATION OF CELLS IN CENTRAL BRAINSTEM

SENSORY PATHWAYS
- SOURCES OF INPUT INCLUDE ASCENDING SENSORY TRACTS, SENSORY CRANIAL NERVES, CEREBELLUM, AND FEEDBACK FROM CEREBRAL CORTEX

Approach to the Comatose Patient

Consciousness is the awareness of self and environment. Unconsciousness, it follows, is its opposite: a lack of awareness of self and environment. States of consciousness and unconsciousness occur along a continuum of varying levels of awareness, where wakefulness and coma represent two extremes.

Behaviorally, coma is the complete lack of awareness of self and environment. Pathologically, it may be due to one of two possible conditions: (1) a bilateral cerebral hemisphere disturbance or (2) a dysfunction of the ARAS.

A logical diagnostic approach in the comatose patient begins with a history of the present illness from friends, relatives, police, or paramedics and a specially tailored neurological examination. Primarily in the basis of the clinical signs elicited by exam, an anatomic localization may then be deduced. Finally, on the basis of primarily historical clues, the clinician must ask what specific pathological process is most likely responsible and what therapeutic intervention is most appropriate.

Fig. 21.3 **Glascow Coma Scale.**

Neurologic Examination

The purpose of the neurologic examination in the stuporous or comatose patient is to define the level of consciousness and to localize the site of the offending lesion.

Levels of consciousness are often described, in order of decreasing intensity, in terms of wakefulness, obtundation, stupor, and coma. Their determination and differentiation are largely subjective. A more objective and reproducible approach is to observe the patient's response to a series of increasingly intense stimuli. The Glasgow Coma Scale is a commonly used method for testing and recording the consciousness level (**Fig. 21.3**).

Localizing the site of the offending lesion in the comatose patient may be reduced to the interpretation of four clinical signs: respiratory pattern, pupillary response, eye movements, and motor response.

BEST EYE OPENING	
4 POINTS	SPONTANEOUS
3	TO VOICE
2	TO PAIN
1	NO RESPONSE

BEST VERBAL	
5 POINTS	ORIENTED
4	CONFUSED
3	INAPPROPRIATE
2	INCOMPREHENSIBLE
1	NO RESPONSE

BEST MOTOR	
6 POINTS	FOLLOWS COMMANDS
5	LOCALIZES PAIN
4	WITHDRAWS TO PAIN
3	DECORTICATE POSTURING
2	DECEREBRATE POSTURING
1	NO RESPONSE

- GLASCOW COMA SCALE IS A WIDELY USED SCORING SYSTEM TO ASSESS LEVEL OF CONSCIOUSNESS

- TOTAL SCORE COMPRISES SUM OF BEST EYE OPENING, BEST VERBAL, AND BEST MOTOR SCORES

- TOTAL SCORE RANGES FROM 3 (worst) TO 15 (normal)

Respiratory Pattern

See **Fig. 21.4.**

Four identifiable patterns may be seen in coma: (1) Cheyne-Stokes respiration is a pattern in which periods of hyperventilation alternate with periods of apnea. There is a gradual increase in the respiratory rate that finally peaks and then gradually decreases, followed by a period of apnea. Cheyne-Stokes respiration is associated with bilateral hemispheric disorders, metabolic disorders, and brainstem disorders above the level of the upper pons. (2) Central neurogenic hyperventilation is a rare pattern of breathing characterized by a sustained, rapid respiratory rate. It is associated with lesions between the low midbrain and upper pons. (3) Apneustic breathing is marked by prolonged pauses at the end of inspiration. It is associated with lesions at the level of the lower pons. (4) Ataxic breathing is a completely irregular respiratory pattern in which deep and shallow breaths occur randomly. It is associated with lesions in the medulla.

Fig. 21.4 **Respiratory patterns in coma.**

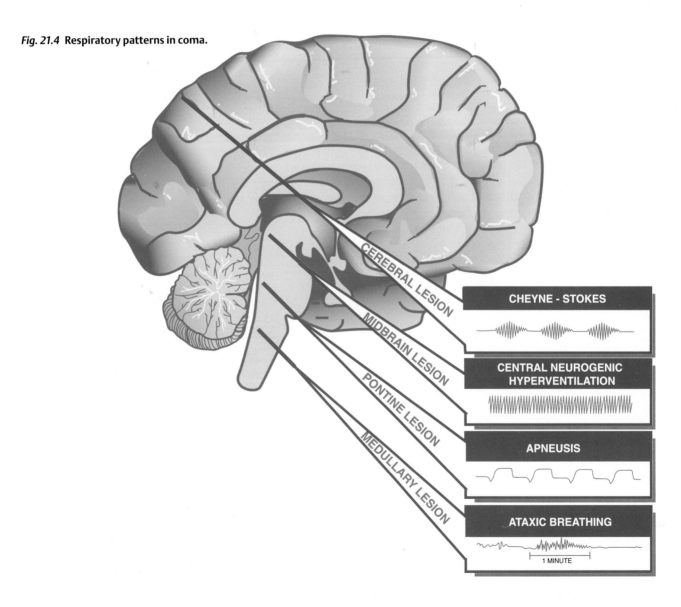

Pupillary Response

See **Fig. 21.5**.

The functional anatomy of the pupillary response is described in Chapter 18. More than any other clinical sign in the comatose patient, an abnormal pupillary response suggests the presence of a structural, rather than a metabolic, lesion. Furthermore, pupillary size and reactivity help localize the site of the structural lesion. Midbrain lesions are associated with pupils that are midposition and fixed (loss of sympathetic and parasympathetic input). Pontine lesions are associated with pupils that are pinpoint (loss of sympathetic input). A unilateral dilated pupil implies herniation of the uncus (medial temporal lobe) through the tentorial opening. This results in compression of the ipsilateral oculomotor nerve (loss of parasympathetic input).

Fig. 21.5 Pupillary response in coma.

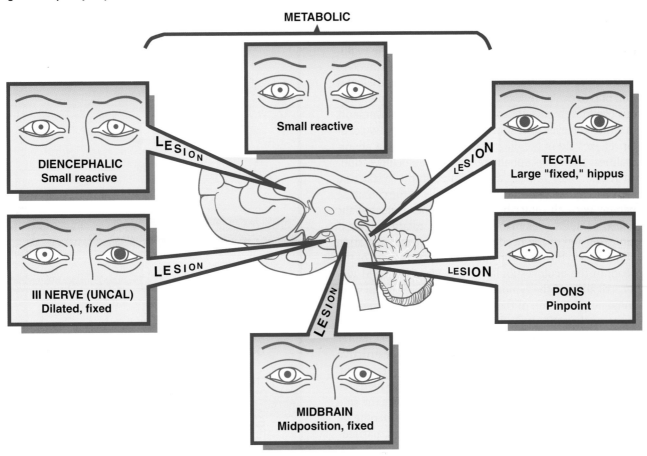

Eye Movements

See **Fig. 21.6**.

The functional anatomy of eye movements and the oculocephalic reflex are described in Chapter 18. The evaluation of eye movements in the comatose patient involves observation of spontaneous eye movements and elicitation of two ocular reflexes. The most common spontaneous eye movements are so-called roving eye movements in which the eyes drift slowly from side to side. Two ocular reflexes aid in the diagnosis of eye movement abnormalities: the oculocephalic reflex and the oculovestibular reflex. These reflexes are inhibited in the awake and alert patient but are conducted normally in the comatose patient with an intact brainstem. In the oculocephalic reflex, or doll's eyes maneuver, lateral rotation or flexion/extension of the head produces conjugate deviation of the eyes in the direction opposite the movement of the head. In the oculovestibular reflex (**Fig. 21.7**), cold water irrigation of the tympanic membrane results in slow conjugate deviation of the eyes toward the irrigated ear. If the oculovestibular reflex is intact, then the lesion is most likely above the brainstem. As described in Chapter 18, eye movement abnormalities result from destructive lesions in the cerebral hemispheres and the brainstem. Hemispheric lesions that involve the frontal eye fields result in conjugate deviation of the eyes away from the side of the associated hemiplegia. They may be overcome by the oculocephalic and oculovestibular reflexes, particularly by the latter, which presents the stronger stimulus. Brainstem lesions produce eye movement abnormalities of two types: (1) lesions of the paramedian pontine reticular formation (PPRF) result in conjugate deviation of the eyes toward the side of the associated hemiplegia, and (2) lesions of the medial longitudinal fasciculus (MLF) result in loss of adduction of the ipsilateral eye. Neither of these brainstem lesions, which localize to the pons, is overcome by oculocephalic or oculovestibular stimulations. In metabolic coma, the oculocephalic and oculovestibular reflexes are maintained early on but are then progressively lost as the level of coma deepens.

Fig. 21.6 Eye movements in coma.

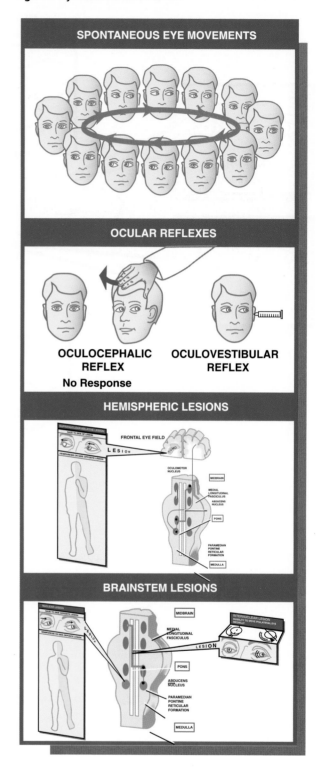

Fig. 21.7 Mechanism of caloric stimulation.

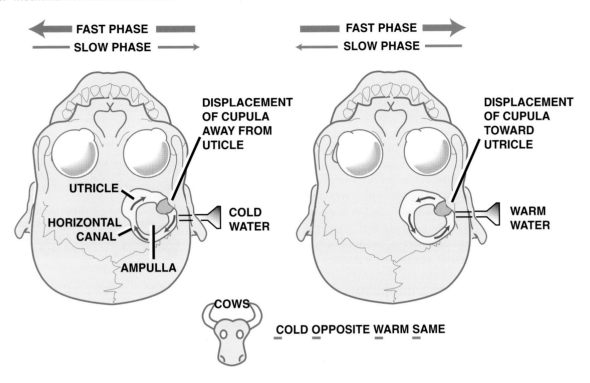

Motor Response

See **Fig. 21.8**.

In the comatose patient, motor function is assessed by observing the motor response to the application of a noxious stimulus. Pressure applied to the supraorbital ridge, the nail bed, or the sternum are easily elicited noxious stimuli associated with a minimum of tissue trauma. Three patterns of responses may be observed: appropriate, inappropriate, and no response. An appropriate response, such as the quick withdrawal of a limb from a noxious stimulus, demonstrates the integrity of the motor pathways that innervate the limb. No response, assuming the integrity of sensory pathways, which is tested by stimulation of both sides of the body, implies a lesion in the motor pathway. This may be unilateral, suggesting a structural lesion in the contralateral cerebral hemisphere or brainstem, or bilateral, suggesting a pontine or medullary lesion. Finally, inappropriate responses, which may occur spontaneously, include decorticate and decerebrate rigidity. *Decorticate posturing* refers to flexion of the arm at the elbow, adduction of the shoulder, and extension of the leg and ankle. It is classically associated with lesions at or above the level of the diencephalon. *Decerebrate rigidity* refers to the extension of the arm, internal rotation at the shoulder and forearm, and leg extension. It is classically associated with lesions at the level of the upper brainstem but may occur in association with massive hemispheric lesions or in the setting of severe metabolic coma.

Fig. 21.8 Motor responses in coma.

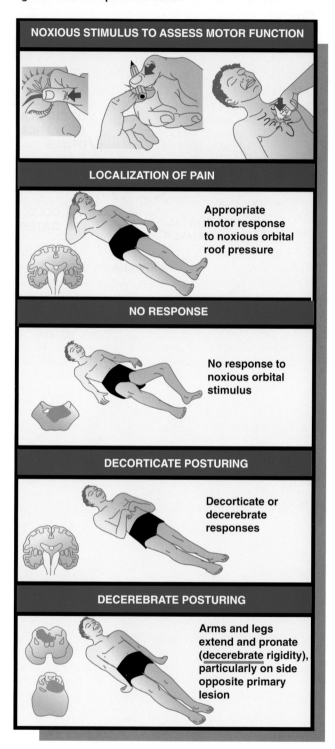

Anatomic Localization of a Lesion Causing Coma

The first step in anatomic localization in the comatose patient is to determine whether the lesion causing coma is structural, which may require emergent neurosurgical intervention, or diffuse and metabolic, which requires appropriate medical management. Structural lesions are identified as supratentorial, depending on their location above or below the tentorium.

Supratentorial Lesions

Supratentorial lesions cause coma by affecting both cerebral hemispheres or by exerting downward pressure that compresses and displaces the diencephalon and midbrain. Compression and displacement of the diencephalon and midbrain are the more common cause. It is recognized by the appearance of a sequence of respiratory, pupillary, ocular, and motor signs that correspond to the rostrocaudal progression of impaired brain function—first diencephalic, then midbrain, pontine, and medullary. Dysfunction below the level of the diencephalon is associated with a poor neurologic recovery.

Downward displacement of brain tissue associated with supratentorial lesions may result in herniation of that tissue through the tentorial opening. Two herniation syndromes, uncal syndrome and central herniation, are described here.

Uncal Syndrome

See **Fig. 21.9**.

For mechanical reasons, expanding temporal lobe lesions tend to cause medial displacement of the uncus and hippocampal gyrus across the edge of the tentorial opening. As a result, the ipsilateral oculomotor nerve is caught between the swollen uncus, and the contralateral cerebral peduncle is compressed against the free edge of the tentorium on the opposite side. Clinically, a unilateral dilated pupil is the earliest sign of uncal herniation. This may be rapidly followed by complete oculomotor nerve paralysis, stupor and coma, loss of oculovestibular responses, and ipsilateral and then bilateral hemiplegia. The contralateral cerebral peduncle lesion causing ipsilateral hemiplegia is known as Kernohan's notch; it is produced by compression of the cerebral peduncle against the free edge of the tentorium on the opposite side.

Fig. 21.9 Uncal syndrome.

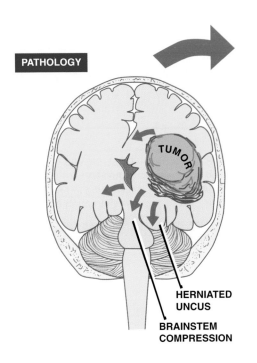

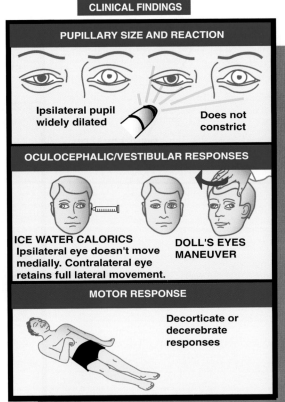

Central Herniation Syndromes

Central herniation involves the downward displacement of the diencephalon and the adjacent midbrain through the tentorial opening. It is early on associated with loss of consciousness because the diencephalon is the first structure encroached upon. Frontal, parietal, and occipital lesions are most commonly responsible. Clinically, central herniation is characterized by a rostrocaudal progression of functional impairment affecting first the diencephalon, then the midbrain, pons, and medulla, in that order. Four stages of rostrocaudal deterioration are identified: (1) the diencephalic stage (**Fig. 21.10**) is characterized by diminished consciousness, Cheyne-Stokes respirations, small pupils with a small range of contraction, normal oculocephalic and oculovestibular responses, and appropriate motor responses to noxious stimuli. (2) The midbrain–upper pons stage (**Fig. 21.11**) is characterized by sustained tachypnea, dilated fixed pupils, impaired oculocephalic and oculovestibular responses, and decerebrate rigidity. (3) The lower pons–upper medulla stage (**Fig. 21.12**) is characterized by rapid shallow or ataxic respirations, midposition fixed pupils, and motor flaccidity. (4) The medullary stage is terminal. It is characterized by periods of apnea associated with an irregular pulse hypotension.

Fig. 21.10 **Central herniation (diencephalic stage).**

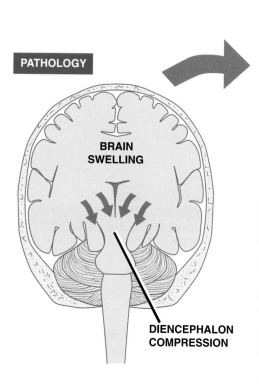

PATHOLOGY

BRAIN SWELLING

DIENCEPHALON COMPRESSION

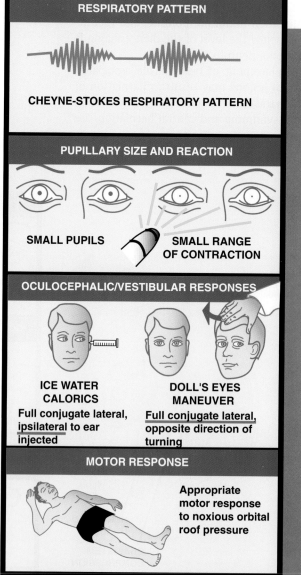

CLINICAL FINDINGS

RESPIRATORY PATTERN

CHEYNE-STOKES RESPIRATORY PATTERN

PUPILLARY SIZE AND REACTION

SMALL PUPILS   SMALL RANGE OF CONTRACTION

OCULOCEPHALIC/VESTIBULAR RESPONSES

ICE WATER CALORICS
Full conjugate lateral, ipsilateral to ear injected

DOLL'S EYES MANEUVER
Full conjugate lateral, opposite direction of turning

MOTOR RESPONSE

Appropriate motor response to noxious orbital roof pressure

Fig. 21.11 **Central herniation (midbrain–upper pons stage).**

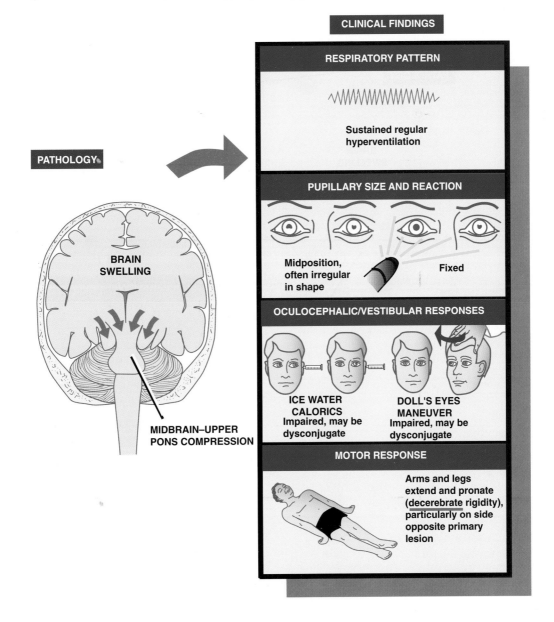

Fig. 21.12 **Central herniation
(lower pons-upper medulla stage).**

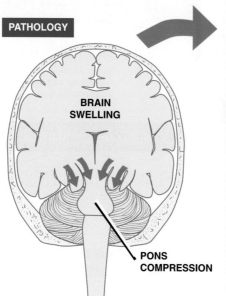

PATHOLOGY

BRAIN
SWELLING

PONS
COMPRESSION

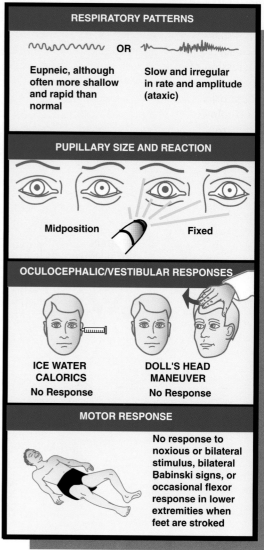

CLINICAL FINDINGS

RESPIRATORY PATTERNS

Eupneic, although
often more shallow
and rapid than
normal

OR

Slow and irregular
in rate and amplitude
(ataxic)

PUPILLARY SIZE AND REACTION

Midposition

Fixed

OCULOCEPHALIC/VESTIBULAR RESPONSES

ICE WATER
CALORICS
No Response

DOLL'S HEAD
MANEUVER
No Response

MOTOR RESPONSE

No response to
noxious or bilateral
stimulus, bilateral
Babinski signs, or
occasional flexor
response in lower
extremities when
feet are stroked

Subtentorial Lesions: Foramen Magnum Herniation

See **Fig. 21.13**.

Subtentorial structural lesions cause clinical deterioration marked by coma and focal brainstem signs. They often develop rapidly and do not exhibit the rostrocaudal progression associated with supratentorial lesions. Rapid progression occurs in part because of the small size of the subtentorial mass.

Pathologically, subtentorial lesions may cause coma by destroying or compressing brainstem tissue. Brainstem compression results from one or more of three pathological mechanisms: (1) direct compression of the midbrain–pontine reticular formation, (2) upward herniation of the cerebellar vermis through the tentorial opening, compressing the midbrain and diencephalon, or (3) downward herniation of the cerebellar tonsils through the foramen magnum, compressing and displacing the medulla.

Clinically, destructive lesions can often be precisely localized by the brainstem signs that accompany the development of coma: (1) midbrain lesions are associated with midposition fixed pupils and long tract motor signs secondary to involvement of the cerebral peduncles. (2) Rostral pontine lesions are associated with pinpoint pupils caused by interruption of sympathetic pathways and internuclear ophthalmoplegia caused by damage to the medial longitudinal fasciculus. (3) Lower pontine lesions are associated with pinpoint pupils and abnormal lateral conjugate gaze secondary to involvement of the paramedian pontine reticular formation. Usually these are accompanied by variable motor signs and an abnormal pattern of respiration.

Upward herniation of the cerebellar tonsils through the foramen magnum causes compression of the medulla with resultant respiratory and circulatory collapse. Coma then results from anoxia secondary to cardiopulmonary failure, rather than medullary compression per se.

Fig. 21.13 **Subtentorial lesions.**

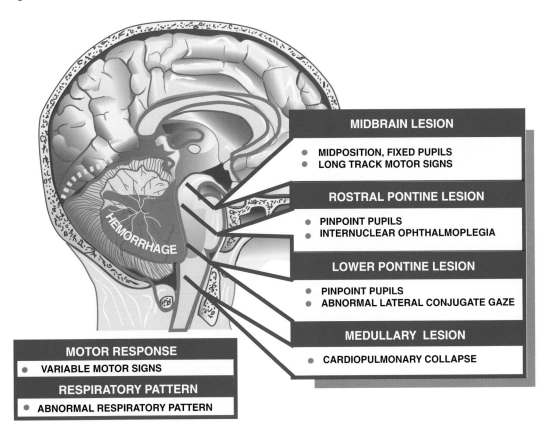

Diffuse Brain Dysfunction (Metabolic Encephalopathies)

See **Fig. 21.14**.

In contrast to the clinical rostrocaudal deterioration of supratentorial lesions and the easily localized signs of subtentorial lesions, the metabolic encephalopathies produce signs of partial dysfunction at many levels of the neuraxis.

The finding of reactive pupils in the presence of widespread brainstem dysfunction is the hallmark of the metabolic encephalopathies.

Hyper- or hypoventilation is usually nonspecific and simply reflects widespread brainstem depression.

The eyes first rove randomly, and, as the coma deepens, they come to rest in the forward position. Tonic conjugate lateral deviation of the eyes suggests the presence of a structural lesion.

Motor abnormalities in the comatose patient with metabolic encephalopathy are of two types: (1) nonspecific changes that progress with deepening of coma from mildly increased tone to decorticate and decerebrate rigidity, and (2) abnormal involuntary movements that are characteristic of metabolic disease. The latter includes tremor, which is coarse and irregular and usually absent at rest; asterixis, which is a flapping movement of dorsiflexed hands that represents sudden, arrhythmic lapses of postural tone; and multifocal myoclonus, which consists of startle-like muscle group contractions that are irregular in rhythm and amplitude, and asymmetric and asynchronous in distribution.

Fig. 21.14 **Diffuse brain dysfunction.**

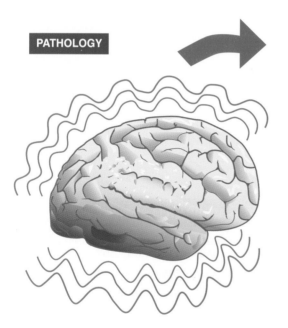

PATHOLOGY

CLINICAL FINDINGS

- **RESPIRATORY PATTERN: NONSPECIFIC HYPOVENTILATION AND HYPERVENTILATION**
- **PUPILLARY SIZE AND REACTION: REACTIVE PUPILS**
- **EYE MOVEMENTS: ROVING EYE MOVEMENTS; OR FORWARD POSITION**
- **MOTOR RESPONSE: NONSPECIFIC; MAY OBSERVE ABNORMAL INVOLUNTARY MOVEMENT**

IV
Fluid-System Anatomy and Function

22 Vascular System

Cerebrovascular diseases are one of the most common neurologic disorders, accounting for nearly 50% of all neurologic patients in a general hospital. Furthermore, stroke is the third leading cause of death among Americans. The clinical manifestation of a cerebrovascular lesion is marked by the sudden onset of a neurologic deficit and is termed a cerebrovascular accident or stroke. Two types of stroke are distinguished by their pathophysiological mechanisms: ischemic stroke (infarct), which is caused by hypoperfusion, thrombosis, or embolism, and hemorrhagic stroke, which is caused by intracranial bleeding.

The often devastating effect of stroke, or cerebral infarction, is in part explained by the fact that neural tissue is so exquisitely sensitive to an interruption in blood flow: brain dysfunction occurs within 8 to 10 seconds of interrupted perfusion, and by 3 to 5 minutes brain damage is permanent. This occurs because the brain is completely reliant on blood flow to provide metabolic substrates (e.g., glucose) and oxygen.

Although the brain constitutes only 2% of the body weight, it requires roughly 17% of the cardiac output and consumes ~20% of the oxygen that is utilized by the body.

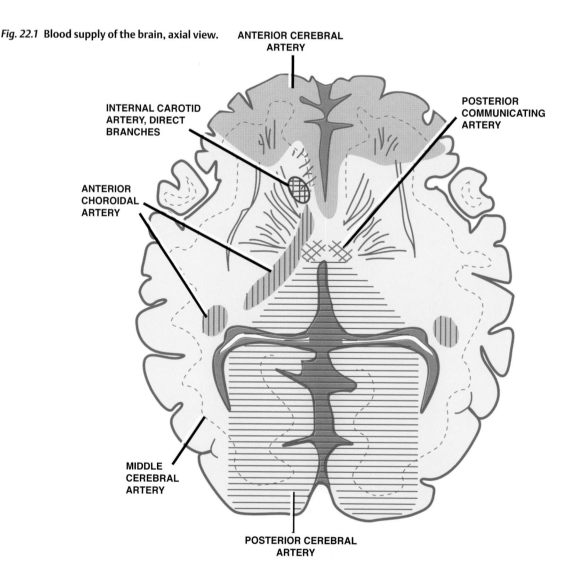

Fig. 22.1 Blood supply of the brain, axial view.

ANTERIOR CEREBRAL ARTERY

INTERNAL CAROTID ARTERY, DIRECT BRANCHES

POSTERIOR COMMUNICATING ARTERY

ANTERIOR CHOROIDAL ARTERY

MIDDLE CEREBRAL ARTERY

POSTERIOR CEREBRAL ARTERY

Due to this high demand and reliance on perfusion for energy production, the brain has developed a system of autoregulation. Autoregulation is the capacity of the brain to maintain cerebral blood flow in the face of systemic hypotension. Autoregulation is primarily determined by metabolic needs but is also increased by systemic blood pressure. For example, both carbon dioxide accumulation and low blood pressure result in cerebral vasodilatation. Therefore, despite the systemic blood pressure (within a specific range of 60 to 160 mm Hg), the brain receives a constant perfusion and energy supply.

This chapter discusses the arterial supply and venous drainage of the brain and spinal cord. Some of the vascular syndromes that result from arterial occlusion are briefly described immediately following the relevant anatomy. A practical approach to localization in the patient with stroke concludes the chapter.

The Blood Supply of the Brain

See **Figs. 22.1, 22.2, 22.3,** and **22.4** and **Table 22.1**.

The arteries of the brain are divided into two systems named after their branches of origin: the internal carotid system and the vertebrobasilar system. An anastomotic connection between these two systems, the circle of Willis, provides a clinically important collateral supply (see later discussion).

The internal carotid system, also known as the anterior circulation, comprises the *internal carotid artery* and its terminal branches, the *anterior and middle cerebral arteries*. Prior to its terminal bifurcation, the (intradural, supraclinoid) internal carotid artery gives rise to the ophthalmic, the *posterior communicating*, and the *anterior choroidal arteries*, in that order.

Fig. 22.2 **Blood supply of the brain, coronal view.**

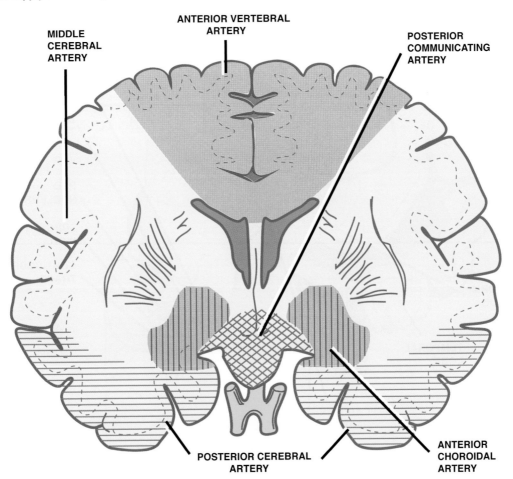

This system supplies the optic nerve and retina; the frontal and parietal lobes, as well as parts of the temporal and occipital lobes; the internal capsule; and the basal ganglia.

The vertebrobasilar system, also known as the posterior circulation, comprises the vertebral and *basilar arteries*. Branches of the vertebral arteries include the meningeal artery, the anterior and posterior spinal arteries, and the posterior inferior cerebellar artery. Branches of the basilar artery include the anteroinferior cerebellar artery, the labyrinthine artery, the pontine arteries, the superior cerebellar artery, and its terminal branch, the posterior cerebral artery.

This system supplies the medial and inferior aspects of the occipital and temporal lobes, the thalamus, the brainstem, the cerebellum, and the upper spinal cord.

Table 22.1 Branches of the Major Cerebral Arteries

Internal Carotid	Vertebral	Basilar
Ophthalmic	Meningeal	Anteroinferior cerebellar
Posterior communicating	Posterior spinal	Labyrinthine
Anterior choroidal	Anterior spinal	Pontine
Anterior cerebral	Posteroinferior cerebellar	Superior cerebellar
Middle cerebral		Posterior cerebral

Fig. 22.3 **Anatomy of internal capsule, basal ganglia, and cerebral peduncle.**

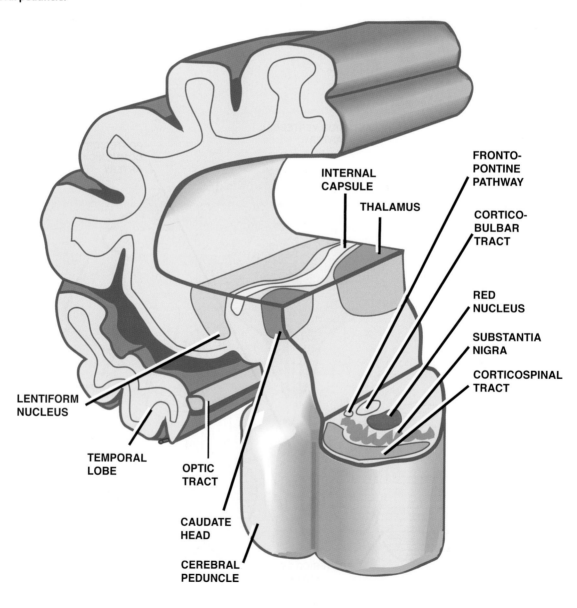

Fig. 22.4 **Blood supply of the deep structures of the hemisphere.**

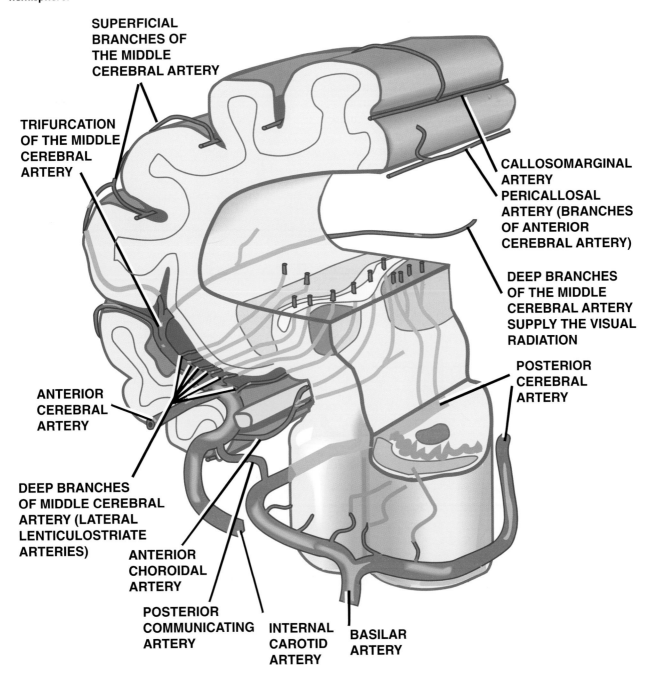

SUPERFICIAL BRANCHES OF THE MIDDLE CEREBRAL ARTERY

TRIFURCATION OF THE MIDDLE CEREBRAL ARTERY

CALLOSOMARGINAL ARTERY PERICALLOSAL ARTERY (BRANCHES OF ANTERIOR CEREBRAL ARTERY)

DEEP BRANCHES OF THE MIDDLE CEREBRAL ARTERY SUPPLY THE VISUAL RADIATION

POSTERIOR CEREBRAL ARTERY

ANTERIOR CEREBRAL ARTERY

DEEP BRANCHES OF MIDDLE CEREBRAL ARTERY (LATERAL LENTICULOSTRIATE ARTERIES)

ANTERIOR CHOROIDAL ARTERY

POSTERIOR COMMUNICATING ARTERY

INTERNAL CAROTID ARTERY

BASILAR ARTERY

The Internal Carotid System

See **Figs. 22.5, 22.6,** and **22.7**.

The internal carotid system supplies the anterior two thirds of the brain.

The *internal carotid artery* (ICA) arises from the bifurcation of the *common carotid artery*. From its origin in the neck to its termination in the cerebrum, the ICA (1) enters the cranial cavity by passing through the carotid canal; (2) travels through the cavernous sinus next to the oculomotor nerve (III), the trochlear nerve (IV), the ophthalmic and maxillary divisions of the trigeminal nerve (VI and V2), and the abducens nerve (VI); (3) penetrates the dura and the arachnoid mater to enter the subarachnoid space; and (4) divides into terminal branches at the medial end of the lateral cerebral sulcus (sylvian fissure).

Fig. 22.5 **Internal carotid artery.**

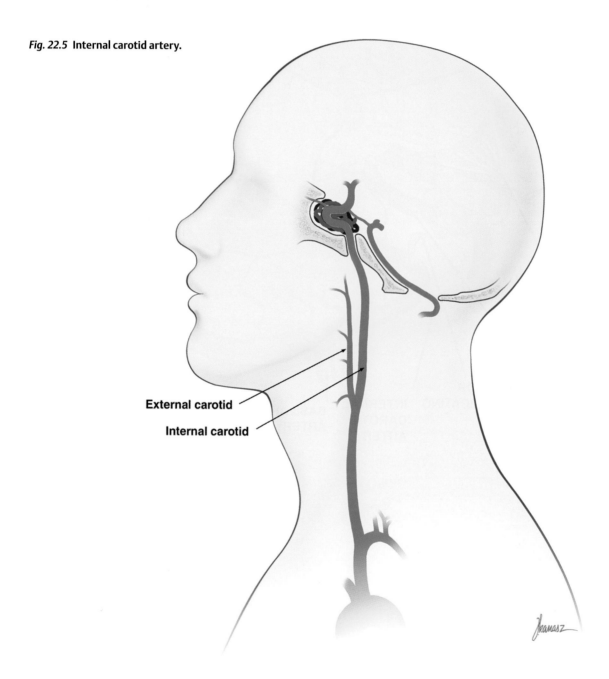

External carotid

Internal carotid

Fig. 22.6 Internal carotid and vertebral artery systems.

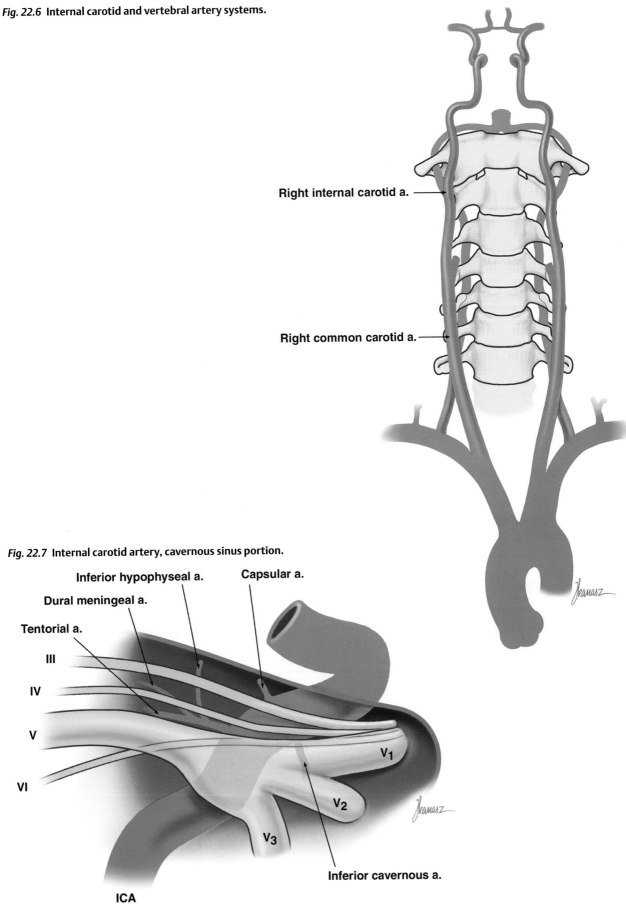

Right internal carotid a.

Right common carotid a.

Fig. 22.7 Internal carotid artery, cavernous sinus portion.

Inferior hypophyseal a.

Capsular a.

Dural meningeal a.

Tentorial a.

III

IV

V

VI

V₁

V₂

V₃

Inferior cavernous a.

ICA

The Five Major Branches of the Internal Carotid Artery

1. The *ophthalmic artery* (**Fig. 22.8**) takes its origin as the ICA emerges from the cavernous sinus to enter the subarachnoid space. It passes through the optic canal and into the orbit, inferolateral in relation to the *optic nerve*. Its major branch is the central retinal artery, which travels in the optic nerve and supplies the neuroretina. The ophthalmic artery forms clinically important anastomoses with branches of the external carotid artery, effectively connecting the internal and external carotid arteries. Occlusion of the ophthalmic artery may cause monocular blindness in the ipsilateral eye.

2. The *posterior communicating artery* (**Fig. 22.9**) arises from the inferolateral wall of the *ICA* near the terminal bifurcation of the ICA. It courses posteriorly above the third nerve to anastomose with the proximal portion of the *posterior cerebral artery*, forming part of the circle of Willis. Many perforators emerge from this artery that supply the posterior hypothalamus, anterior thalamus, posterior limb of the internal capsule, and subthalamus.

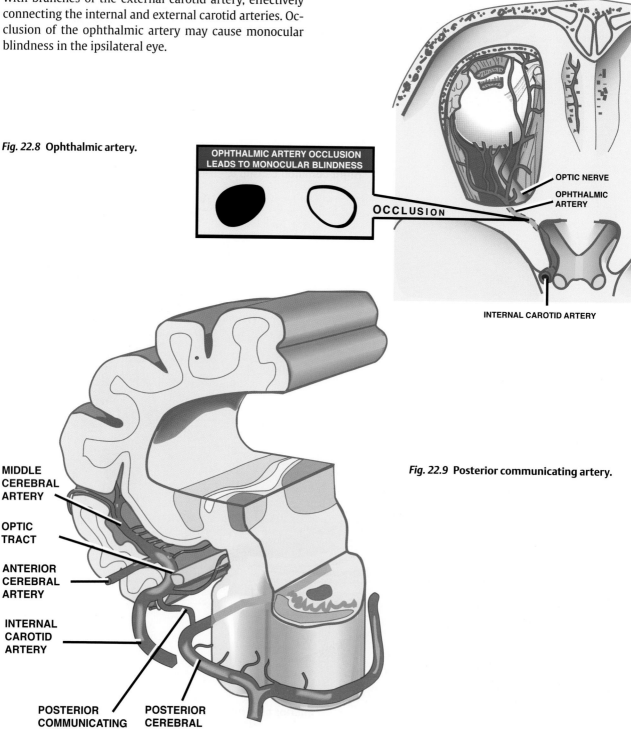

Fig. 22.8 Ophthalmic artery.

OPHTHALMIC ARTERY OCCLUSION LEADS TO MONOCULAR BLINDNESS

OCCLUSION

OPTIC NERVE

OPHTHALMIC ARTERY

INTERNAL CAROTID ARTERY

Fig. 22.9 Posterior communicating artery.

MIDDLE CEREBRAL ARTERY

OPTIC TRACT

ANTERIOR CEREBRAL ARTERY

INTERNAL CAROTID ARTERY

POSTERIOR COMMUNICATING ARTERY

POSTERIOR CEREBRAL ARTERY

Fig. 22.10 **Anterior choroidal artery, coronal view.**

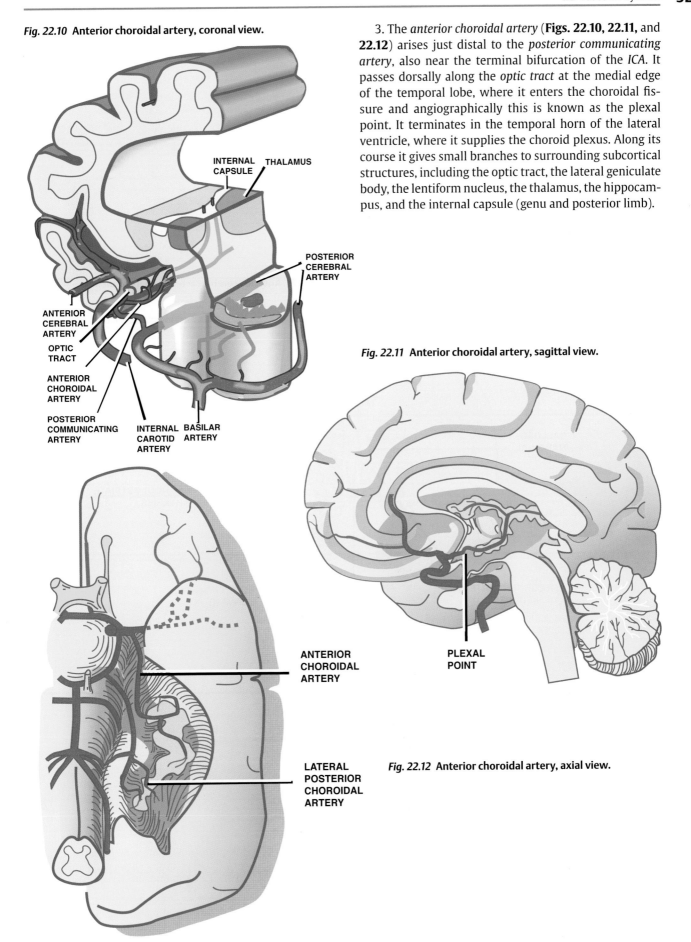

3. The *anterior choroidal artery* (**Figs. 22.10, 22.11,** and **22.12**) arises just distal to the *posterior communicating artery*, also near the terminal bifurcation of the *ICA*. It passes dorsally along the *optic tract* at the medial edge of the temporal lobe, where it enters the choroidal fissure and angiographically this is known as the plexal point. It terminates in the temporal horn of the lateral ventricle, where it supplies the choroid plexus. Along its course it gives small branches to surrounding subcortical structures, including the optic tract, the lateral geniculate body, the lentiform nucleus, the thalamus, the hippocampus, and the internal capsule (genu and posterior limb).

INTERNAL CAPSULE

THALAMUS

POSTERIOR CEREBRAL ARTERY

ANTERIOR CEREBRAL ARTERY

OPTIC TRACT

ANTERIOR CHOROIDAL ARTERY

POSTERIOR COMMUNICATING ARTERY

INTERNAL CAROTID ARTERY

BASILAR ARTERY

Fig. 22.11 **Anterior choroidal artery, sagittal view.**

PLEXAL POINT

ANTERIOR CHOROIDAL ARTERY

LATERAL POSTERIOR CHOROIDAL ARTERY

Fig. 22.12 **Anterior choroidal artery, axial view.**

4. The *anterior cerebral artery* (ACA) (**Figs. 22.13, 22.14,** and **22.15**) is the smaller of the two terminal branches of the ICA. It runs forward and medially above the optic nerve. Before it enters the interhemispheric fissure, it is joined to the ACA of the opposite side by the *anterior communicating artery*. This is also an important aspect of the circle of Willis. The artery then enters the fissure and courses upward and backward on the medial surface of the hemisphere, along the superior aspect of the corpus callosum. The cortical branches of the ACA supply the medial aspect of the frontal and parietal lobes, including the leg area of the pre- and postcentral gyri. The central branches of the ACA (*recurrent artery of Heubner* or *medial striate artery*) penetrate the anterior perforated substance to supply the anteromedial parts of the basal ganglia and anterior limb of the internal capsule.

Fig. 22.13 Anterior cerebral artery and its branches.

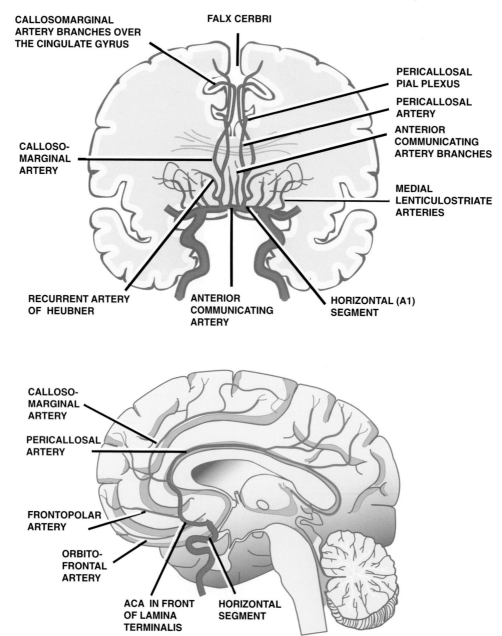

Fig. 22.14 Anterior cerebral artery and its branches.

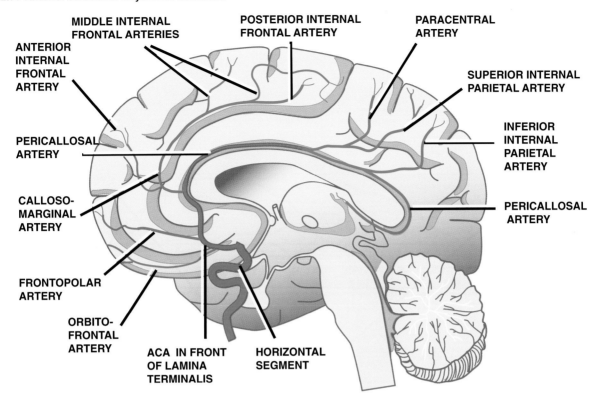

MIDDLE INTERNAL
FRONTAL ARTERIES

POSTERIOR INTERNAL
FRONTAL ARTERY

PARACENTRAL
ARTERY

ANTERIOR
INTERNAL
FRONTAL
ARTERY

SUPERIOR INTERNAL
PARIETAL ARTERY

PERICALLOSAL
ARTERY

INFERIOR
INTERNAL
PARIETAL
ARTERY

CALLOSO-
MARGINAL
ARTERY

PERICALLOSAL
ARTERY

FRONTOPOLAR
ARTERY

ORBITO-
FRONTAL
ARTERY

ACA IN FRONT
OF LAMINA
TERMINALIS

HORIZONTAL
SEGMENT

Fig. 22.15 Anterior cerebral artery occlusion.

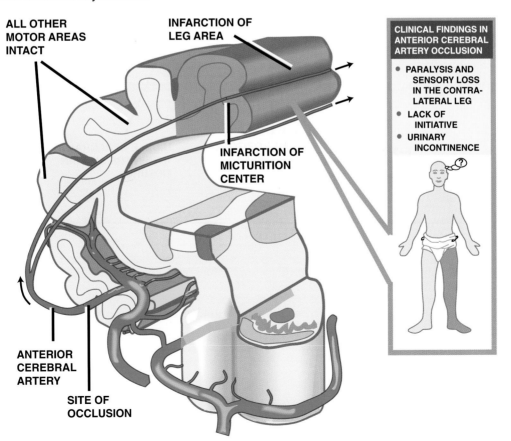

ALL OTHER
MOTOR AREAS
INTACT

INFARCTION OF
LEG AREA

INFARCTION OF
MICTURITION
CENTER

ANTERIOR
CEREBRAL
ARTERY

SITE OF
OCCLUSION

**CLINICAL FINDINGS IN
ANTERIOR CEREBRAL
ARTERY OCCLUSION**

- PARALYSIS AND
  SENSORY LOSS
  IN THE CONTRA-
  LATERAL LEG
- LACK OF
  INITIATIVE
- URINARY
  INCONTINENCE

5. The *middle cerebral artery* (MCA) (**Fig. 22.16**) is the largest of the two terminal branches of the ICA and is considered to be its direct continuation. The artery runs laterally in the lateral cerebral sulcus, where it divides into cortical and central branches.

Fig. 22.16 **Middle cerebral artery.**

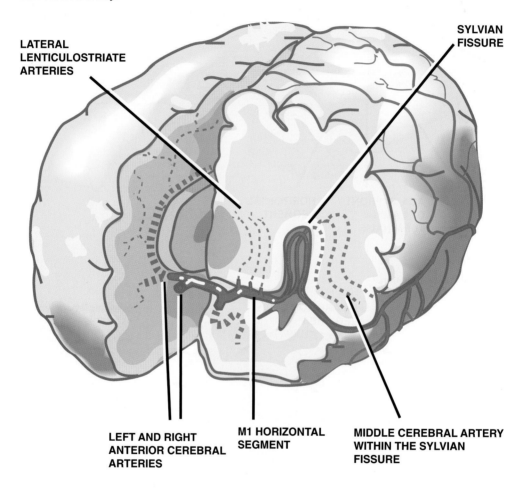

The cortical branches of the MCA supply most of the cortex on the lateral side of the hemisphere (**Fig. 22.4**). A superior division supplies the motor and sensory cortex related to the face and arm and the area of expressive language (Broca's area) of the dominant hemisphere. An inferior division supplies part of the optic tract, the upper part of the optic radiations, and the area of receptive language (Wernicke's area) of the dominant hemisphere. The central branches of the MCA (lenticulostriate arteries) penetrate the anterior perforated substance and supply most of the basal ganglia and internal capsule (**Fig. 22.5**).

Vascular Syndromes Associated with Five Major Internal Carotid Artery Branches

Occlusion of the MCA (or one of its divisions) is the most common cause of ischemic stroke. The vascular syndrome produced depends on the division (or divisions) involved (**Fig. 20.4,** p. 493).

Occlusion of the superior division (**Fig. 22.17**) produces (1) contralateral paralysis of the face and arm due to involvement of the motor cortex, (2) contralateral sensory loss of the face and arm due to involvement of the sensory cortex, and (3) Broca's (expressive) aphasia (dominant hemisphere) due to involvement of the inferior frontal gyrus.

Fig. 22.17 **Superior division occlusion.**

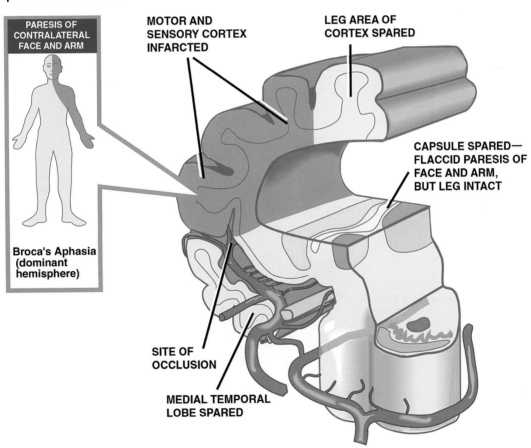

Pure inferior division (**Fig. 22.18**) stroke is a less frequent event. It produces (1) contralateral homonymous hemianopsia due to interruption of the optic tract or radiations; (2) Wernicke's (receptive) aphasia (dominant hemisphere) due to involvement of the posterior superior temporal gyrus; (3) deficient cortical sensory function (e.g., inability to discriminate the form of an object by touch) due to involvement of the primary, secondary, or association sensory cortex; and (4) impaired spatial perception (e.g., lack of awareness of neurologic deficit, and neglect of contralateral limbs and space) due to involvement of the nondominant parietal lobe.

Occlusion of a central branch of the MCA causes contralateral paralysis involving the face, arm, and leg due to involvement of the internal capsule.

Fig. 22.18 Inferior division occlusion.

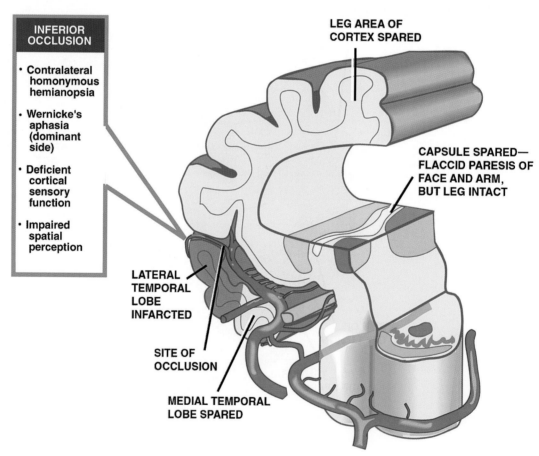

Occlusion of the stem of the MCA (**Fig. 22.19**) results in a clinical syndrome that combines the neurologic deficits caused by cortical and central branch strokes. Thus, ischemic stroke in the distribution of the MCA stem produces hemiplegia and hemianesthesia of the face, arm, and leg on the side opposite the lesion, with variable deficits in language and visual fields.

Fig. 22.19 **Middle cerebral artery occlusion.**

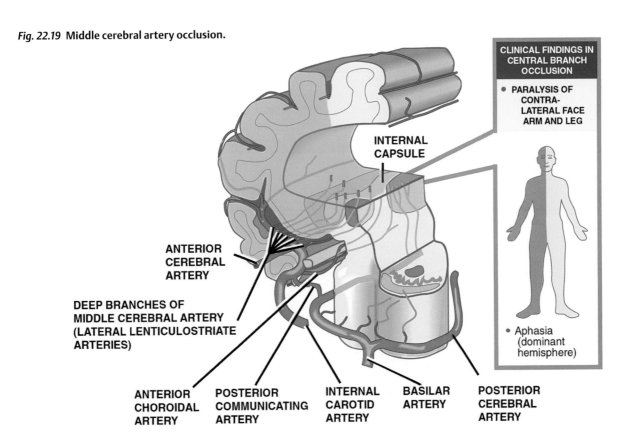

The Vertebrobasilar System

The vertebrobasilar system supplies the posterior one third of the brain.

The *vertebral artery* is the first branch of the subclavian artery (**Figs. 22.20** and **22.21**). Each vertebral artery passes upward in the neck through the transverse foramina of the upper six cervical vertebrae. Unlike the ICA, the vertebral artery gives off multiple muscular and spinal branches in its extracranial ascent. As it enters the cranial cavity through the foramen magnum, the vertebral artery pierces the dura and arachnoid to enter the subarachnoid space.

The paired vertebral arteries then pass anteriorly and medially along the medulla and join to form the *basilar artery* at the pontomedullary junction. The basilar artery continues forward along the midline of the pons and divides into the *posterior cerebral arteries* at the midbrain.

The Four Major Branches of the Vertebral Artery

1. A *meningeal branch* supplies the bone and dura in the posterior cranial fossa.

2. The *posterior spinal artery* supplies the posterior aspect of the caudal medulla and spinal cord.

3. The *anterior spinal artery* supplies the anterior aspect of the caudal medulla and spinal cord.

4. The *posterior inferior cerebellar artery* (PICA) is the largest branch of the vertebral artery. It consists of four segments: the anterior medullary segment, lateral medullary segment, tonsillomedullary segment, and telovelotonsillar segment. It runs a tortuous course between the medulla and the cerebellum to supply the posteroinferior surface of the cerebellar hemisphere, the inferior vermis, the tonsils, the choroid plexus of the fourth ventricle, and the dorsolateral medulla.

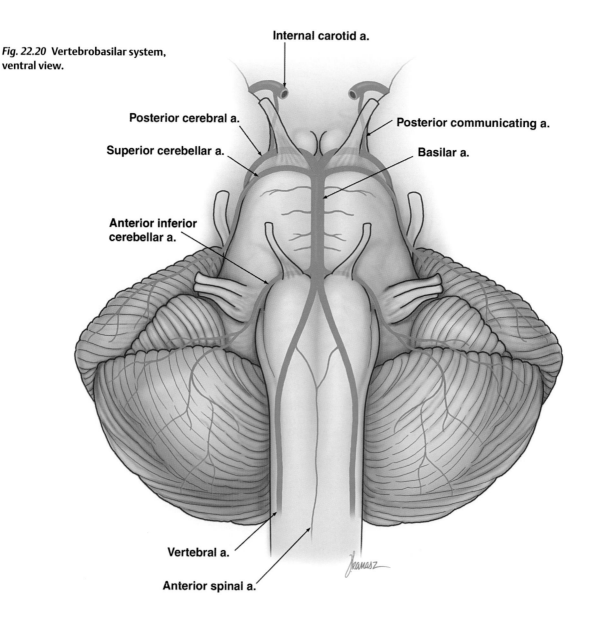

Fig. 22.20 **Vertebrobasilar system, ventral view.**

Internal carotid a.

Posterior cerebral a.

Posterior communicating a.

Superior cerebellar a.

Basilar a.

Anterior inferior cerebellar a.

Vertebral a.

Anterior spinal a.

Fig. 22.21 Vertebrobasilar system. (A) Mid-sagittal view and
(B) lateral view.

A

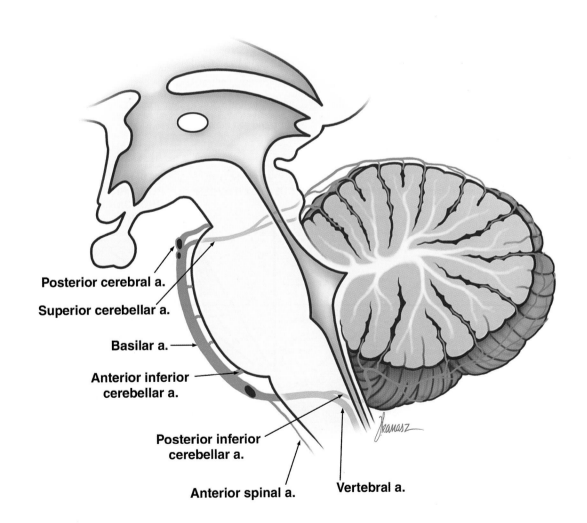

Superior cerebellar a.

Posterior cerebral a.

Basilar a.

Anterior inferior cerebellar a.

Posterior inferior cerebellar a.

Left vertebral a.

Posterior
meningeal branch of vertebral a.

B

Posterior cerebral a.

Superior cerebellar a.

Basilar a.

Anterior inferior
cerebellar a.

Posterior inferior
cerebellar a.

Anterior spinal a.

Vertebral a.

Vascular Syndromes Associated with the Four Major Vertebral Artery Branches

See **Table 22.2**.

Occlusion of the PICA produces the lateral medullary syndrome (Wallenberg syndrome). This syndrome is characterized by (1) dysphagia and dysarthria due to paralysis of the ipsilateral palatal and pharyngeal muscles (nucleus ambiguus); (2) impaired pain and temperature sensation on the ipsilateral side of the face (nucleus and spinal tract of the trigeminal nerve); (3) vertigo, nausea, vomiting, and nystagmus (vestibular nuclei); (4) ipsilateral Horner syndrome (descending sympathetic fibers); (5) ipsilateral gait and limb ataxia (inferior cerebellar peduncle); and (6) impaired pain and temperature sensation of the contralateral side of the body (lateral spinothalamic tract).

The Five Major Branches of the Basilar Artery

1. The *anterior inferior cerebellar artery* is the most caudal branch of the basilar artery. It supplies the anterolateral aspect of the inferior surface of the cerebellar hemisphere and contributes to the central cerebellar nuclei. It also supplies the lateral pons, middle cerebellar peduncle, flocculus, and cranial nerves VII and VIII. It contributes to the internal auditory artery. The upper medulla and lower pons also receive branches from this artery.

2. The *labyrinthine artery* (internal auditory artery) arises from either the basilar artery or the anteroinferior cerebellar artery. It does not supply the brainstem, but rather passes through the internal auditory meatus to supply the inner ear.

Table 22.2 Medial and Lateral Syndromes Common to Vascular Lesions of the Medulla and Pons

Syndrome	Structure	Signs
Lateral	Spinal tract and nucleus of the trigeminal nerve	Impairment of facial pain and temperature sensation (ipsilateral)
	Spinothalamic tract	Impairment of body pain and temperature sensation (contralateral)
	Descending sympathetic fibers	Horner syndrome: ptosis, miosis, anhidrosis (ipsilateral)
	Vestibular nuclei and connections	Nausea, vomiting, vertigo, and nystagmus
	Cerebellar connections	Limb and gait ataxia (ipsilateral)
Medial	Corticospinal tract	Hemiparesis (contralateral)
	Medial lemniscus	Impairment of vibratory and position sensation (contralateral)
	Cerebellar connections (pons)	Limb and gait ataxia (ipsilateral)

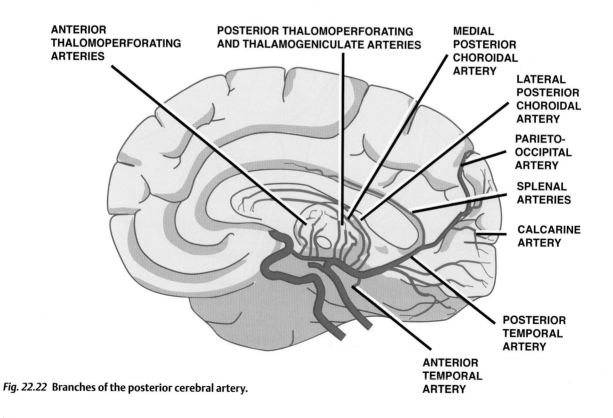

Fig. 22.22 **Branches of the posterior cerebral artery.**

3. The *pontine arteries* are numerous slender branches of the basilar artery that penetrate and supply the pons. Selective occlusion of the basal pons supply interrupts the corticobulbar and corticospinal tracts and results in total paralysis that spares only the eyes. The patient is conscious but immobile in this condition, which is known as the "locked-in" syndrome.

4. The *superior cerebellar artery* arises close to the bifurcation of the basilar artery. It supplies the superior surface of the cerebellar hemisphere as well as contributing branches to the medulla, pons, and midbrain. It provides the major arterial supply to the deep cerebellar nuclei.

5. The *posterior cerebral arteries* (**Figs. 22.22** and **22.23**) constitute the terminal bifurcation of the basilar artery. They arise at the border between the pons and the midbrain. Each posterior cerebral artery receives a posterior communicating artery from the ICA, then curves posteriorly and laterally around the midbrain. Cortical branches at the PCA supply the medial and inferior aspects of the occipital and temporal lobes, including the lower part of the optic radiations, and the visual cortex. Central branches supply the medial midbrain, geniculate bodies, and thalamus.

Fig. 22.23 **Posterior cerebral artery occlusion.**

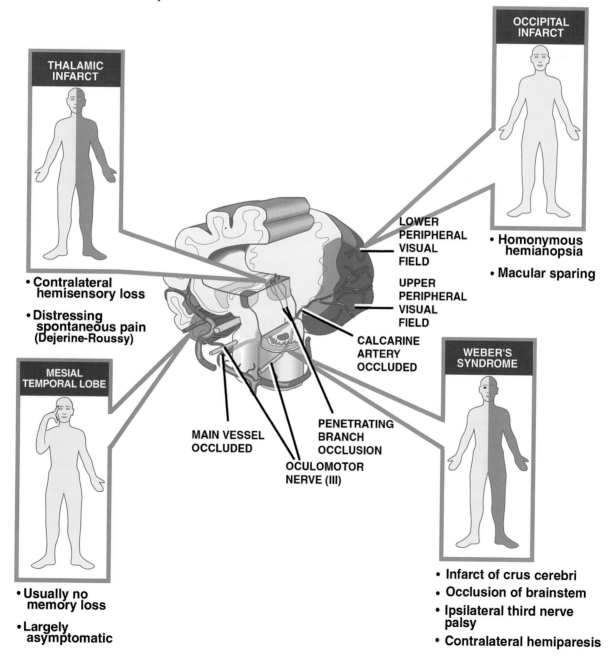

THALAMIC INFARCT

- **Contralateral hemisensory loss**

- **Distressing spontaneous pain (Dejerine-Roussy)**

MESIAL TEMPORAL LOBE

- **Usually no memory loss**

- **Largely asymptomatic**

MAIN VESSEL OCCLUDED

PENETRATING BRANCH OCCLUSION

OCULOMOTOR NERVE (III)

LOWER PERIPHERAL VISUAL FIELD

UPPER PERIPHERAL VISUAL FIELD

CALCARINE ARTERY OCCLUDED

OCCIPITAL INFARCT

- **Homonymous hemianopsia**

- **Macular sparing**

WEBER'S SYNDROME

- **Infarct of crus cerebri**
- **Occlusion of brainstem**
- **Ipsilateral third nerve palsy**
- **Contralateral hemiparesis**

Vascular Syndromes Associated with the Five Major Basilar Artery Branches

See **Table 22.1**.

A great variety of vascular syndromes are produced by occlusion of the posterior cerebral artery. Thalamic involvement produces a "thalamic pain syndrome" or Dejerine-Roussy syndrome marked by contralateral hemisensory loss, dysesthesia, and distressing, spontaneous pain.

Weber's syndrome follows infarction of the crus cerebri and the oculomotor nerve, which results from occlusion of a branch of the posterior cerebral artery that supplies the mediobasal midbrain. Clinically, it consists of contralateral paralysis of the arm and leg (crus cerebri) with ipsilateral ptosis, dilatation of pupil, absent light reflex, and exotropia (oculomotor nerve).

Occlusion of branches to the visual cortex in the occipital lobe causes homonymous hemianopsia with macular visual sparing.

The Circle of Willis

See **Fig. 22.24**.

The circle of Willis is an anastomotic connection between the internal carotid and the vertebrobasilar systems.

It is situated on the base of the brain and is formed by the *anterior communicating* and *anterior cerebral arteries* anteriorly and the *posterior communicating* and *posterior cerebral arteries* posteriorly. It is rarely a complete anatomic circle. Only in ~25% of people is the circle of Willis anatomically "complete" (patent).

The functional significance of the cerebral arterial circle lies in its provision for anastomotic compensatory supply in the event of arterial occlusion. Unfortunately, due to frequent anatomic variations in the circle and atheromatous narrowing of the communicating arteries in the elderly, these anastomoses often fail to avert ischemic stroke.

Other important cerebrovascular anastomoses include connections between the ophthalmic artery and branches of the external carotid artery, and connections between the cortical branches (leptomeningeal) of the anterior, middle, and posterior cerebral arteries.

Circulation to and from the Brain

Venous Return from the Brain

The venous return of blood from the brain passes from veins into venous sinuses. The veins of the brain, which may be divided into superficial and deep cerebral veins, lack valves. They course independently of the arterial system and empty into the venous sinuses, which lie between the periosteal and meningeal layers of the dura. The venous sinuses in turn empty into the internal jugular veins, which exit the cranial cavity through the jugular foramen.

Thus, the venous sinuses channel blood from the cerebral veins into the extracranial venous system.

The superior cerebral veins (10 to 15 in number) collect blood from the convex and medial surfaces of the brain and drain mostly into the superior sagittal sinus, and, to a lesser degree, into the inferior sagittal sinus. The inferior cerebral veins collect blood from the basal surface and ventral parts of the lateral surface of the brain and drain into the basal sinuses, including the cavernous and sphenoparietal sinuses, rostrally, and the petrosal and transverse sinuses, caudally. The venous sinuses may be arbitrarily divided into a posterosuperior group and an anteroinferior group.

Fig. 22.24 **Circle of Willis.**

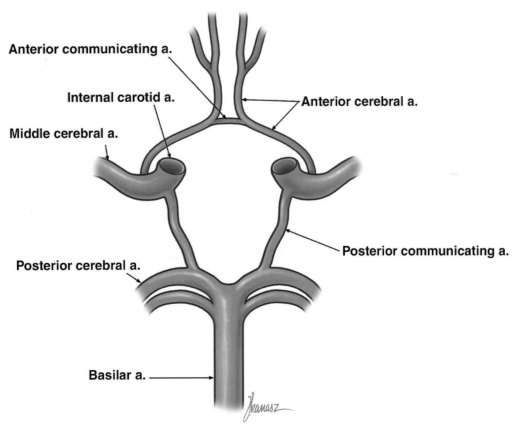

Anterior communicating a.

Internal carotid a.

Middle cerebral a.

Anterior cerebral a.

Posterior communicating a.

Posterior cerebral a.

Basilar a.

There are six venous sinuses in the posterosuperior group (**Fig. 22.25**).

1. The *superior sagittal sinus* runs along the superior margin of the falx cerebri and empties into the confluence of the sinuses. It receives the superior cerebral veins.

2. The *inferior sagittal sinus* runs along the inferior margin of the falx cerebri and continues as the straight sinus after merging with the vein of Galen.

3. The *straight sinus* is carried in the attachment of the falx cerebri to the tentorium cerebelli. Like the superior sagittal sinus, it empties into the confluence of the sinuses.

4. Also drained by the confluence is the *occipital sinus,* which lies within the falx cerebelli.

5. The confluence of the sinuses (along with the superior petrosal sinuses) empties into the *transverse sinuses,* which pass laterally and anteriorly along the attached margin of the tentorium cerebelli in the occipital bone and then inferiorly and medially at the base of the petrous part of the temporal bone to form the sigmoid sinus.

6. The *sigmoid sinus* drains into the internal jugular vein in the jugular foramen.

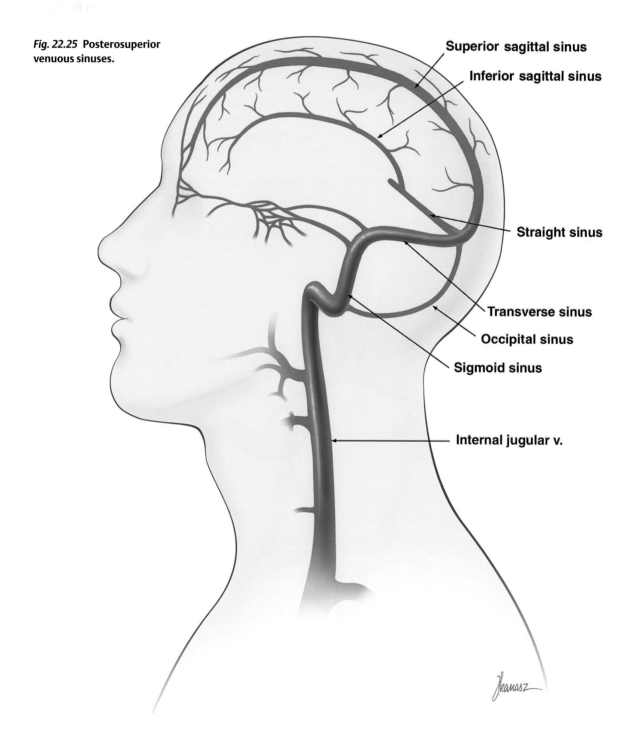

Fig. 22.25 **Posterosuperior venuous sinuses.**

Superior sagittal sinus

Inferior sagittal sinus

Straight sinus

Transverse sinus

Occipital sinus

Sigmoid sinus

Internal jugular v.

There are four venous sinuses in the anteroinferior group (**Fig. 22.26**).

1. The *cavernous sinus* is situated in the middle cranial fossa on the lateral surface of the body of the sphenoid bone and extends from the superior orbital fissure to the petrous portion of the temporal bone. It communicates with its counterpart on the opposite side through the *intercavernous sinus*.

The cavernous sinus drains the inferior and superficial middle cerebral veins (aka the sylvian vein), the ophthalmic vein, and the sphenoparietal sinus and empties into the superior and inferior petrosal sinuses. The cavernous sinus carries cranial nerves III, IV, V1, V2, and VI, as well as the internal carotid artery.

2. The *sphenoparietal sinus* runs along the lesser wing of the sphenoid bone and ends in the cavernous sinus.

3. The *superior* and *inferior petrosal sinuses*, which drain the cavernous sinus, lie on the superior and inferior borders of the petrous portion of the temporal bone. The superior petrosal sinus empties into the transverse and sigmoid sinuses; the inferior petrosal sinus empties directly into the internal jugular vein.

Fig. 22.26 **Anteroinferior venous sinuses.**

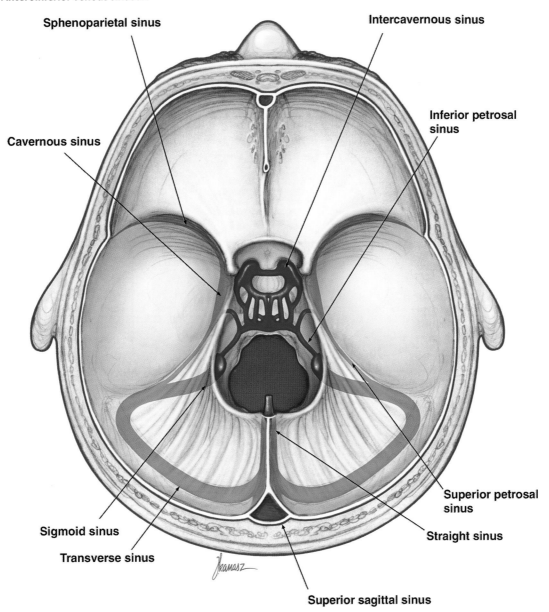

The Three Major Superficial Cerebral Veins

See **Fig. 22.27**.

The superior cerebral vein drains into the *superior sagittal sinus* and the inferior cerebral vein drains into the cavernous sinus. The superficial middle cerebral vein is emptied by the *superior sagittal sinus* (via the superior anastomotic *vein of Trolard*) and by the *transverse sinus* (via the inferior anastomotic *vein of Labbé*).

Fig. 22.27 **Superficial cerebral veins.**

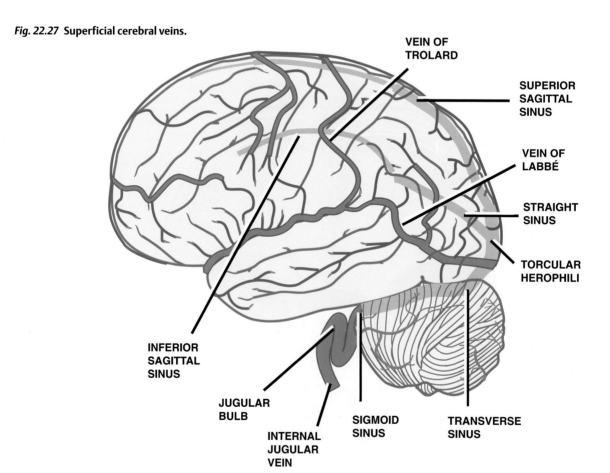

The Three Major Deep Cerebral Veins

See **Figs. 22.28** and **22.29**.

These veins drain the choroid plexus, the periventricular regions, the diencephalon, the basal ganglia, and the deep white matter. The most important of these veins are the paired *internal cerebral veins*, the *basal vein* (*of Rosenthal*), and the great cerebral vein (*vein of Galen*).

The internal cerebral veins and the basal veins join beneath the splenium of the corpus callosum to form the great cerebral vein, which empties into the straight sinus along with the inferior sagittal sinus.

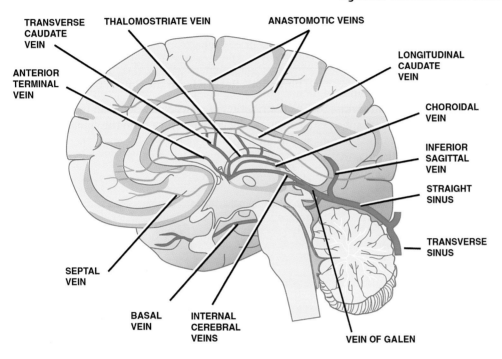

Fig. 22.28 **Internal cerebral veins.**

TRANSVERSE CAUDATE VEIN
THALOMOSTRIATE VEIN
ANASTOMOTIC VEINS
LONGITUDINAL CAUDATE VEIN
ANTERIOR TERMINAL VEIN
CHOROIDAL VEIN
INFERIOR SAGITTAL VEIN
STRAIGHT SINUS
TRANSVERSE SINUS
SEPTAL VEIN
BASAL VEIN
INTERNAL CEREBRAL VEINS
VEIN OF GALEN

Fig. 22.29 **Subependymal veins.**

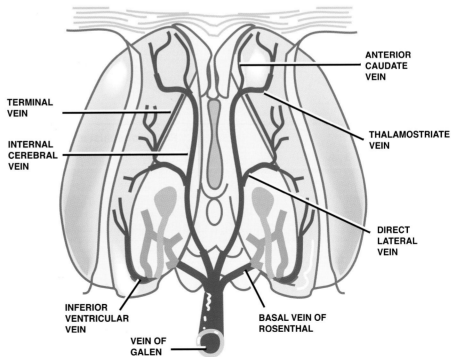

ANTERIOR CAUDATE VEIN
TERMINAL VEIN
INTERNAL CEREBRAL VEIN
THALAMOSTRIATE VEIN
DIRECT LATERAL VEIN
INFERIOR VENTRICULAR VEIN
BASAL VEIN OF ROSENTHAL
VEIN OF GALEN

Circulation to and from the Spinal Cord

The Two Major Arteries That Supply the Spinal Cord

See **Fig. 22.30**.

The spinal cord is supplied by a single *anterior spinal artery* and the *posterior spinal arteries*, both of which originate as descending branches of the *vertebral arteries*.

The anterior spinal artery is formed by an anastomosis of branches from the two vertebral arteries. It runs along the anterior median fissure to supply the anterior two thirds of the spinal cord. The posterior third of the spinal cord is supplied by the paired posterior spinal arteries, which pass down the posterolateral aspect of the cord on either side near the spinal roots.

As reinforcement for the anterior and posterior spinal artery supply, intercostal branches of the thoracic aorta and lumbar branches of the abdominal aorta give off spinal arteries that traverse the intervertebral foramina to enter the vertebral canal. These arteries then divide into anterior and posterior radicular arteries that accompany the ventral and dorsal roots of the spinal nerves.

The radicular arteries contribute to a vascular plexus in the pia mater and anastomose with the anterior and posterior spinal arteries. A great anterior radicular artery, the artery of Adamkiewicz, is a major source of blood supply to the lower two thirds of the spinal cord. It is usually located on the left side in the lower thoracic or upper lumbar region. There are significantly more radicular contributions to the posterior compared with the anterior spinal artery. Therefore, the supply to the anterior two thirds of the cord is tenuous in certain regions of the spinal cord, especially the thoracic cord. This area of the spinal cord is thus vulnerable to infarction in the event that blood supply is compromised, such as may occur during a period of hypoperfusion in the setting of an aortic aneurysm repair.

The Venous Return from the Spinal Cord

The distribution of veins corresponds to the distribution of arteries. The venous return from the spinal cord parallels its arterial supply.

Fig. 22.30 **Spinal arteries.**

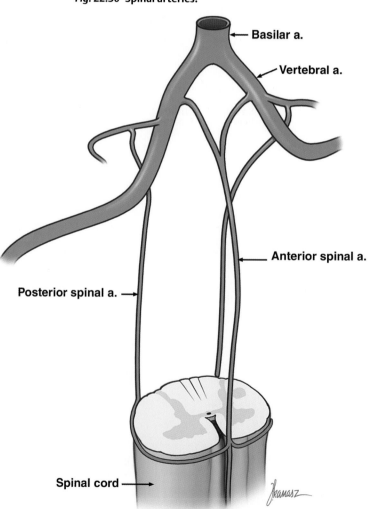

Basilar a.

Vertebral a.

Anterior spinal a.

Posterior spinal a.

Spinal cord

The Approach to the Patient with Stroke

Clinically, stroke presents as a focal neurologic deficit, out of the blue. The clinical features that characterize neurologic syndromes as strokes are (1) acute onset and (2) evidence of damage to a discrete area of the brain. Thus, in approaching the patient with an acute onset neurologic deficit, the initial task is anatomic localization of the dysfunctional CNS region. Clinically speaking, it is to determine if the patient suffered from a focal dysfunction due to an ischemic injury (ischemic stroke) and to initiate appropriate therapy as rapidly as possible. It is essential to rule out the possibility of hemorrhagic injury. The question that underlies the task of localization is What vascular territory has been comprised?

Signs and Symptoms of Anterior and Posterior Circulation Syndromes Present with Characteristic Sets of Signs and Symptoms

See **Tables 22.3** and **22.4**.

The first step in identifying the compromised vascular territory involves determining whether the clinical presentation suggests impairment of the anterior or posterior circulation.

The anterior circulation, or internal carotid artery system, supplies the optic nerve and retina, most of the cerebral cortex, basal ganglia, internal capsule, and optic radiations.

It consists of the internal carotid artery and its three major branches: (1) the ophthalmic artery, the occlusion of which produces monocular blindness in the ipsilateral eye; (2) the anterior cerebral artery, the occlusion of which produces weakness and sensory loss in the contralateral leg; and (3) the middle cerebral artery, the occlusion of which leads to weakness and sensory loss in the contralateral face and arm, contralateral homonymous hemianopsia, and aphasia (in the case of MCA occlusion in the dominant hemisphere).

The posterior circulation, or vertebrobasilar system, supplies the brainstem, cerebellum, thalamus, and parts of the temporal and occipital lobes, including the visual cortex and the optic radiations.

It consists of the vertebral arteries, the basilar artery, and the posterior cerebral arteries. When occluded, branches of these arteries that supply the brainstem produce diplopia, dysarthria, dysphagia, tinnitus, and vertigo (signs and symptoms of various cranial nerve dysfunction). Other posterior circulation signs include an altered level of consciousness (reticular activating system), hemiparesis and hemisensory loss (descending and ascending long tracts), ataxia (cerebellum), hemisensory loss (thalamus), and visual field disturbances (visual cortex and optic radiations).

Anterior Circulation Vascular Syndromes are Clinically Subdivided into Cortical and Subcortial Syndromes

The second step in identifying the comprised vascular territory involves determining whether an anterior circulation syndrome is cortically or subcortically based. The

Table 22.3 Major Structures Supplied by the Anterior and Posterior Cerebral Circulations

Internal Carotid Artery System	Vertebrobasilar Artery System
Optic nerve and retina	Spinal cord
Optic tract and radiations	Brainstem
Basal ganglia	Cerebellum
Internal capsule	Optic tract and radiations
Frontal and parietal cortices, including language area	Thalamus
Parts of temporal and occipital cortices	Parts of the temporal and occipital cortices, including visual cortex

distinction between cortical and subcortical syndromes bears both diagnostic and therapeutic significance. Small, deep subcortical infarcts tend to be hypertensive-related, focusing attention on the management of systemic hypertension (at times in the setting of diabetes and a history of smoking), whereas large cortical infarcts tend to be thrombotic or embolic in origin, focusing attention instead on a search for atherosclerotic disease and potential sources of emboli. There is then potential to perform thrombolysis for the latter group of patients.

Cortical syndromes are primarily distinguished from subcortical ones on the basis of two criteria: (1) the presence of so-called cortical signs and (2) the pattern of neurologic impairment.

Cortical signs refers to neurologic findings localizable to the cerebral cortex. Such findings include (1) disorders of language (e.g., aphasia) and (2) disorders of sensory and motor integration (e.g., agnosia, the failure to perceive the significance of sensory input, and apraxia, the inability to perform complex learned tasks).

Pattern of neurologic impairment refers to the distribution of weakness or sensory loss, which is different in cortical and cortical/subcortical syndromes. Because of the diffuse distribution of the cortical motor and sensory fibers, *most cortically based strokes produce relatively mild hemisyndromes primarily affecting the face and arm* (middle cerebral artery) or leg (anterior cerebral artery). Because motor and sensory fibers converge as they pass through deep subcortical structures, *most subcortically based strokes produce relatively severe hemisyndromes equally affecting the face, arm, and leg* (lenticulostriate arteries).

Thus, in the patient with presumed anterior circulation impairment, further data should be sought regarding the presence of so-called cortical signs and the distribution of neurologic deficits. These findings help distinguish between cortical and subcortical syndromes, which often bear diagnostic, therapeutic, and prognostic significance.

Table 22.4 Clinical Features of Transient Ischemic Attacks (listed in order of frequency)

Internal Carotid Artery Systems	Vertebrobasilar Artery System
Contralateral sensory loss	Vertigo*
Contralateral weakness	Visual field cut
Aphasia*	Drop attacks*
Visual field cut	Dysarthria
Dysarthria	Contralateral sensory loss
	Contralateral weakness
	Diplopia*
	Tinnitus*

*Clinically useful to distinguish between internal carotid artery and vertebral artery system strokes.

Determining the Etiology of Stroke

In approaching the patient with stroke, the first question, here as elsewhere in neurology, is Where is the lesion? In stroke, this question is often asked in terms of vascular distributions: Does the stroke involve the anterior or posterior circulation? If anterior, is it cortical or subcortical? Is the neurologic deficit consistent with a specific arterial territory?

Having resolved these questions, the neurologist must next ask What is the lesion? The possibilities here are threefold: (1) hemorrhage, or rupture and leakage from an intracranial blood vessel; (2) thrombosis, or occlusion of a vessel by a thrombus (i.e., blood clot); and (3) embolism, or occlusion of a vessel by a thrombus dislodged from a more proximal site (artery or heart). The relative likelihood of each of these is suggested by the anatomic diagnosis, and other circumstances such as the stroke's course of onset, the presence of concurrent medical illnesses, and the patient's stroke risk factor profile.

For example, a large stroke of stuttering onset in the distribution of the internal carotid artery in a patient with hypercholesterolemia and diffuse atherosclerosis suggests thrombosis. This is because thrombus formation, which has a predilection for large vessels, typically stutters at onset and is promoted by atherosclerosis.

By contrast, a cortical stroke, maximal at onset, in a patient with a history of chronic atrial fibrillation, suggests embolism. This is because a fibrillating heart is fertile ground for the development of a thrombus that may break loose, travel upstream, and lodge in an intracranial artery, most commonly cortical, to cause a neurologic deficit that is maximal at onset.

Finally, a subcortical stroke associated with headache, nausea, vomiting, and an alteration in consciousness in a patient with severe hypertension suggests hemorrhage. This is because severe hypertension increases the risk of intracranial hemorrhage, which causes headache, nausea, vomiting, and an alteration in consciousness.

23 Cerebrospinal Fluid

The meninges are composed of three connective tissue sheaths that envelope the central nervous system (CNS) and separate it from its bony encasement. From outside in, these are the dura mater, the arachnoid layer, and the pia mater. The cerebrospinal fluid (CSF), a waterlike substance in which the brain is bathed, is contained between the arachnoid layer and the pia mater in the subarachnoid space. There, the fluid serves to help the meninges to support and protect the semisolid brain and spinal cord and to remove metabolic waste products such as carbon dioxide, lactate, and hydrogen ions.

Meninges

Dura Mater

See **Fig. 23.1**.

The tough fibrous dura mater is composed of elongated fibroblasts and collagen fibrils. It contains blood vessels and nerves and is commonly described as comprising two parts, an outer endosteal layer (more properly called *periosteal dura*), which faces the skull, and an inner layer, the *meningeal dura*, which faces the brain. These two dural layers are closely attached to one another, except in certain parts where they separate to form the venous sinuses.

Pia Mater and Arachnoid Mater

The *pia mater* and *arachnoid mater*, which are collectively known as the leptomeninges, are separated from the dura mater by a potential space, known as the subdural space. Developmentally, the pia mater and arachnoid arise as a single layer of mesodermal tissue surrounding the brain and the spinal cord. This layer becomes separated as a fluid-filled space, the CSF-containing subarachnoid space, divides them. The trabeculae that pass between the pia and the arachnoid are remnants of these coverings' common embryological origin.

Although the pia mater adheres to the surface of the brain, closely following the contours of its gyri and sulci, the arachnoid covers only its superficial surface. It follows from this that in certain areas around the brain the pia and arachnoid are separated widely; in such regions are formed cavities called the subarachnoid cisterns (not shown in figure).

Fig. 23.1 Structure of the meninges.

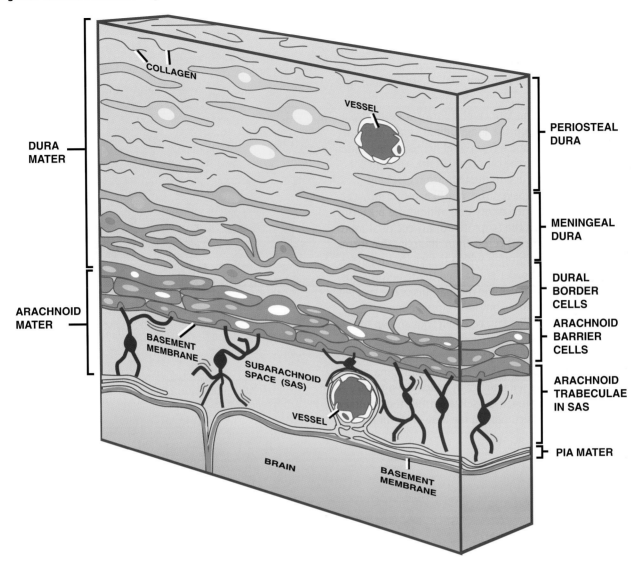

Dural Folds

See **Fig. 23.2**.

The dural folds are created by reflections of the dura mater along the contours of the brain. Three communicating spaces are thus formed in the cranial cavity, two supratentorial and one infratentorial. There are four major dural folds:

1. *Falx cerebri* The falx cerebri forms a vertical partition that runs within the longitudinal cerebral fissure separating the right and left cerebral hemispheres. Anteriorly, it is attached to the crista galli of the ethmoid bone; posteriorly, it is attached to the tentorium cerebelli.

2. *Tentorium cerebelli* The tentlike tentorium cerebelli divides the cranial cavity into middle and posterior fossae and separates the (supratentorial) occipital lobes from the (infratentorial) cerebellum. Its free edge forms the tentorial notch, through which the midbrain passes. Its peripheral fixed border is attached to the petrous portion of the temporal bones and the margins of the grooves for the transverse sinuses on the occipital bone.

3. *Falx cerebelli* The falx cerebelli (not shown in figure) extends vertically for a short distance in the posterior fossa between the cerebellar hemispheres.

4. *Diaphragma sellae* The small diaphragma sellae forms the roof of the sella turcica in which the pituitary is housed. A small opening in the sellae permits the pituitary stalk to pass to its attachment at the base of the brain.

Fig. 23.2 **Dural folds.**

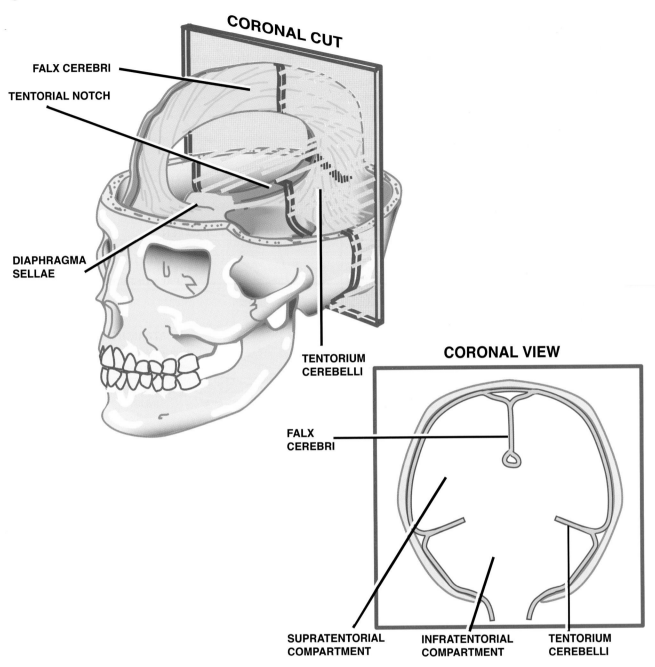

CORONAL CUT

FALX CEREBRI

TENTORIAL NOTCH

DIAPHRAGMA
SELLAE

TENTORIUM
CEREBELLI

CORONAL VIEW

FALX
CEREBRI

SUPRATENTORIAL
COMPARTMENT

INFRATENTORIAL
COMPARTMENT

TENTORIUM
CEREBELLI

Dural Venous Sinuses

See **Fig. 23.3**.

The venous sinuses are formed by the space between the periosteal and meningeal layers of the dura. They are described in Chapter 22. In short, they receive venous blood that is leaving the brain and empty it into the internal jugular veins, which exit the cranial cavity through the jugular foramen.

Fig. 23.3 (A) **Venous sinuses, oblique view.** *(Continued)*

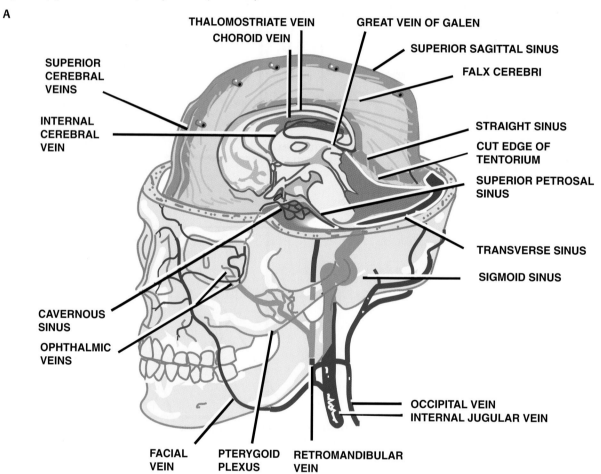

Fig. 23.3 *(Continued)* *(B)* **Venous sinuses, axial view.**

B

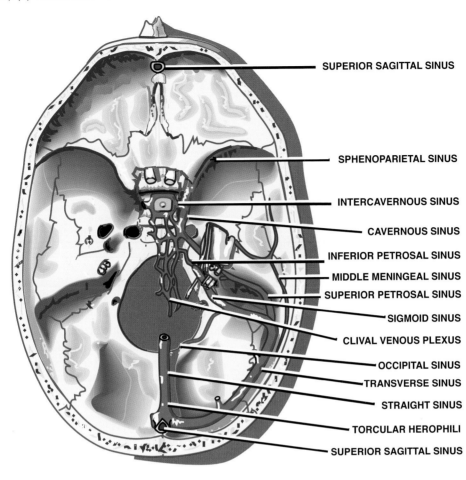

SUPERIOR SAGITTAL SINUS

SPHENOPARIETAL SINUS

INTERCAVERNOUS SINUS

CAVERNOUS SINUS

INFERIOR PETROSAL SINUS

MIDDLE MENINGEAL SINUS

SUPERIOR PETROSAL SINUS

SIGMOID SINUS

CLIVAL VENOUS PLEXUS

OCCIPITAL SINUS

TRANSVERSE SINUS

STRAIGHT SINUS

TORCULAR HEROPHILI

SUPERIOR SAGITTAL SINUS

Subarachnoid Cisterns

See **Fig. 23.4**.

Although they are often described as distinct compartments, the subarachnoid cisterns are in fact not truly anatomically distinct. Rather, these subarachnoid spaces are separated from each other by a trabeculated porous wall with various-sized openings. The contents of the major subarachnoid cisterns are as follows.

Cerebellomedullary Cistern (Cisterna Magna)

This cistern lies between the cerebellum and the medulla. It receives CSF from the fourth ventricle via the median foramen of Magendie and the two lateral foramina of Luschka. The cerebellomedullary cistern contains:

- The vertebral artery and the origin of the posterior inferior cerebellar artery
- The ninth, tenth, eleventh, and twelfth cranial nerves
- The choroid plexus

The Prepontine Cistern

The prepontine cistern surrounds the ventral aspect of the pons. It contains

- The basilar artery and the origin of the anteroinferior cerebellar artery
- The origin of the superior cerebellar arteries
- The sixth cranial nerve

The Cerebellopontine Cistern

The cerebellopontine cistern is situated in the lateral angle between the cerebellum and the pons. It contains

- The seventh and eighth cranial nerves
- The anteroinferior cerebellar artery
- The fifth cranial nerve and the petrosal vein

The Interpeduncular Cistern

The interpeduncular cistern is situated between the two cerebral peduncles. It contains

- The bifurcation of the basilar artery
- Peduncular segments of the posterior cerebral arteries
- Peduncular segments of the superior cerebellar arteries
- Perforating branches of the posterior cerebral arteries
- The posterior communicating arteries
- The basal vein of Rosenthal
- The third cranial nerve, which passes between the posterior cerebral and superior cerebellar arteries

The Crural Cistern

The crural cistern is situated around the ventrolateral aspect of the midbrain. It contains

- The anterior choroidal artery
- The medial posterior choroidal artery
- The basal vein of Rosenthal

The Chiasmatic Cistern

The chiasmatic cistern is situated just ventral to the optic chiasm. It contains

- The anterior aspect of the optic chiasm and optic nerves
- The hypophyseal stalk
- The origin of the anterior cerebral arteries

The Carotid Cistern

The carotid cistern is situated between the carotid artery and the ipsilateral optic nerve. It contains

- The internal carotid artery
- The origin of the anterior choroidal artery
- The origin of the posterior communicating artery

The Sylvian Cistern

The sylvian cistern is situated in the fissure between the frontal and temporal lobes. It contains

- The middle cerebral artery
- The middle cerebral (sylvian) veins
- The fronto-orbital veins
- Collaterals to the basal vein of Rosenthal

The Lamina Terminalis Cistern

The lamina terminalis cistern is situated just rostral to the third ventricle. It contains

- The anterior cerebral arteries (the A1 segment and the proximal A2 segment)
- The anterior communicating artery
- Heubner's artery
- The hypothalamic arteries
- The origin of the fronto-orbital arteries

The Quadrigeminal Cistern

The quadrigeminal cistern is situated dorsal to the midbrain. It contains

- The great vein of Galen
- The posterior pericallosal arteries
- The third portion of the superior cerebellar arteries
- Perforating branches of the posterior cerebral and the superior cerebellar arteries
- The third portion of the posterior cerebral arteries. (These paired arteries approach one another, and then turn posteriorly under the splenium of the corpus callosum. After traveling beneath the corpus callosum, they then bifurcate into two cortical branches, the calcarine and parieto-occipital branches.)

The Ambient Cistern

The ambient cistern is situated along the lateral aspects of the midbrain. It is composed of a supratentorial and an infratentorial compartment. Its supratentorial portion contains

- The basal vein of Rosenthal
- The posterior cerebral artery

Its infratentorial portion contains:

- The superior cerebellar artery
- The fourth nerve

The Lumbar Cistern

The lumbar cistern extends from the conus medullaris (L1–L2) to about the level of the second sacral vertebra. It contains the filum terminale and the nerve roots of the cauda equina. It is from this cistern that CSF is withdrawn during lumbar puncture.

It is of clinical significance that cerebral arteries, veins, and cranial nerves must pass through the subarachnoid space, and that these structures maintain their meningeal investment until around their point of exit from the skull. The optic nerve, for example, is surrounded by subarachnoid space up until its attachment to the eyeball. CSF pressure is thus transmitted to the head of the optic nerve, which may be visualized by the direct ophthalmoscope, as a marker of intracranial hypertension.

Fig. 23.4 **Subarachnoid cisterns.**

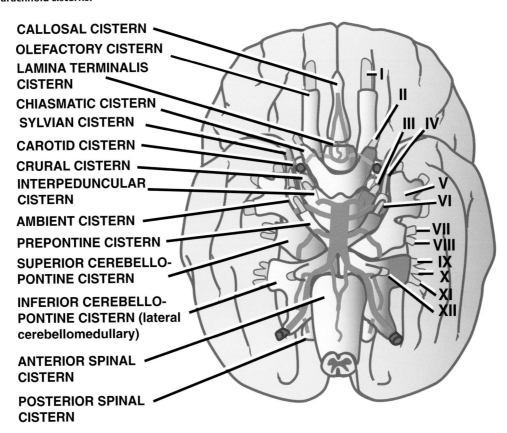

CALLOSAL CISTERN
OLEFACTORY CISTERN
LAMINA TERMINALIS CISTERN
CHIASMATIC CISTERN
SYLVIAN CISTERN
CAROTID CISTERN
CRURAL CISTERN
INTERPEDUNCULAR CISTERN
AMBIENT CISTERN
PREPONTINE CISTERN
SUPERIOR CEREBELLO-PONTINE CISTERN
INFERIOR CEREBELLO-PONTINE CISTERN (lateral cerebellomedullary)
ANTERIOR SPINAL CISTERN
POSTERIOR SPINAL CISTERN

I
II
III IV
V
VI
VII
VIII
IX
X
XI
XII

Cerebrospinal Fluid

See **Fig. 23.5**.

Composition, Volume, and Pressure

CSF is clear and colorless, with a specific gravity of 1.003 to 1.008. It contains up to five lymphocytes per cubic millimeter. The glucose level is roughly two thirds that of blood glucose, and the protein content is low (15 to 45 mg/dL).

The ventricular system and the subarachnoid space together contain ~150 mL of CSF, of which roughly 30 mL is contained in the ventricular system alone. About 500 mL of CSF is formed during a 24-hour period. Normal CSF pressure is 65 to 195 mm water, or 5 to 15 mm Hg.

Formation and Absorption

The formation of CSF is a complex process that is regulated by the choroid plexus. The choroid plexus is a villous structure that invaginates from the ventricular surface into the ventricular CSF. It consists of a core of vascular pia mater, surrounded by epithelium from the ependymal lining of the ventricle.

By contrast, *arachnoid villi*, which are responsible for CSF absorption, invaginate from the subarachnoid space into the dural venous sinuses (**Fig. 35.5A**). Each villus thus consists of a core of subarachnoid space, surrounded by a cellular layer comprising endothelia of the sinus and epithelia of the arachnoid.

Circulation

CSF flows from its origin in the ventricles to its absorption in the venous sinuses (**Fig. 35.5B**), as follows:

1. Forms in the choroid plexi of the *third, fourth,* and *lateral ventricles*

2. Flows from the ventricles into the *cerebellomedullary cistern* via the foramina of the single, midline Magendie and the dual lateral Luschka

3. Circulates in the *subarachnoid space* surrounding the medulla and the spinal cord

4. Flows rostrally through the *pontine,* ambient (not shown in figure), and *interpeduncular cisterns* to reach the superior and lateral surfaces of the cerebral hemispheres

5. Passively diffuses into venous sinuses through the arachnoid villi

Examination

CSF is most readily obtained by lumbar puncture, whereby CSF is withdrawn from the subarachnoid space at the level of the lumbar spine. Examination of the CSF routinely includes the following: (1) measurement of CSF pressure, (2) red and white blood cell count with differential, (3) glucose and protein content, and (4) Gram stain and bacterial culture with sensitivity.

Fig. 23.5 *(A)* Arachnoid villi.
(B) Cerebrospinal fluid circulation.

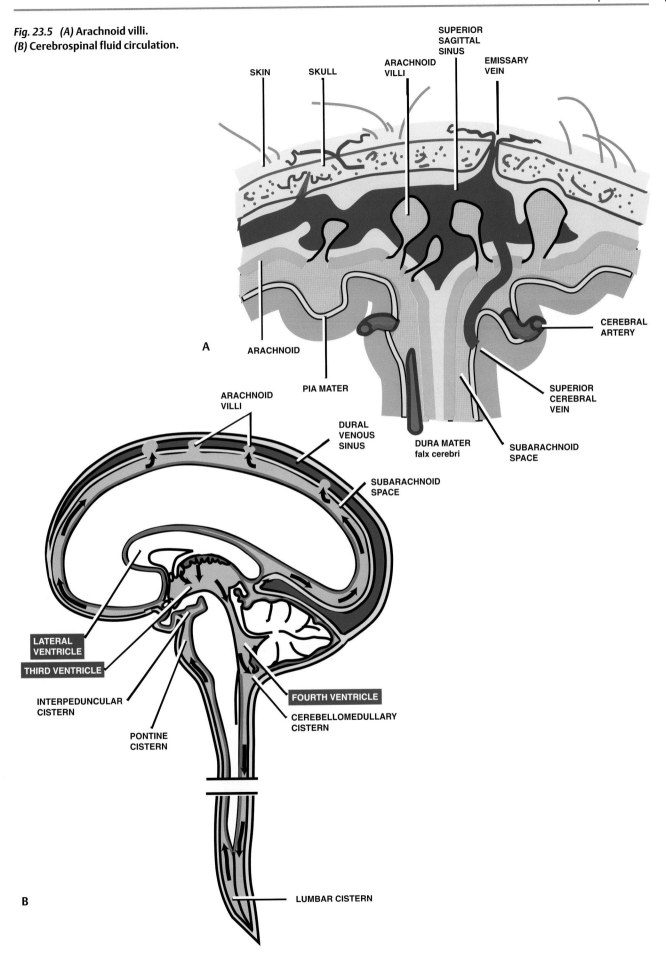

A

SKIN
SKULL
ARACHNOID VILLI
SUPERIOR SAGITTAL SINUS
EMISSARY VEIN
CEREBRAL ARTERY
SUPERIOR CEREBRAL VEIN
SUBARACHNOID SPACE
DURA MATER *falx cerebri*
PIA MATER
ARACHNOID

B

ARACHNOID VILLI
DURAL VENOUS SINUS
SUBARACHNOID SPACE
LATERAL VENTRICLE
THIRD VENTRICLE
FOURTH VENTRICLE
INTERPEDUNCULAR CISTERN
PONTINE CISTERN
CEREBELLOMEDULLARY CISTERN
LUMBAR CISTERN

The Ventricles

Lateral Ventricles

See **Fig. 23.6**.

The *lateral ventricle* comprises a cavity within the telencephalon. During development, this cavity acquires the shape of a flattened **C** with a small tail. For the sake of description, the lateral ventricle is divided into a *anterior horn*, a *body*, an *posterior horn*, and a *inferior horn*. The junction between the body of the lateral ventricle and its *posterior* and *inferior* horns is known as the *atrium* (or trigone).

Because an understanding of the complex topography of the lateral ventricle is instrumental to an understanding of the topography of the brain, its relationship to adjacent structures is described in detail. The structures that are juxtaposed to the walls of the lateral ventricle are as follows (**Figs. 22.7** to **22.13**).

Fig. 23.6 (*A*) Lateral ventricles, lateral view. (*B*) Lateral ventricles, superior view.

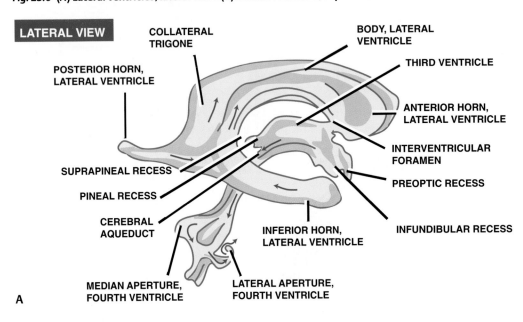

LATERAL VIEW

COLLATERAL TRIGONE

BODY, LATERAL VENTRICLE

THIRD VENTRICLE

POSTERIOR HORN, LATERAL VENTRICLE

ANTERIOR HORN, LATERAL VENTRICLE

INTERVENTRICULAR FORAMEN

SUPRAPINEAL RECESS

PINEAL RECESS

PREOPTIC RECESS

CEREBRAL AQUEDUCT

INFERIOR HORN, LATERAL VENTRICLE

INFUNDIBULAR RECESS

MEDIAN APERTURE, FOURTH VENTRICLE

LATERAL APERTURE, FOURTH VENTRICLE

A

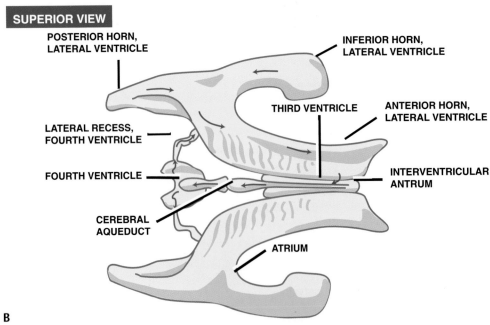

SUPERIOR VIEW

POSTERIOR HORN, LATERAL VENTRICLE

INFERIOR HORN, LATERAL VENTRICLE

THIRD VENTRICLE

ANTERIOR HORN, LATERAL VENTRICLE

LATERAL RECESS, FOURTH VENTRICLE

FOURTH VENTRICLE

INTERVENTRICULAR ANTRUM

CEREBRAL AQUEDUCT

ATRIUM

B

Frontal Horn

See **Fig. 23.7**.

The frontal horn is the part of the lateral ventricle that is located anterior to the foramen of Monro. Its structural borders are as follows:

- Anterior wall: *genu of the corpus callosum*
- Medial wall: *septum pellucidum* and columns of the fornix
- Lateral wall: head of the *caudate nucleus*
- Roof: *genu of the corpus callosum*
- Floor: *rostrum of the corpus callosum*

Fig. 23.7 **Frontal horn, lateral ventricle.**

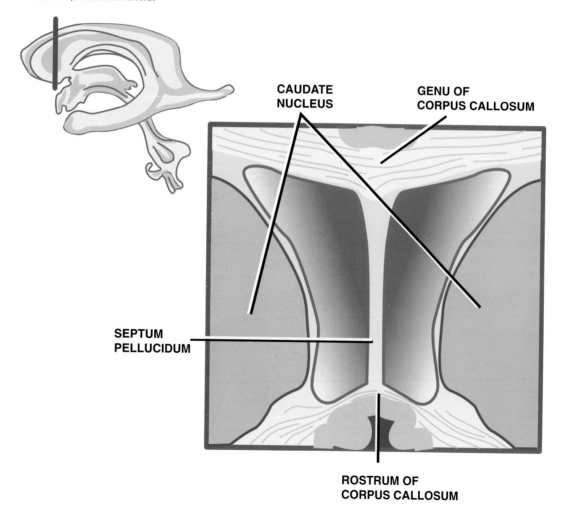

CAUDATE NUCLEUS

GENU OF CORPUS CALLOSUM

SEPTUM PELLUCIDUM

ROSTRUM OF CORPUS CALLOSUM

Body

See **Fig. 23.8**.

The boundaries of the body of the lateral ventricle are the posterior edge of the foramen of Monro, anteriorly, and the point where the septum pellucidum disappears, posteriorly. (Its posterior boundary also marks the point where the corpus callosum and the fornix meet.) The structural borders of the body of the lateral ventricle are as follows:

- Medial wall: *septum pellucidum*
- Lateral wall: *caudate nucleus*
- Roof: *body of the corpus callosum*
- Floor: *thalamus*

Fig. 23.8 **Body, lateral ventricle.**

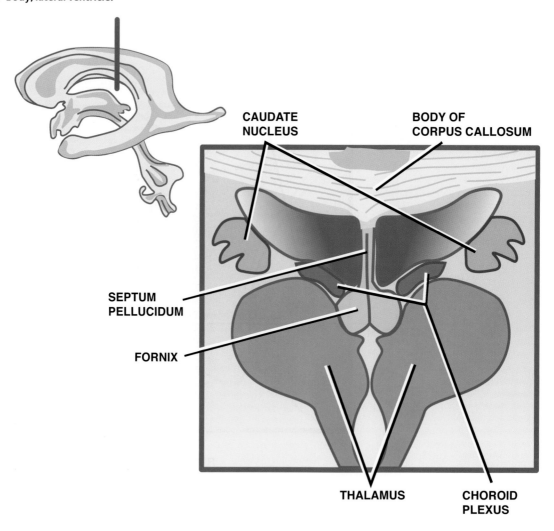

CAUDATE NUCLEUS

BODY OF CORPUS CALLOSUM

SEPTUM PELLUCIDUM

FORNIX

THALAMUS

CHOROID PLEXUS

Atrium and Occipital Horn

See **Fig. 23.9**.

Together these components of the lateral ventricle form a triangular cavity. The apex of this triangle is located in the occipital lobe, and the base of the triangle is located just posterior to the pulvinar. The borders of the atrium and the posterior horn are as follows:

- Anterior wall: crus of the fornix, medially, and pulvinar of thalamus, laterally (not shown in figure)
- Medial wall: formed by two prominences—*forceps major* of the corpus callosum, superiorly, and *calcar avis* (prominence overlying calcarine sulcus), inferiorly
- Lateral wall: caudate nucleus, anteriorly (not shown in figure), and fibers of the *tapetum* (corpus callosum), posteriorly
- Floor: *collateral trigone* (prominence overlying *collateral sulcus*)

Fig. 23.9 **Atrium, lateral ventricle.**

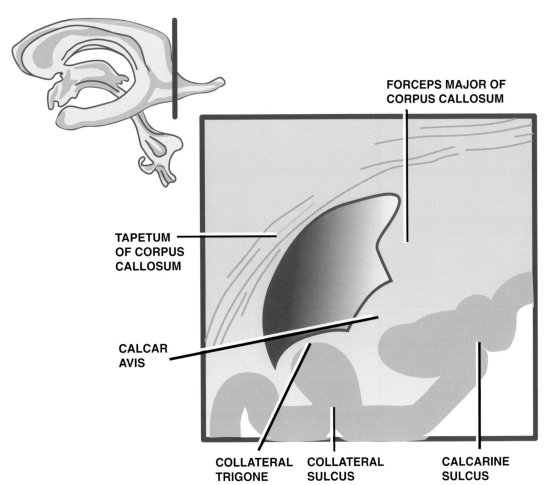

FORCEPS MAJOR OF CORPUS CALLOSUM

TAPETUM OF CORPUS CALLOSUM

CALCAR AVIS

COLLATERAL TRIGONE COLLATERAL SULCUS CALCARINE SULCUS

Temporal Horn

See **Fig. 23.10**.

The temporal horn extends forward from the atrium into the medial part of the temporal lobe. The borders of the temporal horn are as follows:

- Anterior wall: amygdaloid nucleus (not shown in figure)
- Medial wall: *choroidal fissure* (situated between the *thalamus* and the *fimbria of the fornix*)
- Lateral wall: *tapetum* of the corpus callosum
- Roof: thalamus, medially, and tapetum of the corpus callosum, laterally
- Floor: *hippocampus*, medially, and *collateral eminence* (prominence overlying collateral sulcus), laterally

Fig. 23.10 **Temporal horn, lateral ventricle.**

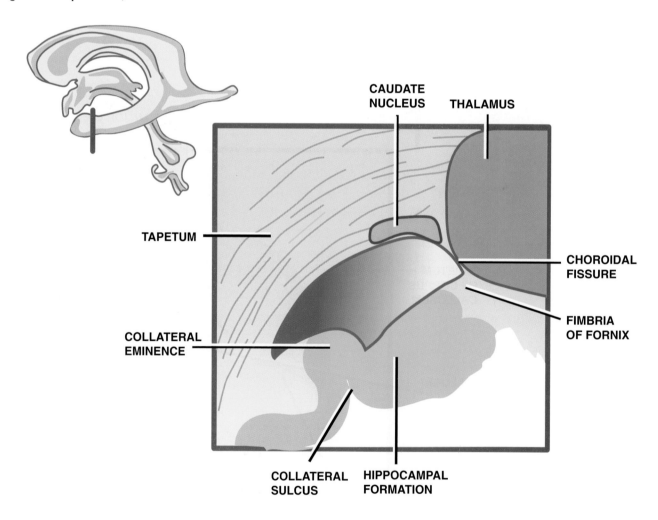

Third Ventricle

See **Fig. 23.11.**

The third ventricle is the cavity of the diencephalon. It communicates rostrally with the lateral ventricle and caudally with the cerebral aqueduct. The walls of the third ventricle are formed by the following structures:

- Anterior wall: *anterior commissure*, superiorly, and *lamina terminalis*, inferiorly
- Posterior wall: from superior to inferior—the *habenular commissure*, the *pineal gland*, and the *posterior commissure*
- Lateral wall: thalamus, superiorly, and hypothalamus, inferiorly
- Roof: *tela choroidea* (the vellum interpositum lies within the two layers of the tela choroidea). Immediately above the tela choroidea is the body of the *fornix*; immediately above the fornix is the *corpus callosum.*
- Floor: *optic chiasm*, anteriorly, and *infundibulum*, posteriorly

Fig. 23.11 **The ventricular system.**

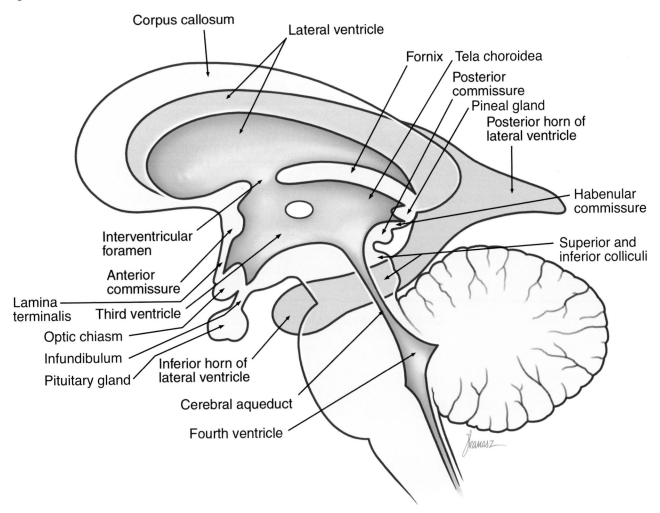

Recesses of the Third Ventricle

See **Fig. 23.12.**

A series of recesses are formed by outpouchings of the structures that border the floor (supraoptic and infundibular recesses) and the posterior wall (pineal and suprapineal recesses) of the third ventricle, as follows:

- *Supraoptic recess*: superior to the optic chiasm
- *Infundibular recess*: in the infundibulum
- *Pineal recess*: in the stalk of the pineal gland
- *Suprapineal recess*: above the pineal recess

Fig. 23.12 **Recesses of the third ventricle.**

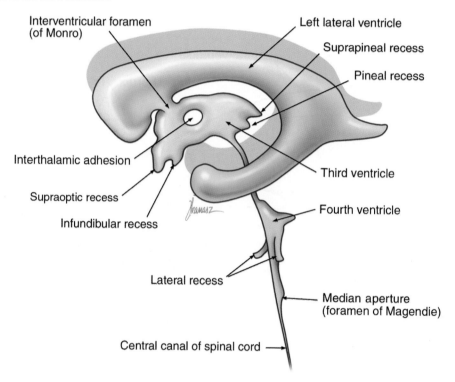

Fourth Ventricle

See **Fig. 23.13**.

The fourth ventricle is a tent-shaped cavity located between the cerebellum and the brainstem. The apex of the tent extends dorsally into the base of the cerebellum. The fourth ventricle communicates rostrally with the cerebral aqueduct, caudally with the cisterna magna (via the foramen of Magendie), and laterally with the cerebellopontine angle cisterns (via the foramen of Luschka). Its borders are formed by the following structures:

- Superior roof: *superior medullary velum*, medially, and the *superior, middle,* and *inferior cerebellar peduncles,* laterally
- Inferior roof: nodule and *inferior medullary velum,* cranially, and *tela choroidea,* caudally
- Floor: dorsal *pons,* rostrally, and dorsal *medulla,* caudally
- Lateral recesses: these consist of pouches formed by the union of the roof and the floor of the fourth ventricle that open through the foramen of Luschka into the cerebellopontine angle cistern

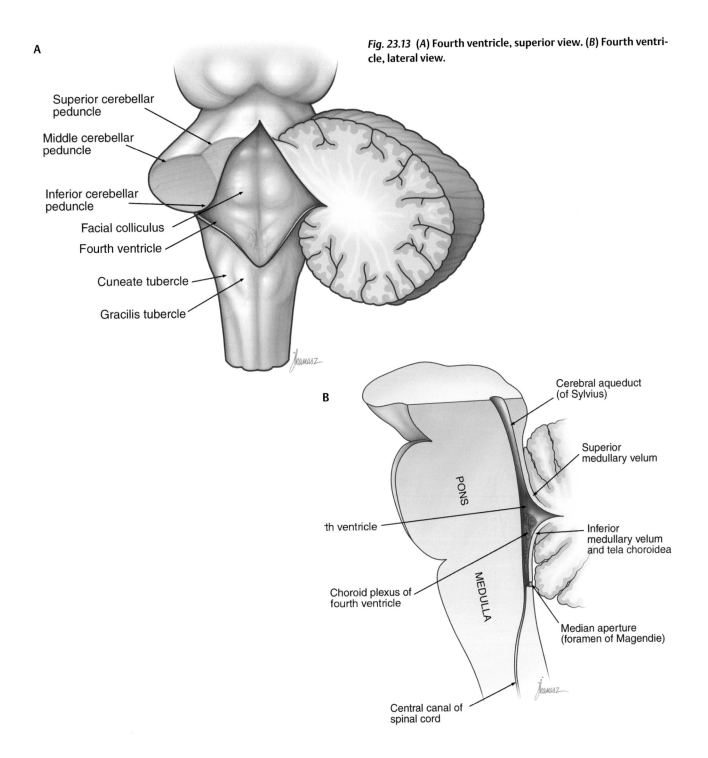

Fig. 23.13 (*A*) Fourth ventricle, superior view. (*B*) Fourth ventricle, lateral view.

Approach to the Patient with Increased Intracranial Pressure

See **Fig. 23.14**.

The cranium constitutes a fixed-volume vault that contains brain tissue, blood, and CSF. Small increases in the volume of these intracranial structures are accommodated by (1) compression of cerebral veins, (2) distention of meninges, and (3) displacement of CSF into the spinal canal. Any increase in volume beyond these modest compensatory measures elevates intracranial pressure exponentially. This is known as the Monro-Kellie doctrine.

Clinical Manifestations

The major signs and symptoms of increased intracranial pressure (**Table 23.1**) include headache, vomiting, papilledema, abducens nerve palsy, decreased level of consciousness, and autonomic changes.

Headache

Characteristically, this is worse in the morning and increased with exertion or Valsalva maneuver (cough, laugh, sneeze). The headache is often generalized or bifrontal in location and of a dull, nonthrobbing quality.

Vomiting

This may be projectile and associated with little or no nausea. For reasons that are unclear, vomiting may provide temporary relief from headaches associated with increased intracranial pressure.

Papilledema

The earliest funduscopic changes include blurring of the nasal disc margins and distention of the retinal veins. Later, venous pulsations may be lost, and flame hemorrhages may appear circumferentially around the disc. Chronic papilledema results in enlargement of the physiological blind spot and concentric diminution of peripheral visual fields. Visual acuity is not usually affected.

Abducens Nerve Palsy

Unilateral or bilateral abducens nerve palsies are common signs of intracranial hypertension. They usually represent "false localizing signs" caused by generalized increased intracranial pressure rather than focal abducens nerve compression.

Depressed Level of Consciousness

This may occur as a result of brainstem compression, affecting the reticular activating system, or generalized increased intracranial pressure. Secondary effects of intracranial hypertension such as hypoxia and ischemia, which also alter the consciousness level, may obscure its cause.

Autonomic Changes

Elevated systemic blood pressure and bradycardia may develop in response to increased intracranial pressure. This response is named the Cushing reflex, after the pioneering American neurosurgeon who described it. The relationship between blood pressure, heart rate, and intracranial pressure is not direct, however, and other causes of systemic hypertension and bradycardia must be considered.

Fig. 23.14

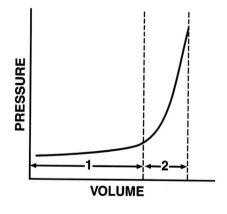

Table 23.1 Clinical Manifestations of Increased Intracranial Pressure

Signs or Symptoms	Characteristics
Headache	Worse in the morning, generalized, dull, nonthrobbing
Vomiting	Often projectile
Papilledema	Blurring of disc margins and distention of retinal veins; loss of venous pulsations; concentric narrowing of visual fields
Abducens nerve palsy	Unilateral or bilateral
Level of consciousness	Depressed
Autonomic changes	Elevated blood pressure with bradycardia (i.e., Cushing reflex)

Major Causes of Increased Intracranial Pressure

Hydrocephalus

See **Fig. 23.15 (A–C)**.

Hydrocephalus is marked by dilation of the cerebral ventricles and an increase in CSF volume. Clinically, patients with hydrocephalus present with signs of intracranial hypertension. The various forms of hydrocephalus, all but one of which are associated with an increase in CSF pressure, are classified as follows:

- *Obstructive hydrocephalus*   This is most common and results from an obstruction to CSF flow inside the ventricular system. It causes dilation of the ventricles proximal to the obstruction while the ventricles to the obstruction distal remain small. Common causes include stenosis of the cerebral aqueduct and fourth ventricular tumor.
- *Communicating hydrocephalus*   In this form of hydrocephalus, no obstruction of CSF flow is evident. All ventricles appear dilated. The cause of hydrocephalus in these cases is obscure. Theoretically, increased CSF production (secondary to a choroid plexus papilloma) or decreased CSF absorption (secondary to subarachnoid hemorrhage or meningitis) may be responsible.
- *Normal pressure hydrocephalus (NPH)*   In this condition, a form of communicating hydrocephalus, hydrocephalus occurs in the absence of elevated intracranial pressure. The ventricular system appears dilated out of proportion to what is expected to occur with aging and brain atrophy. Characteristically, this affects the elderly and results in the clinical triad of gait disturbance, urinary incontinence, and dementia. The cause of NPH is not known.
- *Hydrocephalus ex vacuo*   As a result of cerebral atrophy, passive enlargement of the ventricles may occur without an increase in CSF pressure. The cerebral sulci are not effaced. The clinical picture is that of cerebral atrophy (i.e., dementia), rather than that of intracranial hypertension.

Fig. 23.15 (A) **Obstructive hydrocephalus.**

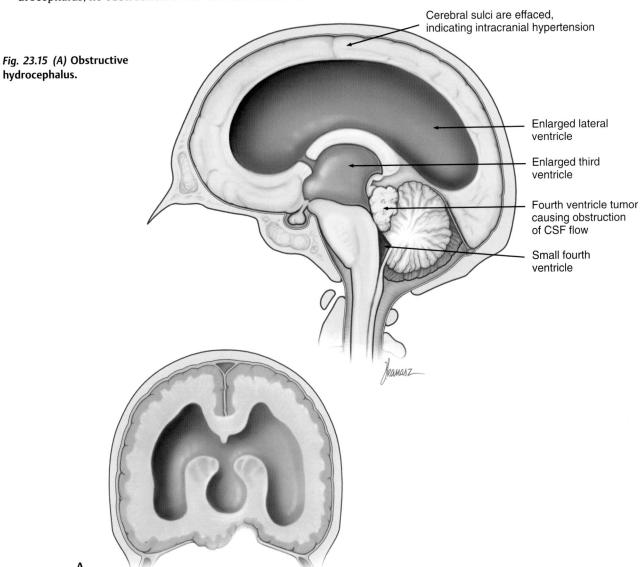

Cerebral sulci are effaced, indicating intracranial hypertension

Enlarged lateral ventricle

Enlarged third ventricle

Fourth ventricle tumor causing obstruction of CSF flow

Small fourth ventricle

A

Brain Edema

Increased intracranial pressure may be related to a diffuse or focal increase in brain tissue water (cerebral edema). This may occur as a result of trauma or infarction or as a response to an intracranial mass (hematoma, infection, or tumor). The clinical picture of cerebral edema is one of focal neurologic deficits and increased intracranial pressure. Two pathophysiological mechanisms are identified:

- *Cytotoxic edema*   Cytotoxic edema consists of cellular injury (neuronal, glial, and endothelial) that results in an increase in intracellular fluid. It predominantly affects the gray matter and is most commonly associated with infarction. There is no response (i.e., decrease in the amount of edema) with the administration of steroids.

- *Vasogenic edema*   This represents increased permeability of brain capillary endothelial cells and a resultant increase in extracellular fluid. It predominantly affects the white matter and is most commonly associated with neoplasms and abscesses. In contrast to cytotoxic edema, vasogenic edema responds exquisitely to steroids.

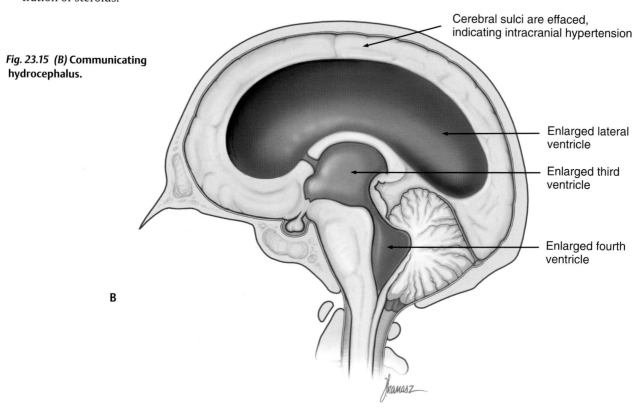

Fig. 23.15 (B) **Communicating hydrocephalus.**

Cerebral sulci are effaced, indicating intracranial hypertension

Enlarged lateral ventricle

Enlarged third ventricle

Enlarged fourth ventricle

B

Intracranial Masses

Intracranial masses such as hematomas, tumors, and abscesses frequently cause mass effect—a shift in intracranial structures—that is exacerbated by surrounding vasogenic edema. As a result of the fixed intracranial volume, such mass effect leads to increased intracranial pressure. Severe displacement of brain tissue produces herniation syndromes, as described next.

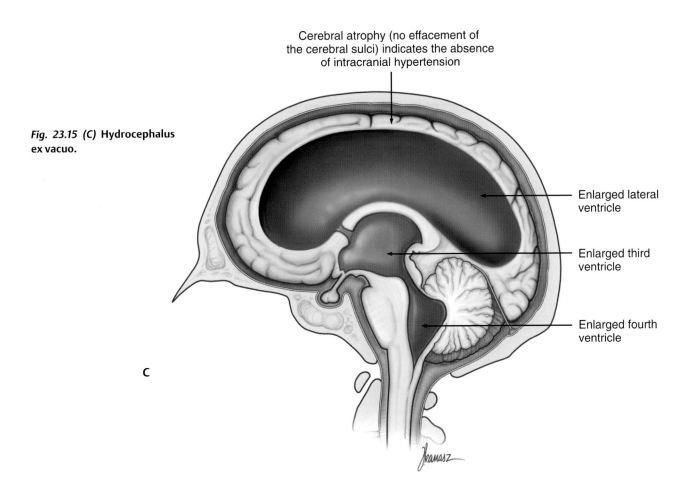

Fig. 23.15 (C) **Hydrocephalus ex vacuo.**

Cerebral atrophy (no effacement of the cerebral sulci) indicates the absence of intracranial hypertension

Enlarged lateral ventricle

Enlarged third ventricle

Enlarged fourth ventricle

C

Herniation Syndromes

See **Fig. 23.16**.

Two major dural folds divide the intracranial cavity into three compartments (see earlier discussion). The tentorium, which lies between the cerebellum and the occipital lobes, separates the cavity into supratentorial and infratentorial compartments. The falx cerebri, which lies between the right and left cerebral hemispheres, separates the supratentorial compartment into right and left halves.

As a result of these divisions and the fixed volume of the skull, a focal cerebral mass elevates intracranial pressure unevenly. Pressure gradients thus form across the three compartments, causing herniation of brain tissue from high to low pressure areas. Three herniation syndromes are identified:

- *Subfalcial herniation*   In this condition, the cingulate gyrus is forced under the falx. There are no known clinical manifestations.

- *Uncal herniations*   In this condition, the uncus (medial temporal lobe) is forced through the incisura, the tentorial opening through which the midbrain passes. The herniating mass compresses the ipsilateral third cranial nerve and ipsilateral cerebral peduncle. This results in ipsilateral third cranial nerve palsy and contralateral hemiparesis. The midbrain may be compressed and shifted enough to compress the contralateral cerebral peduncle against the tentorial edge, producing a false loading sign with ipsilateral third cranial nerve palsy and weakness. This has been described as the Kernohan phenomenon. The key clinical point to remember is that the lesion is always ipsilateral to the third cranial nerve palsy.

- *Tonsillar–foramen magnum herniation*   In this condition, the cerebellar tonsils are forced down into the foramen magnum, usually by increased pressure in the posterior fossa (infratentorial compartment). Medullary compression results in respiratory and cardiovascular collapse and possible arrest, which may be rapid.

Fig. 23.16 **Herniation syndromes.**

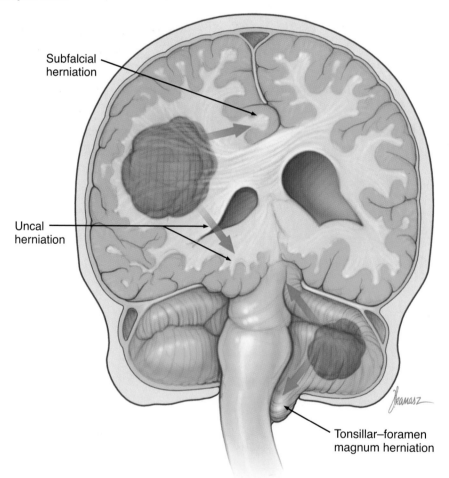

Subfalcial herniation

Uncal herniation

Tonsillar–foramen magnum herniation

Index